NURSING CARE PLANS

Nursing Diagnosis & Intervention

NURSING CARE PLANS
Nursing Diagnosis & Intervention

MICHAEL REESE HOSPITAL AND MEDICAL CENTER

Chicago, Illinois

Department of Nursing

Edited by

Meg Gulanick, RN, MSN, CCRN

Clinical Specialist

Audrey Klopp, RN, MS, CCRN, CS, ET

Clinical Specialist

Sue Galanes, RN, MS, TNS, CCRN

Clinical Specialist

The C. V. Mosby Company

ST. LOUIS • TORONTO • PRINCETON   1986

A TRADITION OF PUBLISHING EXCELLENCE

Editor: Barbara Ellen Norwitz
Developmental editor: Sally Adkisson
Manuscript editors: Sylvia B. Kluth, Maureen Kenison
Book design: Kay M. Kramer
Cover design: Susan Lane
Production: Florence Fansher, Deborah A. Wedemeier

These comprehensive care plans were developed as guidelines for patient care at Michael Reese Hospital and Medical Center and do not constitute standards of care governing a nurse's or an agency's obligation to a patient.

Printed in the United States of America

The C.V. Mosby Company
11830 Westline Industrial Drive, St. Louis, Missouri 63146

Library of Congress Cataloging-in-Publication Data

Main entry under title:

Nursing care plans.

Includes index.
1. Nursing care plans. 2. Nursing—Planning.
3. Diagnosis. I. Gulanick, Meg. II. Klopp, Audrey.
III. Galanes, Sue. IV. Michael Reese Hospital
and Medical Center. [DNLM: 1. Nursing Process.
2. Patient Care Planning. WY 100 N9748]
RT49.N87 1986   610.73   85-29812
ISBN 0-8016-3361-3

GW/VH/VH 9 8 7 6 5 4 3   01/A/055

Contributors[*]

Verda Abernathy, RN, MA, Nurse Clinician, Diabetes Teaching Service

Kathy Alexander, RN, Clinical Nurse III

Josephine C. Anderson, RN, Clinical Nurse IV

Cynthia Antonio, RN, BSN, Clinical Nurse II

Linda Arsenault, RN, MSN, CNRN, Clinical Specialist, Neurosurgery

Margaret Bell, RN, Clinical Nurse III

Bella Biag, RN, BSN, Clinical Nurse III

Caramen Billheimer, RN, BSN, Clinical Nurse III

Denise Birkner, RN, BSN, Clinical Nurse III

Carolyn Bolton, RN, Clinical Nurse II

Janice Borman, RN, MSN, Nurse Manager

Carol Boyd, RN, Clinical Nurse III

Paulette E. Brevard, RN, BSN, Clinical Nurse IV

Monalisa S. Bron, RN, BSN, Clinical Nurse III

Kathryn S. Bronstein, RN, MS, CS, PhD Candidate, Clinical Nurse Specialist, Neurology

Jean L. Burke, RN,C BSN, Clinical Nurse III

Carol Burkhart, RN, BSN, CCRN, Nurse Manager

Virginia Cabongon, RN, BSN

Marian D. Cachero-Salavrakos, RN, BSN, Clinical Nurse III

Urakay Campbell, RN, Clinical Nurse III

Elicita Chaves, RN, Clinical Nurse IV

Vicki Chester, RN, BSN, Clinical Nurse II

Sarah Cohen, RN, Clinical Nurse III

Joanne Coleman, RN, Clinical Nurse III

Dawnetta Collins, RN,C Nurse Manager

Sue A. Conneighton, RN, MSN, Clinical Nurse Specialist

Nancy J. Cooney, RN, BSN, Clinical Nurse IV

Cathy Croke, RN, MSN, Loyola University, Chicago, Illinois

Margaret A. Cunningham, RN, MS, Clinical Specialist, Northwestern Memorial Hospital, Chicago, Illinois

Maria Dacanay, RN, Clinical Nurse III

Marlene T. de la Cruz, RN, BSN, Clinical Nurse III

Leona Dempsey, RN, MSN, CS, Clinical Nurse Specialist, Psychiatric Nursing

Martha Dickerson, RN, MS, CCRN, Coordinator, Nursing Education, Evaluation, and Research

Gail L. Dykstra, RN, Clinical Nurse IV

Linda Escobar, RN, BSN, Clinical Nurse III

Sandra Eungard, RN, BSN, Clinical Nurse II

Martina Evans, RN, BS, Nurse Clinician

Yvonne Evans-Wordell, RN, MSN, Loyola University, Chicago, Illinois

Imelda Fahy, RN, Clinical Nurse IV

Patricia Farrell, RN,C Clinical Nurse II

Ann Filipski, RN, MSN, CS, Clinical Nurse Specialist, Liaison Psychiatry

Susan Galanes, RN, MS, TNS, CCRN, Clinical Nurse Specialist, Critical Care

Diane Gallagher, RN, BSN, Nurse Clinician

Remedios S. Garces, RN, BSN, Nurse Clinician

Lorraine Goodwin, RN, MSN, CS, Education Coordinator, Evanston Hospital, Evanston, Illinois

Cynthia Gordon, RN, BSN, Clinical Nurse III

Deidra Gradishar, RNC BA, Nurse Clinician

Terry Griffin, RN, Nurse Clinician

Meg Gulanick, RN, MSN, CCRN, Clinical Nurse Specialist, Cardiac Rehabilitation

Patricia A. Hannon, RN, Clinical Nurse II

Frankie Harper, RN, Clinical Nurse II

Antoinette Harris-Hardy, RN, BSN, Cardiac Catheterization Nurse

Pam Harston, RN, Plastic Surgery

Patricia Hasbrouck-Aschliman, RN, CCRN, Clinical Nurse IV

Hope Hlinka, RN, Clinical Nurse III

Barbara J. Hobbs, RN, MSN, Administrative Coordinator, Nursing Quality Assurance and Research

Corea Hodge, RN, Clinical Nurse IV

Anita C. Houtsma, RN, Clinical Nurse IV

Doris M. Humphries, RN, BSN, Clinical Nurse IV

Christine Hunt, RN, IAPB Technician

Kathleen Hurst-Delia, RN, BSN, Clinical Nurse III

Florencia Isidro-Sanchez, RN, BSN, Clinical Nurse II

Kathleen Jaffry, RN, Clinical Nurse III

Annie F. Jenkins, RN, Clinical Nurse II

Nola D. Johnson, RN, Nurse Manager

Agnes Jones, RN, Clinical Nurse III

Linda M. Jones, RN, BSN, Clinical Nurse II

Vivian Jones, RN, Clinical Nurse II

Christine Jutzi, RN, BS, Clinical Nurse II

Susan Kansas, RN,C Clinical Nurse II

Karen Kavanaugh, RN, MSN, Clinical Nurse Specialist

Paulette N. Kelleher, RN,C BSN, Clinical Nurse IV

Bernadette Keller, RNC, Clinical Nurse IV

*All contributors are from Michael Reese Hospital and Medical Center unless otherwise specified.

Judith Kenney, RN, MSN, Clinical Nurse III
Cheryl A. King, RN, BSN, Clinical Nurse II
Audrey Klopp, RN, MS, CCRN, CS, ET, Clinical Nurse Specialist and Enterostomal Therapist
Vanida Komutanon, RN, Clinical Nurse III
Mary P. Knoezer, RN, BSN, Clinical Nurse III
Michele Knoll-Puzas, RN,C BS, Nurse Clinician, Pediatrics
Karen Kushibab, RN, BSN, Clinical Nurse III
Susan R. Laub, RN, MEd, CS, Clinical Nursing Supervisor/ Clinical Nurse Specialist, Northwestern Memorial Hospital, Chicago, Illinois
Phyllis Lawlor-Klean, RN, BSN, Clinical Nurse III
Mary Lawson-Carney, RN, Clinical Nurse III
Deborah Lazzara, RN, CCRN, Clinical Nurse III
Dorothy Lewis, RN,C BSN, Clinical Nurse III
Digna Limjoco, RN, Clinical Nurse III
Janet I. Linder, Registered Physical Therapist
Maureen T. Linehan, RN, Consultant/Health Care Information Systems, Peat, Marwick and Mitchell Co., Chicago, Illinois
Chris Loftus, RN, BS, Clinical Nurse III
Lori Luke, RN, Clinical Nurse II
Marilyn Magafas, RN,C BSN, Nurse Manager
Ofelia Mallari, RN, Clinical Nurse III
Mary Martinat, RN, BSN, Clinical Nurse II
Janet McCants, RN, BSN, Clinical Nurse III
Mary Chris McCarthy, RN, BSN, Clinical Nurse III
Patsy McDonald, RN, Clinical Nurse III
Michelle McGhee, RN, BSN, Clinical Nurse II
Ellen T. McSwiney, RN, BSN, Clinical Nurse II
Encarnacion Mendoza, RN, BSN, Clinical Nurse III
Fe Corazon R. Mendoza, RN, BSN, Clinical Nurse III
Janice L. Miller, RN,C MSN, Clinical Nurse Specialist, Pediatrics
Jacqueline Monaco, RN, Clinical Nurse III
Karen Moyer, RN, MS, CCRN, CNA, Director, Critical Care Services, Morton F. Plant Hospital, Clearwater, Florida
Mary Muse, RN,C BSN, Nurse Manager
Denise Myles, RN,C Clinical Nurse III
Lillian Navarrete, RN, Clinical Nurse III
Ruth E. Novitt, RN, MSN, Nurse Clinician, Pediatrics
Joanne O'Connor, RN, BSN, Clinical Nurse II
Manee Omsin, RN, BSN, Clinical Nurse III
Sandra P. Orr, RN, BSN, Clinical Nurse IV
Denise Pang, RN, BSN, Clinical Nurse II
Jane Parker, RNC BAN Nurse Clinician, Labor and Delivery
Lumie L. Perez, RN, BSN, CCRN, Nurse Clinician, Cardiac Rehabilitation
Evangeline Pintang, RN, BSN, Clinical Nurse III
Connie Powell, RN, MSN, Nurse Manager
Linda Powless, RN, CCRN, CNA, Nurse Clinician, Critical Care
Eileen Raebig, RN,C Clinical Nurse III
Vanessa Randle, RN, Clinical Nurse IV
Donna Raymer, RN, BSN, CCRN, Clinical Nurse III

Dorothy Rhodes, RN, Clinical Nurse II
Debby Rickard, RN, BSN, Clinical Nurse III
Yvette Roberts, RN,C BSN, MHA Obstetrics, Jackson Park Hospital, Chicago, Illinois
Carol Ann Rooks, RN, BSN, Staff Nurse, Middlesex General University Hospital, New Brunswick, New Jersey
Linda Rosen-Walsh, RN, BSN, Clinical Nurse III
Mayda T. Roseta, RN, Clinical Nurse II
Ruby Rotor-Cajindos, RN, BSN, Clinical Nurse II
Marilyn Rousseau, RN, Clinical Nurse II
Geraldine Rowden, RN, Clinical Nurse II
Robert Rowlands, RN, Clinical Nurse III
Terri L. Russell, RN, Clinical Nurse III
Laura L. Rybicki, RN, BSN, Clinical Nurse III
Louise Rzeszewski, RN, BSN, Assistant Director, Operating Rooms
Teodorina M. Saez, RN, BSN, Clinical Nurse II
Rosetonia Sapaula, RN, BSN, Clinical Nurse III
Caroline Sarmiento, RN, BSN, Clinical Nurse III
Christa M. Schroeder, RN, MSN, Clinical Nurse Specialist, Hematology/Oncology
Michael K. Schroyer, RN, BSN, CCRN, Nurse Manager
Lydia Serra, RN, Clinical Nurse II
Joanne Shearer, RN, MSN, Loyola University, Chicago, Illinois
Susan Smalheiser, RN, MSN, Clinical Specialist, Nutritional Support Service
Helen Snow-Jackson, RN, BSN, TNS, CEN, Nurse Clinician, Ambulatory and Acute Care
Andrea So, RN, BSN, Clinical Nurse III
Concordia Solita, RN, BSN, Nurse Manager
Rosita Sortijas, RN, BSN, Clinical Nurse II
Kathy V. Stewart, RN, Clinical Nurse II
Linda Marie St. Julien, RN, BSN, Clinical Nurse III
Virginia M. Storey, RN, ET, Enterostomal Therapist, St. Anthony's Hospital, Crown Point, Indiana
Salvacion P. Sulit, RN, BSN, CCRN, Clinical Nurse IV
Jackie Suprenant, RN, BSN, Childbirth Education Specialist
Terry Takemoto, RN, MSN, CCRN, Loyola University, Chicago, Illinois
Apolonia Tinio, RN, BSN, Clinical Nurse II
Christine Todd, RN, Clinical Nurse III
Marisa C. Trybula, RN, BSN, Clinical Nurse IV
Christina L. Valenta, RN, BS, Nurse Clinician, Diabetes
Theresa Vanderhei, RN, Clinical Nurse III
Laura Vieceli-Brooks, RN, BSN, Clinical Nurse II
Malu N. Viloria, RN, BSN, Clinical Nurse III
Marion C. Wallis, RN, CCRN, Clinical Nurse IV
Laura Watanabe, RN, Clinical Nurse II
Margaret Williams, RN, Clinical Nurse III
Katie Wyatt, RN, Inservice Co-ordinator, Operating Rooms
Gloria Young, RN, BS, Clinical Nurse III
Ofelia Zafra, RN, BSN, Clinical Nurse III

Preface

For over a century, nurses at Michael Reese Hospital and Medical Center in Chicago have been committed to providing quality nursing care. Today we are privileged to share with other professionals the fruits of a three-year project to develop comprehensive nursing guides that serve as reference standards from which nurses can individualize patient care based on nursing diagnosis and nursing process. This volume is not meant to serve as a ''cookbook'' but rather as a guide for designing plans of care consistent with each institution's nursing practice. These unique guides* were developed by clinical staff nurses and nurse specialists at Michael Reese Hospital and Medical Center. All contributors are active practitioners, and many are nationally recognized experts in their fields.

Approximately one year after its conception, this project was incorporated into the general requirements of our institution's clinical ladder program. To maintain a consistent standard of quality and to preserve a standardized format, a specific procedure was formulated for development of these care plan guides. Appropriate topics included any nursing diagnosis approved by the North American Nursing Diagnosis Association (NANDA) and any medical disorder or therapeutic intervention with which several nursing diagnoses were commonly associated. No attempts were made to include every NANDA nursing diagnosis or every medical disorder. Instead, guides were developed for the problems and treatments most commonly encountered by the Medical Center's nurses in their daily practice. A clinical resource person (a clinical specialist or nurse clinician with expertise in the content area) was consulted regarding the appropriateness and necessity for the selected care plan topic.

After each nurse drafted the care plan guide, the content was reviewed by the clinical resource person with particular emphasis on identification of independent nursing interventions and use of consistent terminology. Next, a nursing specialist outside the content area reviewed the completed document for clarity. Finally, the care plan guide was submitted for approval by the Standard Care Plan Committee, a subcommittee of the Nurse Specialist Group within the Department of Nursing. (The Nurse Specialist Group consists of clinical specialists/nurse clinicians from each nursing division: ambulatory care, critical care, medicine, obstetrics/gynecology, operating room, pediatrics, psychiatry, special care nursery, and surgery.)

Each care plan includes the following information: actual or potential nursing diagnosis, defining characteristics, etiologies, nursing orders, and expected outcomes. Most of the nursing diagnoses and defining characteristics are expressed in the nomenclature approved by NANDA; however, some original diagnostic labels and defining characteristics are incorporated into care plans at the discretion of the clinical nurse. Several possible etiologies are included for most diagnoses. The nursing orders include ongoing assessment criteria and specific independent nursing interventions. Patient teaching is also integrated into this section. Both process and outcome formats for expected outcomes are utilized, depending on the clinical problem.

These nursing care plan guides have become an indispensable tool at Michael Reese Hospital—for clinical practice, teaching, quality assurance, and research. On clinical units the care plans are utilized in a variety of ways. Some nurses refer to the guides for writing more specific patient care plans. Other nurses use copies of the guides as worksheets for frequently identified diagnoses. The nurse can delete inappropriate interventions and add more specific nursing orders before signing and dating the plan for inclusion in a specific patient's permanent medical record. Some nurses find it helpful to keep the guide in a Kardex file or at the bedside until it is finally incorporated into the patient's chart at the time of transfer or discharge.

These guides have been adopted as a standard by which nurse managers can evaluate nursing practice on their units and as a means to assess learning needs of their staff. Nurse specialists involved in education programs and internships find the guides useful as instructional references because they identify nursing diagnoses associated with common medical/patient problems and exemplify the nursing process in action.

The care plans can be used in a number of ways for quality assurance: as the basis for chart audits when studying nursing interventions and documentation, to determine nursing care for diagnosis related groups (DRGs), and to set comprehensive standards for practice.

Finally, the plans form a framework for developing outcome criteria and testing the efficacy of specific interventions.

Reflecting the clinical expertise of over 160 nurses, this clinical reference is truly one of a kind—developed *by* nurses, *for* nurses.

Meg Gulanick

*Referred to in the individual standard care plans as SCPs.

Contents

CHAPTER ONE

Nursing Diagnoses

Activity Intolerance

DEFINING CHARACTERISTICS	NURSING ORDERS			EXPECTED OUTCOMES
	ASSESSMENT	INTERVENTIONS	PATIENT EDUCATION	

Verbal report of fatigue or weakness
Abnormal heart rate or BP response to activity
Exertional discomfort or dyspnea
Electrocardiographic changes reflecting arrhythmias or ischemia
	A. Assess patient's respiratory status before activity
	  1. Respiratory quality and quantity
	  2. Need for O_2 with increased activity
	B. Assess patient's cardiac function before activity
	  1. Pulse: rate, rhythm, volume
	  2. BP: baseline, orthostatic changes
	  3. Skin: color, temperature, moisture, perfusion
	  4. How Valsalva's maneuver affects heart rate when patient moves in bed
	C. Assess patient's level of mobility (see Standard Care Plan [SCP] in this chapter: Mobility, impaired physical)
	D. Assess nutritional status (see SCP in this chapter: Nutrition, alteration in: less than body requirement)
	E. Assess potential for physical injury with activity
	F. Assess need for ambulation aids
	G. Assess understanding by patient/significant others of change in activity tolerance
		A. Observe and document response to activity
		B. Report
		  1. Rapid pulse (>20 beats over resting rate or 120 BPM)
		  2. Palpitations
		  3. Significant increase in systolic BP (>20 mm Hg)
		  4. Significant decrease in systolic BP (drop of ≥20 mm Hg)
		  5. Dyspnea, labored breathing, wheezing
		  6. Weakness, fatigue
		  7. Chest pain, light-headedness, dizziness, pallor, cold sweats
		C. Assist with ADL as indicated
		D. Provide bedside commode as indicated
		E. Encourage adequate rest periods, especially before ambulation, diagnostic procedures, meals
		F. Refrain from performing nonessential procedures
		G. Anticipate patient's needs (e.g., keep telephone, tissues within reach)
		H. Provide small, frequent meals
		I. Use slow progression of patient activity
		  1. Dangling 10-15 min t.i.d.
		  2. Deep breathing exercises t.i.d.
		  3. Sitting up in chair 30 min t.i.d.
		  4. Walking in room 1-2 min t.i.d.
		  5. Walking in hall 25 feet, then slowly progressing to _____ feet, saving energy for return trip
		J. Encourage active ROM exercises t.i.d. to maintain muscle strength; if further reconditioning needed, confer with rehabilitation medicine personnel
		K. Provide emotional support while increasing activity
			A. Teach patient/significant others signs of physical overactivity
			B. Involve patient/significant others in activity, goal setting, and care planning
			C. Encourage significant others to bring ambulation aides: walker or cane
			D. Teach appropriate use of environmental aides (e.g., bed rails, elevating head of bed when patient gets out of bed, chair in bathroom, hall rails)
			E. Teach ROM exercises
			F. Encourage patient to verbalize concerns about discharge and home environment
			G. Involve patient/significant others in discharge planning
				A. Activity level will be maintained within limits of patient's capabilities
				B. Patient/significant others will verbalize an understanding of
				  1. Signs of overexertion
				  2. Plan for activity progression
				  3. Appropriate use of environmental aids

Originated by **Michael K. Schroyer, RN, BSN, CCRN**
Resource persons: **Meg Gulanick, RN, MSN, CCRN**
   Sue A. Conneighton, RN, MSN

Airway Clearance, Ineffective

DEFINING CHARACTERISTICS	NURSING ORDERS			EXPECTED OUTCOMES
	ASSESSMENT	INTERVENTIONS	PATIENT EDUCATION	
Abnormal breath sounds (rales, rhonchi, wheezes) Change in respiratory rate or depth Cough Cyanosis Dyspnea	A. Assess respirations: note quality, rate, pattern, depth, flaring of nostrils, dyspnea on exertion, evidence of splinting, use of accessory muscles B. Assess changes in orientation and behavior pattern C. Assess changes in vital signs and temperature D. Assess patient's present knowledge base of disease process	A. Position patient with proper body alignment for optimal breathing pattern (if tolerated head of bed at >45 degrees) B. Auscultate lungs for presence of breath sounds every shift (or as needed) C. If abnormal sounds are present, use oropharyngeal or tracheal suction as needed D. Note presence of sputum; assess quantity, color, consistency (may have patient use a sputum container) E. Provide humidity (when appropriate) via bedside humidifier (positioned near patient) and humidified O_2 therapy F. Encourage oral intake/fluids within the limits of cardiac reserve G. Instruct and/or change patient's position (e.g., ambulate, turn every ___ hours) H. Administer medication as ordered (antibiotics, bronchodilators, diuretics), noting effectiveness and side effects I. Assist with oral hygiene q.4h. or as needed J. Maintain adequate airway K. Monitor ABGs; note changes L. Coordinate with respiratory therapy department optimal time for postural drainage and percussion, i.e., at least 1 hour after eating M. Pace activities to avoid fatigue N. Maintain planned rest periods O. Instruct patient to avoid restrictive clothing P. Demonstrate and teach coughing, deep breathing, and splinting techniques	A. Instruct patient on use, frequency, and side effects of medications B. Teach patient about environmental factors that can precipitate respiratory problems C. Explain effects of smoking D. Instruct patient on warning signs of pending/recurring pulmonary problems E. Use pulmonary clinical nurse specialists	A. Patient will demonstrate ability to mobilize secretions or free airway of secretions B. Patient will exhibit an understanding of respiratory health needs 1. Demonstrates correct coughing techniques, etc. 2. Verbalizes or takes correct medications at appropriate times 3. Verbalizes his/her potential environmental hazards 4. Lists warning signs of recurring pulmonary problem and names correct health agency/professionals to contact

Originated by **Lorraine Goodwin, RN, MSN, CS**
Helen Snow-Jackson, RN, BSN, TNS, CEN
Remedios S. Garces, RN, BSN
Janice L. Miller, RN,C MSN

Anxiety/Fear

DEFINING CHARACTERISTICS	NURSING ORDERS			EXPECTED OUTCOMES
	ASSESSMENT	INTERVENTIONS	PATIENT EDUCATION	
Mild anxiety Restlessness Increased awareness Increased questioning **Moderate/severe anxiety** Restlessness Insomnia Glancing about/increased alertness Facial tension/wide-eyed Focus on self Poor eye contact Increased perspiration Anorexia/GI problems Overexcited/jittery Expressed concern Trembling Constant demands **Panic** Dyspnea Palpitations Chest pain Hot/cold flashes Sweating Faintness Trembling/shaking Preoccupied with trivial detail Easily distracted Inability to learn Fear of impending doom Behavior focused on relief; may scream, cry, pray, thrash limbs, run No realistic judgments May assume fetal position	A. Recognize patient's level of anxiety (mild, severe); note any signs and symptoms, especially nonverbal communication B. Assess patient's normal coping patterns (by interview with patient/significant others/physician)	**For mild, moderate, severe anxiety** A. Display confident, calm manner and tolerant, understanding attitude B. Orient to environment C. Establish rapport with patient, especially through continuity of care D. Encourage ventilation of feelings, concerns, and dependency. Listen carefully. Sit down, if possible. Give an unhurried, attentive appearance E. Place in quiet environment; reduce distracting stimuli. Use discretion in conversation in or near room. Remove excess equipment from environment F. Adapt care to patient's routines and needs G. Encourage patient to call on nursing staff when feelings of anxiety or anxiety-provoking situations occur H. Refrain from performing nonessential procedures. Reduce demands placed on patient. Provide rest periods. Minimize number of personnel involved in care I. Support a realistic assessment of the situation; omit false reassurances J. Allow significant others to visit. Explain tests and equipment to them; involve them in care as appropriate K. Use other supportive measures/staff as indicated (e.g., medications, psychiatric liaison, clergy, social services) L. Provide diversional materials (e.g., magazines, books, radio, changing picture in room) M. Monitor changes in level of anxiety; assist in use of usual coping behaviors N. Identify special problems of ''sundowners.'' Keep night light in room; stay with patient as much as possible; use soft music	Encourage patient to ask questions to clear misconceptions. Provide accurate information regarding disease, medications, tests/procedures, and self-care	A. Decreased level of anxiety will be evidenced by 　1. Calm, relaxed appearance 　2. Verbalization of fears/feelings 　3. Restful night B. Patient will verbalize relief from acute distress

Originated by **Meg Gulanick, RN, MSN, CCRN**
Janice Borman, RN, MSN
Leona Dempsey, RN, MSN, CS

Anxiety/Fear—cont'd

DEFINING CHARACTERISTICS	NURSING ORDERS			EXPECTED OUTCOMES
	ASSESSMENT	INTERVENTIONS	PATIENT EDUCATION	

		For panic
		A. Take patient to a quiet area
		B. Administer antianxiety medication as needed
		C. Remain with patient through the attack
		D. Maintain a calm manner
		E. Use short, simple sentences and a firm voice
		F. Give a clear, honest statement about the situation (e.g., "You are having an anxiety attack. Your heart is beating faster because of stress")
		G. After attack is over and patient has rested, ask him/her to describe events preceding attack
		  1. Use concrete questions
		  2. Observe patient for nonverbal cues
		H. Consider focusing patient's energy on a physically tiring task		

Body Image: disturbance in

DEFINING CHARACTERISTICS	NURSING ORDERS			EXPECTED OUTCOMES
	ASSESSMENT	INTERVENTIONS	PATIENT EDUCATION	
Verbal identification of feeling about altered structure/function of a body part Verbal preoccupation with changed body part or function Naming changed body part or function Refusal to discuss/acknowledge change Focusing behavior on changed body part and/or function Actual change in structure/function Refusal to look at, touch, or care for altered body part Change in social behavior (withdrawal, isolation, flamboyancy) Compensatory use of concealing clothing, other devices	A. Assess perception of change in structure/function of body part (also proposed change) B. Assess perceived impact of change on ADL, social behavior, personal relationships, occupational activities C. Note patient's behavior regarding actual or perceived changed body part/function D. Note verbal references to actual or perceived change in body part/function	A. Acknowledge normalcy of emotional response to actual or perceived change in body structure/function B. Help patient identify actual changes C. Help patient identify concerns regarding actual perceived changes D. Encourage verbalization regarding positive or negative feelings regarding actual or perceived change E. Assist patient in incorporating actual changes into ADL, social life, interpersonal relationships, occupational activities F. Encourage use of support groups	Teach patient adaptive behavior to compensate for actual changed body structure/function	Patient will begin to acknowledge feelings about altered structure/function

Originated by **Audrey Klopp, RN, MS, CCRN, CS, ET**

Bowel Elimination, Alteration in: constipation/impaction

DEFINING CHARACTERISTICS	NURSING ORDERS			EXPECTED OUTCOMES
	ASSESSMENT	INTERVENTIONS	PATIENT EDUCATION	
Straining at stools Passage of liquid fecal seepage Frequent but nonproductive desire to defecate Anorexia Abdominal distention Nausea and vomiting Dull headache, restlessness, and depression Fecal incontinence	**Bowel habits** A. Assess home pattern of elimination; compare to present pattern. Include size, frequency, color, and quality B. Evaluate laxative use, type, and frequency **Diet** A. Evaluate usual dietary habits, eating schedule, and liquid intake. Compare with hospital regime B. Assess food preferences **Mobility** A. Assess activity level (prolonged bed rest and lack of exercise contribute to constipation) B. Listen for bowel sounds every shift **Medications** Evaluate current medication usage, which may contribute to constipation **Psychologic factors** A. Evaluate degree of stress during hospitalization B. Assess privacy for elimination (i.e., enforced use of bedpan) C. Evaluate fear of pain D. Assess time limitation	**Dietary considerations** A. Encourage increase bulk in diet e.g., raw fruits, fresh vegetables, (if appropriate) B. Consult dietitian if appropriate C. Encourage patient to eat prunes, prune juices, cold cereals, bean products, etc. (if appropriate) **Fluid intake** Encourage and provide daily fluid intake of 2000-3000 ml/day, if not contraindicated medically **Activity** A. Orient patient to location of bathroom B. Increase patient's physical activity by planning ambulation periods if possible C. Assist with mobility **Fecal evacuation** Provide a regular time, e.g., after breakfast or at patient's usual time **Privacy/comfort** A. Offer a warm bedpan to bedridden patient B. Assist patient to assume a high Fowler's position with knees flexed C. Curtain off the area; allow patient time to relax **Regular exercises** A. Initiate occupational/physical therapy consultation as needed B. Assist with passive/active ROM exercises C. Instruct in isometric abdominal and gluteal exercises unless contraindicated D. Encourage as much patient self-help as possible **Tension-relieving measures** Try to prevent factors that make patient suppress the urge to defecate	Explain to patient/significant others the importance of the following A. Balanced diet that contains adequate bulk, fresh fruits, vegetables B. Adequate fluid intake (8 glasses/day) C. Regular meals D. Regular time for evacuation and adequate time for defecation E. Regular exercise F. Privacy for defecation G. Administration of rectal suppositories, enemas, or laxatives when necessary	A. Relief of constipation/impaction will be evidenced by regular passage of soft, formed stools B. Patient/significant others will verbalize causes of constipation and specific measures that prevent or alleviate the problem

Originated by **Marian D. Cachero-Salavrakos, RN, BSN**
 Resource persons: **Connie Powell, RN, MSN**
 Linda Arsenault, RN, MSN, CNRN

Bowel Elimination, Alteration in: constipation/impaction—cont'd

DEFINING CHARACTERISTICS	NURSING ORDERS		PATIENT EDUCATION	EXPECTED OUTCOMES
	ASSESSMENT	INTERVENTIONS		

	Disease/rectal problems
	A. Assess for hemorrhoids
	B. Check for history of bowel obstruction
	C. Check for history of paralytic ileus
	
	Others ———————
	———————
		Documentation
		Record bowel activity, consistency, color, and quantity
		
		Administration of prescribed agents
		A. Metamucil: increases fluid, gaseous and solid bulk of intestinal contents
		B. Stool softeners: e.g., Colace
		C. Chemical irritants: e.g., castor oil, cascara, Milk of Magnesia. These irritate the bowel mucosa and cause rapid propulsion of contents of small intestines
		D. Suppositories: aid in softening stools and stimulate rectal mucosa; best results occur when given 30 min before usual defecation time or after breakfast
		E. Oil: retention enema to soften stool
		
		Other measures
		A. Digitally remove fecal impaction
		B. For patients who cannot achieve control, employ some technique for stool collection until patient is ready to start training (depending on patient's condition). In addition,
		  1. Check stools regularly
		  2. Keep patient clean, dry, and free of feces
		  3. Provide incontinence pads for patient's use
		  4. Use soap, water, and lotion on buttocks after each BM
		  5. Prevent skin excoriation by proper cleaning after each incontinent BM and by turning the patient q.2h. as needed
		C. Consult with physician, and institute a bowel program as needed, e.g., daily stool softeners and laxative suppositories q.o.d. Also, to minimize rectal discomfort
		  1. Warm sitz bath
		  2. Hemorrhoidal preparations		

Bowel Elimination, Alteration in: diarrhea

DEFINING CHARACTERISTICS	NURSING ORDERS			EXPECTED OUTCOMES
	ASSESSMENT	INTERVENTIONS	PATIENT EDUCATION	

Abdominal pain
Cramping
Frequency of stools
Loose/liquid stools
Urgency
Hyperactive bowel sounds/sensations
	Patterns of elimination/etiologic factors
	Subjective
	A. Patient's report of normal as compared to present pattern
	B. Report of abdominal pain, cramping, frequency, urgency, loose/liquid stools, and hyperactive bowel sensations
	
	Objective
	A. Drugs patient is or has been taking
	B. Diet
	  1. Idiosyncratic intolerances
	  2. Method of food preparation
	  3. Osmolality of tube feedings
	  4. Change in eating schedule
	C. Level of activity
	D. Emotional impact
	  1. Loss of privacy
	  2. Stress
	E. Absorptive capability
	  1. History of previous GI surgery
	  2. GI disease(s)
	  3. History of abdominal radiation
	F. Iatrogenic causes for diarrhea, (e.g., preparation for GI tests, drugs that predispose to diarrhea, pelvic radiation)
	G. For assessment parameters see SCP in this chapter: Fluid volume deficit, actual
		A. Promote normal evacuation
		  1. Give antidiarrheal drugs as ordered
		  2. Provide dietary alterations as allowed
		    a. Bulk (cereals, grains, Metamucil)
		    b. "Natural" antidiarrheals (e.g., pretzels, matzohs, cheese)
		    c. Avoidance of stimulants (e.g., caffeine, carbonated beverages)
		  3. Check for fecal impaction by digital examination
		  4. Minimize emotional impact of illness and hospitalization by providing
		    a. Privacy
		    b. Opportunity for verbalization
		  5. Compensate for malabsorption as much as possible with help of dietitian
		  6. Evaluate appropriateness of physician's x-ray protocols for bowel preparation based on age, weight, condition, disease, and other therapies
		  7. Assist with/administer perianal care after each BM
		  8. See SCP in this chapter: Skin integrity, impairment of: actual and potential
			A. Teach patient those etiologic factors that can be controlled
			B. Teach patient importance of good perianal hygiene following each BM
				A. Etiologic factors will be eliminated as much as possible
				B. Normal (for patient) elimination will be established
				C. Complications of diarrhea will be minimized

Originated by **Audrey Klopp, RN, MS, CCRN, CS, ET**
Virginia M. Storey, RN, ET

Breathing Pattern, Ineffective

DEFINING CHARACTERISTICS	NURSING ORDERS			EXPECTED OUTCOMES
	ASSESSMENT	INTERVENTIONS	PATIENT EDUCATION	

Dyspnea
Shortness of breath
Tachypnea
Fremitus
Cyanosis
Cough
Nasal flaring
Respiratory depth changes
Altered chest excursion
Use of accessory muscles
Pursed-lip breathing/ prolonged expiratory phase
Increased anteroposterior chest diameter
	A. Assess respiratory rate and depth by listening to breath sounds—minimum every shift
	B. Assess for dyspnea and quantify (i.e., note how many words per breath patient can say); relate dyspnea to precipitating factors
	C. Note breathing pattern (i.e., Cheyne-Stokes; Kussmaul)
	D. Note use of muscles used for breathing (i.e., sternocleidomastoid, abdominal, diaphragmatic)
	E. Note retractions, flaring of nostrils
	F. Assess position patient assumes for normal/easy breathing
	G. Assess for changes in orientation, restlessness
	H. Assess skin color, temperature, capillary refill; note central versus peripheral cyanosis
	I. Assess presence of breath sounds every shift
	J. Note changes in activity tolerance
	K. Assess anxiety level
	L. Assess presence of sputum for quantity, color, consistency
		A. Monitor changes in vital signs, especially breathing pattern
		B. Position patient with proper body alignment for optimal breathing pattern. Position patient prefers is _____
		C. Encourage sustained deep breaths by
		  1. Demonstration (emphasizing slow inhaling, holding end inspiration for a few seconds, and passively exhaling)
		  2. Use of incentive spirometer (Place close for convenient patient use)
		  3. Asking patient to yawn, which promotes deep inspiration
		D. Monitor ABGs; note differences
		E. Suction as needed
		F. Pace and schedule activities to avoid dyspnea resulting from fatigue. Present schedule is _____
		G. Check position of portable chest x-ray plate (when needed) so that entire lung field can be examined; check that patient's position allows for optimal lung expansion
		H. Provide reassurance and allay anxiety by staying with patient during acute episodes of respiratory distress
		I. Encourage diaphragmatic breathing for patient with chronic disease
		J. Assist patient with weak or paralyzed abdominal muscles to cough effectively
			A. Explain effects of wearing restrictive clothing
			B. Explain the use of O₂ therapy used for patient
			C. Instruct patient/ significant others in the O₂ therapy to be used at home
			D. Explain environmental factors that may worsen patient's pulmonary condition (e.g., pollen, smoking)
			E. Explain symptoms of a "cold" and impending problems
			F. Teach patient/significant others appropriate breathing, coughing, and splinting techniques
			G. Teach patient how to count own respirations and to relate respiratory rate to activity tolerance
			H. Teach patient when to inhale and exhale while doing strenuous activities
				A. Optimal respiratory status within the limits of the disease will be achieved
				B. Patient will
				  1. Demonstrate breathing exercise
				  2. Discuss potential hazardous and environmental factors
				  3. List warning signs of pulmonary problems
				  4. Demonstrate management of O₂ equipment (if available)

Originated by **Lorraine Goodwin, RN, MSN, CS**
    Helen Snow-Jackson, RN, BSN, TNS, CEN
    Lumie Perez, RN, BSN, CCRN

Cardiac Output, Alteration in: decreased

DEFINING CHARACTERISTICS	NURSING ORDERS			EXPECTED OUTCOMES
	ASSESSMENT	INTERVENTIONS	PATIENT EDUCATION	
Variations in hemodynamic parameters (BP, heart rate, CVP, pulmonary artery pressures, cardiac output, neck veins) Arrhythmias, ECG changes Rales, tachypnea, dyspnea, orthopnea, cough, abnormal ABGs, frothy sputum Weight gain, edema, decreased urine output Anxiety, restlessness, syncope, dizziness, weakness, fatigue Abnormal heart sounds Decreased peripheral pulses, cold clammy skin Confusion, change in level of consciousness	A. Assess physical status as appropriate B. Document changes C. Report significant alterations in 1. Temperature, pulse, respiration, apical/radial pulses, peripheral pulses, cardiac rhythm 2. BP, pulsus paradoxus 3. Heart sounds, murmurs, rubs 4. Jugular venous distention, pulmonary artery pressure 5. Skin color, temperature, moisture 6. Fluid balance, presence of peripheral edema (I & O, weight) 7. Mentation 8. Pain 9. Diagnostic studies (e.g., ECG changes, ABGs, CBC, chest x-ray examination)	A. Administer medication as ordered, noting response and observing for side effects and toxicity B. Maintain optimal fluid balance 1. Administer fluid challenge as ordered, closely monitoring effects 2. Maintain hemodynamic parameters at prescribed levels Heart rate: _____ BP: _____ CVP: _____ Pulmonary capillary wedge pressure/pulmonary artery diastolic: _____ Urine output: _____ 3. Restrict fluid and Na as ordered C. Maintain adequate ventilation/perfusion 1. Place patient in optimal position 2. Administer O_2 as ordered 3. Perform diagnostic studies as indicated/ordered (see Assessment) D. Maintain physical and emotional rest 1. Restrict activity to reduce O_2 demands 2. Provide quiet, relaxed environment 3. Organize nursing and medical care to allow rest periods 4. Monitor progressive activity 5. Administer stool softeners p.r.n. 6. Monitor sleep patterns; administer sedative p.r.n. E. Monitor ECG for rate, rhythm, ectopy, and change in PR, QRS, and QT intervals every _____. If arrhythmia occurs, determine patient response, document; report if significant or not tolerated. Intervene according to protocol F. Monitor therapeutic aids within prescribed protocol (e.g., intraaortic balloon pump, pacemaker)	A. Explain symptoms and interventions for decreased cardiac output related to etiology B. Explain drug regimen, purpose, dose, and side effects C. Explain progressive activity schedule, and signs of overexertion D. Explain diet program	A. Optimal hemodynamic function will be maintained B. Patient will 1. State symptoms and interventions for decreased cardiac output 2. Explain drug/diet regimen 3. Explain progressive activity schedule

Originated by **Meg Gulanick, RN, MSN, CCRN**
Karen Moyer, RN, MS, CCRN, CNA

Comfort, Alteration in: pain

DEFINING CHARACTERISTICS	NURSING ORDERS			EXPECTED OUTCOMES
	ASSESSMENT	INTERVENTIONS	PATIENT EDUCATION	

Patient/significant others report pain
Guarding behavior, protective
Self-focusing, narrowed focus (altered time perception, withdrawal from social or physical contact)
Relief/distraction behavior (e.g., moaning, crying, pacing, seeking out other people or activities; restlessness, irritability, alteration in sleep pattern)
Facial mask of pain
Alteration in muscle tone (listless/flaccid; rigid/tense)
Autonomic responses not seen in chronic, stable pain (e.g., diaphoresis, change in BP, pulse rate, pupillary dilation, increased/decreased respiratory rate, pallor)
	A. Solicit patient's description of pain, documenting in patient's own words
	B. Assess pain characteristics
	  1. Quality (e.g., sharp, burning, shooting)
	  2. Severity (scale 1-10, 10 most severe)
	  3. Location (anatomic description)
	  4. Onset (gradual/sudden)
	  5. Duration (how long, intermittent/continuous)
	  6. Precipitating/relieving factors
	C. Solicit techniques patient believes to be or has found to be helpful in decreasing pain
		A. Anticipate need for analgesics or additional methods of pain relief
		B. Respond immediately to complaint of pain
		C. Eliminate additional stressors or sources of discomfort whenever possible
		D. Give analgesics as ordered, evaluating effectiveness and observing for any signs and symptoms of untoward effects
		E. Use any additional comfort measures whenever appropriate
		  1. Alteration in environment
		  2. Distractional devices
		  3. Relaxation techniques
		  4. Use of physiologic interventions (heat/cold; position change)
		  5. Reassurance and contact
		  6. Positive suggestion
		  7. Use of psychosocial support systems
		  8. Soliciting/using techniques patient believes to be or has found to be helpful
		F. Provide rest periods to facilitate comfort, sleep, and relaxation
		G. Notify physician if interventions are unsuccessful or if current complaint is significant change from past pain or pain relief pattern
			A. Instruct patient to report pain so that relief measures may be instituted
			B. Instruct patient to evaluate and to report effectiveness of measures used
			C. Explain cause of pain/discomfort, if known
			D. Explain rationale for relief measures chosen
			E. Provide anticipatory instruction on pain causes, appropriate prevention, and relief measures
				A. Pain will be relieved or minimized
				B. Patient will verbalize causes and appropriate relief measures for pain

Originated by **Ann Filipski, RN, MSN, CS**
           Janice Borman, RN, MSN
           Susan R. Laub, RN, MEd, CS

Communication, Impaired: aphasia, dysarthria, slurred speech

DEFINING CHARACTERISTICS	NURSING ORDERS			EXPECTED OUTCOMES
	ASSESSMENT	INTERVENTIONS	PATIENT EDUCATION	
Inability to recognize or understand spoken/written words Difficulty in articulating words Inability to recall familiar words, phrases, or names of known persons, objects, and places	Determine the type and degree of aphasia the patient has by assessing the following A. Ability to speak spontaneously B. Ability to understand spoken word C. Ability to understand written word, pictures, gestures	A. Treat patient as an intelligent adult. Explain all diagnostic, therapeutic, and comfort measures before initiating them B. Maintain eye contact with patient when speaking. Stand close, within patient's line of vision, generally midline (patient may have defect in field of vision) C. Keep distractions such as television, radio at a minimum when talking to patient	A. Offer significant others the opportunity to ask questions about patient's communication problem B. Inform patient/significant others of the type of aphasia patient has and how it affects speech, understanding, language skills	A. Communication skills will be maximized B. Patient/significant others will demonstrate understanding of patient's disability and special communications needs as reflected by increased socialization

Originated by **Maria Dacanay, RN**
Resource persons: **Linda Arsenault, RN, MSN, CNRN**
                     Connie Powell, RN, MSN

Continued.

Communication, Impaired: aphasia, dysarthria, slurred speech—cont'd

DEFINING CHARACTERISTICS	NURSING ORDERS			EXPECTED OUTCOMES
	ASSESSMENT	INTERVENTIONS	PATIENT EDUCATION	
	D. Ability to express ideas E. Ability to name objects	D. Anticipate need to decrease feelings of helplessness E. Place call light within reach F. When patient cannot understand spoken word, repeat simple directions until understood. Supplement with gestures if necessary G. When patient cannot identify objects by name, give practice in receiving word images (e.g., point to an object and clearly enunciate its name: ''cup,'' ''pen'') H. Speak slowly and distinctly, repeating key words I. Give concrete directions that the patient is physically capable of doing (e.g., ''Point to ____''; ''Open your mouth''; ''Turn your head'') J. Use short sentences. Ask only one question at a time K. Do not speak loudly unless patient is hard of hearing L. When patient has difficulty with verbal expressions, give practice in repeating words after you. Begin with simple words, then progress. (e.g., ''Yes''; ''No''; ''This is a cup'') M. Encourage patient to speak N. Give ample time to respond. Avoid finishing sentences for patient. Say word slowly and distinctly if help is requested O. Listen attentively when patient attempts to communicate P. Provide with word-and-phrase cards, writing pad, and pencil Q. Provide with list of words patient can say; add new words to it R. If vocabulary is limited to yes and no answers, try to phrase questions so that patient can use these responses S. Orient patient to time by placing a clock and calendar at bedside T. Never talk in front of patient as though he/she comprehends nothing U. Praise patient's accomplishments V. Consult with speech therapist for additional help W. See that patient is well-rested before each session with speech therapist	C. Explain that because of associated brain injury, patient's attention span may be limited D. Encourage patient to socialize with family and friends. Explain that communication should be encouraged despite impairment E. Provide patient with an appointment with a speech therapist F. Inform patient/significant others to seek information about aphasia from American Speech-Language-Hearing Association 10810 Rockwell Pike Rockville, MD 20852	

Fluid Volume Deficit, Actual

DEFINING CHARACTERISTICS	NURSING ORDERS			EXPECTED OUTCOMES
	ASSESSMENT	INTERVENTIONS	PATIENT EDUCATION	
Decreased urine output Concentrated urine Dilute urine Output greater than intake Sudden weight loss Decreased venous filling Hemoconcentration Increased serum sodium Hypotension Thirst Increased pulse rate Decreased skin turgor Decreased pulse volume/pressure Dry mucous membranes Weakness Sunken fontanels Possible weight gain Edema	A. Assess hydration status: skin turgor, mucous membranes, I & O, weight, other: ____ ____ B. Observe for complications of dehydration. Report to physician	A. Monitor strict I & O every ____ hours B. Record daily weight C. Report urine output <30 ml/hour for 2 consecutive hours D. Administer parenteral fluids as ordered, monitoring IV flow rate E. Monitor electrolytes, serum/urine osmolarity, and specific gravity F. Monitor and document patient's vital signs. Report any abnormality	Educate patient/significant others regarding fluids and special diet considerations	Adequate fluid volume and electrolyte balance will be maintained A. Normal electrolytes B. Urine output at least 30 ml/hour C. Balanced I & O D. Normal skin turgor E. Moist mucous membranes F. Normal urine specific gravity

Originated by **Jackie Suprenant, RN, BSN**
       Carol Burkhart, RN, BSN, CCRN
       Maureen T. Linehan, RN

Grieving, Dysfunctional: failure to grieve

DEFINING CHARACTERISTICS	NURSING ORDERS			EXPECTED OUTCOMES
	ASSESSMENT	INTERVENTIONS	PATIENT EDUCATION	

Mild, chronic depression
Withdrawal from friends and/or normal activities
Somatic complaints
"Acting out" behavior
Regression
Guilt or rumination
Constricted affect
Avoidance of affectively charged topics
Patient/significant others report failure to grieve
	A. Assess current affective state
	  1. Observe for presence/absence of emotional distress
	  2. Observe quality/quantity of communication (verbal and nonverbal)
	B. Assess past coping style and mechanisms used in stressful situations
	C. Explore nature of individual's past attitude/relationship with lost object
	D. Assess degree of relatedness with others
		A. Approach individual in unhurried manner
		B. Provide atmosphere of acceptance:
		  1. Listen attentively
		  2. Encourage verbalization of feelings and expression of affect (such as crying)
		  3. Refrain from criticizing
		  4. Provide appropriate reassurance
		  5. Encourage acceptance of individual limitations or differences in means of expression
		C. Communicate comfort with patient's discussion of loss and grief
		D. Recognize variation and the need for individual adjustment to loss and change
		E. Offer feedback regarding patient's expressed feelings
			A. Explain that emotional response to loss is appropriate and commonly experienced
			B. Offer hope that emotional pain will decrease with time
			C. Encourage/facilitate expression of acceptance by significant others
			D. Support others' offers of emotional support to patient
			E. Describe the normal "stages" of grief (denial, anger, bargaining, depression, acceptance)
				A. Patient will be provided with opportunity to discuss loss and, as able, will begin experience of grieving in supportive environment
				B. Patient will verbalize "normalcy" of grief secondary to loss
				C. Patient will identify normal grieving behaviors such as
				  1. Variability in affect
				  2. Ambivalence toward lost object
				  3. Preoccupation with lost object

Originated by **Jean L. Burke, RN,C BSN**
Resource person: **Ann Filipski, RN, MSN, CS**

Continued.

Grieving, Dysfunctional: failure to grieve—cont'd

DEFINING CHARACTERISTICS	NURSING ORDERS			EXPECTED OUTCOMES
	ASSESSMENT	INTERVENTIONS	PATIENT EDUCATION	

	E. Determine degree of insight in present situation
	F. Identify disturbing topics of conversation or experience
	G. Estimate degree of stress currently experienced
	H. Identify actual/potential loss(es)
		F. Support the use of adaptive coping mechanisms
		G. Recognize the need for use of defense mechanisms; avoid personalizing negative expressions of affect
		H. Discuss anticipated/actual loss with patient
		  1. Support realistic assessment of situation
		  2. Explore with patient individual strengths and available resources
		  3. Explore reasons for avoiding discussion of feelings
		  4. Encourage sharing of common problems with others
		I. Initiate referrals to others as appropriate
			F. Reassure that some negative thoughts and feelings are normal
			G. Review common changes in behavior associated with grieving (e.g., change in appetite and sleep and dream patterns) with patient/significant others. Explain that while intensity and frequency will decrease with time, mourning period may continue for some time
			H. Discuss possible tension reduction or normal coping behaviors in grief recovery (e.g., activity with others)
				4. Change in normal physiologic functions (e.g., hunger, activity)

Injury: potential for high-risk fall status

DEFINING CHARACTERISTICS	NURSING ORDERS			EXPECTED OUTCOMES
	ASSESSMENT	INTERVENTIONS	PATIENT EDUCATION	

Previous history of falls
Altered mental status
Presence of medical condition that places patient at risk
Administration of medications that places patient at risk
Need for assistance to get out of bed or to ambulate
Limited ability to perform ADL
Use of assisting devices
Use of mechanical restraints
Test or procedure preparation that affects mental status or ambulation
	Complete the following to identify *high-risk* patients on admission and to reassess as needed
	
	Risk factors
	A. Is patient over 50?
	B. Review following systems. Document any condition that potentially could place patient in risk of falling
	  1. Mental status (e.g., confusion, sundowning)
	  2. Respiratory system
	  3. Cardiovascular system
		Institute and document appropriate safety precautions
		
		Environmental
		A. Place bed in low position
		B. Place side rails up
		C. Place bed brakes on
		D. Place call light within reach
		E. Ensure adequate lighting
		F. Ensure unobstructed walkway
		G. Ensure that patient is able to reach bedside stand
		
		Physical needs
		A. Use assisting devices as appropriate: walkers, canes, wheelchairs
		B. Use patient restraints as documented in policy manual
		C. Establish regular schedule of elimination assistance
		D. Assist patient in ADL and ambulation when necessary
			Teach patient
			A. To use call light
			B. To observe activity restrictions per physician's order
			C. What patient's own responsibility is in preventing falls
				Risk of fall will be minimized

Originated by **Yvonne Evans Wordell, RN, MSN**
Resource persons: **Urakay Campbell, RN**
      Barbara J. Hobbs, RN, MSN

Injury: potential for high-risk fall status—cont'd

DEFINING CHARACTERISTICS	NURSING ORDERS			EXPECTED OUTCOMES
	ASSESSMENT	INTERVENTIONS	PATIENT EDUCATION	
Inability to use call light or to call nurse	4. Musculoskeletal system 5. Renal system 6. GI system 7. Neurologic system **Medications** Is patient receiving any medication that places him/her at risk of falling? **Level of activity** A. What is prescribed level of activity? B. Does patient need assistance to get out of bed? to go to the bathroom? to ambulate? C. Does patient require constant supervision? **History of falls** A. Has patient had any prehospital falls (at work, at home?) B. Has patient ever fallen while in hospital? C. Has patient fallen during current admission? **ADL** Assess patient's level of capability performing routine ADL **Assisting devices** Are special assisting devices prescribed for or used by patient? **Mechanical restraints** Are any mechanical restraints (Posey vest or soft or leather restraints) being used on patient?	E. Advise use of hearing aid and corrective lenses while patient ambulates and when appropriate F. Schedule patient safety checks as necessary or _____ **Psychosocial needs** A. Orient patient to time, place, and person as necessary B. Provide calendar and clock when appropriate		

Continued.

Injury: potential for high-risk fall status—cont'd

DEFINING CHARACTERISTICS	NURSING ORDERS			EXPECTED OUTCOMES
	ASSESSMENT	INTERVENTIONS	PATIENT EDUCATION	
	Test or procedure preparation A. Does preparation interfere with ambulation ability? B. Does patient require assistance to bathroom because of test preparation? **Physical environment** A. Does patient know how to call nurse? B. Is patient able to reach and use call light? **Risk level determination** A. Mild or no risk B. Moderate—can trust patient to call for assistance C. High risk—severe/multiple problems			

Knowledge Deficit

DEFINING CHARACTERISTICS	NURSING ORDERS			EXPECTED OUTCOMES
	ASSESSMENT	INTERVENTIONS	PATIENT EDUCATION	
Questioning members of health care team Verbalizes incorrect/inaccurate information Noncompliance Denial of need to learn Anger/hostility Depression Withdrawal from environment Altered orientation to environment Inability to read, hear, see Physical inability to perform task Performs task incorrectly Expresses frustration or confusion when performing task	A. Assess orientation to person, place, environment B. Assess intellectual ability to learn C. Assess ability to see, hear, and read D. Assess physical ability to perform tasks E. Identify priority of learning need within the overall plan of care F. Assess motivation and willingness of patient/significant others to learn G. Question patient regarding previous experience and health teaching	A. Provide physical comfort for learner B. Provide quiet atmosphere without interruptions C. Establish objectives and goals for learning at the beginning D. Allow learner to identify what is most important to him/her E. Explore attitudes and feelings about change F. Allow for, and support, self-directed, self-designed learning G. Assist the learner in integrating information into daily life H. Allow adequate time for integration of material that is in sharp conflict with existing values or beliefs I. Refer patient to support groups as needed J. Include significant others whenever appropriate	A. Provide explanations at level of understanding of patient/significant others B. Give clear, thorough explanations and demonstrations C. Provide information using various mediums to improve retention of information D. Move from concrete information to abstract concepts E. Provide models for change F. Keep sessions directed at single concept or idea	Patient/significant others will be able to demonstrate _____ or to state _____

Originated by **Martha Dickerson, RN, MS, CCRN**

Knowledge Deficit—cont'd

DEFINING CHARACTERISTICS	NURSING ORDERS			EXPECTED OUTCOMES
	ASSESSMENT	INTERVENTIONS	PATIENT EDUCATION	
Multiple hospitalizations for same problem Frequent exacerbations of illness Development of complications	H. Identify any existing misconceptions regarding material to be taught I. Determine cultural influences on health teaching		G. Keep sessions short to prevent fatigue H. Encourage questions from patient/significant others I. Allow learner to practice new skills; provide immediate feedback on performance J. Provide positive reinforcement of learning K. Allow learner to maintain self-esteem L. Document progress of teaching/learning	

Mobility, Impaired Physical

DEFINING CHARACTERISTICS	NURSING ORDERS			EXPECTED OUTCOMES
	ASSESSMENT	INTERVENTIONS	PATIENT EDUCATION	

Inability to move purposefully within physical environment, including bed mobility, transfer, and ambulation
Reluctance to attempt movement
Limited ROM
Decreased muscle strength, control, or mass
Imposed restrictions of movement including mechanical, medical protocol, and impaired coordination
Verbalization of inability to perform
	A. Assess patient's ability to carry out ADL on daily basis
	B. Assess knowledge patient/significant others have of immobility (what they know, need to know, and their misconceptions)
	C. Assess respiratory rate, rhythm, and amplitude every ____ hours
	D. Auscultate breath sounds every ____ hours
	E. Assess for pulmonary embolism (chest pain, dyspnea, tachycardia, changes in BP)
	F. Assess for developing thrombophlebitis (calf pain, Homans' sign, redness, localized swelling, and rise in temperature)
		A. Encourage and facilitate early ambulation and other ADL when possible. Assist with each initial change—dangling, sitting in chair, ambulation
		B. Obtain adequate assistance of ____people/Hoyer lift when transferring patient to bed, chair, or stretcher
		C. Encourage appropriate use of assisting devices
		D. Turn and position q.2h. or as needed
		E. Maintain limbs in functional alignment (e.g., with pillows, sandbags, or wedges)
		  1. Support feet in dorsiflexed position
		  2. Assist with passive/active ROM exercises every ____ hours
		  3. Turn prone or semiprone once daily unless contraindicated
		F. Use prophylactic antipressure devices (e.g., heel/elbow pads, sheepskin, and special mattresses) as appropriate
		G. Clean, dry, and moisturize skin every ____hours and as needed
			A. Explain progressive physical activity to patient. Help patient/significant others to establish reasonable and obtainable goals
			B. Instruct patient/significant others in importance of position change, ROM, coughing exercises, etc.
			C. Reinforce principles of exercise, emphasizing that joints are to be exercised to the point of pain, not beyond
			D. Encourage verbalization of feelings, strengths, and weaknesses
				Optimal physical mobility will be maintained

Originated by **Linda Arsenault, RN, MSN, CNRN**
    Marilyn Magafas, RN,C BSN
    Karen Moyer, RN, MS, CCRN, CNA

Continued.

Mobility, Impaired Physical—cont'd

DEFINING CHARACTERISTICS	NURSING ORDERS			EXPECTED OUTCOMES
	ASSESSMENT	INTERVENTIONS	PATIENT EDUCATION	
	G. Assess skin integrity. Check for signs of redness, tissue ischemia (especially over ears, shoulders, elbows, sacrum, hips, heels, ankles, and toes) every ___ hours H. Assess nutritional needs as they relate to immobility (possible hypocalcemia, negative nitrogen balance) I. Assess elimination status (usual pattern, present pattern, signs of constipation)	H. Encourage coughing and deep breathing exercises every ___ hours; use suction as needed I. Maintain I & O record as needed; monitor daily consumption J. Encourage liquid intake of 2000-3000 ml/day unless contraindicated K. Monitor and record bowel activity daily L. Keep side rails up and bed in low position M. Consult rehabilitation medicine personnel (after clearance with physician) as appropriate		

Nutrition, Alteration in: less than body requirements

DEFINING CHARACTERISTICS	NURSING ORDERS			EXPECTED OUTCOMES
	ASSESSMENT	INTERVENTIONS	PATIENT EDUCATION	

Loss of weight with or without adequate caloric intake ≥10%-20% *under* ideal body weight
Documented inadequate caloric intake
Caloric intake inadequate to keep pace with abnormal disease/metabolic state
	A. Document patient's actual weight on admission (do not estimate)
	B. Obtain nutritional history as appropriate
		A. Consult dietitian when appropriate
		B. Document appetite, I & O
		  1. Encourage patient participation (daily log)
		  2. Record strict I & O (do not estimate)
		C. Assist patient with meals as needed
		D. Encourage frequent oral ingestion of high calorie/protein foods and fluids
		E. Encourage high-fiber foods; give stool softeners as ordered to promote regular elimination patterns
		F. Obtain weight as ordered, with minimum of 1 weighing each week on all patients
		G. Monitor urine/serum electrolytes, CBC, glucose, and urine sugar/acetone as needed
		H. Encourage exercise
			A. Review and reinforce the following to patient/significant others
			  1. Importance of maintaining adequate caloric intake
			  2. Foods high in calories/protein
			  3. Eating patterns that will promote weight gain and nitrogen balance (e.g., small frequent meals of foods high in calories and protein)
			B. Assist patient/significant others in recognizing regular eating patterns
			C. Educate family in necessity of emotional support
				A. Optimal caloric intake will be maintained
				B. Patient will understand basic nutritional concepts and demonstrate correct eating patterns

Originated by **Jackie Suprenant, RN, BSN**
     Maureen T. Linehan, RN
     Carol Burkhart, RN, BSN, CCRN

Nutrition, Alteration in: more than body requirements

DEFINING CHARACTERISTICS	NURSING ORDERS			EXPECTED OUTCOMES
	ASSESSMENT	INTERVENTIONS	PATIENT EDUCATION	

Weight 10%-20% over ideal weight for height and frame
Sedentary activity level
Reported or observed dysfunctional eating patterns
	A. Perform nutritional assessment as appropriate
	B. Document patient's actual weight on admission (do not estimate)
		A. Consult dietitian or diabetes teaching service when appropriate
		B. Assist patient with selection of appropriate foods from each food group
		C. Encourage patient to keep a daily log of food/liquid ingestion and caloric intake
		D. Encourage water intake
		E. Encourage patient to be more aware of nutritional habits
		  1. To realize the time it takes to eat (encourage putting fork down between bites)
		  2. To focus on eating and to avoid other diversional activities (e.g., reading, television viewing, telephoning)
		  3. To observe for cues that lead to eating (e.g., odor, time, depression, and boredom)
		  4. To eat in the same place as much as possible
		  5. To identify actual need for food
		F. Weigh patient as ordered, at least once a week
		G. Monitor urine/serum electrolytes, CBC, glucose, and urine sugar/acetone as needed
		H. Encourage exercise
			A. Review and reinforce dietitian's teaching regarding
			  1. Four food groups and proper serving sizes
			  2. Caloric content of food
			  3. Methods of preparation
			B. Provide family counseling as needed
			C. Encourage diabetic patients to attend diabetic classes. Review and reinforce principles of dietary management of diabetes
				A. Patient will demonstrate weight reduction over time
				B. Diabetic patient will verbalize the purpose of meal planning in the control of diabetes

Originated by **Jackie Suprenant, RN, BSN**
Carol Burkhart, RN, BSN, CCRN
Maureen T. Linehan, RN

Self-Concept: disturbance in

DEFINING CHARACTERISTICS	NURSING ORDERS			EXPECTED OUTCOMES
	ASSESSMENT	INTERVENTIONS	PATIENT EDUCATION	
Subjective Patient/significant other(s) report change in self-concept **Objective** Change in affect and/or appearance (sadness, anger, irritability, decreased attention to grooming) Change in behavior (e.g., severe or prolonged denial, refusal to participate in care or treatment, withdrawal, decrease in functioning, disproportionate sense of capability) Change in cognitive/intellectual functioning (impaired judgment/thinking; inability to make decisions; poor reality testing) Verbalization of ambivalence, discontent, fears, sense of helplessness, loss of control Focus on the past Self-deprecating remarks	A. Document past level of functioning 　Emotional 　Social 　Interpersonal 　Intellectual 　Vocational 　Physical B. Note quality/quantity of verbalizations regarding self C. Note report by patient/significant others of changes in self-concept D. Assess for evidence of change in behavior (see Defining Characteristics) E. See SCP earlier in this chapter: "Body image: disturbance in"	A. Provide environment conducive to expression of feelings 　1. Make frequent contact in unhurried manner 　2. Avoid excessive focus on physical tasks 　3. Listen in supportive manner 　4. Provide privacy 　5. Allow patient to personalize environment with own belongings and/or familiar persons as appropriate 　6. Convey sense of respect for abilities/strengths in addition to recognizing problems/concerns B. Provide anticipatory guidance to minimize anxiety and fear of the unknown 　1. Explain routines and procedures in plan of treatment 　2. Orient patient/significant others to environment 　3. Use language and terminology patient/significant others can understand 　4. Provide opportunities for questions and verbalization of feelings 　5. Include patient/significant others in planning care whenever possible 　6. Observe response to information, caretakers, and environment 　7. See SCP in this chapter: Anxiety/fear C. Assist in efforts to obtain understanding and mastery of new experiences 　1. Support efforts at maintaining independence, reality, positive self-image, sense of capability, problem solving 　2. Provide realistic appraisal of progress 　3. Reinforce efforts at constructive change 　4. Recognize variations in manner and pace at which each individual attempts to adjust to illness 　5. Encourage involvement in varied activities and interaction with others 　6. Use referral sources (other professionals or lay persons) as appropriate to support coping efforts	A. Discuss "normal" impact of alteration in health status (temporary or permanent) on self-concept B. Reassure patient that such changes frequently result in a variety of emotional/behavioral responses C. Advise of realistic need for additional support in coping with change and stress D. Serve as role model for patient/significant others in healthy expression of feelings/concerns E. See SCP earlier in this chapter: Knowledge deficit	Patient/significant others will acknowledge possible impact of health status on self-concept External sources of anxiety and discomfort will be minimized Patient/significant others will be provided with support in attempts to integrate anticipated actual changes into overall self-concepts and to retain/obtain positive self-image

Originated by **Ann Filipski, RN, MSN, CS**
　　　　　　Susan R. Laub, RN, MEd, CS

Sexual Dysfunction: alteration in sexual functioning

DEFINING CHARACTERISTICS	NURSING ORDERS			EXPECTED OUTCOMES
	ASSESSMENT	INTERVENTIONS	PATIENT EDUCATION	

Verbalization of concern(s) regarding sexual functions
Questions regarding "normal" sexual function
Noncompliance with medications/treatments with known risk of impaired sexual function
Expressed decrease in sexual satisfaction
Decreased self-esteem
Reported change in relationship with partner(s)
Actual/perceived limitation secondary to diagnosis or therapy
Sexually inappropriate behavior within setting
Frequent seeking of confirmation of sexual desirability
	A. Assess/explore patient's/couple's past sexual practices/attitudes
	B. Assess patient's/couple's understanding of sexual therapy and physiology
	C. Identify potential/actual difficulty as to
	    Nature
	    Course
	    Onset
	    Duration
	D. Identify possible/actual causative factors or contributing situational variables
	  1. Anxiety
	  2. Trauma/damage to body part(s)
	  3. Physiologic limitations secondary to disease
	  4. Pain
	  5. Fatigue/decreased activity tolerance
	  6. Effects of medications and/or therapies
	  7. Functional disorders (e.g., psychosis, depression)
	  8. Altered self-concept
	  9. Knowledge deficit
	 10. Situational factors (e.g., unwilling/unavailable partner, lack of appropriate environment)
	 11. Acute illness
		A. Use a relaxed, comfortable manner
		B. Provide atmosphere of acceptance and privacy when discussing sexuality
		C. Offer opportunities to verbalize concerns and convey their normalcy
		D. Encourage patient's/couple's efforts to discuss difficulty and their ideas about possible influencing factors
		E. Discuss both physiologic and emotional influences on sexual functioning
		F. Explore patient's/couple's awareness of and comfort with means of sexual satisfaction besides intercourse
		G. Encourage patient to share concerns/information with partner(s), or involve in sexual health counseling
		H. Consider referral for further workup/treatment
		  1. Primary physician
		  2. Specialized physician
		  3. Psychiatric consultant
		  4. Sexual dysfunction clinic
		I. Consider referral to such professional/lay support groups as
		  1. Sexual Impotence Resolved
		  2. Reach for Recovery
		  3. Ostomates
		  4. Mended Hearts
		  5. Huff & Puff
			A. Provide health teaching regarding "normal" range of sexual functioning and practices throughout life cycle
			B. Use terminology appropriate to patient's level
			C. Consider a variety of teaching strategies (e.g., individual/couple/group instruction, written materials, visual aids)
			D. Teach techniques for modifying limitations/difficulties as appropriate, e.g., change positions, use oxygen-conserving methods, use of nitroglycerin before activity, medication treatment regime, relaxation techniques
				A. Individual/couple will be able to identify factors influencing own sexual functioning
				B. Individual/couple will be provided with support/counseling to enable resumption of sexually satisfying activity

Originated by **Ann Filipski, RN, MSN, CS**

Skin Integrity, Impairment of: actual and potential

DEFINING CHARACTERISTICS	NURSING ORDERS			EXPECTED OUTCOMES
	ASSESSMENT	INTERVENTIONS	PATIENT EDUCATION	

Potential
External
 	
Mechanical factors (shearing forces, pressure, restraint)
Hypothermia/hyper-thermia
Chemical substance
Radiation
Physical immobility
Excretions/secretions
Humidity
 	
Internal
 	
Medication
Altered nutritional/ metabolic state
Altered circulation
Altered sensation
Altered pigmentation
Altered skin turgor
Psychogenic
Immunologic
Skeletal prominence
 	
Actual
 	
Stage I: redness, skin intact
Stage II: blisters
Stage III: necrosis
Stage IV: necrosis involving bones, joints
	A. Assess skin integrity
	  1. Note color, moisture, texture, temperature
	  2. Ask patient about burning or itching
	B. Assess nutritional status
	  1. Diet: amount of intake, number of calories, and use of supplement
	  2. Laboratory data: serum albumin, total protein
	  3. Weight
	C. Assess physical impairments contributing to potential/actual breakdown (e.g., paralysis, sensory deficit)
	D. Assess psychologic conditions contributing to potential/actual breakdown (e.g., depression)
		Potential
		A. Check for signs of tissue ischemia, redness, changes (e.g., pain, numbness) on admission and every ____ hours
		B. Turn q.2h., according to established turning schedule
		C. Provide prophylactic use of pressure-relieving devices (e.g., sheepskin, special mattresses, Stryker boots, elbow pads)
		D. Maintain functional body alignment
		E. Increase tissue perfusion by massaging *around* affected area; *do not* massage reddened areas
		F. Clean, dry, and moisturize skin, especially over bony prominences, b.i.d., or as indicated by incontinence or sweating
		G. Encourage adequate nutrition and hydration
		  1. 2000-3000 calories/day (more if increased metabolic demands)
		  2. Fluid intake of 2000 ml/day unless medically restricted
		  3. Dietitian consult as appropriate
		
		Actual
		A. Determine degree of impairment
		  1. Measure depth and diameter
		  2. Document size and describe surrounding skin in nurses' notes
		
		Stage I
		A. See preventive measures (*Potential);* have they been instituted?
		B. Massage *around* affected areas; avoid reddened areas, since rubbing will damage ischemic skin
		C. Eliminate or minimize pressure or shearing forces; lift *(not pull)* patient in bed
		D. Institute skin protective devices
			A. Teach patient factors important to skin integrity
			  1. Nutrition
			  2. Mobility
			  3. Hygiene
			B. Teach patient early recognition of skin breakdown
			  1. Signs and symptoms
			  2. Reporting
				Potential
				Skin breakdown will not occur
				
				Actual
				Area of breakdown will heal
				Patient will verbalize knowledge of skin care and participate in own care as is feasible

Originated by **Audrey Klopp, RN, MS, CCRN, CS, ET**
    Virginia M. Storey, RN, ET
    Kathryn S. Bronstein, RN, MS, CS, PhD Candidate

Skin Integrity, Impairment of: actual and potential—cont'd

DEFINING CHARACTERISTICS	NURSING ORDERS			EXPECTED OUTCOMES
	ASSESSMENT	INTERVENTIONS	PATIENT EDUCATION	

		Stage II
		A. See preventive measures *(Potential);* have they been instituted?
		B. Leave blisters intact
		C. Protect blister by positioning and by use of Op-site, Stomahesive, or Duoderm
		
		Stage III
		A. See preventive measures *(Potential);* have they been instituted?
		B. Determine depth, presence of infection
		C. Promote healing by using appropriate protocols. Protocol can consist of physical, chemical, nutritional, pharmacologic, surgical intervention. General principles include
		  1. Keeping ulcer surface moist
		  2. Packing cavity tightly
		
		Stage IV
		A. See preventive measures *(Potential);* have they been instituted?
		B. Establish presence of eschar
		C. Proceed with debridement plan
		  1. If possible, try chemical debridement (Elase, Santyl, Debrisan)
		  2. If chemical debridement is impractical, impossible, or unsuccessful, obtain surgical consultation
		D. Once wound is clean, promote granulation through nursing protocol		

Sleep Pattern Disturbance

DEFINING CHARACTERISTICS	NURSING ORDERS			EXPECTED OUTCOMES
	ASSESSMENT	INTERVENTIONS	PATIENT EDUCATION	

Patient/significant others report alteration in "normal" sleep pattern
Restlessness
Lethargy
Insomnia
Irritability
Dozing
Yawning
Early morning awakening
Interrupted sleep
Altered mental status
Difficult to arouse
Change in activity level
Altered facial expression (e.g., blank look, fatigued appearance)
	A. Assess usual/past patterns of sleep in normal environment: amount, bedtime, rituals, depth, length, positions, aids, and interfering agents
	B. Assess patient's perception of cause of sleep difficulty and possible relief measures
	C. Document nursing observations of sleeping and wakeful behaviors
		A. Maintain environment conducive to sleep/rest (e.g., quiet, comfortable temperature, closed door)
		B. Assist patient in observing any previous bedtime ritual
		C. Provide nursing aids to promote rest, relaxation (e.g., back rub, bedtime care, pain relief, comfortable position, relaxation techniques)
		D. Organize nursing care to promote minimal interruption in sleep/rest
		  1. Eliminate nonessential nursing activities
		  2. Prepare patient for necessary anticipated interruptions/disruptions
		E. Establish semblance of "normal" daily routine with periods of activity, rest
		F. Provide soporifics as needed (e.g., milk, avoidance of stimulants such as caffeine or cola beverages and decreased exercise before sleep)
		G. Administer hypnotics as ordered, and evaluate effectiveness
			A. Educate patient/ significant others about need to sleep/rest
			B. Educate patient/ significant others about factors that may facilitate or interfere with sleep/rest
			C. Elicit and facilitate patient exploration of emotional factors that may be interfering with normal sleep pattern. Provide emotional support; encourage verbalization of feelings
				Patient will verbalize increased satisfaction with rest and sleep patterns
				Patient/significant others will begin to identify and correct abnormal sleep patterns

Originated by **Ann Filipski, RN, MSN, CS**
Janice Borman, RN, MSN
Marilyn Magafas, RN,C BSN

Tissue Perfusion, Alteration in: peripheral

DEFINING CHARACTERISTICS	NURSING ORDERS			EXPECTED OUTCOMES
	ASSESSMENT	INTERVENTIONS	PATIENT EDUCATION	

Pain, cramping, ache in extremity
Intermittent claudication (pain or weakness in one or both legs relieved by rest)
Numbness of toes on walking, relieved by rest
Foot pain at rest
Tenderness, especially of toes
Cool extremities
Pallor of toes/foot when leg is elevated for 30 seconds
Dependent rubor (20 seconds to 2 min after leg is lowered)
Decreased capillary refill
Diminished or absent arterial pulses
Shiny skin
Loss of hair
Thickened, discolored nails
Ulcerated areas/gangrene
Edema
Change in skin texture
	A. Assess extremities for color, temperature, texture every _____ , and document
	B. Assess extremities for swelling, edema, ulceration every _____
	C. Assess quality of peripheral pulses, noting capillary refill and dependent changes every _____
	D. If no pulses are noted, assess arterial blood flow using doppler ultrasonic instrumentation (if available)
	E. Assess pain/numbness/tingling as to causative factors, time of onset, quality, severity, relieving factors
	F. Assess for bilateral involvement of extremities
	G. Assess for possible causative factors related to temporary/chronic impaired arterial blood flow
	   Reduced cardiac output
	   Hypovolemia
	   Arterial spasm
	   Embolism/thrombus
	   Vasoconstriction secondary to medications, tobacco, etc.
	   Local or generalized hypothermia
	   Atherosclerosis
	   Circumferential burns
		For acute changes
		A. Evaluate causative factors, initiating corrective measures as appropriate (e.g., reposition extremity, deflate tourniquets, proper use of cooling blanket)
		B. Notify physician of signs of decreased perfusion
		C. Administer analgesic as ordered
		D. Anticipate need for possible embolectomy, heparinization, vasodilator therapy, thrombolytic therapy
		
		For chronic condition
		A. Maintain affected extremity in a dependent position
		B. Keep extremity warm (socks, blankets)
		C. Administer analgesics as ordered
		D. Bathe in warm bath water—never hot
		E. Change position at least every hour
		F. Remove all vasoconstricting factors, e.g., clothing, bandages
		G. Do not elevate bed at the knee gatch
		H. Assist with progressive activity program, noting claudication and signs of overexertion
		I. Evaluate coping responses (e.g., depression, body image problem, fear), and initiate appropriate interventions and consultations as needed
		J. Provide prophylactic pressure-relieving devices as appropriate (e.g., sheepskin, special mattresses, elbow pads, lamb's wool pads between toes, foot cradle)
		K. See SCP in this chapter: Skin integrity, impairment of
			A. Instruct patient on appropriate diagnostic tests: Doppler studies, arteriography
			B. Instruct patient on how to prevent progression of disease and avoid complications
			EFFECTS OF TEMPERATURE
			1. Keep extremities warm. Wear stockings to bed
			2. Keep house/apartment as warm as possible
			3. Wear enough clothes during winter
			4. Never apply hot water bottles or electric pads to feet/legs
			5. Avoid local cold applications
			FOOT CARE
			1. Wash feet daily with warm soap/water. Dry thoroughly by gentle patting. Never rub dry
			2. Trim toenails carefully and only after soaking in warm water. See podiatrist as needed
			3. Lubricate skin to prevent cracking
			4. Wear clean stockings
			5. Do not walk barefoot
			6. Wear correctly fitting shoes
			7. Inspect feet frequently for signs of ingrown toenails, sores, blisters, etc.
			EXERCISE/ACTIVITY
			1. Do not cross legs or keep pillows behind knees
			2. Do not sit for extended time intervals
			3. Begin a daily exercise program to promote collateral circulation
			  a. Walk about half a block after intermittent claudication is experienced, unless otherwise ordered by the physician
			  b. Stop and rest until all discomfort subsides
			  c. Repeat same procedure for total of 30 min, 2 to 3 times/day
				Optimal peripheral tissue perfusion will be maintained

Originated by **Meg Gulanick, RN, MSN, CCRN**

Tissue Perfusion, Alteration in: peripheral—cont'd

DEFINING CHARACTERISTICS	ASSESSMENT	NURSING ORDERS		EXPECTED OUTCOMES
		INTERVENTIONS	PATIENT EDUCATION	
	Indwelling arterial catheters (e.g., intraaortic balloon pump) Rotating tourniquets Constricting casts Malpositioning/ immobility Compartment syndrome		SMOKING Avoid all tobacco, which further decreases an already compromised circulation DIET If atherosclerotic problem exists, provide diet counseling on need for reduction in fats MEDICATION Take prescribed medications, observing for reaction and side effects	

Urinary Elimination, Alteration in Patterns: retention

DEFINING CHARACTERISTICS	NURSING ORDERS			EXPECTED OUTCOMES
	ASSESSMENT	INTERVENTIONS	PATIENT EDUCATION	

Decreased (<30 ml/hour) or absent urinary output for 2 consecutive hours
Frequency
Hesitancy
Urgency
Lower abdominal distention
Abdominal discomfort
	A. Evaluate previous patterns of voiding
	B. Visually inspect lower abdomen for distention
	C. Palpate over bladder for distention
	D. Evaluate time intervals between voidings
	E. Assess amount, frequency, character (color, odor, specific gravity)
	F. Determine balance between I & O
	G. Monitor urinalysis, urine culture, and sensitivity
	H. If indwelling catheter is in situ, assess for patency, kinking
		A. Initiate methods to facilitate voiding
		  1. Encourage fluids. Amount ____/shift. Patient preference: _____
		  2. Restrict fluids after ____ (time)
		  3. Offer cranberry juice daily to keep urine acidic
		  4. Position patient in _____
		  5. Place bedpan/urinal or bedside commode within reach
		  6. Provide privacy
		  7. Try to establish regular voiding schedule every ____
		  8. Have patient listen to sound of running water or place hands in warm water and/or pour warm water over perineum
		  9. Offer fluids before voiding
		  10. Perform Credé's method over bladder
		B. Monitor I & O every ____ hour. Record time, amount, character, circumstances of voiding (i.e., spontaneous, stimulated, or staining)
		C. Administer bethanechol (Urecholine) as ordered (stimulates parasympathetic nervous system to release acetylcholine at nerve endings; increases tone and amplitude of contractions of smooth muscles of urinary bladder)
		SIDE EFFECTS: Rare, following oral administration of therapeutic dose. In small subcutaneous doses: abdominal cramps, sweating and flushing. In larger doses: malaise, headache, diarrhea, nausea, vomiting, asthmatic attacks, bradycardia, lowered BP, atrioventricular block, and cardiac arrest
		D. Institute intermittent catheterization as ordered every ____ hours
		E. Insert retention (Foley) catheter as ordered
		  1. Tape catheter to abdomen (male)
		  2. Tape catheter to thigh (female)
		  3. Cleanse insertion point of catheter every shift with soap and water, and dry thoroughly
		F. Monitor BUN and creatinine levels
		G. Send urine for urinalysis and culture every ____ as ordered
			A. Educate patient/significant others about the importance of adequate intake, i.e., 8-10 glasses of fluids daily
			B. Instruct patient/significant others on measures to help voiding (e.g., regular voiding times, privacy, running water, Credé's method, and intermittent catheter technique)
			C. Instruct patient/significant others on signs and symptoms of overdistended bladder (e.g., decreased or absent urine, frequency, hesitancy, urgency, lower abdominal distention, or discomfort)
			D. Instruct patient/significant others on signs and symptoms of urinary tract infection (e.g., chills and fever, frequent urination or concentrated urine, abdominal or back pain)
				A. Urine output will be appropriate to fluid intake
				B. Patient/significant others demonstrate measures that enhance voiding

Originated by **Doris M. Humphries, RN, BSN**
Resource person: **Linda Arsenault, RN, MSN, CNRN**

CHAPTER TWO

Cardiovascular

DISORDERS

Anaphylactic Shock

NURSING DIAGNOSIS/ PATIENT PROBLEM	DEFINING CHARACTERISTICS	NURSING ORDERS		EXPECTED OUTCOMES
		ASSESSMENT	INTERVENTIONS	
Cardiac output, alteration in: decreased Etiology Severe reactions to drugs, insect bites, diagnostic agents, or food	Hypotension Tachycardia Decreased CVP Decreased pulmonary artery pressures Decreased cardiac output Oliguria Decreased peripheral pulses	Assess physical status every _____ hours and document changes. Report significant increases in the following to physician A. Vital signs including temperature, pulse rate, BP, cardiac rhythm, respiratory rate B. Lung sounds (rales, wheezing, stridor) C. Jugular vein distention, pulmonary pressures D. Skin color, rashes, temperature, moisture E. Changes in level of consciousness or mentation F. Patient's level of anxiety (mild or severe)	A. Delay absorption of drug or substance with forced emesis when appropriate for ingested drugs or food or by applying a tourniquet above injection site or insect bite B. Administer medications per orders (i.e., benedryl, epinephrine, aminophylline), noting responses C. Maintain hemodynamic parameters at prescribed levels Heart rate: _____ BP: _____ CVP: _____ Pulmonary capillary wedge pressure/pulmonary artery pressure: _____ Urine output: _____	Reversal of shock state will be evidenced by A. Response to medications B. Vital sign stability C. Hemodynamic stability
Fluid volume deficit, actual Etiology Shock state	Decreased urine output Concentrated urine Decreased venous filling Hypotension Thirst Tachycardia	A. Assess fluid balance (I & O) every _____ B. Obtain daily weights C. Assess for edema	A. Maintain optimal fluid balance 1. Administer parenteral fluid of _____ at _____ ml/hr as ordered per physician 2. Give fluid challenges as ordered, and closely monitor and record effects B. Refer to SCP in Ch. 1: Fluid volume deficit	Adequate fluid volume will be maintained
Breathing pattern, ineffective: potential Etiology Bronchospasm or laryngeal edema	Dyspnea Wheezing Tachypnea Stridor	A. Monitor respiratory status every _____ B. Monitor ABGs and note changes C. Observe for changes in respiratory status (e.g., increased shortness of breath, tachypnea, dyspnea, wheezing, stridor)	A. Position patient for optimal lung expansion and ease of breathing B. Administer O₂ per orders: _____ C. Instruct patient to breathe deeply and slow down respiratory rate D. Give medications as ordered (e.g., steroids, antihistamines, aminophylline, 1:1000 aqueous epinephrine), and record effects	Adequate ventilation and perfusion will be maintained as indicated by ABGs and regular breathing pattern

Originated by **Chris Loftus, RN, BS**
Resource person: **Susan Galanes, RN, MS, TNS, CCRN**

Anaphylactic Shock—cont'd

NURSING DIAGNOSIS/ PATIENT PROBLEM	DEFINING CHARACTERISTICS	NURSING ORDERS		EXPECTED OUTCOMES
		ASSESSMENT	INTERVENTIONS	
		D. Check breath sounds every _____ and report changes E. Monitor chest x-ray reports	E. Maintain patent airway. Anticipate emergency intubation or tracheostomy	
Urinary elimination, alteration in patterns: potential **Etiology** Decreased renal perfusion	Decreased urine output Decreased venous filling Hemoconcentration from third spacing Increased heart rate Increased BUN and creatinine levels	A. Monitor serum and urine electrolytes and osmolarity. Document changes and notify physician B. Monitor urine output every _____ hours, and notify physician and document C. Monitor daily weights D. Monitor I & O q.1h. E. Monitor laboratory data for elevation in BUN and creatinine levels, acid base imbalances, particularly Na^+ and K^+	A. Administer parenteral fluids as ordered B. See SCP in Ch. 7: Acute renal failure	Maintenance of adequate renal function will be evidenced by A. Normal electrolytes B. Urine output of at least 30 ml/hour
Consciousness, altered levels of: potential **Etiology** Shock and decreased cerebral perfusion	Changes in alertness Changes in orientation Inappropriate responses (verbal) Agitation Lethargy Pupillary changes	A. Obtain neurologic checks every _____ . Report and record any changes B. Observe for seizure activity C. Monitor vital signs every _____	A. Protect patient from possible injuries (seizures, decreased gag reflex) B. Maintain BP at _____ to _____ to increase cerebral perfusion C. Give fluids as ordered to maintain BP D. See SCP in Ch. 3: Consciousness, alteration in level of	Cerebral perfusion will be maintained as evidenced by lack of changes in level of consciousness

Skin integrity, impairment of: potential
Etiology
Allergic reaction
	Urticaria
	Pruritus
	Edema
		A. Observe for signs of flushing (localized or generalized)
		B. Watch for rashes developing; note character: macules, papules, pustules, petechia
		C. Assess for swelling/edema
			A. Give medications as ordered (e.g., Benadryl)
			B. Prevent patient from excessive scratching
			  1. Instruct patient not to scratch
			  2. Clip nails if patient is scratching in sleep
			  3. Mitten hands if necessary
			C. Be prepared for intubation or tracheostomy (if facial edema is present, upper respiratory edema may also occur)
				Urticaria will be resolved, and skin condition will return to normal

Anxiety/fear: potential **Etiology** Alteration in breathing Shock state Another allergic reaction Other possible allergens	Restlessness Withdrawal Indifference Demanding behavior Uncooperative behavior Tachycardia Tachypnea Diarrhea	A. Recognize patient's level of anxiety, and note signs and symptoms B. Assess patient's coping mechanisms	See SCP in Ch. 1: Anxiety/fear	Anxieties and fears will be allayed, and patient will return to normal coping mechanisms

Continued.

Anaphylactic Shock—cont'd

NURSING DIAGNOSIS/ PATIENT PROBLEM	DEFINING CHARACTERISTICS	NURSING ORDERS		EXPECTED OUTCOMES
		ASSESSMENT	INTERVENTIONS	
Knowledge deficit of allergens **Etiology** New condition	Recurrent allergic reactions Unable to identify allergens	Assess patient's knowledge of his/ her condition and allergens	A. Explain symptoms and interventions to help prevent anaphylactic shock B. Instruct patient/significant others what factors could precipitate a recurrence of shock and ways to prevent or avoid these precipitating factors C. Explain environmental factors that may increase risk of anaphylaxis, i.e., certain drugs, bee stings, food D. Instruct patient on use of insect sting kits (containing a chewable antihistamine, epinephrine in prefilled syringe and instructions for use) if they are to be used E. Instruct patient with known allergies to wear medic-alert tags F. Patient/significant others should be made aware that when giving past medical history they should include allergies to certain foods	A. Patient/significant others will be able to state factors that can precipitate a recurrence of anaphylactic shock and know ways to prevent or avoid such factors B. Patient will know how to use insect sting kit before a sting

Angina, Unstable*: acute phase (CCU)

NURSING DIAGNOSIS/ PATIENT PROBLEM	DEFINING CHARACTERISTICS	NURSING ORDERS		EXPECTED OUTCOMES
		ASSESSMENT	INTERVENTIONS	

Comfort, alteration in: pain
 Unstable angina is also called preinfarction angina, acute coronary insufficiency, or crescendo angina. It can represent an impending myocardial infarction
 	
 Etiology
 Myocardial ischemia
	New onset (<60 days) angina; or
	 Changing pattern of previously stable angina; or
	 Angina occurring at rest or with minimal exertion; or
	 Angina occurring during sleep
	 ECG changes
	 A. Normal or depressed ST segment
	 B. ST segment elevation during pain with variant *Prinzmetal's angina*
		A. Solicit patient's description of or absence of pain
		 B. Assess pain characteristics
		   1. Quality: as with stable angina (squeezing, tightening, choking, pressing, burning)
		   2. Location: substernal area, may radiate to extremities (e.g., arms, shoulders)
		   3. Severity: more intense than classic angina pectoris
		   4. Duration: persists longer than 20 min
			A. Maintain strict bed rest to decrease O₂ demands
			 B. Provide therapeutic environment conducive to rest and sleep
			 C. Instruct patient to report pain as soon as it starts (important for diagnosis and easier to treat)
			 D. Respond immediately to complaint of pain
			 E. Administer O₂ as ordered
			 F. Perform ECG immediately during and after episode of pain to evaluate ST changes (to assist in diagnosing cardiac origin of pain and site of coronary artery involvement)
			 G. Give medications as ordered, evaluating effectiveness and observing signs/symptoms of untoward reactions
			   1. Nitrates
			     a. Anticipate IV nitroglycerin drip
				Discomfort will be relieved or minimized

Originated by **Teodorina M. Saez, RN, BSN**
Resource person: **Meg Gulanick, RN, MSN, CCRN**
*Rule out myocardial infarction.

Angina Unstable: acute phase (CCU)—cont'd

NURSING DIAGNOSIS/ PATIENT PROBLEM	DEFINING CHARACTERISTICS	NURSING ORDERS		EXPECTED OUTCOMES
		ASSESSMENT	INTERVENTIONS	
		5. Onset: minimal exertion or during rest or sleep	b. Anticipate large doses to control pain (100-600 mg/min) c. Monitor BP closely (every _____) d. Anticipate fluid challenge to treat hypotension 2. Beta blockers. Observe for side effects (hypotension) H. Anticipate intraaortic balloon pump management if pain and ischemic changes persist despite maximal medical therapy I. Anticipate cardiac catheterization and, depending on results, anticipate coronary artery bypass surgery	
Cardiac output, alteration in: decreased (potential) **Etiology** Prolonged episodes of myocardial ischemia affecting contractility	Variations in hemodynamic parameters (increased/decreased BP, increased heart rate, increased systemic vascular resistance, increased pulmonary artery pressures, abnormal heart sounds [S_3 or S_4], increased jugular venous distention, pulmonary congestion) Arrhythmias, ECG changes (depressed or elevated ST segment) Restlessness, mentation changes	A. Assess hemodynamic status every _____and especially during episode of pain B. Assess for myocardial ischemia (ST changes) on ECG C. Monitor ECG continuously for arrhythmias, especially during episode of pain	A. Anticipate possible progression to myocardial infarction 1. Monitor results of cardiac isoenzymes q.8h. as ordered 2. Monitor frequency, duration, severity, and occurrence of pain B. If symptoms develop, institute SCP in Ch. 1: Cardiac output, alteration in: decreased C. Maintain bed rest to prevent increased O_2 demands D. Anticipate development of life-threatening arrhythmias (tachydysrhythmias or bradydysrhythmias may occur) 1. Anticipate/administer lidocaine for ventricular arrhythmias per protocol 2. If high degree atrioventricular block develops, anticipate atropine/isoproterenol IV and insertion of temporary pacemaker	Optimal cardiac output will be maintained

Continued.

Angina Unstable: acute phase (CCU)—cont'd

NURSING DIAGNOSIS/ PATIENT PROBLEM	DEFINING CHARACTERISTICS	NURSING ORDERS		EXPECTED OUTCOMES
		ASSESSMENT	INTERVENTIONS	
Anxiety/fear **Etiology** Recurrent anginal attacks Increased frequency of attacks Incomplete relief from pain by usual means (nitroglycerin and rest) Fear of impending doom and death Alteration in activity level precipitating chest pain (decreased activity level)	**Mild** Restlessness Increased awareness Increased questioning **Moderate/severe** Restlessness Insomnia Glancing about/increased alertness Facial tension/wide-eyed Focus on self Poor eye contact Increased perspiration Anorexia/GI problems Overexcited/jittery Expressed concern Trembling Constant demands	Assess level of anxiety (mild to severe) and patient's coping patterns	A. Institute SCP in Ch. 1: Anxiety/fear B. Encourage patient to call for nurse when pain or anxiety develops C. Immediately respond to any complaint of pain D. Make every effort to remain at bedside throughout episode of pain E. Check on patient frequently to provide reassurance	Decreased level of anxiety as evidenced by A. Calm, relaxed appearance B. Verbalization of fears and feelings
Knowledge deficit **Etiology** Unfamiliarity with disease process, treatment, recovery	Multiple questions or lack of questioning Verbalized misconceptions	A. Assess present level of understanding by patient/significant others B. Assess physical/emotional readiness for learning by patient/significant others	A. Instruct patient to report pain so that relief measures may be instituted B. Instruct patient to evaluate and report effectiveness of measures used C. Teach patient/significant others 1. Anatomy and physiology of the coronary condition 2. Atherosclerotic process and the implications of angina pectoris 3. Special emphasis on the use of nitroglycerin and its side effects when chest pain occurs D. Remind patient that further teaching will take place after transfer from unit	Patient/significant other will be able to A. Verbalize understanding of anatomy/physiology of unstable angina B. Decide when to seek emergency help C. Develop an understanding of causes and appropriate relief measures for pain

Hypertensive Crisis

NURSING DIAGNOSIS/ PATIENT PROBLEM	DEFINING CHARACTERISTICS	NURSING ORDERS		EXPECTED OUTCOMES
		ASSESSMENT	INTERVENTIONS	
Systemic blood pressure, alteration in: hypertensive crisis **Etiology** Fluid overload Increased metabolic rate Increased resistance by arterial walls Poor compliance with antihypertensive medication treatment plan Toxemia of pregnancy	Systolic >200 mm Hg Diastolic >120 mm Hg Mean arterial pressure >150 mm Hg Weakness Dizziness Severe headache Diplopia Seizure activity	Assess significant alterations in BP in both arms lying, sitting, and with arterial line if present	A. Monitor and record respiratory rate, heart rate, and BP every _____ B. Administer and adjust medications as ordered to maintain BP within prescribed parameters: Systolic: _____ Diastolic: _____ Mean arterial pressure: _____ NOTE: Notify physician if BP is above or below these parameters C. Monitor and record I & O every _____ D. Weigh daily and record E. Maintain head of bed at 30-degree elevation F. Maintain on complete bed rest; instruct patient to change positions gradually G. Explain to patient the necessity of avoiding Valsalva's maneuver 1. Stress importance of exhaling when patient is being positioned 2. Provide stool softener as ordered H. Monitor and notify physician of abnormal serum chemistry values I. Monitor and notify physician of urine specific gravity every _____	Optimal BP will be maintained
Injury, potential for **Etiology** Potential for complication of nitroprusside therapy	**Side effects of nitroprusside** Nausea Sweating Dizziness Hypotension Headache Restlessness Palpitations Tremors Substernal discomfort **Complications** Severe hypotension Thiocyanate accumulation: blurred vision, delirium, hypothyroidism, convulsions, metabolic acidosis, loss of consciousness	Assess for side effects or complications of nitroprusside therapy	A. Administer an IV infusion of nitroprusside, using a motorized pump via piggyback 1. Dose: 0.5 μg/kg/min to 10 μg/kg/min 2. Change solution every _____ 3. Do not mix other drugs in bag or main IV line 4. Cover infusion container with opaque material to exclude light B. Maintain a constant infusion rate of main IV line while nitroprusside via piggyback is infusing to prevent patient from receiving bolus of nitroprusside C. Titrate nitroprusside to maintain prescribed BP ranges. If hypotension occurs, stop nitroprusside immediately, notify physician, and lower head of bed to flat or Trendelenburg's position	Complications of nitroprusside therapy will be decreased

Originated by **Nola D. Johnson, RN**
Resource persons: **Susan Galanes, RN, MS, TNS, CCRN**
Meg Gulanick, RN, MSN, CCRN

Continued.

Hypertensive Crisis—cont'd

NURSING DIAGNOSIS/ PATIENT PROBLEM	DEFINING CHARACTERISTICS	NURSING ORDERS		EXPECTED OUTCOMES
		ASSESSMENT	INTERVENTIONS	
			D. Monitor thiocyanate levels q.72h. as appropriate. Discontinue if level is increased to 10 mg/100 ml and notify physician	
Consciousness, altered levels of: potential **Etiology** Encephalopathy or cerebrovascular accident	Change in alertness, orientation, verbal response, eye opening, motor response, pupillary reaction Memory impairment Impaired judgment Agitation Inappropriate affect Impaired thought process Blurred vision Focal motor weakness	Assess for alteration in level of consciousness/responsiveness every _____	A. Keep oral airway at bedside, and be prepared to protect patient if seizures occur B. Keep side rails up at all times, bed in low position, and a functioning call light within reach C. Reorient patient to environment as needed D. If restraints are needed, position patient on side, *never* on back E. If an alteration in level of consciousness is present, see SCP in Ch. 3: Consciousness, alteration in level of	Optimal state of consciousness will be maintained
Cardiac output, alteration in: decreased (potential) **Etiology** Potential: congestive heart failure	Variations in hemodynamic parameters: heart rate, CVP, pulmonary wedge pressure, urine output Rales, tachypnea, dyspnea, orthopnea, cough, abnormal ABGs, frothy sputum Weight gain, edema Anxiety, restlessness Syncope, dizziness	Assess for signs of decreased cardiac output	See SCP in Ch. 1: Cardiac output, alteration in: decreased (as appropriate)	Optimal cardiac output will be maintained
Renal function, alteration in: potential **Etiology** Increased systemic BP	Urine output <400-600 ml/24 hours Elevated serum BUN, potassium, creatinine, phosphorus levels Low serum calcium level	Assess, monitor, and document A. I & O every _____ B. Daily weights C. Serum BUN, creatinine, and uric acid levels D. Urine specific gravity every _____ hours E. Urinalysis and vanillylmandelic acid (VMA)	A. Notify physician of alterations from normal B. Administer diuretics/fluids as ordered C. See SCP in Ch. 7: Renal failure, acute (as appropriate)	Optimal renal function will be maintained

Hypertensive Crisis—cont'd

NURSING DIAGNOSIS/ PATIENT PROBLEM	DEFINING CHARACTERISTICS	NURSING ORDERS		EXPECTED OUTCOMES
		ASSESSMENT	INTERVENTIONS	
Comfort, alteration in **Etiology** Increased intracranial pressure	Headache Dizziness Nausea, vomiting Restlessness	Solicit patient's description of discomforting factors, documenting in patient's own words	A. Provide rest periods to facilitate comfort, sleep, relaxation B. Provide quiet environment. Keep lights low, noise to minimum. Limit visitors. C. Give medications (e.g., acetaminophen [Tylenol], prochlorperazine [Compazine]) as ordered, evaluating effectiveness and observing for any untoward effects D. Use any additional comfort measures whenever appropriate 　1. Physiologic interventions (e.g., heat/cold, position change) 　2. Positive suggestion 　3. Reassurance and contact E. Notify physician if interventions are unsuccessful or if current complaint is a significant change	Discomfort, as evidenced by patient's verbalization and by relaxed, comfortable appearance, will be minimized
Knowledge deficit **Etiology** Unfamiliarity with disease process, treatment, and procedures	Noncompliance with medications, diet, follow-up care, preventive measures Verbalizes lack of knowledge, asks questions about hypertension	Solicit patient's description and understanding of A. Precipitating events B. Disease process C. Treatment and procedures	A. Explain to patient/significant others 　1. Disease process 　　a. Signs and symptoms of recurrence or progression (headache, diplopia, weakness, faintness, nausea) 　　b. Possible complications 　2. Treatment and procedures 　　a. Importance of decreasing or maintaining a stable weight 　　b. Importance of low fat, low salt diet 　　c. Importance of maintaining proper fluid intake and of limitations such as caffeinated coffee, tea, and alcohol 　　d. Importance of knowing medications, dosages, and times 　　e. Importance of follow-up appointments	Patient/significant others will verbalize a basic understanding of the disease process, procedures, treatments

Mitral Valve Prolapse

NURSING DIAGNOSIS/ PATIENT PROBLEM	DEFINING CHARACTERISTICS	NURSING ORDERS		EXPECTED OUTCOMES
		ASSESSMENT	INTERVENTIONS	
Knowledge deficit of patient/significant others concerning occurrence, physiology, treatment, and complications of disease **Etiology** Unfamiliarity with disease process, treatment, recovery	Asking multiple questions Expressing fears Overly anxious Asking no questions	A. Assess knowledge of patient/significant others B. Assess readiness to learn of patient/ significant others C. Assess emotional and psychologic needs	A. Teach patient about occurrence of disease 1. Fairly common; large number of undiagnosed, asymptomatic people in general population 2. Common in women but also diagnosed in men B. Teach patient of causative factors 1. Etiology usually unknown 2. Can be primary or secondary to previous ischemic heart disease, rheumatic fever, cardiomyopathy, or ruptured chordae tendinae 3. Important to understand that serious heart disease is usually not present, that the symptoms are more a nuisance than significant, and that prognosis for life is excellent C. Teach patient the physiology of the disease: prolapse of one or both valve leaflets into the left atrium D. Inform patient of usual diagnostic procedure (echocardiogram) 1. An echocardiogram is a simple, painless test in which high frequency sound waves are pictured on a screen and recorded 2. Patient is undressed to the waist, and electrodes are applied to each shoulder and right side of stomach 3. A small transducer is moved across the chest to listen to echo waves 4. The test takes only 15-30 min E. Teach patient of the treatment of the disease 1. Beta blockers, calcium blockers a. Need for compliance to prescribed dosages, even when symptom-free b. Side effects of medication 2. Unrestricted activity if patient is symptom-free 3. Self-limitation of activities and stresses that precipitate symptoms	Patient/significant others will verbalize A. Occurrence of disease B. Causative factors C. Physiology of disease D. Diagnostic procedure E. Treatment F. Complications

Originated by **Marilyn Rousseau, RN**
Resource person: **Meg Gulanick, RN, MSN, CCRN**

Mitral Valve Prolapse—cont'd

NURSING DIAGNOSIS/ PATIENT PROBLEM	DEFINING CHARACTERISTICS	NURSING ORDERS		EXPECTED OUTCOMES
		ASSESSMENT	INTERVENTIONS	
			F. Teach patient the possible, but rare, complications of the disease 　1. Mitral regurgitation leading to congestive heart failure 　2. Infective subacute bacterial endocarditis 　　a. Prophylaxis is indicated 　　b. Patient should contact physician for prophylactic antibiotics before any dental procedures (especially teeth cleaning), gynecologic procedures, or other invasive procedures 　　c. It is felt that many common invasive procedures will leave a pathway in which bacteria can travel to the heart 　3. Sudden death	
Cardiac output, alteration in: decreased (potential) **Etiology** Alteration in cardiac rate and rhythm, specifically paroxysmal tachycardia	Palpitations, a sudden, rapid, regular fluttering sensation in the chest Faintness, light-headedness Weakness Shortness of breath Rapid pulse ECG abnormalities	A. Note, record, and report palpitations. Check relationship to activity, diet, and stress B. Assess cardiac status 　1. Pulse rate: rhythm and volume 　2. BP 　3. Skin condition C. Assess respiratory status 　1. Note respiratory rate, quality, need for O_2 　2. Check skin, nailbeds, mucosa for signs of cyanosis D. Check ECG for abnormalities	A. Provide rest in upright position B. Provide emotional and psychologic support C. Check vital signs frequently D. If signs and symptoms of decreased cardiac output occur, see SCP in Ch. 1: Cardiac output, alteration in: decreased	Optimal cardiac output will be maintained

Continued.

Mitral Valve Prolapse—cont'd

NURSING DIAGNOSIS/ PATIENT PROBLEM	DEFINING CHARACTERISTICS	NURSING ORDERS		EXPECTED OUTCOMES
		ASSESSMENT	INTERVENTIONS	

Activity intolerance
Etiology
Imbalance between O_2 supply and demands
Side effects of medications
	Verbal reports of fatigue
	Abnormal heart rate
	Palpitations or BP change in response to activity
	Dyspnea; exertional discomfort
		A. Assess respiratory status before activity
		  1. Quality and rate
		  2. Need for O_2
		B. Assess cardiac status
		  1. Pulse rate, rhythm and volume
		  2. BP
		  3. Skin condition
		C. Assess understanding of changes in activity tolerance of patient/significant others
			A. Observe and document patient's response to activity
			B. Report any changes: rapid pulse, palpitations, elevated BP, dyspnea, fatigue, lightheadedness, dizziness, chest pain, pallor
			C. Encourage rest periods
			D. Encourage patient to refrain from physical activities that precipitate symptoms, i.e., exercise, sports
			E. Provide emotional support when increasing activity
				Patient will resume activities within limits of disease or medications

Comfort, alteration in: pain
Etiology
Myocardial ischemia
	Complaint of chest pain that is nonanginal in character. It is usually prolonged and may be substernal or diffuse. In general, the pain is atypical. It is not specifically related to exertion or stress
	Restlessness
	Irritability
	Facial mask of pain
		A. Note, record, and report type, location, intensity, and length of occurrence of chest pain. Ascertain if pain is related to exertion, eating, or stress conditions
		B. Assess cardiac status
		  1. Note pulse rate, rhythm and volume
		  2. Note BP
		  3. Check skin color, temperature, moisture, perfusion
			A. Permit unrestricted activity if patient is asymptomatic
			B. Encourage rest if pain is exertionally induced
			C. Provide nonstressful environment
			D. Provide psychologic and emotional support by allaying fears of the seriousness of this benign condition
			E. Provide relief of atypical chest pain by administering medications as ordered
				A. Pain will be minimized or relieved
				B. Patient will be assured that the pain does not signify serious disease

Myocardial Infarction: acute phase (1 to 3 days)

NURSING DIAGNOSIS/ PATIENT PROBLEM	DEFINING CHARACTERISTICS	NURSING ORDERS		EXPECTED OUTCOMES
		ASSESSMENT	INTERVENTIONS	
Comfort, alteration in: chest pain **Etiology** Myocardial ischemia/ myocardial infarction (MI)	Patient report and verbalizations (see Assessment criteria) Restlessness, apprehension Moaning, crying Facial mask of pain Diaphoresis Change in vital signs: BP, heart rate, respiratory rate Pallor, weakness Nausea and vomiting Fear and guarding behavior	Assess for characteristics of myocardial pain A. Quality 1. Choking, squeezing, aching, "vise-like" 2. Intense pressure with heaviness 3. Burning 4. Other _____ B. Severity: scale 1-10 (10 most severe) C. Onset: sudden/ constant D. Duration 1. At least 30 min; usually 1-2 hours 2. Residual soreness 1-3 days 3. Pain could be intermittent E. Location 1. Anterior chest, usually substernal 2. May radiate to shoulder, arms, jaw, neck, and epigastrum F. Precipitating factors 1. Physical or emotional exertion 2. May occur at rest G. Other characteristics 1. Not relieved with rest or nitrates	**General** A. Maintain bed rest, at least during periods of pain B. Position patient comfortably, preferably Fowler's position C. Maintain a quiet, relaxed atmosphere; display confident manner D. Allow rest periods for relaxation/sleep E. Offer emotional support in terms of positive reinforcements and encouragements F. If patient complains of pain 1. Report immediately to physician 2. Assess appropriateness of ECG immediately 3. Monitor vital signs 4. Administer O_2 per order 5. Institute medical therapy per order (see Specific interventions following) 6. Reassess response to interventions **Specific** A. Administer morphine sulfate as ordered per unit protocol 1. Monitor baseline vital signs; note changes after morphine 2. Administer IV morphine at increments of 2-5 mg over 5 min 3. Repeat dose until pain is relieved or a total of 10 mg has been given (if vital signs are stable) 4. Monitor closely for side effects of morphine a. Hypotension b. Decreased respirations c. Bradycardia d. Nausea; have naloxone (Narcan) on standby	Prompt relief of chest pain as evidenced by patient's verbalizations and appearance of relief, comfort

Originated by **Cynthia Antonio, RN, BSN**
Resource person: **Meg Gulanick, RN, MSN, CCRN**

Continued.

Myocardial Infarction: acute phase (1 to 3 days)—cont'd

NURSING DIAGNOSIS/ PATIENT PROBLEM	DEFINING CHARACTERISTICS	NURSING ORDERS		EXPECTED OUTCOMES
		ASSESSMENT	INTERVENTIONS	

		2. Not affected by position change or breathing
		3. May be associated with nausea and vomiting, dyspnea, anxiety, diaphoresis, fatigue
			B. Initiate IV nitrates as ordered per unit protocol to relieve current pain or to prevent future episodes of pain
			  1. Monitor BP and heart rate before beginning medication. BP should be at least 100/70 mm Hg
			  2. Prepare in glass bottle with special tubing; note that nitroglycerin (Tridil) should not be infused with any parenteral medication
			  3. Start at low dose, usually 5-10 μg/min through infusion pump
			  4. Titrate dose according to patient's pain and BP at increments of _____
			  5. Check vital signs every 5 min after change in dose and every 15 min thereafter until stable
			    a. Report immediately a BP drop of _____ mm Hg
			    b. Anticipate a fluid challenge
			  6. If patient complains of headache (common side effect), treat with acetaminophen (Tylenol)
			  7. Continually reassess patient's chest pain and response to medication. If no relief from optimal dose of medication, report to physician for assessment for intraaortic balloon pump, thrombolytic treatment, angioplasty, catheterization, bypass surgery	

Comfort, alteration in: nausea/vomiting **Etiology** Nausea and vomiting occur frequently in patients with acute MI (particularly inferior site) and with severe pain, presumably because of the activation of a vagal reflex. Nausea and vomiting are common side effects of opiates	Patient feels sick to stomach and as if he/she has to vomit Retching Straining Expelling gastric contents	A. Assess for signs and symptoms of epigastric distress B. Assess color, consistency, amount of emesis	A. Position patient comfortably in Fowler's position B. Keep emesis basin at bedside C. Record and report contents, color, and amount of emesis D. Administer antiemetics as ordered; prochlorperazine (Compazine) or trimethobenzamide (Tigan) suppositories p.r.n. Assess response E. Note any vasovagal responses from suppositories and straining (bradycardia, dizziness, and light-headedness) F. If no response from antiemetics, report to physician for other remedies	Discomfort associated with nausea and vomiting will be relieved

Myocardial Infarction: acute phase (1 to 3 days)—cont'd

NURSING DIAGNOSIS/ PATIENT PROBLEM	DEFINING CHARACTERISTICS	NURSING ORDERS		EXPECTED OUTCOMES
		ASSESSMENT	INTERVENTIONS	
			G. Offer ice chips as desired H. Offer small but frequent meals as tolerated I. Offer general liquid to soft diet as tolerated J. Provide mouth care/mouth wash as necessary	

Comfort, alteration in: chest pain
Etiology
Pericarditis secondary to acute MI
	Patient's description of pain
	Pericardial friction rub (transient)
	ST segment elevation in most limb and precordial ECG leads without reciprocal ST segment depression
	Fever
		A. Assess characteristics of pericardial pain. Similar to that in MI except pericardial pain
		  1. Increases with deep inspiration, turning of thorax, lying down
		  2. Relieved by sitting up or leaning forward
		  3. Quality
		    a. Sharp, stabbing, knife-like, "pleuritic"
		    b. Moderate to severe, or only an ache (deep or superficial)
		  4. Onset: sudden, 1-3 days after MI
		  5. Duration
		    a. Intermittent or continuous
		    b. May last for days
		    c. Residual soreness
		B. Assess vital signs
		  1. BP—check for pulsus paradoxus
		  2. Heart rate
		  3. Respirations
		  4. Temperature
			A. Position patient comfortably, preferably sitting up in bed 90 degrees or leaning forward propped on a pillow on a side table
			B. Offer assurance and emotional support through explanations about pericarditis. Reinforce that this pain is *not* another "heart attack"
			C. Give medications as ordered, usually aspirin every 6 hours or indomethacin (Indocin) every 8 hours to reduce inflammation around the heart. Give medications on full stomach
			D. Auscultate chest for heart sounds; document presence or change in pericardial rub
			E. Offer pillows to support chest when coughing
				Discomfort will be minimized

Continued.

Myocardial Infarction: acute phase (1 to 3 days)—cont'd

NURSING DIAGNOSIS/ PATIENT PROBLEM	DEFINING CHARACTERISTICS	NURSING ORDERS		EXPECTED OUTCOMES
		ASSESSMENT	INTERVENTIONS	
Cardiac output, alteration in: decreased (potential) **Etiology** Altered preload, afterload, and contractility secondary to A. Acute MI (especially anterior site) affecting pumping ability of the heart B. Papillary muscle rupture, mitral insufficiency C. Ventricular aneurysm	Low urine output, decreased BP; or decreased or increased heart rate Change in mental status Chest pain	A. Assess respirations every shift and p.r.n. for rate, depth, quality, and use of accessory muscles B. Auscultate lungs every shift and p.r.n. for rales and wheezes; report/ record changes C. Assess for heart rate, rhythm, BP, presence of S_3 or S_4, systolic murmur. Record and report changes D. Monitor fluid balance closely (I & O, weight gain, jugular venous distention, edema) E. Assess for restlessness, fatigue, change in mental status F. Monitor ABGs	If signs of left ventricular failure occur A. Initiate O_2 as needed B. Report to physician C. Initiate SCP in Ch. 1: Cardiac output, alteration in: decreased	Optimal cardiac output will be maintained
Etiology A. Electrical instability/irritability secondary to ischemia or necrosis 1. PVC 2. Ventricular tachycardia 3. Idioventricular rhythm 4. Presence of acute ECG changes (increased ST segment) B. Conduction system defects 1. With *inferior* ventricular MI a. Sinus bradycardia b. First- and second-degree heart block c. Wenckebach heart block	Decreased or increased heart rate; decreased BP Change in mental status Weakness, dizziness Restlessness Loss of peripheral pulses Abnormal heart sounds Chest pain Seizure activity Hemodynamic compromise Cardiopulmonary arrest	A. Monitor patient's heart rate and rhythm continuously. Document and report arrhythmias noted 1. Monitor in lead II, observing for left anterior hemiblock (deep S-wave) 2. If anterior MI with left anterior hemiblock, monitor in modified chest lead (MCL_1) for right bundle branch block B. Check vital signs during arrhythmias; note other associated signs and symptoms. Note rate and quality of pulses (see Defining Characteristics)	A. Institute treatment as appropriate and as per protocol 1. Lidocaine/procainamide (Pronestyl) for PVC/ventricular tachycardia 2. Atropine SO_4 for symptomatic bradycardia 3. Isoproterenol/temporary pacemaker for complete heart block 4. Temporary pacemaker for Mobitz type II, new bifasicular bundle branch block 5. Cardioversion for atrial fibrillation, ventricular tachycardia 6. Defibrillation for ventricular fibrillation 7. Precordial thump or CPR as appropriate B. Assess response to treatment and management C. Monitor PR, QRS, and QT intervals (see protocol for care of patients taking type II antiarrhythmics)	A. Risk of complications from arrhythmias will be minimized B. Optimal cardiac output will be maintained

Myocardial Infarction: acute phase (1 to 3 days)—cont'd

NURSING DIAGNOSIS/ PATIENT PROBLEM	DEFINING CHARACTERISTICS	NURSING ORDERS		EXPECTED OUTCOMES
		ASSESSMENT	INTERVENTIONS	

2. With *anterior* ventricular MI
  a. Second-degree heart block—Mobitz type II
  b. Complete heart block
  c. Right bundle branch block
3. With atrial infarct: atrial arrhythmias
		C. Assess ventilation and oxygenation; note change in consciousness		

Anxiety/fear **Etiology** Threat to or change in health status Threat of death Threat to self-concept Change in environment Unmet needs	Tense appearance, apprehension; fear of impending doom Fidgety/listless behavior Restless/unable to relax Repeatedly seeking assurance Signs of denial; disinterest in surroundings Sad expression; crying Slow speech	A. Assess patient's level of anxiety. Note all signs and symptoms, especially nonverbal communication B. Assess patient's normal coping patterns	A. Institute SCP in Ch. 1: Anxiety/fear B. After assessing readiness, explain in simple terms patient's illness (e.g., various aspects of MI); identify and clarify misconceptions C. Foster patient's optimism that recovery is fully anticipated. Offer assurance in realistic manner D. Assist patient to understand that the emotions being felt are normal, anticipated responses to an acute MI E. Establish rest periods between care and procedures F. Provide diversional materials (e.g., newspapers, magazines, music, and television), which can be relaxing and prevent feelings of isolation G. Administer mild tranquilizers/ sedatives as ordered	Patient will be able to manage or cope with emotional stress that accompanies an acute MI
Activity intolerance **Etiology** Generalized weakness Altered mobility Imbalance between O_2 supply and demand	Weakness/fatigue with ADL activity performance Increased heart rate of >15 beats over resting during activity Increased BP >20 mm Hg systolic during activity Decreased BP of >10 mm Hg systolic during activity Chest pain, dizziness Skin color changes/ diaphoresis Dyspnea	Assess patient's respiratory and cardiac status before initiating activity	A. Encourage adequate rest periods, especially before activities (e.g., ADL, visitors, meals) B. Provide emotional support when increasing activity C. Maintain progression of activity as ordered by physician and/or cardiac rehabilitation team by monitoring *cardiac rehabilitation stages* Stage 1. Complete bed rest Stage 2 1. Wash face, hands, personal areas (in bed). Nurse will wash back and legs 2. Use bedside commode with assistance 3. Perform active ROM exercises t.i.d. per protocol	Response/tolerance to activity will be optimal

Continued.

Myocardial Infarction: acute phase (1 to 3 days)—cont'd

NURSING DIAGNOSIS/ PATIENT PROBLEM	DEFINING CHARACTERISTICS	NURSING ORDERS		EXPECTED OUTCOMES
		ASSESSMENT	INTERVENTIONS	
			Stage 3. Dangle 10-15 min t.i.d. Stage 4 1. Perform bath in chair 2. Shave at bedside 3. Sit in chair with legs elevated for 30 min t.i.d. 4. Perform ROM exercises while sitting in chair D. Observe and document response to activity. Report 1. Pulse >15 beats over resting or 120 BPM 2. Palpitations 3. BP increased >20 mm Hg systolic 4. BP decreased >10 mm Hg systolic 5. Dyspnea, weakness 6. Chest pain, dizziness 7. Pale skin color, diaphoresis E. Instruct patient *not* to hold breath while exercising or moving about in bed F. Instruct patient *not* to strain for bowel movement; suggest stool softeners as needed G. Provide light meal (progress from liquids to regular diet as appropriate)	
Knowledge deficit **Etiology** Unfamiliarity with disease process, treatment, recovery	Multiple or lack of questions Confusion over events Expressed need for more information	A. Assess readiness of patient/significant others for teaching/counseling B. Note baseline knowledge	A. Establish good rapport with patient/significant others B. Encourage patient/significant others to ask questions and verbalize concerns C. Provide information on the following (as appropriate), limiting sessions to 10-15 min at a time 1. Positive aspects of the unit (CCU) 2. Diagnosing of MI in CCU (e.g., with ECG, blood tests, scans) 3. Healing process and recovery 4. Cardiac anatomy 5. MI vs angina 6. Risk factors for MI D. Use available teaching tools (e.g., anatomic heart model, brochures, cassette tapes for MI, flip charts) E. Use appropriate resources (e.g., unit nurses, clinical specialists, physician) F. Document teaching G. Inform patient that more extensive teaching sessions will be instituted after transfer to the medical floor	Patient/significant others will verbalize understanding of patient's condition, healing process of the MI, the need for observation in CCU, and diagnosis/treatment of the MI

Myocardial Infarction: intermediate phase (days 4 to 10)

NURSING DIAGNOSIS/ PATIENT PROBLEM	DEFINING CHARACTERISTICS	NURSING ORDERS		EXPECTED OUTCOMES
		ASSESSMENT	INTERVENTIONS	
Knowledge deficit about myocardial infarction and follow-up care **Etiology** Unfamiliarity with disease process, treatment, recovery	Questioning Verbalizing misconceptions Not verbalizing feelings	A. Assess patient's physical and emotional readiness to learn B. Assess patient/significant others' understanding of disease process, recovery process, diet, medications, activity progression, preventive care	A. Plan teaching sessions so patient is not overwhelmed at one time B. Provide environment conducive to learning C. Consult with cardiac rehabilitation clinical specialist regarding appropriate teaching materials (hospital television, heart model, group class, handouts) D. Provide information regarding 1. Coronary artery disease 2. Angina vs myocardial infarction (MI) pain characteristics 3. Immediate treatment for MI 4. Healing process from MI 5. Resuming activities of daily living 6. Risk factor modification 7. Dietary regime 8. Medications 9. Progressive activity/exercise plan a. Home walking program b. Climbing stairs c. Going to the store d. Driving a car e. Sexual activity 10. Coping mechanisms to help adjustment to new or altered life-style 11. Immediate treatment for recurrence of chest pain	Patient/significant other will verbalize understanding of disease state, recovery process, diet, medications, activity, and preventive care
Activity/intolerance **Etiology** Imposed activity restrictions Generalized weakness; deconditioned state Imbalance between O_2 supply and demand Sedentary life-style	Report of fatigue or weakness Abnormal heart rate or BP response to activity Exertional discomfort Dyspnea Chest pain Dizziness Diaphoresis	A. Assess patient's respiratory/cardiac status before activity B. Observe and document response to activity. Report 1. Pulse >20 beats over resting, or 120 BPM 2. Palpitations 3. BP increases >20 mm Hg 4. BP decreases >10 mm Hg 5. Dyspnea, weakness 6. Chest pain, dizziness 7. Skin color changes, diaphoresis	A. Encourage adequate rest periods, especially before activities B. Monitor active ROM exercise t.i.d. to maintain muscle strength C. Provide emotional support when increasing activity D. Maintain progression of activity as ordered by cardiac rehabilitation team, physician **Cardiac rehabilitation stages** **Stage 3:** Date _____ Dangle 10-15 min t.i.d. Feed self **Stage 4:** Date _____ Partial bath in chair; shave self; sit in chair 30 min t.i.d. **Stage 5:** Date _____ Partial bath at sink; bathroom privileges; up in chair whenever desired; walk in room **Stage 6:** Date _____ Self morning care; walk in hall 150 feet t.i.d.	Optimal activity tolerance will be maintained

Originated by **Meg Gulanick, RN, MSN, CCRN**

Myocardial Infarction: intermediate phase (days 4 to 10)—cont'd

NURSING DIAGNOSIS/ PATIENT PROBLEM	DEFINING CHARACTERISTICS	NURSING ORDERS		EXPECTED OUTCOMES
		ASSESSMENT	INTERVENTIONS	
			Stage 7: Date _____ Sit in hall; walk 300 feet t.i.d. **Stage 8:** Date _____ Walk 600 feet t.i.d. **Stage 9:** Date _____ Stair climbing with cardiac rehabilitation nurse	
Self-concept, disturbance in: body image, self-esteem, role performance (potential) Etiology Physiologic limitations secondary to disease Change in body function Possible change in life-style (job, physical activity) Increased amount of disease-related symptoms Change in health status Threat of death	Refusal to accept rehabilitative efforts Inappropriate attempts to direct own treatment Signs of grieving: crying, despair, anger Refusal to participate in self-care Self-destructive behavior Withdrawal from social contacts Focus on past strength, function Feelings of helplessness, hopelessness, powerlessness Preoccupation with change or loss Inability to accept positive reinforcement Nonparticipation in therapy Change in self-perception of role Change in usual patterns of responsibility	A. Assess contributing factors B. Assess present coping status C. Assess meaning of the loss/change for patient/significant other	A. Encourage verbalization of feelings B. Clear up any misconceptions and provide reliable information C. Assist person to accept help from others D. Identify outlets that foster feelings of personal achievement and self-esteem E. While being realistic, point out positive changes in person's condition F. For deeper depression problems, make appropriate referrals	Patient will verbalize positive expressions of continued self-worth
Comfort, alteration in: chest pain (potential) Etiology Myocardial ischemia/ infarction Pericarditis	Patient report and verbalizations of pain Restlessness, apprehension Facial mask of pain Diaphoresis Change in vital signs (BP, heart rate, respiratory rate) Pallor, weakness Fear and guarding behavior	A. Assess characteristics of pain, differentiating between myocardial infarction and pericarditis (see SCP, this chapter: Myocardial infarction—acute phase), and between stable and unstable angina (see SCP, this chapter: Unstable angina—acute phase) B. Assess hemodynamic response to pain	A. Instruct patient to report pain so relief measures can be instituted B. Maintain bed rest, at least during periods of pain C. Position comfortably, preferably Fowler's position D. Maintain a quiet and relaxed atmosphere; display confident manner E. Administer medications as ordered, noting effectiveness and side effects F. If *nonpericardial* chest pain is not relieved within 15 to 30 min 1. Report immediately to physician 2. Assess appropriateness of immediate ECG 3. Monitor vital signs 4. Administer O_2 per order 5. Institute medical therapy per order	Pain will be alleviated or minimized

Myocardial Infarction: intermediate phase (days 4 to 10)—cont'd

NURSING DIAGNOSIS/ PATIENT PROBLEM	DEFINING CHARACTERISTICS	NURSING ORDERS		EXPECTED OUTCOMES
		ASSESSMENT	INTERVENTIONS	

			6. Stay with patient to provide support and reassurance
			7. Anticipate need for IV
			G. *If pericardial pain* is noted
			  1. Position patient comforta-bly, preferably sitting up in bed 90 degrees or leaning forward propped on a pillow set on a side table
			  2. Offer assurance and emo-tional support
			  3. Reinforce that this pain is *not* another "heart attack"
			  4. Give medications as or-dered, usually aspirin q.6h. or indomethacin (Indocin) q.8h. to reduce inflamma-tion around the heart; give medications on full stomach
			  5. Auscultate chest for heart sounds and document pres-ence or change in pericardi-al rub	

Cardiac output, alter-ation in: decreased (potential)
Etiology
Altered preload
Altered afterload
Altered contractility
Altered heart rate sec-ondary to left ven-tricular dysfunction, myocardial ischemia
	Low urine output
	Decreasing BP, in-creasing or decreas-ing heart rate
	Cutaneous sign of va-soconstriction
	Change in mental status
	Dizziness
	Weakness, fatigue
	Restlessness
	Abnormal heart sounds
	Abnormal lung sounds
	Neck vein distention
	Edema
	Chest pain
		Assess physical status closely, document changes, report sig-nificant changes in parameters
		A. Arterial BP, or-thostatic changes, pulsus paradoxus, heart rate
		B. Apical/radial pulses; peripheral pulses (strength, equality)
		C. Heart sounds
		D. Lung sounds
		E. Jugular venous distention
		F. Mentation
		G. Urine output
		H. Skin color, tem-perature
			A. Administer routine cardiac medications as ordered; ob-serve for side effects and tox-icity
			B. Maintain optimal fluid intake
			
			C. Monitor I & O every _____
			D. Monitor daily weights
			E. If signs of left ventricular failure are noted
			  1. Initiate O_2 as needed
			  2. Report to physician
			  3. Initiate SCP in Chapter 1: Cardiac output, alteration in: decreased
				Optimal hemodynam-ic status will be maintained

Cardiac output, alter-ation in: decreased (potential) **Etiology** Cardiac dysrhythmias (atrial, junctional, ventricular) second-ary to ischemia, electrolyte imbal-ance, altered electri-cal conduction/ rhythm/rate	Irregular heart rate Tachycardia/bradycar-dia Decreasing/increasing K^+ levels Hypoxia	A. Monitor heart for rate, rhythm, and ectopy every _____ B. If telemetry ECG monitoring is available, continu-ously monitor ECG for rate, rhythm, abnormal-ity, and change in PR, QRS, and QT intervals if appro-priate C. Observe for ab-normalities in car-diac electrolytes	A. If arrhythmia occurs, determine patient response, document, and report if significant or symptomatic B. Have antiarrhythmia drugs readily available C. Treat arrhythmias according to medical orders or protocol, and evaluate response	Optimal cardiac rhythm and cardiac output will be main-tained

Cynthia Whyte

Pulmonary Edema, Acute

NURSING DIAGNOSIS/ PATIENT PROBLEM	DEFINING CHARACTERISTICS	NURSING ORDERS		EXPECTED OUTCOMES
		ASSESSMENT	INTERVENTIONS	

Gas exchange, impaired
Etiology
Pulmonary-venous congestion
Alveolar-capillary membrane changes
	Restlessness
	Irritability
	Inability to move secretions
	Pink, frothy sputum
	Hypercapnea
	Hypoxia
	Cough
	Rales
	Dyspnea
	Cyanosis
		A. Assess respiratory rate, depth; presence of shortness of breath; use of accessory muscles
		B. Assess breath sounds in all lung fields noting aeration, presence of rales, wheezes
		C. Assess sputum/ tracheal secretions noting color, consistency, quantity
		D. Assess baseline ABGs
			A. Monitor and document changes in respiratory status continuously during acute phase, then every _____
			B. Provide O_2 as needed to maintain Po_2 at _____
			C. Obtain and monitor serial ABGs
			  1. Routinely every _____
			  2. 20-30 min after a change in O_2/drug treatment
			D. If ABGs are expected to be drawn more frequently than at four 1-hour intervals, suggest appropriateness of an arterial line
			E. Position patient for optimal breathing pattern (high Fowler's; feet dangling at bedside)
			F. Encourage slow, deep breaths as appropriate
			G. Assist with coughing or suctioning p.r.n.
			H. Assist with positioning for optimal lung expansion for chest x-ray examination
			I. Administer prescribed medication carefully
			  1. If diuretics are used, monitor K^+ levels, I & O, need for Foley catheter
			  2. If morphine sulfate is used, monitor respiratory rate; observe for bradycardia, nausea. Keep naloxone (Narcan) available
			  3. If aminophylline is used, monitor ventricular rate and frequency of ectopics closely. Monitor aminophylline levels p.r.n.
				Patient will have improved ventilation and oxygenation as seen by
				A. Return of respiratory rate to baseline (16-22/min)
				B. Verbalization of ease of breathing
				C. Clear breath sounds on auscultation
				D. Blood gas values within patient's normal range
				  pH _____
				  Pco_2 _____
				  Po_2 _____
				  Saturation _____

Cardiac output, alteration in: decreased
Etiology
Increased preload
Increased afterload
Decreased contractility
Combined etiologies
	Variations in hemodynamic parameters (BP, heart rate, CVP, pulmonary artery pressure, cardiac output, neck veins, urine output, peripheral pulses)
	Arrhythmias/ECG changes
	Weight gain, edema, ascites
	Nausea, vomiting
	Abnormal heart sounds
	Anxiety, restlessness
		A. Assess hemodynamic parameters (see Defining Characteristics)
		B. Assess skin color, temperature, moisture, peripheral edema
		C. Assess fluid balance, weight gain
		D. Assess heart sounds, noting murmurs, gallops, S_3, S_4
		E. Assess heart rate, rhythm (both apical and radial)
			A. Monitor patient's physical state as appropriate, documenting changes and reporting significant alterations
			B. Anticipate need for hemodynamic monitoring. If ordered
			  1. Prepare patient for insertion of Swan-Ganz catheter
			  2. Assemble equipment per unit routine
			  3. Use D5W for peripheral lines
			  4. Use central ports for medication infusion. Keep on infusion pumps to maintain patency of lines
				Optimal cardiac output will be seen by
				A. Heart rate/BP within patient's normal range
				B. Warm, dry skin
				C. PAWP <30 mm Hg
				D. Absence of arrhythmia
				E. Absence of restlessness/confusion
				F. Urine output >30 ml/hour

Originated by **Nancy J. Cooney, RN, BSN**
Resource person: **Meg Gulanick, RN, MSN, CCRN**

Pulmonary Edema, Acute—cont'd

NURSING DIAGNOSIS/ PATIENT PROBLEM	DEFINING CHARACTERISTICS	NURSING ORDERS		EXPECTED OUTCOMES
		ASSESSMENT	INTERVENTIONS	
	Dizziness, weakness, fatigue	F. Assess mentation, noting restless-ness, confusion	5. Monitor pulmonary artery (PA), pulmonary artery wedge (PAW) waveforms closely. If PAW correlates within 10% of pulmonary artery end-diastolic pressure (PAEDP), monitor PAEDP instead of PAW 6. If PAW readings change more than 10% from pre-vious readings, recheck all lines, recalibrate system. Report to physician as needed 7. Refer to SCP in Ch. 2: Swan-Ganz catheterization C. If increased preload is the etiol-ogy, anticipate use of rotating tourniquets, nitrates, or diu-retics 1. If rotating tourniquets are used 　a. Apply per unit routine 　b. Avoid using extremity with IV line 　c. Monitor peripheral pulses every 15 min 　d. Do not inflate cuff lon-ger than 45 min 　e. At the end of use, re-move one cuff at a time (every 15 min) 2. If nitrates are used 　a. Prepare IV nitrate in glass bottle using special tubing 　b. Evaluate need to prepare as a multiple concentra-tion: _____ 　c. Initiate dose at _____ 　d. Titrate nitrate to PAW of _____ or until desired effect: _____ 　e. Observe patient for hy-potension. If this occurs, stop medication immedi-ately, lower head of bed as appropriate, and noti-fy physician. Anticipate need for pressor/fluid treatment 3. Position patient for optimal reduction of preload (high Fowler's position, dangling feet at bedside) 4. If diuretics are used, see preceding nursing diagnosis: Gas exchange, impaired	

Continued.

Pulmonary Edema, Acute—cont'd

NURSING DIAGNOSIS/ PATIENT PROBLEM	DEFINING CHARACTERISTICS	NURSING ORDERS		EXPECTED OUTCOMES
		ASSESSMENT	**INTERVENTIONS**	
			D. If increased afterload is the etiology, anticipate measures for afterload reduction 1. If nitroprusside (Nipride) is used a. Make certain patient has a clear, audible BP by cuff. If not, evaluate need for arterial line b. Prepare nitroprusside per unit routine (1) Infuse per IMED/ IVAC pump (2) Titrate dose 0.5-10 μg/kg/min (3) Do not infuse with any other medicines (4) Protect from sunlight (5) Anticipate potential side effects: hypotension, sweating, nausea, confusion c. Confer with physician regarding the desired hemodynamic goals e.g., heart rate _____ d. Monitor hemodynamic parameters every 5-10 min until stable e. Monitor thiocyanate levels p.r.n. E. If arrhythmia is the etiology 1. Monitor continuously for arrhythmias 2. Administer prescribed digoxin/verapamil per unit protocol 3. Monitor patient's electrolytes, especially K$^+$ levels F. If hypotension is a related problem 1. Evaluate need for central line 2. Anticipate use of pressor agents 3. If dopamine/dobutamine (Dobutrex) is prescribed a. Titrate dose 0.5-20 μg/kg/min for *dopamine* b. Titrate dose 0.5-10 μg/kg/min for *dobutamine* c. Keep phentolamine (Regitine) on standby d. Anticipate potential side effects: tachycardia, decreased urine output (with high doses) e. If necessary, dopamine and dobutamine may be infused through the same line	

Pulmonary Edema, Acute—cont'd

NURSING DIAGNOSIS/ PATIENT PROBLEM	DEFINING CHARACTERISTICS	NURSING ORDERS		EXPECTED OUTCOMES
		ASSESSMENT	INTERVENTIONS	
Anxiety/fear **Etiology** Dyspnea Excessive monitoring equipment Increased staff attention	Restlessness Increased awareness Increased questioning Avoids looking at equipment Constant demands, complaining Uncooperative behavior	Assess patient's level of anxiety and normal coping pattern	A. Remain with patient during periods of acute respiratory distress B. Promote an environment of confidence and reassurance C. Anticipate need and use of morphine sulfate D. Institute SCP in Ch. 1: Anxiety/fear	Reduction in anxiety will be seen by A. Calmer, relaxed state B. Verbalization of fears C. Restful night
Comfort, alteration in **Etiology** Dyspnea Prolonged bed rest Fatigue Uncomfortable therapeutic interventions	Complaints of thirst Diaphoresis Pain; dyspnea Restlessness Uncomfortable feeling from face mask or Foley catheter	A. Assess patient's level of comfort, noting both verbal/nonverbal communication B. Assess the characteristics of patient's discomfort	A. Position patient in preferred position B. Offer frequent backrubs and massages C. Turn patient from side to side every _____ hours as tolerated by respiratory status D. Keep extra pillows available; use pillows to help prop patient upright E. Obtain egg crate mattress/flotation pad as needed F. Keep patient's linens dry G. Provide frequent oral hygiene every _____ H. Provide ice chips to lessen complaints of thirst and dry mouth. Maintain accurate I & O records I. Monitor ABGs closely, so patient can be switched from face mask to nasal cannula as soon as possible	Patient will be as comfortable as possible as seen by A. Verbalization of comfort B. Appearance of improved comfort
Injury, potential for: infection **Etiology** Increased pulmonary congestion Increased use of invasive equipment	Elevated temperature WBC count increased Foul-smelling sputum or urine Phlebotic area above IV site Redness, swelling, tenderness at catheter insertion site	A. Assess patient's IV sites, noting any incidence of redness, soreness, drainage B. Assess all indwelling catheters for patency, cleanliness C. Assess patient's temperature, CBC every _____	A. Monitor patient's IV site and IV tubing per unit protocol B. Change tubing, bottles, site per unit protocol C. For central lines, examine IV site more frequently, every _____ D. Remove unnecessary IV lines as soon as possible E. If patient has Swan-Ganz catheter or arterial line, encourage physician to change lines q.72h. F. If infection is suspected, send tip of catheter for culture G. Encourage patient to cough and deep breathe every _____ hours while awake H. If suctioning is needed, use aseptic technique I. Monitor patient's secretions; obtain cultures p.r.n. J. Monitor patient's temperature per unit protocol. If temperature is >38.5° C, notify physician immediately; prepare for possible blood culture, and repeat temperature q.1-2h.	Occurrence of infection will be minimized

Continued.

Pulmonary Edema, Acute—cont'd

NURSING DIAGNOSIS/ PATIENT PROBLEM	DEFINING CHARACTERISTICS	NURSING ORDERS		EXPECTED OUTCOMES
		ASSESSMENT	INTERVENTIONS	
			K. Administer antibiotics as prescribed, remembering to check for possible allergies and incompatibility with other medicines L. Administer antipyretics as prescribed	
Knowledge deficit **Etiology** New equipment New environment New medications/ treatments	Questioning Verbalized misconceptions Lack of questions	A. Assess understanding of patient/significant others about the need for increased monitoring, invasive equipment, understanding of pulmonary edema (treatment in acute phase) B. Assess physical and emotional readiness for learning of patient/significant others	A. During acute phase of illness explain only *necessary* treatments and procedures to patient B. Keep all information simple and brief C. Include significant others in explanations, reassuring them that more information will be explained once patient is through the acute phase D. Document all areas of explanations in nursing notes, including patient/significant others response to explanations	Patient/significant others will verbalize and understand A. The need for the increased monitoring equipment in the unit B. Rationale regarding treatment of pulmonary edema

Thrombophlebitis

NURSING DIAGNOSIS/ PATIENT PROBLEM	DEFINING CHARACTERISTICS	NURSING ORDERS		EXPECTED OUTCOMES
		ASSESSMENT	INTERVENTIONS	
Circulation, interruption of: peripheral **Etiology** Venous stasis Injury to vein Hypercoagulability	A. Superficial (rarely involved): heat, pain, swelling, tenderness on palpation of posterior calf (Pratt's sign), induration along the length of affected vein B. Deep vein (most often involved): may be asymptomatic, severe pain, fever, chills, malaise, possible swelling, cyanosis of affected part, loss of sensation	A. Assess patient every _____ for signs and symptoms of superficial and deep vein thrombosis B. Assess pain as to causative factors, time of onset, quality, radiation, severity C. Check laboratory values reflecting coagulation profile (e.g., PT, PTT) D. Be aware of results of blood flow studies E. Report to physician any abnormalities in assessment	Minimize the possibility of embolus by A. Encouraging and maintaining bed rest, with the affected extremity elevated B. Applying elastic stockings or bandage wraps as ordered C. Applying warm soaks to relieve pain and inflammation as ordered D. Administering analgesics as ordered/indicated by assessment E. Administering and monitoring anticoagulant therapy as ordered (heparin/warfarin [Coumadin]) F. Observing for side effects of anticoagulant therapy (see Nursing Diagnosis: Gas exchange, impaired) G. Making sure heparin is administered in minidrip tubing and Buretrol	Incidence of embolization will be minimized

Originated by **Gloria Young, RN, BS**
Resource persons: **Audrey Klopp, RN, MS, CCRN, CS, ET**
    Carol Burkhart, RN, BSN, CCRN

Thrombophlebitis—cont'd

NURSING DIAGNOSIS/ PATIENT PROBLEM	DEFINING CHARACTERISTICS	NURSING ORDERS		EXPECTED OUTCOMES
		ASSESSMENT	INTERVENTIONS	

			H. Maintain adequate hydration
			  1. Encourage oral fluids
			  2. Regulate IV infusions as scheduled
			  3. Document patient's I & O	

Knowledge deficit **Etiology** Unfamiliarity with pathology, treatment, prevention	Multiple questions Lack of questions Misconceptions	A. Assess patient's level of understanding B. Assess patient's readiness for learning	A. Instruct patient to avoid rubbing or massaging calf to prevent breaking off clot, which may circulate as embolus B. Recommend properly applied elastic stockings, and instruct patient in importance of wearing them to increase venous return C. Encourage early ambulation of surgical patients; encourage leg exercises for bedridden patients, if not contraindicated, to prevent stasis D. Instruct patient to avoid long periods of sitting with legs crossed E. Inform patient of signs and symptoms of thrombophlebitis to avoid recurrence F. Inform patient to report promptly to the physician any symptoms of abnormal bleeding	Patient will verbalize a basic understanding of the signs and symptoms of thrombophlebitis and the importance of reporting symptoms promptly. Patient will be able to use appropriate measures for prevention

Gas exchange, impaired: actual/potential
Etiology
Dislodgement of thrombus (embolus)
	Cyanosis
	Dyspnea
	Tachypnea
	Substernal, sharp chest pain
	Palpitations
	Tachycardia
	Hemoptysis
	Diaphoresis
	Engorged neck veins
	Anxiety
	Restlessness
	Sense of impending doom
		A. Assess patient every ____ for signs and symptoms of pulmonary embolus
		B. Monitor vital signs every ____
		C. Check laboratory values, i.e., ABGs, chest x-ray, ECG, PT, PTT, every ____ hours
		D. Auscultate breath sounds every ____
		E. Document observations
		F. Report to physician
		BP: <____ or >____
		Pulse: <____ or >____
		CVP: <____ or >____
		ECG changes: ____
		Chest x-ray results: ____
			A. Elevate head of bed
			B. Administer O_2 at ____L/min
			C. Provide emotional support
			  1. Create nonstressful environment
			  2. Administer sedatives as ordered
			D. Maintain anticoagulant therapy as outlined in Nursing Diagnosis: Circulation, interruption of: peripheral
			E. Prepare the patient for transfer to ICU (if transfer impending)
			  1. Explain transfer to patient/ significant others
			  2. Offer reassurance
			  3. Accompany patient to unit
				Incidence of recurrence or extension of thromboembolism will be minimized, and gas exchange will be maximized

Continued.

Thrombophlebitis—cont'd

NURSING DIAGNOSIS/ PATIENT PROBLEM	DEFINING CHARACTERISTICS	NURSING ORDERS		EXPECTED OUTCOMES
		ASSESSMENT	INTERVENTIONS	
Injury, potential for **Etiology** Heparin therapy	**Too much heparin** Bleeding from IV sites, drains, wounds Petechiae, purpura, hematoma Bleeding from mucous membranes GI, GU bleeding Bleeding from respiratory tract PTT 2½ times normal **Too little heparin** Continued evidence of further clot formation (newly developed signs of pulmonary embolus or peripheral thromboemboli) PTT not at desired level	Note adverse effects of heparin therapy A. Note any increase in bleeding from IV sites (e.g., GI and GU tracts, respiratory tract wounds) B. Observe for development of new purpura, petechiae, or hematomas C. Inquire about bone and joint pain D. Observe for mental status changes	**Too much heparin** A. Check PTT; notify physician B. Reevaluate heparin dose **Too little heparin** A. Check to make sure infusion is not interrupted (e.g., infiltrated IV, malfunctioning infusion device) B. Check PTT; notify physician C. Reevaluate heparin dose	Risk of injury will be minimized

THERAPEUTIC INTERVENTIONS

Cardiac Catheterization

NURSING DIAGNOSIS/ PATIENT PROBLEM	DEFINING CHARACTERISTICS	NURSING ORDERS		EXPECTED OUTCOMES
		ASSESSMENT	INTERVENTIONS	
Knowledge deficit **Etiology** Precatheterization: un- familiarity with car- diac catheterization	Expresses a need for information Multiple questions Lack of questions Increase in anxiety level	A. Assess patient's knowledge of heart anatomy, disease, and cardi- ac catheterization B. Assess readiness to learn of patient/ significant others	A. Use appropriate materials (e.g., booklets, television, film, heart model) for teaching patient B. Provide information concerning 1. Heart anatomy and physi- ology 2. Patient's heart problem (valve disease, coronary ar- tery disease, _____) 3. Cardiac catheterization a. Indications b. Precatheterization prepa- rations c. Procedure itself d. Postcatheterization care C. Include family in teaching plan as appropriate D. Be in room when catheteriza- tion team evaluates patient (as appropriate). Interpret physi- cian's information (as appropri- ate)	The patient will ver- balize a basic under- standing of heart anatomy, disease, and cardiac cathe- terization procedure
Circulation, interrup- tion of: potential **Etiology** Postcatheterization: arterial vasospasm	Decrease or absence of peripheral pulses Lessening in tempera- ture of affected ex- tremity Presence of mottling, pallor, rubor, or cy- anosis in affected extremity	Assess and monitor extremity for occlu- sion over four 30-min periods and then q.1h. until sta- ble A. Assess presence and quality of pulses distal to catheter insertion site (radial pulse for brachial site; dorsalis pedis for femoral site) B. If dorsalis pedis pulse is being monitored, mark site with "X" C. Assess the color, temperature, and capillary refill of affected extremity	A. Document presence and quality of pulses every _____ B. Notify physician of decrease in quality or absence of pulses 1. Obtain Doppler ultrasonic reading, if possible, to check for decrease in pulses 2. Prepare for possibility of embolectomy 3. Prepare to heparinize if or- dered	Risk of complications from spasm will be minimized

Originated by **Patricia Farrell, RNC**
Resource person: **Meg Gulanick, RN, MSN, CCRN**

Continued.

Cardiac Catheterization—cont'd

NURSING DIAGNOSIS/ PATIENT PROBLEM	DEFINING CHARACTERISTICS	NURSING ORDERS		EXPECTED OUTCOMES
		ASSESSMENT	INTERVENTIONS	
Injury, potential for **Etiology** Bleeding	Significant bleeding noted on dressing Apprehension and restlessness Hematoma at site of insertion Increased heart rate, increased respiratory rate, decreased BP	Assess insertion site and dressing every _____ for signs of bleeding	A. Maintain bed rest for 6 hours or _____ B. Do not elevate head of bed >45 degrees for 6 hours C. If femoral site is used, keep bandaged leg straight for _____ hours D. Avoid sudden movements with affected extremity to facilitate clot formation and wound closure at insertion site **For bleeding** A. Circle date, time and amount of drainage B. Estimate blood loss C. Reinforce dressing; apply pressure to site D. Apply sandbag (10 pounds) to bleeding site E. Notify physician if bleeding is significant F. Monitor vital signs, Hb and Hct as appropriate	Risk of bleeding will be minimized
Fluid volume deficit **(mild/severe)** **Etiology** Dye-induced diuresis Restricted intake before procedure	Nervousness and apprehension Poor skin turgor Dry, sticky mucous membranes Decrease in urine output Decrease in BP; increase in heart rate and respiratory rate Pale, cool, clammy skin	Assess and monitor hydration status, mental status, skin, and hemodynamic status	A. Maintain strict I & O for several hours after catheterization B. Anticipate frequent use of urinal/bedpan for several hours after catheterization. Keep urinal within reach C. Push oral fluids as tolerated D. Keep water pitcher/juices or _____ at bedside on return of patient E. Institute IV fluids as ordered, monitoring flow rate F. If patient requires nitrates, monitor BP closely, anticipating drop in BP and need for additional fluids	Potential dehydration will be minimized

Cardiac Catheterization—cont'd

NURSING DIAGNOSIS/ PATIENT PROBLEM	DEFINING CHARACTERISTICS	NURSING ORDERS		EXPECTED OUTCOMES
		ASSESSMENT	INTERVENTIONS	
Anxiety/fear **Etiology** Unknown outcome of cardiac catheterization	Increased questioning Increased irritability Restlessness Anger Withdrawal	Assess patient's level of anxiety	A. Institute SCP in Ch. 1: Anxiety/fear B. Be with patient when physician returns to reinforce and explain information. Provide emotional support as needed	Reduction in anxiety will be evidenced by calm, relaxed state

Comfort, alteration in
Etiology
Incision
Restricted movement
Myocardial ischemia
	Patient complaints of discomfort
	Restlessness and increased anxiety
	Increased irritability
	Maintains rigid, non-moving positions
		A. Solicit patient's description of pain
		B. Assess pain characteristics
		  1. Quality
		  2. Severity
		  3. Location
		  4. Onset
		  5. Duration
		  6. Precipitating factors or relieving factors
			For incisional pain
			A. Check incision for hematoma formation
			B. Medicate as ordered
			C. Give reassurance
			D. Use additional comfort measures whenever appropriate
			E. Assist patient in changing position (within limitations)
			F. Use distractional devices when applicable
			G. Provide reassurance and emotional support
			H. Notify physician if interventions are unsuccessful
			
			For anginal pain
			A. Notify physician of pain
			B. Give medications (nitroglycerin) as ordered. Monitor BP closely, anticipating drop in BP and need for additional fluids
			C. If pain is unrelieved within 5 min
			  1. Call physician immediately for further assessment and medical intervention
			  2. Anticipate need for ECG
				Patient will verbalize that discomfort is decreased or more manageable

Coronary Artery Bypass: intermediate postoperative care

NURSING DIAGNOSIS/ PATIENT PROBLEM	DEFINING CHARACTERISTICS	NURSING ORDERS		EXPECTED OUTCOMES
		ASSESSMENT	INTERVENTIONS	
Gas exchange, impaired **Etiology** Altered O_2-carrying capacity of blood Alveolar-capillary membrane changes Altered blood flow	Dyspnea, shortness of breath Abnormal breath sounds Decreased oxygenation on serial ABGs (PO_2, saturation) Abnormal chest x-ray film	A. Inspect chest for respiratory rate and rhythm every ____ B. Auscultate breath sounds every ____ for adventitious sounds C. Monitor ABGs and chest x-ray film as needed	A. Encourage use of incentive spirometer 10 times each hour as tolerated B. Demonstrate and teach coughing, deep breathing, and splinting techniques. Encourage cough and deep breathing 10 times each hour while patient is awake C. Assist with splinting of chest for more effective coughing D. Provide pain medication p.r.n. to optimize effective cough and deep breathing E. Provide fluids or vaporizer to assist in loosening secretions F. Provide rest periods between breathing/coughing exercises G. Provide O_2 therapy as ordered. Use nasal cannula during meals if necessary; use portable O_2 while patient is ambulating H. Turn, reposition, ambulate patient per cardiac rehabilitation protocol to mobilize secretions	Optimal gas exchange will be maintained

Comfort, alteration in: pain
Etiology
Surgical incisions
	Patient or significant others verbalize pain
	Protective decreased physical activity
	Restlessness, irritability, altered sleep pattern
	Facial mask of pain
	Alteration in muscle tone, (listlessness, flaccidity/rigidity, tenseness)
		Assess characteristics of pain, differentiating between incisional pain and myocardial (see SCP in Ch. 1: Comfort, alteration in: pain)	**For incisional pain**
			A. Anticipate need for analgesics, especially before activities
			B. Administer medications as ordered, evaluating effectiveness and observing for side effects
			C. Use additional comfort measures when appropriate
			  1. Heating pad
			  2. Distraction techniques
			  3. Relaxation techniques
			D. Provide rest periods to facilitate comfort and relaxation
			E. Instruct patient to report pain so relief measures can be instituted
				Incisional pain will be alleviated or minimized

Originated by **Antoinette Harris-Hardy, RN, BSN**
Resource person: **Meg Gulanick, RN, MSN, CCRN**

Coronary Artery Bypass: intermediate postoperative care—cont'd

NURSING DIAGNOSIS/ PATIENT PROBLEM	DEFINING CHARACTERISTICS	NURSING ORDERS		EXPECTED OUTCOMES
		ASSESSMENT	INTERVENTIONS	
Activity intolerance **Etiology** Generalized weakness	Reluctant to attempt movement Limited ROM Decreased muscle strength, control, or mass	A. Assess patient's respiratory/cardiac status before activity B. Observe and document response to activity. Report 1. Pulse >20 beats over resting or 120 BPM 2. Palpitations 3. BP increases >20 mm Hg (systolic) 4. BP decreases >10 mm Hg (systolic) 5. Dyspnea, weakness 6. Chest pain, dizziness 7. Skin color, diaphoresis	A. Provide bedside commode as indicated B. Encourage adequate rest periods, especially before activities C. Monitor active ROM exercises t.i.d. to maintain muscle strength D. Provide emotional support when increasing activity E. Maintain progression of activity as ordered by cardiac rehabilitation team **Cardiac rehabilitation stages** *Stage 3:* (date) _____ Dangle 10-15 min t.i.d.; feed self *Stage 4:* (date) _____ Partial bath in chair; shave self; sit in chair 30 min t.i.d. *Stage 5:* (date) _____ Partial bath at sink; bathroom privileges; chair as desired; ambulate in room *Stage 6:* (date) _____ Self-care (AM); ambulate in hall 150 feet t.i.d. *Stage 7:* (date) _____ Sit in hall; walk 300 feet t.i.d. *Stage 8:* (date) _____ Walk 600 feet t.i.d. *Stage 9:* (date) _____ Stair climbing with cardiac rehabilitation nurse	Increased tolerance to activity will be evidenced
Cardiac output, alteration in: decreased (potential) **Etiology** Altered preload Altered afterload Altered contractility Altered heart rate	Low urine output Decreasing BP, increase/decrease in heart rate Decreasing or absent pulse Cutaneous sign of vasoconstriction Change in mental status Weight gain, edema Dizziness Weakness, fatigue Restlessness Abnormal heart sounds Abnormal lung sounds Neck vein distention	Assess physical status closely, document changes, report significant changes in parameters A. Arterial BP, orthostatic changes, pulsus paradoxus, heart rate B. Apical/radial pulses; peripheral pulses (strength, equality) C. Heart sounds D. Lung sounds E. Jugular venous distention F. Mentation G. Urine output H. Skin color, temperature	A. Administer routine cardiac medications as ordered; observe for side effects and toxicity B. Maintain optimal fluid intake C. Administer O_2 as ordered D. Monitor I & O every _____ E. Monitor daily weight	Optimal hemodynamic status will be maintained

Continued.

Coronary Artery Bypass: intermediate postoperative care—cont'd

NURSING DIAGNOSIS/ PATIENT PROBLEM	DEFINING CHARACTERISTICS	NURSING ORDERS		EXPECTED OUTCOMES
		ASSESSMENT	INTERVENTIONS	
Cardiac rhythm (atrial, junctional, ventricular rhythms): alteration in (potential) **Etiology** Ischemia Electrolyte imbalance Altered electrical conduction/rhythm/rate	Irregular heart rate Tachycardia/bradycardia Decreasing/increasing K$^+$ levels Hypoxia	A. Monitor heart for rate, rhythm, and ectopy every ____ B. If ECG monitoring is available, continuously monitor ECG for rate, rhythm, abnormality, and change in PR, QRS, and Q-T intervals if appropriate C. Observe for abnormalities in cardiac electrolytes	A. If arrhythmia occurs, determine patient response, document, and report if significant or symptomatic B. Have antiarrhythmics readily available C. Treat arrhythmias according to medical orders or protocol D. If bradyarrhythmias occur, anticipate use of pacemaker generator with connection to external pacing wires	Baseline cardiac rhythm will be maintained
Circulation, interruption of: peripheral (potential) **Etiology** Saphenous vein grafting Bed rest/immobility	Edema, swelling of affected parts Coolness, pallor of lower extremities Tenderness of affected extremities Pain, tingling, numbness	A. Assess posterior, tibial, and pedal pulses daily B. Note color and temperature of extremities and presence of edema or pain every ____	A. Apply TED hose *especially* to affected extremity to promote venous return 1. TED hose should be removed daily to adequately assess extremity 2. As activity increases, TED hose can be removed at night B. Ambulate to promote venous return C. Assist patient with active ROM exercises 2-3 times daily per cardiac rehabilitation protocol	Adequate peripheral circulation will be maintained
Injury, potential for: infection **Etiology** Surgical intervention	Febrile Increased WBC count Redness, swelling, drainage from incision site Excessive tenderness at site of incision	Assess incisional sites daily (chest and donor leg) for signs and symptoms of infection	A. Maintain aseptic technique during procedures B. Keep incision dry and clean using mild soap and water 1. 4 × 4 bandages are used to cover incision during postoperative days 1 and 2 2. Incision usually kept uncovered after third postoperative day unless drainage is noted C. Monitor temperatures routinely D. If pacing wires (external) are still present 1. Be careful not to apply increased amount of tension 2. Keep pacing wire tips in syringes at all times	Occurrence of infection will be decreased

Coronary Artery Bypass: intermediate postoperative care—cont'd

NURSING DIAGNOSIS/ PATIENT PROBLEM	DEFINING CHARACTERISTICS	NURSING ORDERS		EXPECTED OUTCOMES
		ASSESSMENT	**INTERVENTIONS**	

Knowledge deficit
Etiology
Unfamiliarity with disease process, treatment, and recovery
	Not verbalizing feelings
	Questioning
	Verbalizing misconceptions
		A. Assess patient's physical and emotional readiness to learn
		  1. Receptive
		  2. Eager
		  3. Asking questions
		  4. Not fatigued or in pain
		B. Assess level of understanding of bypass procedure, recovery process, diet, medications, activity progression, and preventive care by patient/significant others
			A. Involve significant others in patient education and care
			B. Plan teaching sessions so patient is not overly informed at one time
			C. Coordinate teaching with cardiac rehabilitation clinical specialist to use appropriate teaching materials (e.g., hospital television programs on bypass surgery and heart care; heart model; group class; medication handouts)
			D. Provide information regarding
			  1. Bypass surgical procedure
			  2. Coping mechanisms to help adjustment to new or altered life-style
			  3. Dietary intake compatible with therapeutic and personal goals
			    a. Restricted foods
			    b. Reason for diet
			    c. How to maintain adequate dietary intake
			  4. Activity pattern compatible with therapeutic and personal goals
			    a. Signs and symptoms of overexertion
			    b. Gradual increase in activity level (including sexual activity)
			  5. Pharmacologic regimen compatible with goals
			    a. Name, dose, method
			    b. Reason for taking medications
			    c. Side effects of medications
			  6. Preventive care
			    a. Risk factors of heart disease
			    b. Effects of smoking and alcohol on heart
			    c. Incisional care
			    d. Use of TED hose for 1 month at home
			E. Document teaching
				Patient/significant others will be able to communicate an understanding of disease state, bypass procedure, recovery process, diet, activity, medications, and preventive care

Intraaortic Balloon Pump

NURSING DIAGNOSIS/ PATIENT PROBLEM	DEFINING CHARACTERISTICS	NURSING ORDERS		EXPECTED OUTCOMES
		ASSESSMENT	INTERVENTIONS	

Cardiac output, alteration in: decreased (potential)
 Etiology
 Balloon or pump malfunction, secondary to
   Loss of or poor hemodynamic or ECG signals
   Arrhythmias/paced rhythms
   Inappropriate timing/inadequate diastolic augmentation
   Kinked catheter
   Low helium
   Balloon catheter leak/rupture/malposition
	Variations in hemodynamic parameters (BP, pulmonary artery pressure, cardiac output, heart rate, pulmonary artery wedge pressure, left atrial pressure)
	 Arrhythmias, ECG changes
	 Abnormal heart sounds
	 Abnormal lung sounds
	 Restlessness, mentation changes
		A. Assess hemodynamic status every _____
		 B. Assess for myocardial ischemia: chest pain, ST-T wave changes on ECG
		 C. Assess and maintain clear ECG tracing with upright QRS segment to ensure proper balloon triggering. If paced rhythm, assess that triggering is from *R* wave, not paced spike
		 D. Assess and maintain clear arterial pressure waveform. Balloon must inflate at dicrotic notch and deflate before systole
		 E. Assess and maintain good pulmonary pressure tracings
			A. Observe for cardiac arrhythmias continuously. If tachycardia results in inadequate augmentation, pumping ratio may be adjusted to 1:2 as appropriate
			 B. Keep alarms turned on at all times
			 C. Monitor timing of inflation/deflation every _____
			 D. Document in chart arterial pressure tracing with balloon on and off
			   1. At insertion of balloon
			   2. Routinely every ___ hours
			   3. When any change in tracing occurs
			 E. Keep catheter system visible at all times. Keep tubing connections tight and catheter free of kinks
			 F. If technical problems resulting in hemodynamic compromise should occur
			   1. Institute intraaortic balloon pump troubleshooting procedure per protocol
			   2. Notify medical and surgical physicians and pump technician
			   3. Anticipate cardiovascular decompensation, titrate cardiotonic drugs, and maintain pressure
			   4. Remain composed and reassuring to patient
				Hemodynamic parameters will be in desired range

Comfort, alteration in **Etiology** Insertion of balloon and subsequent restriction in movement	Complaint of pain Restlessness, irritability Facial mask of pain	Assess quality, quantity, location of pain, associated manifestations, precipitating and relieving factors	A. Anticipate need for comfort B. Provide comfort measures: position change, back rubs, distraction techniques, analgesics as ordered C. Position to maintain correct body alignment; support dependent parts with pillows D. Provide rest periods to facilitate comfort E. Instruct patient to report pain and effectiveness of intervention	Patient will be as comfortable as possible

Originated by: **Salvacion P. Sulit, RN, BSN, CCRN**
Resource persons: **Meg Gulanick, RN, MSN, CCRN**
                Christine Hunt, RN
                Linda Powless, RN, CCRN, CNA

Intraaortic Balloon Pump—cont'd

NURSING DIAGNOSIS/ PATIENT PROBLEM	DEFINING CHARACTERISTICS	NURSING ORDERS		EXPECTED OUTCOMES
		ASSESSMENT	INTERVENTIONS	

Circulation, interruption in: peripheral (potential)
Etiology
Presence of catheter
Catheter displacement
Thrombus from platelet aggregation on balloon catheter
	A. Extremity
	  1. Decrease or absence of pulse
	  2. Cool/discolored extremity
	  3. Tingling, numbness or pain
	B. Subclavian
	  1. Change in level of consciousness
	  2. Loss of radial pulse
	  3. X-ray catheter position too high
	C. Renal
	  1. Flank pain
	  2. Decrease in output
	  3. X-ray catheter position too low
	D. Mesentery
	  1. Abdominal pain/distention
	  2. GI bleeding
	  3. Acidosis
	  4. Catheter position too low on x-ray film
		A. Assess and record quality of peripheral pulses, color and temperature of extremity to be cannulated, before insertion of balloon catheter
		B. Monitor pulses, color and temperature of cannulated extremity over four 30 min periods, then every 1 hour. Mark site of pedal pulses with "X"
		C. Monitor for local pain, numbness, and tingling in cannulated extremity that may signify ischemia
		D. Observe for signs and symptoms of obstruction of subclavian, renal, or mesenteric artery. If noted, call physician, document catheter position on x-ray examination, and anticipate repositioning
			A. Ensure proper anticoagulation for duration of balloon pumping by monitoring clotting time and administering prescribed medication and fluids
			B. Apply TED hose to unaffected leg
			C. Perform ROM exercise to arms and unaffected leg q.2-4h.
			D. Maintain safety measures to prevent catheter displacement
			  1. Keep cannulated leg straight
			  2. Do not raise head of bed more than 30 degrees
			  3. Weigh carefully on portable bed scale
			E. Do not decrease pumping rate lower than 1:4 and limit time to _____
			F. Should balloon pumping cease for longer than ____, manually inflate/deflate catheter several times every 10 min
				Adequate blood flow to affected extremity and general circulation will be maintained

Injury, potential for: aortic dissection or injury
Etiology
Trauma during insertion
Movement of balloon tip
	Arterial injury
	Hypotension
	Tachycardia
	Pain or discomfort in lower back
	Hematoma at or near insertion site
	Decreased Hct/Hb
	Decrease urine output
	Abdominal pain/distention
	Change in acid-base
		Assess for signs and symptoms of aortic dissection or injury. If this occurs, notify physician	If injury or rupture occurs
			A. Administer blood replacement as ordered
			B. Anticipate cardiovascular decompensation
			  1. Prepare emergency medication
			  2. Anticipate emergency surgery
			C. Provide emotional support to patient
				Risk for injury will be minimized

Injury, potential for **Etiology** Alteration in coagulation (decreased platelets)	Abnormal coagulation studies Petechiae Hematuria Guaiac positive stool/ nasogastric drainage	Assess/monitor daily CBC, PTT, PT, platelets. Report to physician any abnormalities	A. Administer platelets as necessary B. Observe for swelling/hematoma at the insertion site C. Observe for other signs of bleeding: petechiae/hematuria/ and guaiac positive stool/nasogastric drainage	Potential for thrombocytopenia and consequent bleeding tendency will be prevented or minimized

Continued.

Intraaortic Balloon Pump—cont'd

NURSING DIAGNOSIS/ PATIENT PROBLEM	DEFINING CHARACTERISTICS	NURSING ORDERS		EXPECTED OUTCOMES
		ASSESSMENT	INTERVENTIONS	
Anxiety/fear **Etiology** Insertion of/presence of balloon catheter Dependence on proper functioning of balloon pump Continuous noise of pumping Alteration in body image Inability to control environment Gravity of illness; fear of pain/death	Restlessness Vigilant watch over equipment Afraid to sleep Complaining/uncooperative behavior Withdrawal	Assess level of anxiety and normal coping patterns of patient and significant others	A. Institute SCP in Ch. 1: Anxiety/fear B. Stay with patient as much as possible C. Explain purpose/functioning of balloon and pump as appropriate D. Prepare patient at times balloon is turned down to listen to heart, record baseline pressure, etc. E. Provide continuity of care by staff members who are competent and experienced in functioning of pump F. Avoid unnecessary conversations about pump function in front of patient G. Allow patient as much control of environment as possible (e.g., bathing preference, meal times) H. Minimize noise in room I. Offer television or music as appropriate	Decreased anxiety level for patient/significant others will be evidenced by A. Calmer, relaxed appearance B. Verbalization of fears/feelings C. Restful night
Knowledge deficit **Etiology** New procedure/equipment	Questioning Verbalized misconceptions Lack of questions	A. Assess level of understanding about the balloom pump by patient/significant others B. Assess physical/ emotional readiness for learning by patient/significant others	A. Take time to provide environment conducive to learning. Give an unhurried appearance. Advise distracting personnel to leave the room B. Provide information regarding 1. Rationale for balloon use 2. Insertion procedure 3. Ongoing care related to balloon C. Include significant other in teaching D. Refer to cardiac nurse specialist or cardiac surgeon for more specific questions	Patient/significant others will verbalize an understanding of the rationale behind insertion of balloon and use of pump

Intraaortic Balloon Pump—cont'd

NURSING DIAGNOSIS/ PATIENT PROBLEM	DEFINING CHARACTERISTICS	NURSING ORDERS		EXPECTED OUTCOMES
		ASSESSMENT	INTERVENTIONS	
Mobility, impaired physical **Etiology** Bed rest Leg catheter Critical physical condition	Inability to purposefully move within the physical environment (patient on bed rest) Limited ROM (affected leg must be kept straight)	A. Assess respiratory rate, rhythm, heart sounds every ___ hour(s) B. Assess for signs of pulmonary embolism C. Assess skin integrity for signs of redness and tissue ischemia	A. Reposition patient q.2h. to either side or back. Use pillow support to maintain proper leg alignment B. Perform ROM exercises to arms, unaffected leg, and ankle of affected leg q.2-4h. C. Use footboard or boot or shoe to prevent foot drop D. Use egg crate, foam or air mattress on bed E. Maintain dry skin F. Apply lotion and massage around pressure areas q.4-8h. G. Encourage coughing, deep breathing exercises q.2h. when appropriate H. Use incentive spirometer q.i.d. I. Monitor ABGs and chest x-ray films as appropriate J. Use oropharyngeal or tracheal suction p.r.n. K. See SCP in Ch. 1: Mobility, impaired physical	Complications of immobility will be absent or minimized
Injury, potential for (high risk for infection) **Etiology** Invasive procedures and long-term catheter insertion in femoral area	Febrile Elevated WBC Redness, drainage, swelling, tenderness at catheter insertion site	A. Monitor temperature q.4h. If febrile, take temperature q.2h. Notify physician. Obtain culture as ordered B. Monitor WBC every ___	A. Keep femoral dressing dry and intact B. Ensure that surgical assistant/nurse changes catheter insertion site dressing daily and p.r.n. Monitor site for redness, drainage, and tenderness C. Maintain any other catheters and tubes per unit protocol	Risk for infection will be minimized
Sleep pattern disturbance **Etiology** Increased nursing and medical care Noise from balloon, etc. Sleep deprivation	Subjective complaints Restlessness Lethargy Dozing Interrupted sleep Altered mental status Irritability	Assess sleep pattern over past few days	If lack of meaningful sleep is a problem, institute SCP in Ch. 1: Sleep pattern disturbance	Patient will verbalize satisfaction with rest and sleep patterns

Pediatric Cardiac Surgery with Extracorporeal Circulation: immediate postoperative care

NURSING DIAGNOSIS/ PATIENT PROBLEM	DEFINING CHARACTERISTICS	NURSING ORDERS		EXPECTED OUTCOMES
		ASSESSMENT	INTERVENTIONS	
Fluid volume deficit **Etiology** Use of extracorporeal circulation alters clotting factors and platelet function Hemorrhage from surgical suture line	Variations in hemodynamic parameters: increase in heart rate (HR) and respiratory rate (RR); decrease in BP, left atrial pressure (LAP), central venous pressure (CVP), and right atrial pressure (RAP); decrease in pulses, perfusion, and capillary refill Increase in chest tube drainage Widening of mediastinum on x-ray film Decreased urine output Hb below 10 Hct below 30 Platelets below 100,000 PT above 14 PTT above 38	A. Observe and document changes in HR, BP, LAP, RAP, CVP, and RR B. Observe and document changes in perfusion, pulses, and capillary refill 1. Monitor perfusion level q.1h. or ____, and document 2. Check capillary refill (normal: 2-4 seconds) 3. Check brachial, radial, and pedal pulses (normal: 3-4 plus) C. Observe and document changes in chest tube drainage D. Observe and document changes in Hb, platelets, PT, and PTT E. Observe and document changes of mediastinum on x-ray film. Monitor serial chest x-ray studies as ordered. Note for widening mediastinum, and notify physician if present F. Document accurate I & O q.1h. or ____ hour. Include amounts of blood withdrawn for laboratory values. Measure and record urine output q.1h. Note color, consistency, dipstick results, and specific gravity. Notify physician for urine out-	A. Maintain hemodynamic parameters HR 100 to 150 or ____ to ____ BP systolic 80 to 120 or ____ to ____ BP diastolic 50 to 70 or ____ to ____ LAP 10 to 14 or ____ to ____ RAP 10 to 16 or ____ to ____ CVP 10 to 16 or ____ to ____ Notify physician of deviations B. Monitor chest tube drainage q.1h. or every ____ hours, and document 1. Gently strip chest tubes every hour (note decreases in HR, LAP, RAP, and CVP, which denote increased intrathoracic pressures) 2. Note color, temperature, amount, and consistency of drainage; notify physician of drainage 5-10 ml/kg/hour or ____ ml ____ kg ____ hour 3. Maintain water-sealed chest drainage at 20 cm H_2O wall suction or ____ cm as ordered C. Draw Hb, Hct, platelets, PT, PTT every ____ hour as ordered by physician. Notify of abnormal changes. D. Administer blood products, fresh frozen plasma, or platelets as ordered via Harvard pump to ensure accurate infusion time E. Maintain accurate account of the availability of blood and blood products	Vital organ and tissue perfusion will be maintained

Originated by **Kathleen Hurst-Delia, RN, BSN**
Resource persons: **Linda Powless, RN, CCRN, CNA**
                     Susan Galanes, RN, MS, TNS, CCRN

Pediatric Cardiac Surgery with Extracorporeal Circulation: immediate postoperative care—cont'd

NURSING DIAGNOSIS/ PATIENT PROBLEM	DEFINING CHARACTERISTICS	NURSING ORDERS		EXPECTED OUTCOMES
		ASSESSMENT	INTERVENTIONS	
		put below _____ ml/hour (note normal urine output >1 ml/kg/ hour) G. Record amount, pH, and hematest of nasogastric drainage q.12h. or every _____ H. Administer antacids as ordered by physician		
Cardiac output, alteration in: decreased **Etiology** Low cardiac output syndrome may occur as a result of extracorporeal circulation and surgical procedure	Decreases in BP, perfusion, peripheral pulse, and capillary refill Increased HR, RR, LAP, RAP, CVP Decreased urine output Metabolic acidosis	A. Observe and document changes in HR, BP, LAP, RAP, CVP, RR, perfusion, capillary refill, and pulses B. Assess and document changes in ABGs C. Assess and document urine output. Administer diuretics as ordered by physician (note standard pediatric doses: mannitol 0.5-1.0 gm/kg; furosemide [Lasix] 1-2 mg/kg)	A. Maintain hemodynamic parameters HR _____ to _____ BP _____ to _____ LAP _____ to _____ RAP _____ to _____ CVP _____ to _____ Notify physician of deviations B. Administer vasopressor drugs as ordered by physician 1. Use Harvard pump to ensure accuracy 2. Mix vasopressors in solution ordered by physician 3. Administer drugs through central line to ensure potency 4. Keep drug calculations at bedside to decrease errors when changing drip rates: desired amount (μg/kg) $\times$ 60 min/hour $\div$ standard concentration C. Monitor serial ABG as ordered by physician; notify if signs of metabolic acidosis occur	Maintenance of cardiac output will be adequate to perfuse vital organs
Cardiac rhythm, alteration in **Etiology** Use of extracorporeal circulation alters electrolyte balances Surgical procedure may interfere with conduction system	Premature atrial contractions Junctional escape beats or rhythm Supraventricular tachycardias Atrioventricular dissociation	Assess baseline rhythm and monitor ECG continuously. Note and document changes by obtaining rhythm strips. Notify physician of changes	A. Obtain baseline rhythm strip q.12h. or _____ hours B. Connect pacemaker to pacing wires, and set parameters per physician's orders. Use gloves when handling pacing wires so as not to fibrillate patient. Note usual initial settings—rate 100, mA 3, sensitivity at 1.5, set on demand mode C. Administer resuscitative drugs as ordered by physician. Note standard pediatric doses Epinephrine 0.1-0.2 mEq/kg via IV (0.01 mg/kg); intra- cardiac 0.01-0.02 ml/kg	Optimal cardiac rhythm will be maintained

Continued.

Pediatric Cardiac Surgery with Extracorporeal Circulation: immediate postoperative care—cont'd

NURSING DIAGNOSIS/ PATIENT PROBLEM	DEFINING CHARACTERISTICS	NURSING ORDERS		EXPECTED OUTCOMES
		ASSESSMENT	INTERVENTIONS	
			Sodium bicarbonate 1-2 mEq/kg via IV Atropine 0.01 mg/kg via IV Calcium chloride 20-50 mg/ kg via IV slowly Lidocaine 2% 1 mg/kg D. Administer digitalis preparations as ordered by physician. Note that two people should check dosage against orders as well as actual calculation of amount to be given to ensure accuracy. Serum K$^+$ should be 4.0-4.5	
Fluid composition, alteration in: potential **Etiology** Electrolyte imbalance	ECG changes, widening QRS, ST changes, and atrioventricular blocks Seizure or tremor activity Na below 130 or above 142 K below 4.0 or above 5.0 Cl below 98 or above 115 Ca below 9.0 or above 11.0 Glucose below 90 or above 150 BUN above 20 Creatinine above 1.8	A. Observe and document ECG changes. Monitor ECG for changes, document, and notify physician B. Observe and document for changes in mentation or seizure activity. Assess level of consciousness/responsiveness every ____ or as indicated C. Determine contributing factors to any change (e.g., anesthesia, medications) D. Observe and document serial laboratory data. Monitor Na, K, Cl, glucose, Ca, BUN and creatinine q.4h. or ____ hour as ordered by physician. Notify of abnormalities	A. Maintain adequate electrolyte balance by administration of desired electrolytes as ordered by physician. Hypertonic solutions may be used to correct Na and Cl deficiencies. K and Ca may be corrected by administration of K$^+$ 1 mEq/3 kg or ____; CaCl 50-100 mg/kg or ____ as ordered by physician (note K and CaCl are usually given via central IV over 1 hour to ensure accuracy) B. Maintain adequate glucose levels with administration of D10 as ordered by physician. Use Chemstrips to determine serum glucose q.1h. or ____ hour as ordered and document C. Obtain blood specimens using the minimal amount that can be sent as a specimen. Nettleson capillary tubes, which hold 0.25 ml blood, may be used NOTE: Na, K, Cl, Ca use four capillary tubes; glucose: one capillary tube on ice; BUN, creatinine: two capillary tubes	Fluid balance will be maintained

Pediatric Cardiac Surgery with Extracorporeal Circulation: immediate postoperative care—cont'd

NURSING DIAGNOSIS/ PATIENT PROBLEM	DEFINING CHARACTERISTICS	NURSING ORDERS		EXPECTED OUTCOMES
		ASSESSMENT	INTERVENTIONS	

Breathing pattern/gas exchange, alteration in: requiring use of ventilator
 Etiology
 Surgical procedure requiring extracorporeal circulation
 Patients who are under the effects of anesthesia
	Hypoinflated or hyperinflated chest expansion
	 Asymmetric chest expansion
	 Rales, rhonchi, wheezes, dyspnea, tachypnea
	 Decreased perfusion and capillary refill
	 Circumoral, vascular, or peripheral cyanosis
	 Increased gastric dilation
	 ABG:
	   pH below 7.38 or above 7.50
	   P_{CO_2} below 33 or above 44
	   P_{O_2} below 75
	   O_2 saturation below 92
		A. Assess and document chest expansion and breath sounds q.1h. Note the presence or absence of rales, rhonchi, or wheezes
		 B. Assess and document perfusion level, capillary refill, and presence or absence of cyanosis
		 C. Observe and document changes in ABGs
			A. Maintain adequate mechanical ventilation
			   1. Ventilator settings per physician's orders
			     Volume set ____ (note tidal volume 10-15 ml/kg)
			     FIO_2 _____
			     Rate _____
			     Continuous positive airway pressure _____
			     NOTE: Physiologic continuous positive airway pressure for pediatric use is 2 cm/H_2O
			   2. Draw and record ABGs 20 min after each ventilator change and every ____ hour as ordered by physician; notify of any abnormal changes. Document tidal volume at time of obtaining specimen
			   3. Administer sedation as ordered by physician
			 B. Maintain pulmonary hygiene
			   1. Gentle tracheal suctioning q.1h. or every ____ hour using appropriately sized suction catheter. Turn head slightly to facilitate cleansing of bronchial tree
			   2. Loosen tracheal secretions by instillation of 0.5-1 ml sterile normal saline lavage
			   3. Hyperventilate, hyperinflate, and hyperoxygenate lungs by using 100% O_2 per air-mask-bag unit (Ambu bag). Inflate lungs gently, noting chest expansion and allowing for expiration. Document resistance if any. Notify physician of any deviations in chest excursion
			   4. Suction oral cavity after endotracheal (ET) suctioning. Document amount, color, and consistency of secretions obtained
				Respiratory status will be maximized as evidenced by adequate oxygenation of life systems and patient's response to ventilatory support changes

Continued.

Pediatric Cardiac Surgery with Extracorporeal Circulation: immediate postoperative care—cont'd

NURSING DIAGNOSIS/ PATIENT PROBLEM	DEFINING CHARACTERISTICS	NURSING ORDERS		EXPECTED OUTCOMES
		ASSESSMENT	INTERVENTIONS	
			C. Maintain placement and patency of nasogastric tube D. Monitor serial chest x-ray films as ordered by physician for ET tube placement E. Place additional ET tube of the same size along with placement setup at bedside for emergency reintubation F. As needed, use soft restraints on extremities or place sandbags on either side of patient's head to prevent accidental ET dislodgement	
Body temperature: alteration in **Etiology** Hypothermia used in conjunction with extracorporeal circulation	Temperature <37° (rectal) Skin cool with decreased perfusion and capillary refill Tachycardia or heart block	Assess and document perfusion, skin temperature, and capillary refill	A. Monitor rectal temperature continuously. Verify probe accuracy by checking patient's temperature with glass thermometer q.4h. B. Monitor and document changes in skin temperature, perfusion, and capillary refill q.1h. or every ___ hour. Notify physician of changes C. Continuously monitor ECG, document changes, and notify physician of changes. Keep pacemaker on standby D. Increase body temperature to ___ as ordered by physician. Use extra blankets or warm packs as needed. Protect skin against burns by providing a layer of protection between patient's skin and warming apparatus	Adequate body temperature will be maintained
Consciousness, altered levels of: potential **Etiology** Fluid volume deficit Change in cardiac output Electrolyte imbalance Altered body temperature	Change in alertness, orientation, eye opening, motor response Agitation Inappropriate affect Glasgow Coma Scale less than 11	A. Assess level of consciousness and responsiveness every ___ hour B. Assess more frequently if any deterioration C. Determine contributing factors to any change	If signs of an alteration in level of consciousness are present, see SCP in Ch. 3	Optimal level of consciousness will be maintained
Anxiety in family members **Etiology** Decreased knowledge of surroundings and events related to postoperative care Separation during surgery	Unable to concentrate on explanations being given Unable to touch child Crying and nervous appearance	Assess family's knowledge of postoperative care	A. Orient family to environment B. Encourage members to verbalize feelings C. Encourage family's use of support services D. Show concern for family's feelings E. Encourage family to call about patient's condition	Anxiety level will be decreased as evidenced by A. Calm appearance B. Ability to express concern in a calm manner C. Understanding of environment D. Child's acceptance of touch without fear

Swan-Ganz Catheterization

NURSING DIAGNOSIS/ PATIENT PROBLEM	DEFINING CHARACTERISTICS	NURSING ORDERS		EXPECTED OUTCOMES
		ASSESSMENT	INTERVENTIONS	
Cardiac arrhythmias (PVCs), potential for **Etiology** Irritation of ventricular endocardium by catheter during insertion/repositioning Migration of catheter from pulmonary artery to right ventricle Excessive looping of catheter in right ventricle	Palpitation Dizziness and fainting Shortness of breath Arrhythmia seen on oscilloscope	A. Document baseline arrhythmias precatheterization, noting frequency and type B. Observe cardiac monitor continuously for arrhythmias during and after catheter positioning C. Monitor catheter position on chest x-ray daily and whenever arrhythmias occur, or inform physician of need for x-ray examination D. Assess insertion site, and note length of inserted catheter (check markings) E. Monitor pulmonary artery waveform closely, observing for change to right ventricle F. Assess and document the amount of air needed to wedge catheter (amount increases as catheter migrates to right ventricle, or catheter will not wedge)	A. Have lidocaine bolus and crash cart available B. Maintain appropriate positioning of extremity to prevent malposition of catheter C. If arrhythmias occur 1. Assess patient for complaints of dizziness, palpitations, light-headedness, shortness of breath 2. Document rhythm strip and notify physician 3. Observe contributing factors that may have potentiated arrhythmias (e.g., patient/ catheter position; other medical problems) 4. Treat arrhythmias as indicated	Occurrence of ventricular arrhythmias will be minimized
Injury, potential for: pulmonary artery infarction or hemorrhage **Etiology** Continuous or prolonged wedging of catheter; overinflation of balloon; migration of catheter to pulmonary capillary as seen on x-ray film	Patient complains of shortness of breath Hemoptysis	A. Monitor pulmonary arterial pressure waveform continuously B. Monitor pulmonary artery position of catheter on x-ray, or notify physician of need to determine position of catheter	A. Watch waveforms during wedge inflation; inject only enough air to obtain pulmonary artery wedge pressure B. Do not inflate balloon past recommended volume. Document amount used C. Leave balloon *deflated* after wedging D. Monitor pulmonary artery diastolic pressure instead of wedge pressure when both values are correlated E. Do not forcefully flush catheter when in wedge position	Patient will have decreased susceptibility to pulmonary artery damage as evidenced by A. No prolonged periods of wedging as seen on monitor B. Prompt interventions if catheter remains wedged

Originated by **Patricia Hasbrouck-Aschliman, RN, CCRN**
 Resource persons: **Janice L. Miller, RN,C MSN**
 Meg Gulanick, RN, MSN, CCRN
 Susan Galanes, RN, MS, TNS, CCRN

Continued.

Swan-Ganz Catheterization—cont'd

NURSING DIAGNOSIS/ PATIENT PROBLEM	DEFINING CHARACTERISTICS	NURSING ORDERS		EXPECTED OUTCOMES
		ASSESSMENT	INTERVENTIONS	

			F. If catheter appears permanently wedged
			  1. Verify that cause is not false wedge pressure waveform, as with dampening or other technical problems
			  2. Have patient take deep breaths, raise arm, turn on left side, cough to attempt to unwedge
			  3. Determine catheter/balloon position on chest x-ray or inform physician of need
			  4. Notify physician immediately to pull back catheter to pulmonary artery	

Injury, potential for: electrical shock **Etiology** Direct low resistance pathway of current through catheter to heart Current leakage Improperly grounded electrical equipment Frayed cords, exposed wires Wet skin or bed area Invasive catheters	PVCs, ventricular tachycardia, ventricular fibrillation produced by microshock	Assess environment for electrical safety	Maintain electrical safety standards when rendering care to high risk patients A. Use as few electrical devices as needed B. Substitute battery-operated machines when possible C. Keep bed linen dry D. Ground electrical equipment	Risk of electrical shock will be minimized
Injury, potential for: pneumothorax **Etiology** Use of subclavian insertion site Patient movement during insertion	Shortness of breath Decreased breath sounds on affected side Unequal thoracic wall movement Shift of trachea toward unaffected side	A. Assess breath sounds, respiratory pattern, and chest movement before and immediately after insertion B. When checking for catheter placement on x-ray, note lung expansion	A. Keep patient still during procedure. Provide sedatives, local anesthesia, and reassurances as needed B. Provide optimal positioning of insertion area (back/shoulder/subclavian region) C. If any symptoms of pneumothorax are noted, refer to physician and anticipate chest tube insertion	Occurrence of pneumothorax will be minimized
Injury, potential for: infection **Etiology** Invasive monitoring; indwelling catheter; manipulation of catheter or connecting tubing; prolonged use of catheter	Redness at site Swelling Change in local temperature Foul drainage Fever	A. Check insertion site every ____ for signs of infection B. Assess vital signs every 2 hours	A. Change IV tubing every ____ B. Change IV dressing every ____ using sterile technique C. Apply antiseptic ointment or ____ to site D. Use caps on all ports of stopcock E. Encourage removal of catheter or change of insertion site every 3 days F. If infection occurs, notify physician for removal of catheter and culturing treatment	Occurrence of infection will be minimized

Swan-Ganz Catheterization—cont'd

NURSING DIAGNOSIS/ PATIENT PROBLEM	DEFINING CHARACTERISTICS	NURSING ORDERS		EXPECTED OUTCOMES
		ASSESSMENT	INTERVENTIONS	

Comfort, alteration in: potential
 Etiology
 Thrombophlebitis
 Venous stasis
 Dependent edema
 Catheter irritation
 Difficult/traumatic insertion
	Report of discomfort
	 Restlessness
	 Irritability
	 Limited movement of extremity
	 Tenderness, swelling at insertion site
	 Edema of extremity
		A. Check insertion site/extremity q.4h. or ____ for signs of inflammation or discomfort
		 B. Check extremity for swelling or dependent edema. Compare with unaffected extremity
			A. Assist during insertion so catheter positioned smoothly and rapidly
			 B. Maintain optimal position of extremity. Elevate distal portion of extremity
			 C. Avoid tight bandaging of affected extremity. Use occlusive but nonconstricting dressing
			 D. Promote circulation to affected extremity by performing active/passive ROM, noting limitations of catheter
			 E. Encourage removal of catheter or change of insertion site every 3 days whenever possible
			 F. If pain, phlebitis, or inflammation occurs
			   1. Facilitate removal of catheter
			   2. Apply warm compresses
			   3. Elevate extremity
			   4. Give pain medication p.r.n.
				Patient will have minimal discomfort in affected extremity as evidenced by verbalization of comfort

Knowledge deficit of patient/significant others
 Etiology
 Newness, complexity, and urgency of procedure
	Asking several questions
	 Overly anxious
	 Inability to talk about procedure
	 Asking no questions
		A. Assess current level of knowledge
		 B. Assess learning capabilities of patient/significant others
			A. Provide patient/significant others with information regarding Swan-Ganz catheter
			   1. Purpose
			   2. Procedure
			   3. Complications
			   4. Ongoing care
			   5. Duration
			 B. Reinforce previous learning
			 C. Encourage questions
			 D. Develop family rapport
				Patient/significant others will state why the Swan-Ganz catheter is needed

Transvenous Pacemaker, Permanent

NURSING DIAGNOSIS/ PATIENT PROBLEM	DEFINING CHARACTERISTICS	NURSING ORDERS		EXPECTED OUTCOMES
		ASSESSMENT	INTERVENTIONS	
Cardiac output, decrease: potential **Etiology** Ventricular arrhythmias caused by ventricular irritation from pacing electrode (lead) Cardiac tamponade resulting from myocardial perforation Permanent pacemaker malfunction caused by A. Lead displacement B. Battery fault or depletion C. Lead fracture D. Changing myocardial threshold E. Competitive rhythms F. Malfunctioning generator circuitry G. Faulty connection between lead and pulse generator H. Improperly set pacemaker parameters	Signs of hemodynamic compromise (hypotension; decrease in measured cardiac output; decrease in urine output; confusion; restlessness; dizziness; chest pain; cool skin) and/ or congestive heart failure Palpitations Significant decrease (5% to 10%) in heart rate from present parameter Stokes-Adams syndrome "Runaway" pacemaker (pacer tachycardia) Ventricular arrhythmias Loss of sensing Loss of capture Failure to fire Decrease in amplitude of pacemaker artifact Change in configuration of paced QRS Signs of cardiac tamponade (jugular vein distention; elevated central venous pressure; pulsus paradoxus; quiet heart sounds; signs of decreased cardiac output)	**If ECG monitored** A. Assess for proper pacemaker function 1. Capture 2. Sensing 3. Firing 4. Amplitude of pacemaker artifact 5. Configuration of paced QRS B. Assess for pacemaker induced arrhythmias **If unmonitored** A. Assess apical and radial pulses every _____ B. Assess patient's hemodynamic status and for signs of congestive heart failure routinely every _____ **If ventricular arrhythmias or pacemaker malfunction occurs** Assess patient for hemodynamic status and for signs of congestive heart failure routinely every ___ (see Defining Characteristics) **If myocardial perforation is suspected** Assess for signs of cardiac tamponade (see Defining Characteristics)	A. Check operative note for 1. Type of pacemaker (programmable, ventricular demand, AV sequential, etc.), and prescribed parameters B. Monitor chest x-ray and ECG studies after patient returns from OR, and _____ as ordered C. If ECG monitored 1. Keep alarms on at all times 2. Record rhythm strips a. Routinely every _____ b. If any malfunction is noted c. After changes in pacemaker parameters D. If *pacemaker malfunction* is noted: 1. Evaluate adequacy of patient's own rhythm 2. If patient is not monitored, call for 12-lead ECG 3. Monitor for signs of hemodynamic compromise and/ or congestive heart failure 4. Notify physician 5. Initiate basic life support measures as needed 6. Prepare IV isoproterenol for standby 7. Prepare for temporary pacemaker insertion and other advanced life support measures as needed 8. If pacemaker is programmable, have the programmer brought to the bedside 9. Anticipate possible return to OR E. If *failure to sense* is noted 1. Monitor chest x-ray study to check for position of the electrode 2. Observe for diaphragmatic contraction (hiccups) and intercostal or abdominal muscle twitching 3. Turn patient on left side 4. Observe for rapid ventricular arrhythmias secondary to pacemaker competition F. If *loss of capture* is noted 1. See *E: 1, 2, 3, 4* 2. Assess for factors that increase myocardial threshold (myocardial ischemia, fibrosis at tip of the electrode, electrolyte imbalance, acidosis, and some antiarrhythmic drugs)	Optimal cardiac output will be maintained

Originated by **Terry Takemoto, RN, MSN, CCRN**
Resource person: **Meg Gulanick, RN, MSN, CCRN**

Transvenous Pacemaker, Permanent—cont'd

NURSING DIAGNOSIS/ PATIENT PROBLEM	DEFINING CHARACTERISTICS	NURSING ORDERS		EXPECTED OUTCOMES
		ASSESSMENT	INTERVENTIONS	

			G. If *myocardial perforation* is suspected
			  1. Monitor chest x-ray film for electrode placement
			  2. Monitor closely for signs of cardiac tamponade
			  3. Anticipate need for possible pericardiocentesis
			H. If hemodynamic compromise is noted, see SCP in Chapter 1: Cardiac output, alteration in: decreased	

Mobility, impaired physical **Etiology** Imposed restriction of activity Reluctance to attempt movement because of pain or fear of injury	Verbalization of inability to perform Limited ROM Complaints of shoulder joint stiffness and pain Muscle weakness, especially of upper extremity on operative side	While patient is on bed rest (usually 24 to 48 hours after insertion): A. Auscultate breath sounds every _____ , and assess respiratory rate, rhythm every _____ B. Assess skin integrity; check for signs of redness or tissue ischemia every _____ C. Assess for developing thrombophlebitis (increased temperature, redness, swelling, calf pain) every _____ D. Assess for pulmonary embolism every _____ (chest pain, shortness of breath, tachycardia, increased BP) E. Observe for signs of discomfort F. Assess for conditional deterrents to mobility	While patient is on bed rest A. Explain necessity for imposed activity restriction B. Encourage patient to turn every 1 to 2 hours but not to right side C. Assist with active ROM exercises to nonaffected extremities t.i.d. D. Provide passive ROM to shoulder on *operative* side t.i.d. E. Assist patient in using affected extremity to perform ADL; however, caution patient against raising arm over head until instructed to do so F. Encourage patient to cough and deep breathe every hour while awake; incentive spirometry may be used when appropriate G. Administer pain medication as ordered and institute other measures for promotion of pain relief H. Allow patient to verbalize feelings of fear or pain. Render emotional support, and teach as needed to decrease reluctance to move extremity on operative side I. If bed rest will be prolonged, institute prophylactic use of antipressure devices (e.g., eggcrate mattress)	Complications of immobility will be absent or minimized

Comfort, alteration in
Etiology
"Frozen" shoulder
Insertion of permanent pacemaker
Self-imposed restriction of movement of extremity on operative side
Lead displacement
	Patient/significant other reports discomfort
	Requests pain medication
	Restlessness, irritability
	Guarded or withdrawn behavior
	Pallor, increased BP, or diaphoresis
	Crying
	Grimacing
		A. Observe for objective signs of discomfort (e.g., crying, grimacing)
		B. Assess characteristics of source of discomfort including quality, quantity, location, onset, associated manifestations, precipitating and relieving factors
			A. Anticipate need for pain relief and administer analgesics as ordered
			B. Provide comfort measures
			  1. Back rubs
			  2. Gentle massage to shoulder on operative side
			  3. Heating pad to shoulder as ordered
			  4. Relaxation techniques to decrease muscle tension
			C. Instruct patient to report discomfort
				Discomfort will be relieved or minimized

Continued.

Transvenous Pacemaker, Permanent—cont'd

NURSING DIAGNOSIS/ PATIENT PROBLEM	DEFINING CHARACTERISTICS	NURSING ORDERS		EXPECTED OUTCOMES
		ASSESSMENT	INTERVENTIONS	

	Reluctance to move
	Splints wound with hands
	Limited ROM of shoulder on operative side
	Hiccuping (diaphragmatic contraction); intercostal or abdominal muscle twitching
		C. Assess for hiccups or muscle twitching
		D. Solicit information about effectiveness of pain-relief measures the patient has used in the past
			D. Instruct patient to report effectiveness of interventions
			E. Discuss reasons for self-imposed restriction of movement of extremities on affected side, and teach as needed
			F. If hiccups or muscle twitching are noted
			  1. Notify physician
			  2. Explain to patient this may be caused by lead displacement
			  3. Arrange for chest x-ray examination to check for lead placement and anticipate repositioning
			G. Use SCP in Ch. 1: Comfort, alteration in	

Knowledge deficit
Etiology
New procedure/equipment
	Questioning
	Verbalized misconceptions
	Lack of questions
	Inappropriate behavior
		A. Assess patient's level of understanding about the pacemaker
		B. Assess patient's readiness for learning
			A. Provide environment conducive to learning
			B. Utilize appropriate teaching materials
			  1. Pacemaker equipment
			  2. Manufacturer's pamphlet
			  3. "Enjoy a Fuller Life with Your Pacemaker," an in-hospital television program
			C. Include significant others in teaching
			D. Document teaching
			E. Refer patient to clinical nurse specialist or physician for further information as needed
			F. Provide the following teaching as needed
			
			Preoperatively
			A. Basic anatomy and physiology of the normal conduction system
			B. Function and use of the pacemaker
			C. Insertion procedure
			
			Postoperatively
			A. Activity limitations
			  1. Bed rest for _____ hours as ordered
			  2. Avoid any over-the-head motion of the arms for _____ days
			  3. Avoid turning to right side for _____ days
			B. Notify nurse of any wetness, discoloration, loose dressing
			C. Notify nurse of any dizziness, headache, confusion, shortness of breath, chest pain, muscle twitching, or hiccups
			D. Need for chest x-ray examination and 12-lead ECG
				Patient will
				A. Verbalize an understanding of rationale for pacemaker insertion
				B. Verbalize an understanding of rationale for activity limitations

Transvenous Pacemaker, Permanent—cont'd

NURSING DIAGNOSIS/ PATIENT PROBLEM	DEFINING CHARACTERISTICS	NURSING ORDERS		EXPECTED OUTCOMES
		ASSESSMENT	INTERVENTIONS	
			Prior to discharge A. How to take and record pulse daily B. Need for regular follow-up care C. Type of pacemaker that was inserted (programmable, chamber[s] paced, synchronous or asynchronous) D. Brand name of pacemaker ____ E. Model number _____ F. Pacing rate _____ G. Normal pulse range ____ to ____ H. Pacemaker battery should last ____ years. Replacement of battery requires approximately 3 days hospitalization I. Signs and symptoms of pacemaker malfunction 1. Dizziness 2. Shortness of breath 3. Chest pain 4. Edema and increase in weight 5. Hiccups or muscle twitching 6. Change in heart rate less than ____ or greater than ____ J. Signs and symptoms of infection at insertion site 1. Redness 2. Soreness 3. Drainage 4. Swelling 5. Fever 6. Chills K. Notify physician of any signs and symptoms of pacemaker malfunction or infection at insertion site L. Wound care for insertion sites M. Always carry an I.D. card with type and model of pacemaker N. Alert any dentist or physician to presence of pacemaker O. Personnel at airport screening area should be made aware that patient has a pacemaker that may trigger the alarm P. Most household appliances and office and shop equipment that are in good repair can be used safely, including 1. Televisions or radios 2. Toasters, electric can openers, or blenders	

Continued.

Transvenous Pacemaker, Permanent—cont'd

NURSING DIAGNOSIS/ PATIENT PROBLEM	DEFINING CHARACTERISTICS	NURSING ORDERS		EXPECTED OUTCOMES
		ASSESSMENT	INTERVENTIONS	
			3. Washers, dryers, or electric stoves	
			4. Hair dryers or shavers	
			5. Heating pads and electric blankets	
			6. Gardening equipment	
			7. Electric brooms or vacuum cleaners	
			8. Microwave ovens can be used by patients with newer model pacemakers (check with physician or manufacturer's owner manual)	
			9. Copy machines or electric typewriters	
			10. Light metalworking and woodworking tools	
			Q. Avoid equipment that contains powerful magnets or emits high-frequency electrical signals	
			1. Diathermy or electrocautery equipment	
			2. High current, industrial machinery	
			3. Radio and television station transmitting equipment	
			R. If interference with pacemaker function is suspected	
			1. Turn off the equipment or move away from it	
			2. The pacemaker will resume normal function without permanent effects	
			S. Instruct patient that pacemaker company representatives can make home visits to determine possible sources of electrical interference	
			T. Most activities can be resumed	
			1. Traveling or driving a car	
			2. Sex	
			3. Swimming, bowling, fishing, hunting, or golfing	
			4. Working	
			U. Avoid contact sports (e.g., football, basketball)	

Transvenous Pacemaker, Permanent—cont'd

NURSING DIAGNOSIS/ PATIENT PROBLEM	DEFINING CHARACTERISTICS	NURSING ORDERS		EXPECTED OUTCOMES
		ASSESSMENT	INTERVENTIONS	
Anxiety/fear Etiology Insertion/presence of permanent pacemaker Dependence on proper functioning of pacemaker Alteration in body image caused by loss of normal cardiac function or cosmetic appearance of generator and incision line	Excessive concern over the function of the pacemaker Increased questioning Restlessness Withdrawal or indifference Increase or self-imposed decrease in activity Afraid to sleep at night Verbal expression of feelings of loss, fear/anxiety, or negative feelings about the body Refusal to look at or touch the incision or pulse generator site Overexposure or hiding of the incision or pulse generator site Refusal to learn about pacemaker, participate in care of the incision, or follow instructions about wound care or activity limitations	A. Assess level of anxiety B. Assess normal coping patterns	A. Explain all procedures before they are performed B. Allow patient to verbalize his concerns C. Correct knowledge deficits D. Institute measures to promote adequate sleep E. Preoperatively involve patient in decision making for optimal generator placement F. Request consultation from clergy, social service, or liaison nurse when appropriate G. Institute SCP in Ch. 1: Anxiety/fear	Decreased level of anxiety will be evidenced by A. Calm, relaxed appearance B. Verbalizations of less anxiety and fear C. Restful night

Potential for injury: infection
Etiology
Alteration in skin integrity caused by permanent pacemaker insertion
	Febrile
	Redness, drainage, edema, induration, or excessive tenderness at incision line
	Elevated WBC with left shift
		A. Assess insertion site for signs of infection (see Defining Characteristics): healing, intact sutures, hematoma, skin breakdown over pulse generator site
		B. Monitor WBC count every _____
		C. Monitor temperature every _____ and as needed
		D. Assess amount and characteristics of Hemovac drainage if present
			A. Keep dressing dry and intact
			B. Change dressing using sterile technique every _____ as per infection control policy until skin closure is complete
			C. If Hemovac is in place, record output q.8h. and as necessary, and report excessive drainage
			D. Encourage a high protein, high calorie diet unless contraindicated to facilitate wound healing
			E. Administer antibiotics as ordered
			F. Before discharge, teach patient
			  1. Signs/symptoms of infection
			  2. Wound care
				Risk for infection will be minimized

Transvenous Pacemaker, Temporary

NURSING DIAGNOSIS/ PATIENT PROBLEM	DEFINING CHARACTERISTICS	NURSING ORDERS		EXPECTED OUTCOMES
		ASSESSMENT	INTERVENTIONS	
Cardiac output, alteration in: decreased (potential) **Etiology** Temporary pacemaker malfunction secondary to Improperly set pacemaker parameters Displaced pacemaker lead (catheter) Broken wire Poor electrical connections Battery exhaustion Malfunctioning generator circuitry Unsafe environment Changing myocardial threshhold Competitive rhythms	Loss of pacemaker capture Loss of pacemaker sensing Loss of firing of pacemaker Significant decrease in heart rate Signs of hemodynamic compromise (i.e., hypotension, confusion, decrease in cardiac output, restlessness, cool skin, decrease in urine output)	A. Assess that prescribed pacemaker parameters are maintained (rate, mA, mode, sensitivity) B. Monitor ECG continuously for appropriate pacemaker function 1. Sensing 2. Capturing 3. Firing C. If pacemaker is on standby, ensure that pacemaker capture is checked daily and as needed by physician by overriding of the spontaneous rhythm D. Assess for pacemaker-induced arrhythmias E. Assess that patient is in an electrically safe environment 1. All electrical equipment is properly grounded 2. Environment is dry 3. "Exposed" electrode terminals are insulated in rubber glove 4. Patient in non-electric bed F. If signs of pacemaker malfunction occur, assess patient's hemodynamic status every _____	A. Keep alarms turned on at all times B. Document spontaneous and paced rhythms during physician rounds 1. Daily or _____ 2. When changes in pacer parameters are instituted C. If pacemaker malfunction is noted (especially if not easily corrected by steps *D, E,* and *F* below) 1. Evaluate adequacy of patient's own rhythm 2. Monitor vital signs 3. Notify physician 4. Prepare IV isoproterenol for standby D. If *failure to sense* is noted 1. Check that power switch is turned on 2. Check that dial is *NOT* on "asynchronous" 3. Check for loose connections 4. Reposition limb of body 5. Notify physician of need to adjust sensitivity dial 6. Check position of lead by chest x-ray examination 7. If problem is not corrected and patient's rate is adequate, evaluate whether the pacemaker should be turned off (standby) E. If *loss of capture is noted* 1. Check all possible connections 2. Turn patient on left side to facilitate optimal lead placement 3. Increase mA and evaluate effectiveness for capture F. If *loss of firing* is noted 1. Check that power switch is turned on 2. Check "pace" needle on pacemaker box to see that it is fluctuating back and forth 3. If needle is not "pacing," replace batteries in generator 4. Check all possible connections 5. Check for electrical interference 6. Replace generator as needed	Optimal cardiac output will be maintained

Originated by **Marisa C. Trybula, RN, BSN**
Resource person: **Meg Gulanick, RN, MSN, CCRN**

Transvenous Pacemaker, Temporary—cont'd

NURSING DIAGNOSIS/ PATIENT PROBLEM	DEFINING CHARACTERISTICS	NURSING ORDERS		EXPECTED OUTCOMES
		ASSESSMENT	INTERVENTIONS	
Mobility, impaired physical **Etiology** Imposed restriction secondary to pacemaker insertion	Reluctance to attempt movement Limited ROM Verbalization of inability to perform activities	A. Auscultate breath sounds every ＿＿ and assess respiratory rate, rhythm every ＿＿＿＿ B. Assess skin integrity. Check for signs of redness or tissue ischemia every ＿＿＿＿ C. Assess for developing thrombophlebitis (e.g., increased temperature, redness, swelling, calf pain) every ＿＿ D. Assess for pulmonary embolism every ＿＿ (e.g., chest pain, shortness of breath, tachycardia, increased BP)	A. Turn and position q.2h., but instruct patient *not* to turn on right side B. Assist with active ROM exercises to nonaffected extremities t.i.d. C. Assist patient with modified ROM to extremity with lead insertion t.i.d. D. Instruct patient *not* to raise arm over head if pacemaker lead is in the antecubital fossa E. Institute prophylactic use of antipressure devices F. Encourage cough and deep breathing q.1h. while patient is awake G. Assist patient to dangle after 24 hours if pacemaker lead is in the antecubital fossa H. Ensure that patient maintains strict bed rest with head of bed elevated less than 30 degrees if pacemaker lead is inserted per femoral vein	Complications of immobility will be absent or minimized
Knowledge deficit **Etiology** New procedure/equipment	Questioning Verbalized misconceptions Lack of questions Inappropriate behavior	A. Assess patient's level of understanding about the pacemaker B. Assess patient's readiness for learning	A. Provide environment conducive to learning B. Use appropriate teaching materials 　1. Temporary pacemaker flip chart 　2. Pacemaker equipment C. Give patient explanations regarding 　1. Function and use of a pacemaker 　2. Insertion procedure 　3. Activity restrictions 　4. Ongoing care related to the temporary pacemaker D. Include significant others in teaching as appropriate E. Document teaching F. Refer to cardiac clinical specialist and physician with more specific questions	Patient will verbalize an understanding of rationale for use of temporary pacemaker, insertion procedure, and follow-up nursing care

Continued.

Transvenous Pacemaker, Temporary—cont'd

NURSING DIAGNOSIS/ PATIENT PROBLEM	DEFINING CHARACTERISTICS	NURSING ORDERS		EXPECTED OUTCOMES
		ASSESSMENT	INTERVENTIONS	
Anxiety/fear **Etiology** Insertion/presence of temporary pacemaker Dependence on proper functioning of pacemaker Threat to self-concept, especially if patient is pacer-dependent and will need a permanent pacemaker	Patient concern over equipment Increased questioning Restlessness Withdrawn, indifferent, uncooperative Afraid to sleep at night	A. Assess level of anxiety B. Assess patient's normal coping patterns	A. Institute SCP in Ch. 1: Anxiety/fear B. Establish rapport with patient through continuity of care C. Encourage ventilation of feelings/concerns D. Orient to environment, pacemaker equipment E. Adapt care to patient's needs F. Stay with patient as much as possible G. Provide accurate information regarding purpose/function of pacemaker H. Reassure patient when weaning off pacemaker and especially when terminating	Decreased level of anxiety as evidenced by A. Calm, relaxed appearance B. Verbalization of fear/concerns C. Restful night
Comfort, alteration in **Etiology** Insertion of temporary pacemaker Subcutaneous irritation by catheter Subsequent restriction in movement of extremity Lead displacement	Patient/significant other reports discomfort Restlessness, irritability Guarded behavior Pallor, increased BP, diaphoresis Hiccupping (diaphragmatic contraction); intercostal or abdominal muscle twitching	A. Assess discomfort characteristics such as quality, severity, location, onset, associated manifestations, precipitating and relieving factors B. Assess for hiccups or muscle twitching	A. Anticipate need for comfort B. Provide comfort measures: position change, back rubs, analgesics as ordered C. Turn and position; support dependent parts with pillows D. During dressing change, pad the underside of the generator box with 4 × 4 bandages and wrap securely without constricting circulation E. Instruct patient to report pain F. Instruct patient to report effectiveness of intervention G. Explain cause of pain/discomfort H. Use SCP in Ch. 1: Comfort, alteration in I. If hiccups or muscle twitching are noted, call physician to evaluate lead placement. Anticipate need to reposition lead	Patient will be as comfortable as possible
Injury, potential for: high risk for infection **Etiology** Invasive procedure	Febrile Redness, drainage, swelling, tenderness at catheter site Elevated WBC	A. Assess catheter site for any pain, redness, moisture, drainage, or bleeding B. Monitor WBC every _____ C. Monitor temperature q.4h. and as needed	A. Keep dressing dry and intact B. Change dressing q.48h. or as needed per infection control policy C. Monitor length of time pacemaker is in place and report to physician after 72 hours	Occurrence of infection will be minimized

CHAPTER THREE

Neurologic/Neurosurgical

DISORDERS

Cerebral Artery Aneurysm: preoperative/unclipped

NURSING DIAGNOSIS/ PATIENT PROBLEM	DEFINING CHARACTERISTICS	NURSING ORDERS		EXPECTED OUTCOMES
		ASSESSMENT	INTERVENTIONS	
Tissue perfusion, alteration in: cerebral **Etiology** Subarachnoid hemorrhage Ruptured aneurysm Vasospasm Cerebral edema	Severe headache (unlike anything experienced before) Unconsciousness— transitory or lasting Nuchal rigidity Mental confusion, drowsiness Seizures Transitory or fixed neurologic signs (numbness, speech disturbance, paresis) Hypertension, which may accentuate or aggravate any vascular weakness, although it is not necessarily a causative factor in the development or rupture of an aneurysm	A. Complete an initial assessment of patient's presenting signs and symptoms. (Time of onset is important in assessing time of initial bleed and subsequent hemorrhages, and it may determine type of treatment instituted) B. Complete a baseline assessment of neurologic status and deficits C. Assess for seizure activity, noting 1. Time of onset 2. Localization of seizure 3. Postictal state	Administer anticonvulsants as ordered A. Dilantin: Give *slow* IV push (not faster than 50 mg/min). *Cannot* be given in D5W (precipitation occurs). Must be given slowly to avoid cardiac arrhythmias/arrest B. Valium: Give *slow* IV infusion. Also monitor heart rate and BP	Maximal cerebral perfusion will be achieved
Consciousness, altered levels of **Etiology** Vascular spasm Hemorrhage or rebleed Cerebral edema	Change in alertness, orientation, verbal response, eye opening, motor response Memory impairment Impaired judgement Agitation Inappropriate affect Impaired thought processes Glasgow Coma Scale <11	See SCP in Ch. 3: Consciousness, alteration in level of		Optimal state of consciousness will be maintained
Systemic blood pressure, alteration in (potential) **Etiology** Alteration in autoregulation	Systolic BP <100 or >150 mm Hg Diastolic BP <60 or >90 mm Hg Mean BP <90 or >100 mm Hg	Closely monitor BP and other hemodynamics (CVP, PCWP, cardiac output)	A. Provide bed rest and quiet environment by closing doors to rooms, keeping lights low and noise level to minimum, and limiting visitors. Provide private room if possible B. Administer antihypertensives as ordered; keep BP between ____ systolic and ____ diastolic or ____ mean arterial pressure. NOTE: Sodium nitroprusside may be used initially. Change to oral antihypertensives requires caution (possibility of sudden hypotension with methyldopa or clonidine therapy)	Maximal cerebral perfusion and minimal risk of rebleed will be effected

Originated by **Carol Ann Rooks, RN, BSN**
Resource person: **Linda Arsenault, RN, MSN, CNRN**

Cerebral Artery Aneurysm: preoperative/unclipped—cont'd

NURSING DIAGNOSIS/ PATIENT PROBLEM	DEFINING CHARACTERISTICS	NURSING ORDERS		EXPECTED OUTCOMES
		ASSESSMENT	INTERVENTIONS	
Knowledge deficit Etiology Unfamiliarity with pathology, treatment, and prevention of rebleed	Multiple questions Lack of questions Misconceptions	A. Assess level of understanding B. Assess readiness for learning	A. Explain possible causes of hypertension to patient/significant others B. Explain to patient/significant others rationale for limitation of length and frequency of visits C. Explain to patient/significant others the need to avoid nicotine (nicotine has vasospastic effect on blood vessels and thus increases risk of hemorrhage or vasospasm) D. Explain necessity to avoid Valsalva's maneuver. Stress importance of exhaling when being pulled up in bed and avoiding coughing and straining at stool. Provide stool softener if necessary E. Teach patient/family limitatons of diet and stress management 1. Diet: low salt, low fat 2. Stress: understanding the causs of stress and ways to prevent/cope with it	Patient will understand diagnostic process, treatment, and prevention of rebleed
Injury, potential for Etiology Complications of antifibrinolytic therapy	Deep vein thrombosis Dehydration as a result of volume contraction Pulmonary emboli Side effects of aminocaproic acid (Amicar) therapy: headache, dizziness, nausea, tinnitus, cramps, skin rash, diarrhea, malaise	A. Monitor patient for side effects of drug. Monitor coagulation studies B. Monitor for signs/symptoms of 1. Deep vein thrombosis: pain in lower extremities, positive Homans' sign, increased extremity circumference, increased temperature 2. Dehydration: decreased CVP (<5 cm H_2O, poor skin turgor, dry mucous membranes) 3. Pulmonary emboli: dyspnea, tachycardia, wheezing, chest pain, hemoptysis, right axis deviation	A. Administer antifibrinolytic agents as ordered (inhibits fibrinolysis; prevents clot degradation and the potential for rebleed) • Aminocaproic acid: Initial dose 5 g orally or by *slow* IV infusion followed by 1-1.25 g hourly. Total daily dose approximately 36 g B. Replace fluid, as ordered, for dehydration C. Explain purpose of drug therapy to patient/significant others D. Explain possible side effects of drug to patient/significant others	Risk of complications of antifibrinolytic therapy will be minimized

Continued.

Cerebral Artery Aneurysm: preoperative/unclipped—cont'd

NURSING DIAGNOSIS/ PATIENT PROBLEM	DEFINING CHARACTERISTICS	NURSING ORDERS		EXPECTED OUTCOMES
		ASSESSMENT	INTERVENTIONS	
		on ECG. If pulmonary infarct occurs, pleural effusion, friction rub, and fever may be noted		
Mobility, impaired physical **Etiology** Prolonged bed rest	Inability to move purposefully within the physical environment Decreased muscle strength Impaired coordination Limited ROM	See SCP in Ch. 1: Mobility, impaired physical		Optimal physical mobility will be maintained

Consciousness: alteration in level of

DEFINING CHARACTERISTICS	NURSING ORDERS			EXPECTED OUTCOMES
	ASSESSMENT	INTERVENTIONS	PATIENT EDUCATION	
Change in alertness, orientation, verbal response, eye opening, motor response (see neurologic flow sheet) Memory impairment Impaired judgment Agitation Inappropriate affect Impaired thought processes Glasgow Coma Scale <11	A. Assess level of consciousness/responsiveness every ＿＿ or as indicated B. Assess more frequently if any deterioration C. Determine contributing factors to any change (e.g., anesthesia, medications, awakening from sound sleep, not understanding questions) D. Assess understanding by patient/significant others of events surrounding change in level of consciousness E. Assess potential for physical injury F. Assess vital signs, especially respiratory status every ＿＿	A. Record serial assessments B. Report/record any change or deterioration C. Keep side rails up at all times, bed in low position, and functioning call light within reach D. If restraints are needed, patient must be positioned on *side*, *never on back* E. Reorient to environment as needed F. Explain all nursing activities before initiating G. Protect patient from possible injury (seizure disorders, decreased corneal reflex, decreased blink, decreased gag reflex, *airway*) H. Avoid contributing to confusion/disorientation by agreeing with misinterpretations I. Use calendars, television, radio, clocks, lights to help with reorientation	A. Call neurologic resource personnel if instructions are needed B. Involve patient/significant others in goal setting and care planning C. Encourage significant others to bring in things familiar to patient, e.g., pictures, pajamas D. Consult rehabilitation medicine and social service departments as needed E. Encourage and support verbalization by patient and significant others	Optimal state of consciousness will be maintained

Originated by **Marilyn Magafas, RN,C BSN**
 Karen Moyer, RN, MS, CCRN, CNA
 Kathryn S. Bronstein, RN, MS, CS, PhD Candidate
 Linda Arsenault, RN, MSN, CNRN

Dysphagia

NURSING DIAGNOSIS/ PATIENT PROBLEM	DEFINING CHARACTERISTICS	NURSING ORDERS		EXPECTED OUTCOMES
		ASSESSMENT	INTERVENTIONS	
Nutritional status, alteration in: less than body requirements **Etiology** Dysphagia (difficulty in swallowing)	Drooling Loss of appetite Pocketing food Weight loss Choking during meals Regurgitation of food/ fluid through nares	A. Swallowing 1. Assess presence/absence of gag and cough reflexes 2. Assess strength of facial muscles 3. Assess for residual food in mouth after eating 4. Assess regurgitation of food/ fluid through nares 5. Assess choking while eating/ drinking B. Nutritional status 1. Inquire about food and fluid preferences 2. Observe for drooling or complaint about appetite C. Weight loss 1. Assess patient's admission weight and compare to normal range for age and height 2. Inquire about weight gain/ loss over past few weeks/ months 3. Document amount of weight loss since diagnosed 4. Evaluate 24-hour oral I & O 5. Compare normal caloric requirements and body weight to present	A. Encourage intake of food patient can swallow; provide small frequent meals and supplements B. Instruct patient not to talk while eating C. Encourage patient to chew thoroughly and eat slowly D. Consult the dietitian when appropriate E. Maintain patient in high Fowler's position during and after meals F. Encourage high/low calorie diet that includes all food groups, as appropriate G. Document appetite and fluid intake (2-3 L/day) H. Document weight biweekly I. Prepare environment so that it will be well-ventilated, uncluttered, and cheerful without distraction J. Schedule pain medication, dressing changes, and personal hygiene before meals, and at a pace that does not overly fatigue the patient K. Place suction machine at bedside L. Clean and insert dentures before each meal M. Tell the patient what kind of food you are giving him/her before each spoonful N. Proceed slowly, giving small amounts; whenever possible, alternate servings of liquids and solids to help prevent foods from being left in the mouth O. Check to see if food is being pouched; if so, encourage patient to turn head to the unaffected side and manipulate tongue to the paralyzed side to clean out any residual food P. Encourage patient to feed self as soon as possible Q. If oral intake is not possible or proves inadequate, initiate alternative feedings such as nasogastric feedings, gastrostomy feedings, hyperalimentation	Patient will receive adequate nutritional intake as evidenced by A. Stabilization of weight/weight gain B. Normal serum electrolyte level C. Normal total protein and albumin levels

Originated by **Patsy McDonald, RN**
Resource persons: **Connie Powell, RN, MSN**
   Linda Arsenault, RN, MSN, CNRN

Continued.

Dysphagia—cont'd

NURSING DIAGNOSIS/ PATIENT PROBLEM	DEFINING CHARACTERISTICS	NURSING ORDERS		EXPECTED OUTCOMES
		ASSESSMENT	INTERVENTIONS	
		D. Dehydration 　1. Assess tissue turgor, mucous membrane, muscular weakness, and tremors 　2. Evaluate serum electrolyte reports, total protein, and albumin levels for imbalances		
Breathing pattern, ineffective **Etiology** Pulmonary aspiration	Dyspnea Shortness of breath Tachypnea Fremitus Cyanosis Cough Nasal flaring Respiratory depth changes Altered chest excursion Use of accessory muscles Pursed-lip breathing/ prolonged expiratory phase Increased anteroposterior diameter	Assess for presence of Defining Characteristics	A. Maintain patent airway B. Assist and teach patient to maintain position best suited for optimal lung expansion C. See SCP in Ch. 1: Breathing pattern, ineffective	Maintenance of respiratory status will be evidenced by A. Normal respiratory rate for age B. Absence of dyspnea C. Absence of use of accessory muscles D. Absence of central cyanosis E. Presence of breath sounds, which will be documented
Knowledge deficit **Etiology** New problem (dysphagia) New nutritional needs	Inability to practice good nutritional habits Multiple questions Lack of questions	Assess the following A. Swallowing difficulty and cause B. Patient's ability to feed self C. Family knowledge D. Nutrition knowledge	A. Discuss with and demonstrate to the patient/significant others the following 　1. Avoidance of certain foods or fluids 　2. Seat patient upright while eating 　3. Allow time to eat slowly and chew thoroughly 　4. Provide high-calorie meals 　5. Use fluids to help facilitate passage of solid foods 　6. Monitor patient for weight loss or dehydration (fluid intake should equal 2-3 L/ day; a weight loss of 5 pounds/week over 2 weeks should be reported to physician) B. Facilitate dietary counseling from hospital dietitian C. Inform the patient/significant others of the problem and how it affects swallowing D. Provide name and telephone number of primary nurse and physician and information on when to call E. Discuss feelings about body image and changes in life-style	Patent and significant others will verbalize/demonstrate an understanding of the adequate nutritional intake as evidenced by nutritional maintenance after discharge

Low Back Pain

NURSING DIAGNOSIS/ PATIENT PROBLEM	DEFINING CHARACTERISTICS	NURSING ORDERS		EXPECTED OUTCOMES
		ASSESSMENT	INTERVENTIONS	

Alteration in neurologic status
 Etiology
 Disk herniation (herniated nucleus pulposus)
 Spinal stenosis
 Osteoarthritis
 Mechanical instability
 Back trauma
 Infection
 Metastatic cancer
	Low back pain
	 Radiating pain into lower extremities
	 Paresthesia
	 Weakness in lower extremity
	 Bladder/bowel incontinence
	 Decreased/absent deep tendon reflex
	 Limited straight leg raising
		A. Evaluate history/ onset
		   1. Injury/spontaneous
		   2. Work related
		   3. Unknown
		 B. Assess neurologic and vascular status of lower extremities every _____
		   1. Pulses
		   2. Temperature
		   3. Movement and strength
		   4. Sensation
		   5. Equality of foot strength
		   6. Pratt's symptom, Homans' sign
		   7. Reflexes (knee, ankle, Babinski)
		 C. Assess bladder/ bowel functioning
		   1. I & O
		   2. Dribbling
		   3. Incontinence
		   4. Rectal sphincter tone
		 D. Inquire about previous episodes, hospitalization, and treatment
		   1. Bed rest
		   2. Pelvic traction
		   3. Transcutaneous nerve stimulation
		   4. Heat/massage
		   5. Exercise program
		   6. Medications
		 E. Inquire about previous tests, dates, and results, if known
		   1. Myelogram
		   2. CAT scan
		   3. Electromyogram
		   4. Lumbosacral x-ray studies
		   5. Sedimentation rate
			A. Reinforce need for bed rest as indicated
			 B. Provide bedside commode or assist patient to bathroom as needed
			 C. Anticipate need for pain medication/muscle relaxants as ordered, and document effects
			 D. Apply pelvic traction: _____ pounds every _____ hours _____ times/day as ordered
			 E. Apply heating pad with setting on low heat every _____ as ordered
			 F. Position Gatch bed with knee elevated about 10-20 degrees to relieve sciatic stretch
			 G. Assist patient with application of lumbosacral corset, if appropriate
			 H. Monitor motor strength, reflexes, sensory status every _____ for improvement or deterioration
			 I. Instruct and encourage deep breathing exercises every _____ : quad sets (isometric contraction of anterior thigh muscles with knee in extension), ankle ROM, toe movement
			 J. Send patient to physical therapy via stretcher if indicated
				Potential for relief of pain and return of optimal neurologic functioning will be achieved

Originated by **Vicki Chester, RN, BSN**
 Resource person: **Linda Arsenault, RN, MSN, CNRN**

Continued.

Low Back Pain—cont'd

NURSING DIAGNOSIS/ PATIENT PROBLEM	DEFINING CHARACTERISTICS	NURSING ORDERS		EXPECTED OUTCOMES
		ASSESSMENT	INTERVENTIONS	
		F. Inquire about previous surgery for low back pain 　1. Chemonucleolysis 　2. Lumbar laminectomy 　3. Fusion G. Inquire about location of pain/radiation 　1. Location 　2. Aggravating factors 　3. Alleviating factors		
Comfort, alteration in **Etiology** Low back pain Disk herniation Muscle spasm, strain	**Subjective** Complaints of discomfort **Objective** Decreased physical activity Slow guarded movement Irritability, restlessness, altered sleep pattern Palpable muscle spasm	A. Evaluate for subjective/objective signs of discomfort B. Inquire about previous episodes, hospitalization, and treatment	If characteristics are present, see SCP in Ch. 1: Comfort, alteration in	Pain will be relieved or discomfort minimized as evidenced by verbalization of improved comfort
Mobility, impaired physical **Etiology** Pain Muscle weakness Imposed bed rest	Difficulty with movement and position changes; inability to move Reluctance to attempt movement Limited ROM Decreased muscle strength	A. Evaluate for signs of alteration in mobility B. Assess for potential complications of immobility (e.g., phlebitis, pulmonary embolism, altered skin integrity)	If signs of altered mobility are present, refer to SCP in Ch. 1: Mobility, impaired physical	Minimal complications or early detection of potential complications associated with immobility will be effected
Knowledge deficit **Etiology** Unfamiliarity of causes of low back pain and rehabilitation of the back	Multiple questions Misconceptions	Evaluate patient's knowledge about A. Body mechanics (bending from waist, lifting objects, rotation of spine) B. Cause of low back pain (if known) ＿＿＿＿＿＿＿＿ C. ADL D. Discharge instructions	A. Discuss causes of low back pain (repeated stress on lower back, i.e., poor body mechanics) B. Define disk herniation C. Discuss symptoms of disk herniation (lower back pain, radiation of pain, weakness, changes in sensation) D. Discuss recommended alterations in life-style 　1. When to return to work 　＿＿＿＿＿＿＿＿ 　When to resume driving 　＿＿＿＿＿＿＿＿ 　2. Date and time of follow-up appointment ＿＿＿＿＿ 　＿＿＿＿＿＿＿＿	The patient/significant others will be able to verbalize/demonstrate understanding of low back pain, potential causes, and recommended modifications in ADL

Low Back Pain—cont'd

NURSING DIAGNOSIS/ PATIENT PROBLEM	DEFINING CHARACTERISTICS	NURSING ORDERS		EXPECTED OUTCOMES
		ASSESSMENT	INTERVENTIONS	
			3. Name and telephone number of physician _____ _____	
			4. Recreational restrictions _____ _____	
			E. Discuss exercises for muscle strengthening	
			1. Isometric abdominal and gluteal muscles to begin ____ weeks following discharge	
			2. Flexion-extension exercises to be initiated per physician's instructions	
			F. Discuss the following ADL guidelines with the patient	
			1. Sleeping: Recommend a firm mattress. Sleeping on the side with knees and hips flexed is preferable to sleeping on the back or abdomen	
			2. Bathing: Showers are preferable to tub baths. If tub baths are important to the patient, instruct how to avoid flexing the lower back when getting in and out of the tub	
			3. Bending: Instruct patient to squat rather than bend at waist	
			4. Lifting: When physician allows resumption of lifting (recommend not more than 20 pounds), instruct patient to squat, hold object close to body, straighten knees and *never* to lift anything heavy above the waist	
			5. Reaching: Instruct patient not to reach or strain to pick up an object; to rise to the level required; and to avoid movements such as bending backward, twisting to reach the telephone, or crouching over desk	
			6. Sexual activities: Recommend abstinence for about 3 weeks. Then for about 8-12 weeks, the patient should assume the underlying position with a pillow under the buttocks. An alternative is for the woman to lie on her side with knees bent with the man lying behind and facing her back	
			7. If lower back pain occurs, instruct patient to go to bed and rest his/her back	

Meningitis: adult

NURSING DIAGNOSIS/ PATIENT PROBLEM	DEFINING CHARACTERISTICS	NURSING ORDERS		EXPECTED OUTCOMES
		ASSESSMENT	INTERVENTIONS	
Consciousness, altered level of: potential Etiology Inflammation of the meninges	Meningeal signs Fever Rash Seizures Vomiting	A. Assess patient for meningeal signs 1. Nuchal rigidity 2. Headache 3. Pain with flexion of neck 4. Kernig's sign 5. Brudzinski's sign 6. Photophobia 7. Hyperirritability B. Assess for any neurologic deficits 1. Change in level of consciousness 2. Cranial nerve paresis 3. Seizure activity	A. See SCPs in this chapter: Consciousness: alteration in level of; Seizure activity B. Document baseline neurologic status C. Administer antiobitics and antiemetics as ordered D. Isolate patient if appropriate, e.g., viral meningitis (24-48 hours after start of therapy)	Alteration in level of consciousness will be minimized
Comfort: alteration in Etiology Meningeal irritation	Hyperalgesia Shaking, chills Irritability Headache	Assess patient (see Defining Characteristics)	A. Restrict visitors B. Reduce noise in environment C. Keep room darkened D. Maintain complete bed rest E. Administer analgesics as ordered F. See SCP in Ch. 1: Comfort, alteration in	Patient will be resting comfortably
Fluid volume deficit: potential Etiology Reduced level of consciousness Lack of oral intake Fever	Poor skin turgor Increased urine specific gravity Decreased urine output Change in mental status	A. Assess patient (see Defining Characteristics) B. Assess medications for dehydrating agents, e.g, mannitol	A. See SCP in Ch. 1: Fluid volume deficit B. Monitor I & O C. Replace fluids orally, intravenously, or nasogastrically as ordered D. Carefully document any changes in BP	Optimal fluid volume will be maintained
Nutrition, alteration in: less than body requirements (potential) Etiology Reduced oral intake Vomiting	Weight loss Loss of appetite	A. Assess patient (see Defining Characteristics) B. Assess oral intake and tolerance for food C. Assess weight loss based on serial weights	A. In acute phase, administer IV infusions as ordered B. If able to tolerate food, offer small quantities of bland food C. Provide nasogastric feedings as needed D. Weigh every 2 days	Weight loss will be minimized and nutritional requirements maintained
Knowledge deficit Etiology Lack of prior similar experience	Probing questions Request for information	A. Assess current knowledge base of patient/significant others B. Assess readiness for learning	A. Discuss need for calm, quiet environment and restriction of visitors B. Discuss course prognosis as appropriate C. Identify exposed contacts, and refer for prophylactic treatment if appropriate D. See SCP in Ch. 1: Knowledge deficit	Patient will understand disease process and activity restrictions

Originated by **Kathryn S. Bronstein, RN, MS, CS, PhD Candidate**

Multiple Sclerosis

NURSING DIAGNOSIS/ PATIENT PROBLEM	DEFINING CHARACTERISTICS	NURSING ORDERS		EXPECTED OUTCOMES
		ASSESSMENT	INTERVENTIONS	
Mobility, impaired physical **Etiology** Decreased motor strength Tremors Spasticity secondary to multiple sclerosis	Unsteady gait Dizziness Spasticity Weakness of extremities Incoordination Intention tremor Paraparesis	A. Assess the patient's gait, muscle strength, weakness, coordination, and balance B. Inquire about falls, use of assistive devices, and any decrease in muscle strength	A. Encourage ambulation with assistance/supervision B. Schedule rest periods to decrease fatigue C. Consult physical therapist and occupational therapist for use of assistive/ambulatory devices and ADL evaluation D. Encourage self-care as tolerated. Assist when necessary E. Avoid rushing patient F. Place belongings within reach G. Use adaptive techniques and equipment from occupational therapy department. These may include 1. Wrist weight 2. Using proximal rather than distal muscles of upper extremities 3. Adaptive equipment such as stabilized plates and non-spilling cups 4. Stabilization of extremity and training patient to use trunk and head to compensate for impaired function H. Encourage stretching exercises daily I. Administer antispasmodics as ordered	Optimal mobility will occur
Sensory-perceptual alteration: visual **Etiology** Multiple sclerosis	Diplopia Blurred vision Nystagmus Visual loss Scotomas (blind spots)	Assess for visual impairment and its effect on ADL	A. Orient patient to environment B. Place objects within reach C. Provide an eye patch for diplopia, and encourage alternating patch from eye to eye D. Instruct patient to rest eyes when fatigue is noticed E. Advise of availability of large-type reading materials and talking books F. Place call light within reach with side rails up and bed in a low position G. Place sign over the bed, and indicate visual impairment in chart and Kardex	Optimal visual ability with a minimal risk of injury will be attained

Originated by **Corea Hodge, RN**
Resource persons: **Linda Arsenault, RN, MSN, CNRN**
Connie Powell, RN, MSN

Continued.

Multiple Sclerosis—cont'd

NURSING DIAGNOSIS/ PATIENT PROBLEM	DEFINING CHARACTERISTICS	NURSING ORDERS		EXPECTED OUTCOMES
		ASSESSMENT	INTERVENTIONS	
Urine elimination, alteration in patterns: retention/incontinence **Etiology** Neuromuscular impairment secondary to multiple sclerosis	Frequency Urgency Hesitancy Abdominal distention Pain	Inquire about symptoms of frequency, urgency, abdominal distention, pain, and recurrent urinary tract infections	A. Measure urine output, and catheterize for residual urine as indicated. NOTE: Residual urine >100 ml predisposes patient to urinary tract infections B. Initiate individualized bladder training program: Instruct patient about Credé's methods, intermittent catheterization, signs and symptoms of urinary tract infection, time voiding C. Recommend vitamin C and liberal intake of cranberry juice to acidify urine and reduce bacterial growth D. See SCP in Ch. 1: Urinary elimination, alteration in patterns: retention	Minimal risk of developing urinary tract infections will be achieved
Bowel elimination, alteration in: constipation **Etiology** Spinal cord involvement	Straining at stools Frequent but nonproductive desire to defecate Abdominal distention Hemorrhoids Small, hard stool	Evaluate bowel habits	A. Initiate bowel training program as needed B. Encourage high fluid intake (≥2000 ml/day) and bulk diet C. See SCP in Ch. 1: Bowel elimination, alteration in: constipation	Regular bowel elimination will be achieved
Skin integrity, impairment of: potential **Etiology** Sensory changes	Hypalgesia Paresthesia Loss of position sense	A. Assess skin integrity B. Inquire about areas of the body with decreased sensation	A. Avoid heat, cold, and pressure B. Instruct patient to test bath water with unaffected extremity C. Instruct patient to look at foot placement when ambulating (for decreased position sense) D. See SCP in Ch. 1: Skin integrity, alteration in: potential	Absence of skin breakdown, burns, or decubitus formation will be achieved
Self-concept, disturbance in: body image/ loss of self-esteem **Etiology** Physical and psychosocial changes	Anxiety Depression Noncompliance Poor eye contact Refusal to participate in care/treatment Fears regarding level of independence	A. Assess quality and quantity of verbalizations about self-image B. Observe for changes in behavior and/or level of functioning C. Note patient/significant others report of change in self-concept	A. Make frequent patient contact in an unhurried manner B. Provide an opportunity for the patient to ask questions and talk about feelings C. Include the patient in the planning of care D. Support the patient's efforts at maintaining independence E. Use referral sources (e.g., liaison psychiatry service) when appropriate to facilitate the patient's attempts at coping	External source of discomfort and anxiety will be minimized

Multiple Sclerosis—cont'd

NURSING DIAGNOSIS/ PATIENT PROBLEM	DEFINING CHARACTERISTICS	NURSING ORDERS		EXPECTED OUTCOMES
		ASSESSMENT	INTERVENTIONS	

Knowledge deficit
Etiology
Unfamiliarity with the disease process and management
	Verbalization of misconceptions
	Questioning
	Noncompliance
		Assess patient/significant others knowledge of disease, exacerbations, remissions, and medical regimen	A. Reassure patient/significant others that majority of patients with multiple sclerosis do not become severely disabled
			B. Instruct patient/significant others when to contact health team e.g., urinary symptoms; exacerbations; motor, sensory, visual disturbances
			C. Offer referral for counseling services when indicated
			D. Instruct patient/significant others about
			  1. Purpose of steroid therapy (decreases edema and acute inflammatory response within evolving plaque)
			  2. Side effects such as sodium retention, fluid retention, pedal edema, hypertension, gastric irritation
			  3. Measures to control side effects such as low sodium diet, daily weighing, elevating legs, support hose, monitoring blood pressure, antacids, adequate rest, and avoiding contact with persons with infectious disease
			  4. Importance of maintaining as normal an activity level as possible
			  5. Avoidance of hot baths (increases metabolic demands and may increase weakness)
			  6. Sleeping in a prone position to decrease flexion spasms
			  7. Need to inspect areas of impaired sensation for serious injuries
				Patient/significant others will verbalize an understanding of the disease process, medications used, and adverse effects

Myasthenia Gravis: acute crisis phase

NURSING DIAGNOSIS/ PATIENT PROBLEM	DEFINING CHARACTERISTICS	NURSING ORDERS		EXPECTED OUTCOMES
		ASSESSMENT	INTERVENTIONS	

Muscle weakness
Etiology
Myasthenic/cholinergic crisis secondary to alteration in transmission of acetylcholine across the neuromuscular synapse preventing the nerve impulse
	Myasthenic crisis
	Dysphagia with potential for aspiration
	Diplopia and ptosis
	Generalized weakness with rapid fatigability
	Dyspnea
	Difficulty speaking, often with a nasal quality
	Restlessness
	Difficulty chewing
	
	Cholinergic crisis
	Same as above with the addition of
	  Muscular fasciculations
	  Increase in bronchial secretions
	  Nausea/vomiting
	  Abdominal cramping with diarrhea
	  Increase in tearing and perspiration
		Assess patient's ability to speak, swallow; presence of ptosis and diplopia; degree of proximal muscle strength; presence of cough and gag reflexes; especially patient's respiratory status (rate, depth, excursion, presence of shortness of breath/dyspnea)	A. Check for dysphagia before giving any oral medications or before meals. Hold medications and meal with any questionable dysphagia or lack of gag/cough reflex, and notify physician
			B. Check for presence of diplopia and ptosis at least each shift and as needed
			C. Check hand grasp and degree patient is able to raise arms/legs, at least q.6h. and whenever changing anticholinesterase dosage (usually ½-1 hour after administration) to monitor the effectiveness and to prevent a cholinergic crisis. Record length of time patient is able to hold position. Notify physician of decrease in strength, especially after dosage change. Have patient count from one upward, and record point at which speech becomes unintelligible
			D. Maintain levels of anticholinesterase by giving medications exactly on time. Observe for signs and symptoms of overdosage (see Defining Characteristics), since patient's needs may fluctuate day to day
			E. Assist patient with ADL as needed, and plan activities around periods of optimal strength (usually 1-2 hours after anticholinesterase dose)
			F. Monitor respiratory status q.2h. and as needed (see SCP in Ch. 1: Airway clearance, ineffective)
			G. Place patient in room near nursing station
			H. Prevent precipitating factors in crisis such as infection, overdosage, emotional crisis, and plan frequent rest periods
			I. Use resources as appropriate, e.g., physical therapy (splints/Stryker boots as needed). Turn q.2h. if patient lacks strength
			J. Instruct patient to inform nursing staff or physician of change in muscle strength or respiratory difficulty after receiving anticholinesterase medication
				Complications of muscle weakness will be minimized as evidenced by
				A. Prevention of aspiration
				B. Prevention of cholinergic crisis
				C. Maintenance of optimal muscle strength

Originated by **Donna Raymer, RN, BSN, CCRN**
Resource persons: **Susan Galanes, RN, MS, TNS, CCRN**
            Kathryn S. Bronstein, RN, MS, CS, PhD Candidate

Myasthenia Gravis: acute crisis phase—cont'd

NURSING DIAGNOSIS/ PATIENT PROBLEM	DEFINING CHARACTERISTICS	NURSING ORDERS		EXPECTED OUTCOMES
		ASSESSMENT	INTERVENTIONS	

Airway clearance, ineffective
Etiology
Inability to clear secretions because of weakness of respiratory muscles resulting from myasthenic or cholinergic crisis and/or intubation
	Abnormal breath sounds
	Inadequate ABGs as evidenced by change in patient's baseline
	Weak, nonproductive cough
	Increased airway pressures
	Shallow respirations
	Tachypnea/bradypnea
	Cyanosis
	Complaints of shortness of breath and/or dyspnea
		A. Establish patient's baseline
		  1. Respiratory rate
		  2. Depth of respirations
		  3. Breath sounds
		  4. Use of respiratory muscles and/or accessory muscles
		B. Monitor forced vital capacity (FVC) and tidal volume as ordered, and notify physician of significant change, e.g., FVC <1.0
		C. Assess for neurologic change, e.g., increase in drowsiness, confusion, agitation, or anxiety, which may indicate respiratory acidosis or hypoxemia
			A. Auscultate lungs q.4h. and as needed for presence of, or change in, breath sounds
			B. If abnormal, perform nasotracheal suctioning, or suction via endotracheal tube if present (use sterile technique)
			C. Draw ABGs as ordered or with significant change in respiratory status. Notify the physician
			D. Reposition patient q.2h. to mobilize secretions
			E. Maintain patent airway
			F. Avoid any *unnecessary* activities that increase fatigue (especially during crisis)
			G. Coordinate activities and respiratory treatments to correspond with peak action of medication, such as neostigmine (Prostigmin) and pyridostigmine (Mestinon)
			H. Have suction equipment and emergency intubation equipment readily available
			I. Instruct patient in the need to breathe deeply and to cough during periods of optimal strength to prevent complications of respiratory infections
			J. Explain all procedures and alarms (especially ventilator alarms)
				Patient's respiratory status will be within normal limits as evidenced by
				A. Regular respiratory rate
				B. Normal breath sounds
				C. Absence of shortness of breath or dyspnea
				D. Absence of use of accessory respiratory muscles
				E. Normal temperature
				F. FVC >1.0
				G. Absence of any neurologic changes
				H. Lungs free of secretions or patient able to mobilize secretions
				I. ABGs within normal limits for patient

Anxiety/fear **Etiology** Fear of unknown and inability to express fears and needs Impaired verbal communication	Restlessness Tachypnea, tachycardia Alteration in BP Dilated pupils Withdrawal Fear of sleep	A. Assess patient's level of anxiety and understanding of illness B. Assess patient's normal coping patterns (by interviewing patient/significant others)	A. Have some form of communication system for patients with severe dysarthria and/or tracheal tubes (e.g., paper/pencil; letter, number, picture board; or blinking of eyes to indicate yes/no) B. Encourage patient who is able to speak to ventilate his/her feelings C. Have call light readily available at all times D. Explain all procedures to patient beforehand E. Explain to patient reason for ventilator alarming (one of patient's biggest fears is a malfunctioning ventilator) F. Reassure patient with endotracheal intubation that he/she will be able to speak after extubation	Decrease in anxiety will be evidenced by A. Normal vital signs B. Relaxed appearance without signs of restlessness C. Normal pupils D. Normal airway pressure E. Normal sleeping pattern

Continued.

Myasthenia Gravis: acute crisis phase—cont'd

NURSING DIAGNOSIS/ PATIENT PROBLEM	DEFINING CHARACTERISTICS	NURSING ORDERS		EXPECTED OUTCOMES
		ASSESSMENT	INTERVENTIONS	
Nutrition, alteration in: less than body requirements (potential) **Etiology** Inability to swallow or chew because of weakness of bulbar muscles Lack of appetite resulting from side effects of anticholinesterase medications (i.e., abdominal cramping, nausea, vomiting, and diarrhea)	Loss of weight Lack of appetite Choking or gagging when attempting to swallow Absence of gag reflex Complaints of nausea/ vomiting Diarrhea	A. Assess patient's ability to swallow and chew B. Assess for presence of nausea, vomiting, abdominal cramping, or diarrhea	A. Check patient's ability to chew and swallow before meals. Withhold meal if necessary. Plan meal around peak action of medication (usually 1 hour after dose) B. Give patient who has difficulty in chewing a soft or liquid diet C. Give atropine or anticholinergic drug (i.e., Donnatal) as ordered to decrease side effects of anticholinesterase medication (be aware that anticholinergic drugs can mask the symptoms of overdosage and therefore can precipitate a cholinergic crisis) D. Instruct patient in side effects of anticholinesterase and anticholinergic medications E. Encourage patient to eat well-balanced diet when possible and to space meals during periods of optimal muscular strength F. Instruct patient to report any significant changes in swallowing ability G. If patient is intubated or unable to swallow effectively, see SCP in Ch. 1: Nutrition, alteration in: less than body requirement	Optimal nutritional requirements will be maintained
Knowledge deficit **Etiology** Unfamiliarity with disease process, treatment	Multiple questions Lack of questions Misconceptions	Assess knowledge base and readiness for learning of patient/significant others	A. Instruct patient in difference between cholinergic and myasthenic crisis (see Defining Characteristics) B. Teach patient the factors precipitating a crisis and how to avoid them C. Instruct patient in signs and symptoms of pending or recurring pulmonary problems and how to avoid precipitating factors (e.g., avoiding those with upper respiratory infection/ smokers)	Patient will effectively demonstrate knowledge of disease process, cholinergic/ myasthenic crisis, precipitating factors, and good pulmonary care

Normal Pressure Hydrocephalus (NPH)*

NURSING DIAGNOSIS/ PATIENT PROBLEM	DEFINING CHARACTERISTICS	NURSING ORDERS		EXPECTED OUTCOMES
		ASSESSMENT	INTERVENTIONS	
Thought processes, alteration in **Etiology** Physiologic changes secondary to Past history of subarachnoid hemorrhage Inflammatory process Remote head injury Decreased brain resiliency	Dementia Decreased recent memory Slowness of speech or paucity of speech Impaired judgment	A. Evaluate premorbid behavior B. Assess long-term memory, recent memory attentiveness, attention span, and retention of information C. Assess orientation to person, time, place D. Assess speech pattern (often slow speech, use of few words in response to questions, and little spontaneity) E. Assess affect and behavior (often apathetic, flat affect with decreased insight into illness)	A. Reorient to surroundings as necessary B. Provide a clock/calendar for room C. Explain treatments and nursing care slowly and simply, asking the patient to repeat the explanation D. Allow the patient time to answer questions	Maximal communication and orientation will be achieved
Injury, potential for (self-harm) **Etiology** Physiologic changes related to NPH	Spastic gait Ataxia Urinary incontinence Mental status changes	A. Evaluate gait, ambulation, safety needs B. Assess posture, balance, coordination C. Evaluate premorbid pattern of elimination	A. Apply soft restraints (e.g., Posey vest) as needed, especially at night B. Maintain bed in low position with all side rails up C. Assist patient in ambulating from bed to chair or to bathroom. Number of people needed to assist: _____ D. Minimize environmental barriers such as chairs E. Place needed articles within reach (e.g., water, call light, glasses, tissues) F. Encourage/assist with ROM exercises G. Establish a program for urinary elimination 1. Keep urinal/bedpan within reach of patient 2. Offer urinal/bedpan to patient every ____ hours 3. Encourage ample fluids: ____ ml every day 4. Limit fluid intake after ____ PM H. Evaluate skin integrity daily with special attention to bony prominences and shins of legs where patient may have bumped into objects I. Consult physical therapist, dietitian as ordered/needed	Risk of falls and injury and altered skin integrity will be minimized

Originated by **Corea Hodge, RN**
Resource person: **Linda Arsenault, RN, MSN, CNRN**
*Also referred to as occult hydrocephalus, communicating hydrocephalus, and hydrocephalic dementia.

Continued.

Normal Pressure Hydrocephalus (NPH)—cont'd

NURSING DIAGNOSIS/ PATIENT PROBLEM	DEFINING CHARACTERISTICS	NURSING ORDERS		EXPECTED OUTCOMES
		ASSESSMENT	INTERVENTIONS	
Knowledge deficit **Etiology** Uncertain course of disease, diagnosis, test, and treatment	Questioning Verbalization of misconceptions	Evaluate understanding by patient/significant other of disease process, diagnostic tests, treatments, and outcome	A. Explain disease process (altered brain fluid absorption with consequent changes in ability to walk, behavior, memory, speech, and control of urination) B. Instruct family regarding communication with patient, safety needs, and need for frequent offering of urinal/bedpan C. Explain diagnostic tests to patients and family and repeat explanations as necessary 1. CAT scan 2. Lumbar puncture 3. Skull films D. Provide patient/significant others with booklet of shunting procedure E. Discuss signs and symptoms of shunt malfunction 1. Increased mental deterioration 2. Increased gait disturbance 3. Urinary incontinence	Patient/significant others will be able to verbalize or demonstrate understanding of disease process

Parkinsonism

NURSING DIAGNOSIS/ PATIENT PROBLEM	DEFINING CHARACTERISTICS	NURSING ORDERS		EXPECTED OUTCOMES
		ASSESSMENT	INTERVENTIONS	
Mobility, impaired physical **Etiology** Neuromuscular impairment Decreased strength and endurance	Tremors Muscle rigidity Decreased ability to initiate movements (akinesis) Impaired coordination of movements Limited ROM Impaired ability to carry out ADL Postural disturbances	A. Evaluate baseline activity level B. Assess ability to carry out ADL on a daily basis C. Assess posture, coordination, resting tremors, and poverty of movements	A. Maintain side rails in up position B. Allow sufficient time for ADL C. Encourage and allow sufficient time for hygiene and self care; assist as needed D. Supervise and assist with ambulation at least three times/day E. Encourage patient to lift feet and take large steps while walking F. Remove environmental barriers while patient is ambulating G. Encourage ROM to all joints twice daily H. Consult with physical and occupational therapists regarding aids that may facilitate ADL and safe ambulation	Optimal level of functioning and minimal complications of immobility will be achieved

Originated by **Marian D. Cachero-Salavrakos, RN, BSN**
Resource persons: **Connie Powell, RN, MSN**
        Linda Arsenault, RN, MSN, CNRN

Parkinsonism—cont'd

NURSING DIAGNOSIS/ PATIENT PROBLEM	DEFINING CHARACTERISTICS	NURSING ORDERS		EXPECTED OUTCOMES
		ASSESSMENT	INTERVENTIONS	
Communication, impaired: verbal **Etiology** Dysarthria	Difficulty in articulating words Monotonous voice tones Slow, slurred speech	Evaluate patient's ability to communicate	A. Allow time for the patient to articulate B. Encourage patient to read out loud C. Encourage face and tongue exercises D. Consult speech therapist if indicated E. Place call light and other articles (tissues, water, glasses) within reach F. Avoid speaking loudly unless patient is hard of hearing G. Maintain eye contact with the patient when speaking H. See SCP in Ch. 1: Communication, impaired: verbal	Alternative methods of communication will be facilitated and maximal communication skills will be realized

Nutrition, alteration in: less than body requirements
Etiology
Dysphagia
	Difficulty swallowing
	Choking spells
	Drooling
	Regurgitation of food/ fluids through the nares
		A. Assess patient for degree of swallowing difficulty
		  1. Fluids
		  2. Solids
		B. Assess nutritional status
		  1. Height
		  2. Weight
			A. Supervise patient during meals
			B. Record I & O
			C. Allow time for meals; avoid rushing the patient
			D. Place patient in a high Fowler's position for eating and drinking
			E. Place the suction machine at the bedside for emergency use
			F. Encourage fluids of 2000 ml/ day
			G. Consult with the dietitian for needed changes in diet consistency and for caloric counts
			H. Assist with oral hygiene after meals
			I. Consult with the speech therapist to evaluate swallowing
			J. Weigh the patient three times/ week
				Adequate caloric and fluid intake will be achieved

Breathing pattern, ineffective **Etiology** Decreased muscle strength Decreased chest area	Dyspnea Shortness of breath Tachypnea Cough Cyanosis Altered chest excursion	A. Evaluate respiratory rate and depth pattern every _____ B. Assess for dyspnea C. Assess for changes in orientation and restlessness D. Assess for skin color, temperature, and capillary refill E. Assess breath sounds every _____	See SCP in Ch. 1: Breathing pattern, ineffective	Respiratory status within the limitation of disease as evidenced by A. Normal respiratory rate for age B. Absence of dyspnea C. Absence of use of accessory muscles D. Absence of central cyanosis

Continued.

Parkinsonism—cont'd

NURSING DIAGNOSIS/ PATIENT PROBLEM	DEFINING CHARACTERISTICS	NURSING ORDERS		EXPECTED OUTCOMES
		ASSESSMENT	INTERVENTIONS	
Bowel elimination, alteration in: constipation, diarrhea **Etiology** Drug therapy Inactivity	Straining at stools Passage of liquid fecal seepage Abdominal distention Fecal incontinence	A. Assess home pattern of elimination and compare to present pattern B. Evaluate usual dietary habits, eating schedule, intake of liquid and food C. Assess activity level (prolonged bed rest, lack of exercise contribute to constipation) D. Listen for bowel sounds every shift E. Evaluate current medications that may contribute to constipation/diarrhea	See SCP in Ch. 1: Bowel elimination, alteration in: constipation/ diarrhea	A. Any possible etiologic factors that may contribute to constipation/diarrhea will be minimized B. Constipation/diarrhea will be relieved as evidenced by regular passage of soft, formed stools
Urinary elimination, alteration in patterns: retention (potential) **Etiology** Drug therapy	Decreased (<30 ml/ hour) or absent urinary output for 2 consecutive hours Frequency, hesitancy, urgency, and incontinence Lower abdominal distention Urinary tract infections	A. Evaluate previous pattern of voiding B. Inspect lower abdomen for distention C. Evaluate time intervals between voiding D. Assess amount, frequency, character, color, odor, specific gravity E. Evaluate current medications that may contribute to urinary problems F. Evaluate I & O	See SCP in Ch. 1: Urinary elimination, alteration in patterns: retention (potential)	A. Optimal pattern of urine elimination is maintained B. Risk of overdistention of bladder with resultant infection will be minimized
Self-concept, disturbance in **Etiology** Changes in body image Dependence	Minimal eye contact Self-deprecating statements Anger Expression of guilt	A. Assess patient's perception of self B. Assess patient's level of anxiety C. Assess normal coping pattern D. Evaluate support system	A. Encourage patient to verbalize fears and concerns B. Consider effect of loss on significant persons, and include in discussion C. Explore strengths and resources with patient D. Avoid overprotection of the individual; promote social interaction as appropriate E. Clarify patient's misconceptions and provide accurate information F. Provide privacy as needed	Patient will recognize self-maligning statements and will begin to verbalize positive expression of self-worth

Parkinsonism—cont'd

NURSING DIAGNOSIS/ PATIENT PROBLEM	DEFINING CHARACTERISTICS	NURSING ORDERS		EXPECTED OUTCOMES
		ASSESSMENT	INTERVENTIONS	

Knowledge deficit
Etiology
Uncertain cause of disease and treatment
	Multiple questions
	Lack of questions
	Apparent confusion over condition
		A. Evaluate understanding by patient/significant others of disease process, diagnostic tests, treatments, and outcomes
		B. Assess anxiety level of patient/ significant other
			A. Encourage communication with family/significant others
			B. Involve family/significant others in care and instructions
			C. Reinforce physician's explanation of disease, causes, symptoms, and treatments
			D. Discuss feelings about these symptoms
			  1. Tremors
			  2. Drooling of saliva
			  3. Slurred speech
			E. Encourage independence and avoid overprotection by permitting patient to do things for self
			  1. Self-care
			  2. Feeding
			  3. Dressing
			  4. Ambulation
			F. Discuss with patient, family/ significant others
			  1. Medication
			    a. Dosage, frequency, administration, action, and toxic effects: orthostatic hypotension, nausea and vomiting, abnormal involuntary movements, changes in mental status, and shortness of breath
			    b. Those to be taken with meals
			    c. Limitation of high protein foods such as milk, meat, fish, cheese, eggs, peanuts, grains, and soybeans for patients taking levodopa
			  2. Diet
			    a. High caloric, soft diet
			    b. Cutting food for patient
			    c. Placing utensils within easy reach
			    d. Using blender for thick foods
			    e. Use of brace for severe tremors occurring during meals
			    f. Maintaining intake of 2000 ml of liquid daily unless contraindicated
			    g. Offering frequent, small feedings
			    h. Using straws and bibs for excessive drooling
			    i. Instructing patient to swallow slowly and take small bites of food
				Patient/significant others will demonstrate understanding of the patient's disability and special needs with regard to
				A. Disease process
				B. Activity, exercises, and ambulation
				C. Medication
				D. Diet
				E. Elimination

Continued.

Parkinsonism—cont'd

NURSING DIAGNOSIS/ PATIENT PROBLEM	DEFINING CHARACTERISTICS	NURSING ORDERS		EXPECTED OUTCOMES
		ASSESSMENT	INTERVENTIONS	

			3. Activity
			  a. Planned rest periods
			  b. Passive and active ROM exercises to all extremities
			  c. Encouraging family/significant others to participate in physical therapy exercises of stretching and massaging of muscles
			  d. Encouraging daily ambulation outdoors but avoidance of extreme hot and cold weather
			  e. Encouraging the patient to practice lifting feet while walking, using heel-toe gait, and swing deliberately while walking
			  f. Avoidance of sitting for long periods of time
			  g. Encouraging the patient to dress daily, avoiding clothing with buttons (using zippers instead) and shoes with laces or snaps
			  h. Diversional activities depending on extent of tremors and disability: reading, watching television, hobbies
			  i. Preventing falls by clearing walkways of furniture and scattered rugs and providing side rails on stairs
			4. Speech therapy. Instruct patient to speak slowly and practice reading aloud in an exaggerated manner
			5. Oral hygiene. Perform q.2-4h. and p.r.n. (especially in drooling) and have tissues accessible to patient
			6. Elimination
			  a. Instituting voiding measures as needed
			  b. Instituting bladder control program as needed
			  c. Raised toilet seats with side rails at home to facilitate sitting or standing
			  d. Avoiding constipation; encouraging fluids, use of natural laxatives (prune juices and roughage) and stool softeners as needed	

Seizure Activity

NURSING DIAGNOSIS/ PATIENT PROBLEM	DEFINING CHARACTERISTICS	NURSING ORDERS		EXPECTED OUTCOMES
		ASSESSMENT	INTERVENTIONS	

Injury, potential for
Etiology
Seizure activity
Postictal state
Altered level of consciousness
Impaired judgment
	Increased rhythmic motor activity, jerking of arms and legs
	Repetitive psychomotor activity
	Tonic-clonic movements
	Change in alertness, orientation, verbal response, eye opening, motor response
	Aspiration of oral secretions
		A. Assess frequency, duration, and type of seizure activity
		B. Note the following
		  1. Change in level of consciousness
		  2. Patient's preceding seizure activity
		  3. Where seizure started
		  4. Epileptic cry
		  5. Automatism
		  6. Length of seizure
		  7. Head and eye turning
		  8. Pupillary reaction
		  9. Associated falls
		  10. Foam from mouth
		  11. Urinary or fecal incontinence
		  12. Cyanosis
		  13. Postictal state
		  14. Any postseizure focal abnormality (e.g., Todd's paralysis)
			A. Document observations and frequency of seizures; notify physician
			B. Roll patient to side to prevent aspiration
			C. If patient is in bed
			  1. Pad side rails
			  2. Remove sharp objects from bed
			  3. Keep bed in low position
			D. If patient is on floor, remove furniture (or other potentially harmful objects) from area
			E. Do not restrain patient
				Potential for physical injury will be minimized

Health maintenance, alteration in **Etiology** Perceptual and/or cognitive impairment Lack of fine motor ability Lack of material resources Physiologic derangement	Inadequate serum anticonvulsant levels (below therapeutic range) Intake altered to the degree of affecting medication intake Vomiting Demonstrated inability to take or obtain medications	A. Assess perceptual and cognitive abilities B. Note alterations in fine motor ability C. Inquire as to material resources that would influence ability to obtain medications: money or transportation D. Assess for presence/history of prolonged vomiting	A. Monitor blood levels of anticonvulsants every _____ B. Administer anticonvulsants as ordered during hospitalization C. Suggest to physician alternate routes if patient is vomiting D. Involve significant others/ friends/social support in solving home care needs, where appropriate	Therapeutic level of anticonvulsant will be maintained

Originated by **Kathryn S. Bronstein, RN, MS, CS, PhD Candidate**

Continued.

Seizure Activity—cont'd

NURSING DIAGNOSIS/ PATIENT PROBLEM	DEFINING CHARACTERISTICS	NURSING ORDERS		EXPECTED OUTCOMES
		ASSESSMENT	INTERVENTIONS	
Self-esteem, disturbance in: potential **Etiology** Seizure activity Dependence on medications	Nonparticipation in therapy Lack of responsibility for self-care Self-destructive behavior Lack of eye contact	A. Assess patient's feelings about self and disease B. Assess perceived implications of disease and need for long-term therapy	A. Encourage ventilation of feelings B. Incorporate family and significant others in care plan C. Assist patient and others in understanding nature of disorder D. Dispel common myths and fears about convulsive disorders	Effect of convulsant disorder on self-esteem will be minimized

Knowledge deficit
 Etiology
 Lack of exposure
 Information misinterpretation
 Unfamiliarity with information resources
	Verbalization of problem
	 Inappropriate or exaggerated behavior
	 Request for information
	 Statement of misconception
		A. Assess knowledge of patient/significant others concerning disease and treatment
		 B. Assess readiness for learning
			A. Discuss disease process and therapeutic prescription, e.g., drugs, interactions, side effects
			 B. Review with patient need for medication and schedule
			   1. Right medication at right time and dosage
			   2. Drug levels
			   3. Danger of seizure activity with abrupt withdrawal
			 C. Educate patient for safety measures
			   1. Driving
			   2. Swimming with companion
			   3. Medic-Alert tag
			   4. Home safety
			 D. Refer to Epilepsy Foundation
			 E. See SCP in Ch. 1: Knowledge deficit
				Patient will understand and be able to verbalize disease process, treatment, and safety measures

THERAPEUTIC INTERVENTIONS

Craniotomy: postoperative care

NURSING DIAGNOSIS/ PATIENT PROBLEM	DEFINING CHARACTERISTICS	NURSING ORDERS		EXPECTED OUTCOMES
		ASSESSMENT	INTERVENTIONS	
Tissue perfusion, alteration in: cerebral **Etiology** Cerebral edema Intracranial bleed Cerebral ischemia/infarction Increased intracranial pressure Metabolic abnormalities	Changed level of consciousness Changed pupillary size, reaction to light, deviation Focal or generalized motor weakness Presence of pathologic reflexes (Babinski) Seizures Increased BP and bradycardia Changed respiratory pattern	A. Assess and document baseline level of consciousness: pupillary size, position, reaction to light; motor movement and strength of limbs; and vital signs B. See SCP in Ch. 3: Consciousness, altered levels of C. Compare current assessment to previous assessments D. Check head dressing for signs of drainage and for presence of drains (intraventricular drains; self-contained bulb suction and drainage system, e.g., Jackson-Pratt); check other catheters for monitoring intracranial pressure: _____ E. Assess understanding by patient/significant others of current events, postoperative expectations, monitoring equipment, need for frequent assessment F. Assess laboratory data: CBC, electrolytes, glucose G. Assess current medications, and compare to preoperative medications, with specific attention to thyroid replacement, anticonvulsants, and steroids	A. Monitor neurologic status and vital signs every _____ B. Report any deterioration in level of consciousness, pupillary size and reactivity, progression of motor weakness, and check Systolic BP < ____ > ____ Diastolic BP < ____ > ____ Pulse < ____ > ____ Respirations < ____ > ____ Temperature > ____ NOTE: Report and maintain normothermia with tepid sponge/antipyretics or hypothermia blanket as ordered. Turn blanket off at temperature of _____ C. Evaluate contributing factors to change in responsiveness, and reevaluate in 5-10 min to see if change persists as a result of such factors as anesthesia, medications, awakening from sound sleep, not understanding questions D. Check craniotomy dressings for drainage; circle and reinforce as needed. Evaluate amount of drainage in external drains. Do *not* allow any drainage collector to fall below bed level, and do *not* connect to wall suction E. Maintain head of bed at ____ (usually elevated to 30 degrees). If patient has altered level of consciousness and is receiving tube feeding, maintain head elevation during feedings. Clamp tube during transport F. Turn and reposition patient on side, with head supported in neutral alignment, every 2 hours. Avoid neck flexion/rotation to prevent venous outflow obstruction and increased intracranial pressure G. Reorient patient to environment as needed H. If soft restraints are needed, position patient on side, *never on back*	Optimal cerebral perfusion will be maintained

Originated by **Robert Rowlands, RN**
Resource person: **Linda Arsenault, RN, MSN, CNRN**

Continued.

Craniotomy: postoperative care—cont'd

NURSING DIAGNOSIS/ PATIENT PROBLEM	DEFINING CHARACTERISTICS	NURSING ORDERS		EXPECTED OUTCOMES
		ASSESSMENT	INTERVENTIONS	
			I. Avoid nursing activities that may trigger increased intracranial pressure excursions (straining, strenuous coughing, positioning with neck in flexion, head flat) J. Monitor CBC, electrolytes, and ABGs. Report ABGs: $Pao_2 < 80$ $Pco_2 > 45$ CBC: hct <30 Electrolytes: Na $< 130 > 150$ Glucose < 80 or > 200 K. Evaluate for lash reflex. If patient has difficulty closing eye (cranial nerve VII palsy), administer artifical tears (methylcellulose drops) every _____	
Fluid volume deficit: potential **Etiology** Diabetes insipidus	Urine output >200 ml for 2 consecutive hours Urine sp gr <1.001 Thirst Increased serum Na >145 mEq/L Increased serum osmolarity >300	Assess patient for fluid volume deficit	A. Monitor I & O every _____ hours with specific attention to fluid volume infused over output 1. Check urine sp gr every _____ hours 2. Report urine output >200 ml/hour for 2 consecutive hours and/or urine sp gr ≤ 1.001 B. Replace fluid output: _____ _____ C. Administer vasopressin (Pitressin) as ordered every _____ D. See SCP in Ch. 1: Fluid volume deficit E. Monitor serum and urine electrolytes and osmolarity	Optimal fluid volume will be maintained
Fluid volume, alteration in: excess **Etiology** Syndrome of inappropriate antidiuretic hormone secretion Free H_2O excess	Changed sensorium Decreased serum Na <130 Decreased serum osmolarity <285 Increased urine Na	A. Assess patient for fluid volume excess B. Monitor I & O every _____	A. Monitor serum and urine electrolytes and osmolarity every __ B. Restrict PO/IV fluids to ____ /hour ____ /shift C. Weigh patient every _____ D. Other: _____ _____ _____	Optimal fluid balance will be maintained
Mobility, impaired physical: potential **Etiology** Decreased level of consciousness Weakness/paralysis of extremities	Inability to purposefully move within the physical environment Decreased muscle strength Impaired coordination; verbalization of inability to perform Limited ROM	Assess for alteration in mobility. If present, see SCP in Ch. 1: Mobility, impaired physical. Exception: Do not position patient in prone or semiprone position (increases intrathoracic pressure and may increase intracranial pressure)		Optimal level of mobility will be achieved

Craniotomy: postoperative care—cont'd

NURSING DIAGNOSIS/ PATIENT PROBLEM	DEFINING CHARACTERISTICS	NURSING ORDERS		EXPECTED OUTCOMES
		ASSESSMENT	INTERVENTIONS	
Airway clearance, ineffective **Etiology** Decreased level of consciousness	Abnormal breath sounds Change in rate, depth of respirations, tachypnea Cough, cyanosis, dyspnea Change in respiratory rhythm	Assess for signs of ineffective airway clearance	A. See SCP in Ch. 1: Airway clearance, ineffective NOTE: Nasotracheal suctioning is contraindicated for patients having surgery proximal to frontal sinuses (i.e., pituitary tumor, basal frontal meningioma, basal skull fracture) B. See SCP in Ch. 1: Breathing pattern, ineffective	Airway will be free of secretions
Injury, potential for: seizures **Etiology** Intracranial bleed Infarction Tumor Trauma	Focal and/or generalized seizures with/ without loss of consciousness	Observe for seizure activity. Record and report observations A. Note time and signs of attack B. Observe parts involved: order of involvement and character of movement C. Check deviation of eyes; note change in pupillary size D. Assess airway and respiratory pattern E. Note tonic-clonic stages F. Assess postictal state (e.g., loss of consciousness, alertness, airway)	A. Maintain patient safety, i.e., pad side rails, protect head from injury B. Maintain airway postictal state. Turn patient on side, suction as needed C. Maintain minimal environmental stimuli 1. Noise reduction 2. Curtains closed 3. Private room (when available/advisable) 4. Dim lights D. Administer anticonvulsants as indicated E. Evaluate understanding by patient/significant others of medications (dosage, use, and side effects)	Risk of seizures will be minimized
Knowledge deficit **Etiology** New procedures and treatments	Patient/significant others verbalizing questions and concerns	Assess patient/significant others for knowledge base and readiness for teaching	A. Discuss change in body image related to head dressing and loss of hair, potential for and duration of facial edema B. Discuss need for monitoring equipment C. Explain unit visiting hours and reasons for restrictions D. Instruct in deep breathing and leg exercises E. Explain use of medications such as dexamethasone (Decadron), anticonvulsants, antibiotics F. Discuss need for frequent assessment, reorientation, etc. G. Encourage significant others to participate in reorientation, rehabilitation, etc. H. Reinforce discussion of neurologic definitions/progress given by physician to significant others	Patient/significant others will verbalize understanding of postoperative expectations and experiences

CHAPTER FOUR

Pulmonary

DISORDERS

Bronchial Asthma: pediatric

NURSING DIAGNOSIS/ PATIENT PROBLEM	DEFINING CHARACTERISTICS	NURSING ORDERS		EXPECTED OUTCOMES
		ASSESSMENT	INTERVENTIONS	

Airway clearance, in-effective
Etiology
Constriction of bron-chioles
Allergies
	Irritability
	Retractions
	Grunting
	Stridor
	Nasal flaring
	Wheezing
		A. Assess vital signs every _____
		B. Note color changes (lips, buc-cal mucosa, nail beds)
		C. Look for and doc-ument signs of re-spiratory dysfunc-tion common to the pediatric pa-tient
		  1. Irritability
		  2. Retractions
		  3. Grunting
		  4. Stridor
		  5. Nasal flaring
		  6. Wheezing
		D. Evaluate breath sounds every _____
		E. Monitor laborato-ry work
		  1. Theophylline level
		  2. ABGs
		  3. CBC
		  4. Electrolytes
			A. Keep head of bed elevated to help with expansion of lungs
			B. Keep patient as calm as pos-sible
			C. Check that respiratory treat-ments are given as ordered; no-tify the respiratory therapist if need arises
			  1. Encourage patient to cough, especially after treatments
			  2. Give O$_2$ as ordered
			D. Give medications and IV fluids as ordered
			E. Use appropriate clinical re-sources
			F. See SCP in Ch. 1: Airway clearance, ineffective
				Respiratory dysfunc-tion will be mini-mized as evidenced by
				A. Vital signs within normal limits for age
				B. Respiratory rate, pattern, depth, and quality within nor-mal limits
				C. Minimal wheezing
				D. Good color
				E. No visible signs of dysfunction
				F. Laboratory values within normal lim-its for age/weight

Fluid volume, deficit: potential **Etiology** Decreased fluid intake Increased respiratory distress Diaphoresis	Complaints of thirst Complaints of dryness to lips, mouth Decreased skin turgor Increased specific gravity Decreased urine output Sunken eyes Sunken fontanel in in-fant Lack of tears in infant	A. Monitor vital signs every _____ B. Measure I & O every _____ C. Assess specific gravity _____ D. Monitor electro-lytes E. Assess skin turgor every _____ F. Monitor weight every _____ G. Assess sputum for color, tenacity, liquification, amount	A. Encourage oral intake as toler-ated B. Maintain IV infusion at proper rate C. Keep water pitcher/juices at bedside D. Offer bedpan at frequent inter-vals	Hydration will be maintained as evi-denced by A. Urine output at least 30 ml/hour B. Adequate oral, IV intake C. Skin turgor, mu-cous membranes, specific gravity within normal limits D. Bronchial secre-tions liquified and easily expecto-rated

Originated by **Kathleen Jaffry, RN**
Resource person: **Michele Knoll-Puzas, RN,C BS**

Bronchial Asthma: pediatric—cont'd

NURSING DIAGNOSIS/ PATIENT PROBLEM	DEFINING CHARACTERISTICS	NURSING ORDERS		EXPECTED OUTCOMES
		ASSESSMENT	INTERVENTIONS	
Anxiety **Etiology** Change in health status Change in environment Respiratory distress	**Subjective** "I'm scared" Complaints of inability to breathe **Objective** Restlessness Apprehensiveness Insomnia Increased heart rate Frequently asking for someone to be in room Diaphoresis	Assess anxiety level every ____ including A. Vital signs B. Respiratory status C. Irritability D. Apprehension E. Orientation	A. Help relieve respiratory distress as soon as possible B. Explain all procedures to patient before starting C. Make patient as comfortable as possible 　1. Be available 　2. Reassure the patient D. Provide quiet, diversional activities E. Explain importance of remaining as calm as possible F. Explain that a nurse will always be available if needed G. Explain need for all treatments given and rationale	Decreased anxiety as evidenced by A. Calmer, relaxed appearance B. Rational behavior C. Respiratory function within normal limits
Comfort, alteration in **Etiology** Excessive exertion of accessory respiratory musculature as a result of acute asthma attack	Complaints of pain when breathing Complaints of inability to get comfortable Restlessness Position of patient Insomnia Increased respiratory distress	A. Monitor respiratory distress every ____ and make any changes B. Monitor patient's inability to relax C. Monitor any complaints of pain every ____ (degree, location, length) D. Note changes in activity tolerance	A. Make patient as comfortable as possible 　1. Raise head of bed 　2. Position with pillows 　3. Hold/rock in upright position B. Be available to 　1. Answer questions simply 　2. Explain procedures C. Provide medications as ordered D. Explain need to remain as calm as possible E. Explain need to inform nurses of any discomfort	Relief of discomfort or decrease of pain will be evidenced by verbalization and appearance of relief of pain
Knowledge deficit **Etiology** Chronicity of disease Long-term medical management	Absence of questions Anxious Inability to answer questions properly Ineffective self-care	A. Assess knowledge of disease process B. Assess knowledge of medications C. Evaluate self-care activities 　1. Preventive care 　2. Home management of acute attack	A. Explain disease to patient/ significant other B. Teach signs and symptoms of asthma attack and importance of early treatment for impending attack C. Reinforce need for taking prescribed medications as ordered D. Reinforce what is to be done in an asthma attack 　1. Home management 　2. When to come to emergency room 　3. Prevention E. Reinforce need of keeping follow-up appointments F. Refer to social services if needed G. Refer to support groups if needed	Patient/significant other will verbalize knowledge about disease and its management

Chronic Obstructive Pulmonary Disease (COPD)

NURSING DIAGNOSIS/ PATIENT PROBLEM	DEFINING CHARACTERISTICS	NURSING ORDERS		EXPECTED OUTCOMES
		ASSESSMENT	INTERVENTIONS	
Airway clearance, ineffective **Etiology** Hyperplasia and hypertrophy of the mucous-secreting glands Increased mucous production in the bronchial tubes Decreased ciliary function Thick secretions Decreased energy and fatigue Bronchospasm	"Smoker's cough" Coarse rales over the larger airways Persistent cough for months Copious amount of secretions Wheezing Loud, prolonged expiratory phase	A. Assess characteristics of secretions Quantity Consistency Color Odor B. Assess patient's hydration status and condition of Skin turgor Mucous membranes Tongue C. Assess patient's physical strength D. Evaluate results of pulmonary function tests	A. Auscultate lungs every _____ B. Assist in mobilizing secretions by 1. Increasing room humidification 2. Administering mucolytic agents in conjunction with respiratory therapist (as ordered), e.g., Mucomyst, SSKI (potassium iodide solution) 3. Performing chest physiotherapy, e.g., postural drainage, percussion, vibration C. Encourage increased fluid intake to 1½ to 2 L/day unless contraindicated D. Approximate and record the amount of the secretions E. Monitor accurate I & O F. Administer cough medications as ordered G. Perform nasotracheal suctioning as indicated H. Assist with bronchoscopy as needed I. Demonstrate effective coughing; splint chest for comfort	Airway will be freed of secretions
Gas exchange, impaired **Etiology** Obstruction in air flow during expiration causing increased dead space	Altered I:E ratio (prolonged expiratory phase) Active expiratory phase; use of accessory muscles of breathing Decreased vital capacity (VC) Increased residual volume (RV) and functional residual capacity (FRC) Hypoxemia/hypercapnia $P_{CO_2} > 55$ mm Hg $P_{O_2} < 55$ mm Hg Tachycardia Restlessness Diaphoresis Headache Lethargy Confusion Cyanosis Increase in rate and depth of respiration Increase in BP	A. Assess for altered breathing patterns and increased work of breathing Rate and depth Chest excursions B. Assess for signs and symptoms of hypoxemia/hypercapnia	A. Promote a more effective breathing pattern for better gas exchange by 1. Positioning properly for optimal breathing 2. Teaching patient to use pursed-lip breathing 3. Teaching patient to use abdominal breathing patterns B. Administer bronchodilators as ordered 1. Monitor for therapeutic and side effects 2. Monitor blood levels C. Monitor ABGs every _____ D. Assist in performing pulmonary function tests as needed E. Administer low-flow O_2 as necessary	Hypoxemia will be minimized

Originated by **Lumie Perez, RN, BSN, CCRN**
Joanne O'Connor, RN, BSN
Resource person: **Terry Takemoto, RN, MSN, CCRN**

Chronic Obstructive Pulmonary Disease (COPD)—cont'd

NURSING DIAGNOSIS/ PATIENT PROBLEM	DEFINING CHARACTERISTICS	NURSING ORDERS		EXPECTED OUTCOMES
		ASSESSMENT	INTERVENTIONS	
Nutrition, alteration in: less than body requirements **Etiology** Increased metabolic need because of an increase in work of breathing Poor appetite resulting from fever, dyspnea, and fatigue	Body weight 20% or more under ideal for height and frame Lack of interest in food Alteration in ability to taste Caloric intake inadequate for metabolic demands of disease state Muscle weakness Decrease in muscle tone	A. Assess patient's caloric requirement B. Assess patient's caloric intake C. Assess for possible cause of poor appetite (see Etiology)	A. Compile a diet history, including preferred foods and dietary habits B. Consult and work with the dietitian to estimate caloric requirements C. Offer small feedings at frequent intervals of nutritious soft foods/liquids D. Assist the patient with meals E. Record amount of food intake (calorie count) F. Give frequent oral care G. Instruct patient to avoid very hot/cold foods, gas producing foods, carbonated beverages H. Plan activities to allow for rest before eating I. Substitute nasal prongs for O_2 mask during mealtime	Optimal nutritional status will be maintained
Infection, potential for **Etiology** Retained secretions (serve as a good medium for bacterial growth) Poor nutrition Impaired pulmonary defense system secondary to COPD Use of respiratory equipment	Fever, chills Change in characteristics of sputum (consistency, color, amount, odor) Increase in cough Elevated WBC Abnormal breath sounds Rales, wheezing, shortness of breath Signs of right-sided heart failure Nausea, vomiting, diarrhea Anorexia	A. Assess patient for signs and symptoms of infection (see Defining Characteristics) B. Assess nutritional status	A. Encourage effective coughing and deep breathing exercises B. Encourage increase in fluid intake unless contraindicated C. Assist with nebulizer treatment and physiotherapy D. Ensure that O_2 humidifier unit is properly maintained E. Empty room humidifiers daily (never add new water to old water) F. Promote early discharge to minimize contact with infected patients G. Place patient in a room with noninfectious patient	Risk for infection will be minimized
Activity intolerance **Etiology** Imbalance between O_2 supply and demand	Verbal report of fatigue or weakness Abnormal heart rate and BP response to activity Exertional discomfort or dyspnea	A. Assess patient's level of mobility B. Assess patient's respiratory status	Refer to SCP in Ch. 1: Activity intolerance	Optimal activity tolerance will be maintained

Continued.

Chronic Obstructive Pulmonary Disease (COPD)—cont'd

NURSING DIAGNOSIS/ PATIENT PROBLEM	DEFINING CHARACTERISTICS	NURSING ORDERS		EXPECTED OUTCOMES
		ASSESSMENT	INTERVENTIONS	
Knowledge deficit **Etiology** Newly diagnosed Denial Ineffective teaching/ learning in past	Display of anxiety/ fear Noncompliance Inability to verbalize health maintenance regime Repeated acute exacerbations Development of complications Misconceptions about health status Multiple questioning or none at all	A. Assess learner's readiness to learn B. Assess environmental, social, cultural, and educational factors that may influence teaching plan C. Assess knowledge base	A. Establish common goals B. Instruct patient in basic anatomy and physiology of the respiratory system, with attention to structure and air flow C. Discuss how the disease process related to signs and symptoms the patient is experiencing. Introduce the following words: mucous, spasm, narrowing, obstruction, elasticity, trapping, inflammation D. Discuss purpose and method of administration for each medication E. Discuss appropriate nutritional habits F. Discuss concept of energy conservation. Encourage 1. Resting as needed during activities 2. Avoiding overexertion/fatigue 3. Sitting as much as possible 4. Alternating heavy and light tasks 5. Carrying articles close to body 6. Organizing all needed equipment at beginning of activity 7. Working slowly G. Discuss signs/symptoms of infection; prevention of infection. Encourage patient to seek prompt medical intervention if signs and symptoms of infection occur H. Discuss harmful effects of smoking (refer to Lung Association, Cancer Society pamphlets for information on how to stop smoking) I. Encourage the use of community health care resources/self-help groups concerned with COPD (refer to Lung Association teaching pamphlets for additional information) J. Explain purpose for and technique of pulmonary toilet exercises	Patient will verbalize understanding of disease process and treatment regimes

Chronic Obstructive Pulmonary Disease (COPD)—cont'd

NURSING DIAGNOSIS/ PATIENT PROBLEM	DEFINING CHARACTERISTICS	NURSING ORDERS		EXPECTED OUTCOMES
		ASSESSMENT	INTERVENTIONS	
			Breathing exercises *Exercise 1*. Purpose: to strengthen the muscles of respiration • Technique: Lie supine, with one hand on chest and one on abdomen. *Inhale* slowly through mouth, raising abdomen against hand. Chest should not move. *Exhale* slowly through pursed lips while contracting abdominal muscles and moving abdomen inward *Exercise 2*. Purpose: to develop slowed, controlled breathing • Technique: Walk, stop to take a deep breath, exhale slowly while walking *Exercise 3*. Purpose: to decrease air trapping and airway collapse • Technique for pursed lip breathing: Inhale slowly through the nose. Exhale twice as slowly as usual through pursed lips **Cough** Lean forward; take several deep breaths with pursed lip method. Take last deep breath, and cough with open mouth during expiration, while simultaneously contracting abdominal muscles **Chest physiotherapy/pulmonary postural drainage** Purpose: to facilitate expectoration of secretions and prevent waste of energy Demonstrate correct methods for postural drainage: positioning, percussion, vibration **Hydration** Discuss importance of maintaining good fluid intake to decrease viscosity of secretions. Recommend 1½ to 2 L/day **Humidity** Discuss various forms of humidification to prevent drying of secretions	

Epiglottitis: pediatric ICU

NURSING DIAGNOSIS/ PATIENT PROBLEM	DEFINING CHARACTERISTICS	NURSING ORDERS		EXPECTED OUTCOMES
		ASSESSMENT	INTERVENTIONS	

Injury, potential for: airway obstruction
Etiology
Inflammation
Edema of epiglottis
	Dysphagia
	Drooling
	Dyspnea
	Respiratory distress
	Restlessness
	Elevated temperature
	Increased WBCs
	Cough
	Positive throat culture for *Haemophilus influenzae* type B
		A. Assess respiratory rate every _____
		B. Auscultate breath sounds every _____
		C. Assess for respiratory distress
		  1. Retractions
		  2. Stridor
		  3. Anxiety
		  4. Cyanosis
		  5. Nasal flaring
		  6. Use of accessory muscles
		D. Monitor WBC
		E. Assess results of throat and blood cultures
		F. Check any x-ray film results
		G. Monitor ABG results
			A. Notify physician of any changes in respiratory status
			B. Support child in a high Fowler's position
			C. Administer humidified O_2 at a rate of ____ L/min
			D. Prepare child for x-ray studies as needed
			E. Assist in intubation as necessary
			F. Institute suctioning of airway
			G. Maintain good handwashing technique
			H. Administer antipyretics for temperature greater than ____ as ordered
			I. Sponge child with tepid water for temperature greater than _____
			J. Apply cooling mattress for temperature greater than _____
			K. Administer antibiotics as ordered
				A. Child's airway will remain patent
				B. Child will maintain adequate oxygenation

Fluid volume deficit: potential **Etiology** Respiratory distress Inability to maintain oral intake	Thirst Drooling Inability to swallow Tachypnea Increased sensible fluid loss	See SCP in Ch. 1: Fluid volume deficit	A. Monitor vital signs every _____ B. Weigh daily C. Monitor I & O every ____ hours D. Administer IV fluids at a rate of _____ ml/hour	Adequate fluid and electrolyte balance will be maintained

Anxiety/fear (of the child)
Etiology
Trauma of hospitalization
	Anxiety
	Afraid to sleep
	Constant talking, asking questions, and bargaining
	Crying
	Clinging
		A. Assess child for separation anxiety
		  1. Protest
		  2. Fear
		B. Monitor for presence of fears
		  1. Afraid of strangers
		  2. Unfamiliar surroundings
		C. Assess child for previous experiences and coping behaviors
			A. Orient child to unit
			B. Introduce yourself by name
			C. Provide accurate information at the appropriate level of understanding
			D. Maintain consistent caretakers
			E. Encourage parents to be at bedside as much as possible
			F. Encourage parent participation in child's care
			G. Provide comfort measures as necessary
			H. Provide toys appropriate for age
				Child will demonstrate trusting behaviors toward caretakers as evidenced by
				A. Cooperation with procedures
				B. Friendliness
				C. Ability to play

Originated by **Patricia Hasbrouck-Aschliman, RN, CCRN**
Resource persons: **Ruth E. Novitt, RN, MSN**
              Janice L. Miller, RN,C MSN

Epiglottis: pediatric ICU—cont'd

NURSING DIAGNOSIS/ PATIENT PROBLEM	DEFINING CHARACTERISTICS	NURSING ORDERS		EXPECTED OUTCOMES
		ASSESSMENT	INTERVENTIONS	

Sleep pattern disturbance
Etiology
Respiratory distress and fear
	Irritability
	Confusion/disorientation
	Poor eating
	Inappropriate response to stimuli
	Decreased attention span
		A. Assess any changes in level of consciousness
		  1. Difficulty in arousing
		  2. Altered response to stimuli
		  3. Confusion or disorientation
		B. Note any changes in mood
		C. Assess work of breathing
		  1. Retractions
		  2. Comfort
			A. Decrease amount of stimuli
			B. Decrease distractions by medical and nursing staff
			C. Promote sleep activities
			  1. Decreased light
			  2. Decreased noise
			  3. Home rituals (clean pajamas, brushing teeth, prayers)
			D. Provide comfort measures
			  1. Head elevated
			  2. Good body alignment
			  3. Massage
			  4. Warm bath
				Child will get adequate rest

Anxiety/fear (of the family) **Etiology** Illness of child Lack of knowledge about illness	Constant demands Excess talking Continuous questions Withdrawal Pacing Hand wringing	A. Assess degree of stress and ability to cope B. Assess level of understanding about child's illness and hospitalization C. Assess degree of involvement in child's care D. Assess previous experience with coping to illness and hospitalization	A. Encourage parental expression of feelings about illness and hospitalization B. Establish good rapport C. Spend social time with parents D. Reassure and support parents E. Encourage parent interaction with child and participation in child's care F. Offer factual information G. Clarify misconceptions H. Evaluate effect of interventions by observing positive parent/ child interaction behaviors	Parents' fear/anxiety will be decreased as a result of the use of appropriate coping mechanisms

Pneumonia

NURSING DIAGNOSIS/ PATIENT PROBLEM	DEFINING CHARACTERISTICS	NURSING ORDERS		EXPECTED OUTCOMES
		ASSESSMENT	INTERVENTIONS	

Airway clearance, ineffective
 Etiology
 Increased production of sputum in response to respiratory infection
 Decreased energy and increased fatigue resulting from prolonged immobilization, cardiac failure, postoperative effect of general anesthesia, chronic illness, depression of CNS, excessive intake of alcohol
 Aspiration
	Abnormal breath sounds, e.g., rhonchi, bronchial breath sounds
	 Decreased breath sounds over affected areas
	 Cough
	 Dyspnea
	 Cyanosis
	 Change in respiratory status
	 Infiltrates on chest x-ray film
		A. Assess breath sounds
		 B. Assess respiratory movements and use of accessory muscles
		 C. Monitor chest X-ray reports
		 D. Monitor sputum Gram's stain and culture and sensitivity reports
			A. Assist patient with coughing and deep breathing, splinting as necessary to improve coughing
			 B. Encourage patient to cough and avoid suppressing the cough reflex unless cough is frequent and nonproductive, resulting in hypoxemia
			 C. Use positioning to facilitate the ability to clear secretions
			 D. Use the respiratory therapy department for chest physiotherapy and nebulizer treatments, as appropriate
			 E. Use humidity to loosen secretions (humidified O_2 or a humidifier at bedside)
			 F. Maintain adequate hydration (fluids are lost from diaphoresis, fever, and tachypnea)
			   1. Encourage oral fluids
			   2. Administer IV fluids as ordered
			 G. Administer medication (e.g., antibiotics, expectorants) as ordered, noting effectiveness
			 H. Institute suctioning of airway as needed to remove sputum and mucous plugs
			 I. Use nasopharyngeal/oropharyngeal airway as needed
			 J. Anticipate possible need for intubation if patient's condition deteriorates
				Airway will be freed of secretions

Gas exchange, impaired
 Etiology
 Collection of mucus in airways
	Dyspnea
	 Decreased Pa_{O_2}
	 Increased Pa_{CO_2}
	 Cyanosis
	 Tachypnea
	 Air hunger
	 Tachycardia
	 Pallor
	 Decreased activity tolerance
	 Restlessness
	 Disorientation/confusion
		A. Assess respiratory status
		   Rate
		   Depth
		   Breath sounds
		   Pattern of respiration
		 B. Assess skin color and capillary refill
		 C. Assess for changes in orientation and increasing restlessness
		 D. Assess for changes in activity tolerance
		 E. Monitor changes in vital signs
		 F. Monitor ABGs, and note differences
			A. Notify physician if patient's condition worsens
			 B. Pace activities to patient's tolerance
			 C. Maintain O_2 administration device as ordered per physician. NOTE: Avoid high concentrations of O_2 in patients with COPD
			 D. Anticipate the need for intubation and, possibly, mechanical ventilation if patient's condition worsens
			 E. See SCP in this chapter: Mechanical ventilation (as needed)
				Patient's gas exchange will be enhanced

Originated by **Martha Dickerson, RN, MS, CCRN**
    Susan Galanes, RN, MS, TNS, CCRN

Pneumonia—cont'd

NURSING DIAGNOSIS/ PATIENT PROBLEM	DEFINING CHARACTERISTICS	NURSING ORDERS		EXPECTED OUTCOMES
		ASSESSMENT	INTERVENTIONS	

Temperature regulation, alteration in
Etiology
Invading bacterial/ viral organisms
	Elevated temperature
	Elevated WBC
	Tachycardia
	Chills
	Positive sputum culture report
	Changing character of sputum
		A. Elicit patient's description of illness including
		  1. Onset
		  2. Chills
		  3. Chest pain
		  4. Medications. NOTE: Patients receiving high dosages of corticosteroids have a reduced resistance to infections
		  5. Recent exposure to illness
		  6. Alcohol, tobacco, or drug abuse
		  7. Chronic illness
		B. Assess vital signs
		C. Monitor Gram stain, sputum, culture and sensitivity reports
		D. Monitor WBC
			A. Use appropriate therapy for elevated temperature: antipyretics, cold therapy
			B. Obtain fresh sputum for Gram stain/culture and sensitivity, as ordered
			  1. Instruct patient to expectorate into sterile container. Be sure the specimen is coughed up (i.e., not saliva)
			  2. If patient is unable to effectively cough up a specimen, use sterile nasotracheal suctioning with a Lukens' tube
			C. Administer prescribed antimicrobial agent(s)
			D. Continue to monitor temperature. NOTE: Continued fever may be caused by
			  1. Drug allergy
			  2. Drug-resistant bacteria
			  3. Superinfection
			  4. Inadequate lung drainage
			E. Isolate patient as necessary following review of culture and sensitivity results
				Infection will be minimized as evidenced by
				A. Normal temperature
				B. Negative culture report following appropriate therapy

Comfort, alteration in: pain
Etiology
Respiratory distress
Coughing
	Complaints of discomfort
	Guarding
	Withdrawal
	Moaning
	Facial grimace
	Irritability
	Anxiety
	Tachycardia
	Increased BP
	Increased temperature
		A. Assess complaints of discomfort
		B. Determine quality, severity, location, onset, duration, and precipitating factors for patient's discomfort
			A. Teach patient to verbalize any complaints of discomfort
			B. Examine patient for any objective signs of discomfort
			C. Administer appropriate medications to treat the cough
			  1. Do not suppress a productive cough; but do use moderate amounts of analgesics to relieve pleuritic pain
			  2. Use cough suppressants and humidity for a dry, hacking cough
			D. Administer analgesics as ordered and as needed. Encourage patient to take analgesics before discomfort becomes severe
			E. Evaluate effectiveness of medications. Use additional measures to relieve patient discomfort, including positioning and relaxation
			F. See SCP in Ch. 1: Comfort, alteration in
				Patient's discomfort will be relieved

Consciousness, altered levels of: potential Etiology Cerebral hypoxia Meningitis Delirium tremens (DTs)	Decreasing Pao_2 Change in alertness, orientation, verbal response Agitation Restlessness Irritability	Assess for presence of defining characteristics, and, if present, notify physician	A. For a decrease in Pao_2, see Gas exchange, impaired B. Refer to SCP in Ch. 3: Consciousness, alteration in level of C. If appropriate, see SCP in Ch. 3: Meningitis	Alteration in level of consciousness will be minimized

Continued.

Pneumonia—cont'd

NURSING DIAGNOSIS/ PATIENT PROBLEM	DEFINING CHARACTERISTICS	NURSING ORDERS		EXPECTED OUTCOMES
		ASSESSMENT	INTERVENTIONS	
Anxiety/fear: potential **Etiology** Debilitated condition Air hunger Isolation (if needed)	Restlessness Constant demands Uncooperative behavior Withdrawal Indifference Afraid to sleep	Assess for signs of anxiety (see Defining Characteristics)	See SCP in Ch. 1: Anxiety/fear	Patient will display a calm, relaxed appearance

Nutrition, alteration in: less than body requirements (potential)
 Etiology
 Intake less than metabolic needs
 Increased metabolic needs
 Decreased intake
	Anorexia
	 Loss of weight
	 Decreased caloric intake
		A. Document patient's actual weight
		 B. Obtain nutritional history
		 C. Obtain baseline laboratory values
		   1. Serum total protein
		   2. Serum albumin
		   3. Serum osmolarity
		   4. Vitamin assays (as appropriate)
		   5. Mineral and trace element levels (as appropriate)
			A. Maintain bed rest to decrease metabolic needs
			 B. Increase activity as patient tolerates
			 C. Provide high protein/high carbohydrate diet
			 D. Provide small, frequent feedings
			 E. Administer vitamin supplements as ordered
			 F. Administer enteral supplements and parenteral nutrition as ordered
			 G. See SCP in Ch. 1: Nutrition, alteration in: less than body requirements
				Optimal nutritional status will be maintained

Knowledge deficit
 Etiology
 New condition and procedures
 Unfamiliarity with disease process and transmission of disease
	Questions
	 Confusion about treatment
	 Inability to comply with treatment regimen, including any appropriate isolation procedures
	 Lack of questions
		A. Determine understanding by patient/significant others of disease process, complications, and treatment regimen
		 B. See SCP in Ch. 1: Knowledge deficit
			A. Provide information to patient/ significant others in teaching sessions regarding the need to
			   1. Maintain natural resistance to infection through adequate nutrition, rest, and exercise
			   2. Avoid contact with people with upper respiratory infections
			   3. Obtain immunizations against influenza for the elderly and chronically ill
			   4. Use pneumococcal vaccine for those at greatest risk
			     a. Elderly patients with chronic systemic disease
			     b. Patients with COPD
			     c. Patients with sickle cell anemia
			     d. Patients who have had a splenectomy
			     e. Patients who have had a pneumonectomy and are immunosuppressed
			 B. Encourage patient/significant others to ask questions
			 C. Evaluate understanding of information following teaching sessions
			 D. Observe for compliance with treatment regimen
				Patient and significant others will demonstrate understanding of disease process, compliance with treatment regimen, and any isolation procedures

Pulmonary Embolism

NURSING DIAGNOSIS/ PATIENT PROBLEM	DEFINING CHARACTERISTICS	NURSING ORDERS		EXPECTED OUTCOMES
		ASSESSMENT	INTERVENTIONS	

Gas exchange, impaired
Etiology
Decreased perfusion to lung tissue
	Increased alveolar dead space
	Hypoxemia
	Increased alveolar-arterial (A-a) gradient
	Increased physiologic shunting
	Dyspnea/tachypnea
	Respiratory rate of 30 or more per minute
	Deep chest-cage breathing
	Hypocapnea (PCO_2 level < 35 mm Hg)
	Chest x-ray film reflecting atelectasis
	Rales
	Decreased breath sounds over involved areas of lungs
	Bronchial or tubular breath sounds
	Pleural friction rub
	Whispered pectoriloquy
	Chest pain (pleuritic)
	Elevated temperature
		A. Assess for alteration in lung function
		  1. Hypoxemia
		    a. Tachycardia
		    b. Restlessness
		    c. Diaphoresis
		    d. Headache
		    e. Lethargy/ confusion
		    f. Skin color changes
		  2. Atelectasis
		    a. Diminished chest expansion
		    b. Limited excursion of the diaphragm
		    c. Bronchial/ tubular breath sounds
		    d. Rales
		    e. Tracheal shift to affected side
		  3. Work of breathing
		    a. Increase in rate and depth of respiration
		    b. Increase in use of accessory breathing muscles
		    c. Decrease in number of words patient is able to say between each breath
		B. Assess characteristics of pain: quantity, quality, location, precipitating factors, relieving factors
		C. Assess for fever
			A. Auscultate lungs every _____
			B. Monitor ABGs every _____
			C. Administer O_2 as indicated
			D. Position patient to
			  1. Maintain optimal lung perfusion. When patient is positioned on side, *affected* area should not be *dependent*
			  2. Optimize diaphragmatic excursion
			E. Pace and schedule activities to conserve energy
			F. Administer pain medication as indicated
			G. Use nursing measures to maintain normal body temperature
			H. Obtain specimens for culture for temperature >102° (rectal)
				Optimal gas exchange will be maintained

Originated by **Lumie Perez, RN, BSN, CCRN**
Resource person: **Terry Takemoto, RN, MSN, CCRN**

Continued.

Pulmonary Embolism—cont'd

NURSING DIAGNOSIS/ PATIENT PROBLEM	DEFINING CHARACTERISTICS	NURSING ORDERS		EXPECTED OUTCOMES
		ASSESSMENT	INTERVENTIONS	

Anxiety/fear
Etiology
Threat of death
Change in health status
Overall feeling of being very sick
Multiple laboratory tests
Increased attention of medical personnel
Increasing respiratory difficulty
	Verbalization of fear
	Restlessness, inability to relax
	Multiple questions
	Tremors, shakiness
	Increase in heart rate, BP, and respiratory rate
	Tense/anxious appearance
	Crying
	Withdrawal
	Denial
		A. Assess level of anxiety
		B. Assess patient's normal coping mechanisms
			A. Convey sense of empathic understanding through the appropriate use of silence and touch
			B. Encourage patient to ventilate feelings of anxiety/fear
			C. Provide reassurance and comfort
			D. Support previously effective coping mechanisms
			E. Organize activities to provide for periods of rest
			F. Decrease sensory stimulation
			  1. Dim lights when appropriate
			  2. Remove unnecessary equipment from room
			  3. Limit visitors and telephone calls
			G. Explain reasons for multiple laboratory tests and increased medical personnel attention
			H. Consult physician for possible pharmacologic therapy
			I. See SCP in Ch. 1: Anxiety/fear
				Decrease in anxiety level will be evidenced
				A. Calm, relaxed appearance
				B. Verbalization of feelings

Knowledge deficit
Etiology
New medical condition
	Expresses inaccurate perception of health status
	Verbalizes a deficiency in knowledge
	Multiple questions or none at all
		A. Assess learning ability
		  1. Level of education
		  2. Ability to read
		  3. Language understood
		B. Assess or determine present knowledge of illness
		  1. Severity
		  2. Prognosis
		  3. Risk factors
		  4. Therapy
		C. Assess patient's readiness for learning
		  1. Past acute stage of illness
		  2. Expression of desire to learn
			A. Inform patient/significant others of the following
			  1. Etiology of the problem
			  2. Effects of pulmonary embolus on body functioning
			  3. Common risk factors
			    a. Immobilization
			    b. Trauma: hip fracture, major burns
			    c. Certain heart conditions
			    d. Oral contraceptives
			B. Instruct patient/significant others on medications, their actions, dosages, and side effects
			C. Discuss and provide patient with a list of signs and symptoms of excessive anticoagulation
			  1. Easy bruising
			  2. Severe nosebleed
			  3. Black stools
			  4. Blood in the urine or stools
			  5. Joint swelling and pain
			  6. Coughing up blood
			  7. Severe headache
			D. Discuss and provide patient with a list of what to avoid when taking anticoagulants
			  1. Using a blade razor to shave (electric razor is preferred)
			  2. Taking new medications without consulting physician, pharmacist, or nurses
			  3. Eating foods high in vitamin K (e.g., dark green vegetables, cauliflower, cabbage, bananas, tomatoes)
			  4. Ingesting aspirin or other salicylates
				Patient will understand
				A. Importance of medications
				B. Signs of excessive anticoagulation
				C. Means to reduce risk of bleeding and recurrence of emboli

Pulmonary Embolism—cont'd

NURSING DIAGNOSIS/ PATIENT PROBLEM	DEFINING CHARACTERISTICS	NURSING ORDERS		EXPECTED OUTCOMES
		ASSESSMENT	INTERVENTIONS	
			E. Discuss and provide patient with a list of measures to minimize recurrence of emboli 1. Taking medicines as prescribed 2. Keeping appointments for medical checkups and blood tests 3. Performing leg exercises as advised, especially during long automobile and airplane trips 4. Not crossing legs 5. Use of TED stockings if ordered 6. Maintaining adequate hydration	
Cardiac output, alteration in: decreased (potential) **Etiology** Right-sided heart failure resulting from pulmonary hypertension Left-sided heart failure secondary to right-sided heart failure	**Right-sided heart failure** Accentuated pulmonic component of S_2 Splitting of S_2 Engorged neck veins, positive hepatojugular reflex Increased CVP readings Palpable liver and spleen Altered coagulation values ECG changes associated with right atrial hypertrophy Atrial arrhythmias Pedal edema Weight gain **Left-sided heart failure** Fine rales (bases of the lungs) Increased pulmonary artery wedge pressure Presence of S_3; gallop rhythms Frothy secretions Dyspnea Tachycardia Cough Wheezing Orthopnea Hypoxemia Respiratory acidosis ECG changes associated with left atrial hypertrophy	Assess for signs and symptoms of right-sided heart failure and left-sided heart failure (see Defining Characteristics)	A. Monitor lung sounds every _____ B. Monitor heart sounds every _____ C. If ECG is monitored, observe for ECG changes every _____ D. If patient has Swan-Ganz catheter, record hemodynamic pressures every _____; report any abnormal values to physician as appropriate E. Assist in assuming comfortable position for optimal breathing F. Weigh daily G. If edema is present, see SCP in Ch. 1: Skin integrity, impairment of H. Administer medications as ordered I. Administer O_2 as indicated J. Anticipate the following 1. Mechanical ventilation (see SCP in this chapter: Respiratory failure) 2. Insertion of arterial lines 3. Insertion of Swan-Ganz catheter (SCPs in Ch. 2: Pulmonary edema; Swan-Ganz catheter) 4. Anticoagulant therapy 5. Thrombolytic therapy 6. Vena caval interruptions 7. Pulmonary embolectomy (rarely done) K. If decreased cardiac output becomes a problem, see SCP in Ch. 1: Cardiac output, alteration in: decreased	Optimal cardiac output will be maintained

Continued.

Pulmonary Embolism—cont'd

NURSING DIAGNOSIS/ PATIENT PROBLEM	DEFINING CHARACTERISTICS	NURSING ORDERS		EXPECTED OUTCOMES
		ASSESSMENT	INTERVENTIONS	
Injury, potential for: bleeding **Etiology** Bleeding secondary to anticoagulant/ thrombolytic therapy	Petechiae, purpura, hematoma Bleeding from catheter insertion sites GI, GU bleeding Bleeding from respiratory tract Bleeding from mucous membranes Decreasing Hb and Hct	A. Assess for signs and symptoms of internal bleeding (see Defining Characteristics) B. Assess patient for high-risk condition 1. Liver disease 2. Kidney disease 3. Severe hypertension 4. Cavitary tuberculosis 5. Bacterial endocarditis	A. Minimize complications by 1. Being aware of contraindications for thrombolytic therapy a. Recent surgery b. Recent organ biopsy c. Paracentesis/thoracentesis d. Pregnancy e. Recent stroke f. Recent or active internal bleeding 2. Instituting precautionary measures a. Using only compressible vessels for IV sites b. Compressing IV sites for at least 10 min and arterial sites for 30 min c. Discontinuing anticoagulants and antiplatelet aggregates before thrombolytic therapy d. Limiting physical manipulation of patients e. Padding side rails of restless patient f. Providing gentle oral care g. Avoiding IM injections h. Drawing all laboratory blood specimens through the external line B. Observe patient at all times for signs of bleeding 1. Keep dressings of IV and arterial sites visible 2. Use adhesive tape that is not waterproof 3. Check IV infusion site every _____ C. Estimate and record any blood loss D. Monitor laboratory results of coagulation studies every _____ E. Monitor Hb and Hct every _____ F. Send specimen for type and cross-match as ordered	Risk for bleeding will be minimized

Respiratory Failure, Acute: secondary to chronic obstructive pulmonary disease (COPD)

NURSING DIAGNOSIS/ PATIENT PROBLEM	DEFINING CHARACTERISTICS	NURSING ORDERS		EXPECTED OUTCOMES
		ASSESSMENT	INTERVENTIONS	
Breathing pattern, ineffective **Etiology** Hypoxia Acidosis Obstructed airway and poor ventilation secondary to retention of secretions Pulmonary infections Congestive heart failure resulting from pulmonary hypertension and edema	Shortness of breath Retention of CO_2 O_2 below 50 mm Hg Increased restlessness and irritability Tachycardia Dyspnea Tachypnea Cyanosis Respiratory depth changes Wheezing frequently and increased severity of coughing. As respiratory insufficiency increases in severity, a decrease in level of consciousness may occur	A. Review respiratory health history B. Assess for a productive cough, including amount expectorated, frequency, color, etc. C. Monitor and record vital signs every ___ and notify physician if out of prescribed range BP: ___ to ___ Respiratory rate: ___ to ___ Pulse: ___ to ___. Note any irregularity of pulse D. Observe for any changes in patient's respiratory status Rate: _____ Depth: _____ Changes heard during auscultation: _____ Respiratory effort: _____ E. Observe for signs of hypoxia such as cyanosis, dyspnea, increased pulse, changes in level of consciousness or restlessness F. Observe for signs of increased P_{CO_2} such as asterixis or tremors G. Observe for intercostal retractions and marked use of accessory muscles H. Auscultate lungs every ___ and note breath sounds, observing for wheezing, rales, or rhonchi	A. Administer O_2 as needed NOTE: With patients with severe COPD, give O_2 slowly and in small amounts B. Monitor ABGs carefully and notify physician of abnormalities pH ___ to ___ Pao_2 ___ to ___ $Paco_2$ ___ to ___ HCO_3 ___ to ___ C. Position patient with proper body alignment for optimal breathing pattern. The preferred position is _____ _____ D. Maintain adequate airway, positioning patient to prevent mechanical obstruction from tongue E. Pace activities to avoid fatigue F. Maintain planned rest periods	Adverse changes in breathing pattern will be minimized as evidenced by A. Normal breath sounds B. Absence of dyspnea on exertion C. Adequate ventilation

Originated by **Linda Marie St. Julien, RN, BSN**
Resource person: **Susan Galanes, RN, MS, TNS, CCRN**

Continued.

Respiratory Failure, Acute: secondary to chronic obstructive pulmonary disease (COPD)—cont'd

NURSING DIAGNOSIS/ PATIENT PROBLEM	DEFINING CHARACTERISTICS	NURSING ORDERS		EXPECTED OUTCOMES
		ASSESSMENT	INTERVENTIONS	
Airway clearance, ineffective: potential **Etiology** Respiratory failure requiring intubation	Rales Rhonchi Wheezes Cough Dyspnea	Assess significant alterations in breath sounds such as rhonchi, wheezes	A. Instruct and/or change patient's position q.2h. to mobilize secretions B. Provide humidity (when appropriate) via bedside humidifier/ humidified O$_2$ therapy C. Instruct patient to deep breathe adequately and to cough D. Use nasotracheal suction for patients who cannot clear their secretions as necessary E. When necessary prepare for 1. Intubation a. Lower the bed b. Make sure Ambu bag is at bedside c. Obtain anesthetic to be used for nonemergency intubations d. Have a 20 cc syringe available for balloon inflation e. Instruct the patient who is awake and alert, since explanation is essential for total cooperation 2. Postintubation a. Auscultate lungs for bilateral breath sounds b. Obtain chest x-ray study following intubation to determine ET tube placement c. Stay with patient to allay anxiety d. Institute suctioning via ET tube as necessary	Airway will be free of secretions
Injury, potential for: infection **Etiology** Pulmonary invasive techniques for treatment of COPD	Increased WBC Increased temperature Change in bronchial secretions: amount, thickness, and change in color	A. Monitor and document temperature every ___ and notify physician of temperature >___ NOTE: If the patient is receiving steroid therapy, infections may be more difficult to detect B. Monitor WBC level and notify physician of abnormalities C. Observe patient secretions for color, thickness, and amount. Notify physician of any abnormalities D. Monitor sputum cultures and sensitivities	A. Use conscientious bronchial hygiene, good handwashing techniques, and sterile suctioning NOTE: Most infections are transmitted via hospital personnel B. Administer mouth care every ___ and as needed, e.g., Cepacol, lemon glycerine mouth swabs, Chloraseptic mouth spray C. Institute suctioning of airway every ___ and as needed (accumulations of secretions could lead to an invasive process) D. Maintain the patient's personal hygiene, nutrition, and rest to increase natural defenses E. Send culture and sensitivity of sputum every ___ as ordered per physician	Risk of infection will be minimized

Respiratory Failure, Acute: secondary to chronic obstructive pulmonary disease (COPD)—cont'd

NURSING DIAGNOSIS/ PATIENT PROBLEM	DEFINING CHARACTERISTICS	NURSING ORDERS		EXPECTED OUTCOMES
		ASSESSMENT	INTERVENTIONS	
Consciousness, altered levels of: potential **Etiology** Increased Pa_{CO_2} and/ or decreased Pa_{O_2}	Restlessness Anxiety Confusion Somnolence	A. Observe and document 1. Increased restlessness 2. Increased anxiety 3. Confusion 4. Somnolence B. Check pupils every ____ or as needed for sluggishness C. Obtain initial BP, and monitor serial BP (may be elevated and become hypotensive with progressive changes)	If alteration in level of consciousness is present, refer to SCP in Ch. 3	Optimal level of consciousness will be maintained
Anxiety/fear **Etiology** Threat of death Change in health status Change in environment Change in interaction patterns Unmet needs	Restlessness Diaphoresis Pointing to his/her throat (possibly unable to speak) Uncooperative behavior Withdrawal Watches equipment vigilantly	Assess patient for any signs that could indicate increased fear or increased anxiety	A. If patient is unable to speak because of respiratory status 1. Provide pencil and pad to write 2. Establish some form of nonverbal communication if patient is too sick to write B. Keep the patient in touch with reality by 1. Explaining mechanical ventilation 2. Explaining alarm systems on monitors and ventilators 3. Reassuring patient of your presence to assist him/her C. Display a confident, calm manner and tolerant, understanding attitude D. Allow family/significant others to visit and involve them in the care E. Use other supportive measures as indicated, e.g., medications, psychiatric liaison, clergy, social services	Absence or decrease in fear and anxiety will be evidenced
Knowledge deficit **Etiology** Unfamiliarity with disease process and treatment	Multiple questions Lack of concern Anxiety Noncompliant of medication/health care orders, e.g., smoking	A. Evaluate patient's perception and understanding of disease process B. Assess patient's knowledge regarding O_2 therapy, deep breathing, and coughing	A. Encourage patient to verbalize feelings and questions B. Explain to patient the disease process and correct any misconceptions C. Discuss the need for monitoring equipment and frequent assessments D. Explain all tests and procedures before they occur E. Explain the necessity of O_2 therapy, including its limitations F. Instruct patient to deep breathe and cough effectively	Patient will verbalize understanding of the disease process, procedures, and treatment

Tuberculosis (TB): active

NURSING DIAGNOSIS/ PATIENT PROBLEM	DEFINING CHARACTERISTICS	NURSING ORDERS		EXPECTED OUTCOMES
		ASSESSMENT	INTERVENTIONS	
Breathing pattern, ineffective **Etiology** Decreased total lung capacity Increased metabolism as a result of high fever Frequent productive cough and hemoptysis Nervousness, fear of suffocation	Increased work of breathing: tachypnea, use of accessory muscles, diaphoresis, tachycardia Purulent or bloody expectoration Increased anxiety, nervousness, fear, or anger secondary to dyspnea and/or isolation	A. Assess patient's respiratory status: note depth, rate, and character of breathing every _____ B. Check for increased work of breathing C. Assess patient's cough: note character (weak, hard, productive, or nonproductive) D. Assess nature of secretions; note color, amount, consistency E. Auscultate lungs for presence of breath sounds and abnormal breath sounds every _____ F. Monitor vital signs q.4h.; note time of temperature spikes	A. Administer O₂ as ordered B. Push fluids; provide humidification in room C. Induce sputum with ultrasonic nebulizer if needed and ordered	Optimal respiratory status within the limits of the disease will be achieved

Nutrition, alteration in: less than body requirements
Etiology
Chronically poor appetite
	Body weight below standard for height, age, and sex
	Weight loss >10% body weight
	Reduced arm muscle circumference
	Diminished serum albumin and leukocyte levels
		A. Assess nutritional status through diet history, physical examination on admission
		B. Assess for possible causes of undernutrition
		C. Assess laboratory values
		  1. Serum albumin
		  2. Serum protein
		  3. Leukocyte count
		  4. Urine protein
		  5. Urine glucose on admission and every _____
		D. Obtain admission weight and daily weight thereafter
		E. Record arm muscle circumference and tricep skinfold measurement weekly for 3 weeks
		F. Perform skin test for anergy
			A. See SCP in Ch. 1: Nutrition, alteration in: less than body requirements
			B. Explain the importance of good nutrition while taking TB medications
			C. Instruct patient about diet/nutrition supplements
				Optimal nutritional status will be maintained

Prepared by **Annie F. Jenkins, RN**
Resource person: **Remedios S. Garces, RN, BSN**

Tuberculosis (TB): active—cont'd

NURSING DIAGNOSIS/ PATIENT PROBLEM	DEFINING CHARACTERISTICS	NURSING ORDERS		EXPECTED OUTCOMES
		ASSESSMENT	INTERVENTIONS	
Knowledge deficit **Etiology** Unfamiliarity with disease process and treatment	Patient verbalizes incorrect information Patient states lack of understanding/asks questions Evidence of noncompliance with therapeutic regimen related to lack of or incorrect information	A. Assess knowledge level about TB B. Assess patient for readiness and interest to learn topics related to TB	A. Teach patient the following about TB 1. Detection 2. Transmission 3. Signs/symptoms 4. Treatment and length of therapy 5. Prevention 6. Importance of compliance to therapy 7. Health regimen to follow after discharge a. Clinic appointments b. How and where to get medications c. ADL d. Resource telephone numbers B. Reinforce respiratory isolation techniques 1. Keep sputum cup at bedside 2. Dispose of old secretions properly 3. Use mask; cover mouth when coughing 4. Keep door to room closed at all times 5. Keep tissues at bedside	Patient will verbalize basic knowledge about TB
Noncompliance to therapeutic regimen **Etiology** Patient value system: health and spiritual beliefs and cultural influences Patient and provider relationships	TB reactivation shown on chest x-ray and sputum examination Poor nutritional status: signs of undernutrition Drug-resistant organism seen in culture Verbal cues by patient/ significant others of noncompliance	Assess patient for evidence of noncompliance A. Weight loss B. Increased coughing C. Thick green-gray purulent sputum D. Alcohol abuse E. Drug-resistant organism on culture	A. Identify causes of noncompliance B. Institute respiratory isolation C. Send sputum for culture D. Reeducate patient E. Make TB clinic referral for supervised therapy F. Arrange for visiting nurse G. Enroll patient in TB follow-up program H. Arrange for social service involvement	Patient will describe factors that cause him/her to alter prescribed treatment plan

THERAPEUTIC INTERVENTIONS

Jet Ventilation

NURSING DIAGNOSIS/ PATIENT PROBLEM	DEFINING CHARACTERISTICS	NURSING ORDERS		EXPECTED OUTCOMES
		ASSESSMENT	INTERVENTIONS	
Gas exchange, impaired (requiring mechanical jet ventilation) **Etiology** Adult respiratory distress syndrome Barotrauma Aspiration pneumonitis	Hypercapnea Hypoxia Abnormal ABGs Presence of increased intrathoracic pressures (measured by esophageal balloon and manometer) Low pulmonary compliance exhibited by high peak pressures ($\geq$55 cm H_2O)	A. Assess respiratory rate, rhythm, and character every _____ B. Auscultate lungs every ____ to check for aeration both before and after jet ventilation is begun C. Observe for abnormal breathing patterns (Cheyne-Stokes, Kussmaul, sternal retractions) D. Assess level of consciousness and level of anxiety E. Assess skin color (presence/absence of cyanosis), temperature, capillary refill, and peripheral perfusion F. Monitor vital signs every ____, watching for increased central venous pressure, and increased pulmonary capillary wedge pressure (PCWP), decreased BP, and decreased cardiac output. Notify physician if these occur G. Monitor for complaints of pain, which may increase respirations making it more difficult to ventilate patient. Assess location and duration	A. Administer O_2 as ordered and indicated B. Obtain informed consent for jet therapy if possible C. Prepare patient for intubation with Hi-Lo multi-lumen cuffed ET tube (National Catheter Co.) NOTE: Hi-Lo multi-lumen cuffed ET tube outer diameter is ½ size larger than conventional ET tubes, e.g., 7.5 Hi-Lo single lumen cuffed ET tube = 7.0 Hi-Lo multi-lumen cuffed ET tube 1. Administer sedation or neuromuscular blocking agent as ordered e.g., diazepam (Valium), pancuronium (Pavulon), or succinylcholine 2. Provide comfort measures/reassurance (verbal and nonverbal contact) 3. Obtain baseline status before institution of therapy (PCWP, cardiac output, and ABGs) as ordered D. Maintain adequate blood volume, treating any sources of hemorrhage or changes in vascular compartments with appropriate fluids as ordered (i.e., blood, crystalloid, colloid) E. Combine nursing actions (i.e., bath, bed, and dressing changes) to minimize energy expended by patient, and allow frequent periods of rest F. Provide frequent attendance since there are few alarms on present jet system to detect patient disconnect or low volumes. Be prepared to use Ambu bag in case of emergency failure of machinery or an acute change in the patient's condition	Optimal respiratory status will be maintained pH: _____ PaO_2: _____ $PaCO_2$: _____ HCo_3: _____ Saturation: _____

Originated by **Carol Ann Rooks, RN, BSN**
Resource person: **Susan Galanes, RN, MS, TNS, CCRN**

Jet Ventilation—cont'd

NURSING DIAGNOSIS/ PATIENT PROBLEM	DEFINING CHARACTERISTICS	NURSING ORDERS		EXPECTED OUTCOMES
		ASSESSMENT	INTERVENTIONS	
		H. Monitor ABGs frequently or as indicated (i.e., after changes in FIo$_2$, rate, drive pressure, or continuous positive airway pressure) I. Monitor cardiac output as indicated or ordered, especially after ventilator changes or changes in patient's condition	NOTE: Ambu-bag ventilation may be difficult because of decreased compliance and elasticity G. Administer antibiotics and medications as ordered H. Administer pain relievers as ordered, and provide other comfort measures as needed	

Airway clearance, ineffective
Etiology
Presence/irritation by ET tube
Secretions
Drying of mucosa
Decreased energy and fatigue
	Abnormal breath sounds
	Change in rate, depth, and character of respirations
	Tachypnea
	Cough
	Cyanosis
	Dyspnea or shortness of breath
		A. Assess for alteration in airway clearance
		B. Assess ET tube placement and adequacy of cuff to prevent air leakage every ___
		  1. Underinflation may cause aspiration of oral secretions
		  2. Overinflation of cuff may obliterate perfusion to left or right bronchus *resulting* in deterioration of ABGs
		  3. Notify respiratory therapist to check cuff pressure every ___
		  4. Notify physician if there are any problems with ET tube maintenance (e.g., placement, suctioning, cuff)
			Institute aseptic suctioning of airway as needed to prevent airway obstruction
			A. Potential for mucous plug is present because of drying of mucosa from high frequency (respiratory therapist will maintain humidification)
			B. Jet ventilator must be turned off or disconnected during suctioning; otherwise increased airway resistance may increase potential for pneumothorax
			C. Be aware that the respiratory therapist will use Ambu bag or "sigh" q.1h., with the jet off, to prevent atelectasis or atrophy of respiratory muscles as a result of low tidal volumes
				Airway will be free from secretions

Continued.

Jet Ventilation—cont'd

NURSING DIAGNOSIS/ PATIENT PROBLEM	DEFINING CHARACTERISTICS	NURSING ORDERS		EXPECTED OUTCOMES
		ASSESSMENT	INTERVENTIONS	
Skin integrity, impairment of: potential **Etiology** Prolonged bed rest	Immobility Sensory deficit Altered vasomotor tone and/or altered nutritional state resulting in possible skin breakdown (reddened epidermis or deeper layers of skin or muscle)	Assess bony prominences for signs of threatened or actual breakdown of skin every _____	A. Institute changes in position carefully because of limitations in length of ventilator tubing (which is designed to minimize compressible volume, increasing efficiency). Changes in position may change ability to ventilate patient but should be made every _____ B. Institute prophylactic use of pressure-relieving devices C. See SCP in Ch. 1: Skin integrity, impairment of (as needed)	Skin integrity will be maintained
Knowledge deficit **Etiology** New equipment New environment	Increased frequency of questions posed by patient and significant others Inability to correctly respond to questions asked by medical personnel	A. Evaluate understanding by patient/significant others of patient's overall condition and the need for jet ventilation B. Evaluate readiness for learning by patient/significant others	A. Explain all procedures to patient *before* performing them, especially during period of intubation and initial start of jet ventilation B. Provide reassurance of safety of jet ventilatory system C. Orient and reorient patient to ICU surroundings, routines, equipment alarms, and noises D. Include significant others in explanations of the jet therapy E. Allow patient to ventilate feelings through alternative methods of communication (sign language, written messages, alphabet board) F. Explain methods/procedures of "weaning off" jet. Be aware that sedation, which may have been used before the jet therapy, may need to be reinstituted during weaning process. Reassure that sedation is not meant as a means of punishment but may provide an easier transition to conventional ventilation and eventual extubation	Patient/significant others will demonstrate understanding of rationale for jet ventilation

Mechanical Ventilation

NURSING DIAGNOSIS/ PATIENT PROBLEM	DEFINING CHARACTERISTICS	NURSING ORDERS		EXPECTED OUTCOMES
		ASSESSMENT	INTERVENTIONS	
Gas exchange/breathing pattern, alteration in: requiring mechanical ventilation **Etiology** Pneumonia Chronic obstructive pulmonary disease (COPD) Acute respiratory distress syndrome (ARDS) Tuberculosis Pulmonary embolus Pulmonary edema Airway obstruction Drug overdosage Diabetic coma Uremia Various CNS disorders Smoke inhalation Aspiration	pH <7.35 or >7.45 PO_2 <50-60 $PCO_2 \geq$ 50-60 (depending on pH) Decrease in available Hb resulting in a decreased O_2 content Copious amounts of secretions Changes in mental status Increased or decreased respiratory apnea Inability to maintain airway, i.e., emesis, depressed gag, depressed cough Tracheal edema	A. Monitor vital signs every ____, and notify physician if out of prescribed range BP ____ to ____ Temperature ____ to ____ Heart rate ____ to ____ Respiratory rate ____ to ____ (note patient baseline vs) B. Assess lung sounds per auscultation every ____ (Note rhonchi, rales, wheezing, diminished breath sounds) C. Assess breathing pattern: Cheyne-Stokes respirations, Kussmaul's respirations, labored respirations, apnea, sternal retractions, pursed lip breathing, Biot's breathing, stridor, and paradoxical respirations D. Observe ABGs for any abrupt changes and deteriorations in pH, O_2, CO_2, etc. Normal ranges: pH 7.35-7.45 PO_2 80-90 torr PCO_2 35-45 torr O_2 sat 85%-98% O_2 content 16-23 vol % HCO_3 23-29 mEq/ L Base excess 0 ± 2 mEq/L E. Observe for changes in mental status and level of consciousness (is patient becoming anxious?)	A. Maintain patient's airway before intubation 1. Encourage patient to cough and deep breathe 2. Use nasotracheal suction every ____ and as needed 3. See SCP in Ch. 1: Airway clearance, ineffective 4. Provide O_2 therapy as ordered and indicated 5. Notify respiratory therapist of ordered respiratory treatment B. Prepare the equipment necessary for intubation, including 1. ET tubes of various sizes; note size used 2. Benzoin and waterproof tape or other methods for securing ET tube 3. 20-cc syringe for inflating balloon 4. Local anesthetic agent, e.g., Cetacaine spray, cocaine, lidocaine (Xylocaine) spray or jelly, and cotton tip applicators 5. Sedation as prescribed by physician 6. Stylet 7. Magill forceps 8. Laryngoscope and blades 9. Ambu bag and mask 10. Suction equipment 11. Oral airway if patient is being orally intubated 12. Bilateral soft wrist restraints 13. Notify respiratory therapist to bring a mechanical ventilator C. To alleviate anxiety, explain to patient why intubation is necessary D. Sedate patient per physician's orders E. Place patient in a supine position, hyperextending the neck, aligning the patient's oropharynx, posterior nasopharynx, and trachea F. Assist physician in determining good ET tube position following intubation 1. Inflate cuff until no audible leaks are heard	Alteration in gas exchange will be minimized as evidenced by A. Adequate ABGs B. Regular respirations C. Baseline mental status D. Normal skin color E. Normal Hb and electrolytes F. Patent airway

Originated by **Michelle McGhee, RN, BSN**
Resource person: **Susan Galanes, RN, MS, TNS, CCRN**

Continued.

Mechanical Ventilation—cont'd

NURSING DIAGNOSIS/ PATIENT PROBLEM	DEFINING CHARACTERISTICS	NURSING ORDERS		EXPECTED OUTCOMES
		ASSESSMENT	INTERVENTIONS	
		F. Assess skin color, checking nailbeds and lips for cyanosis G. Observe laboratory data, especially noting changes in Hb, electrolytes, and blood glucose H. If patient has hemodynamic monitoring, assess pressures every ____, and notify physician if out of prescribed ranges. Pulmonary artery systolic: ____ to ____ Pulmonary artery diastolic: ____ to ____ Pulmonary artery mean: ____ to ____ Pulmonary capillary wedge: ____ to ____ Central venous: ____ to ____	NOTE: Overinflation of cuff increases incidence of tracheal erosions 2. Ausculate for bilateral breath sounds during use of Ambu bag 3. Observe for abdominal distention NOTE: Abdominal distention is indicative of *gastric* intubation 4. To prevent patient from biting down on ET tube, insert oral airway for patient who is orally intubated 5. Assist in securing ET tube (if in proper placement per examination) 6. Institute aseptic suctioning of airway 7. Place patient on mechanical ventilator with setting as ordered per physician 8. Obtain chest x-ray film for ET tube placement 9. Apply bilateral soft wrist restraints as needed, explaining to patient reason for use. Although all patients do not require restraints, many do	
Airway clearance, ineffective Etiology Intubation	Copious secretions Abnormal breath sounds Dyspnea	A. Assess breath sounds every ____ and as needed B. Note quantity, color, consistency, and odor of sputum	A. Institute suctioning of airway every ____ and as needed B. Turn patient q.2h. to mobilize secretions C. Use sterile saline instillations during suctioning as needed to help facilitate the removal of tenacious sputum	Airway will remain patent
Communication, impaired: verbal Etiology Intubation	Patient unable to communicate verbally because of intubation Difficulty in being understood with nonverbal methods Increasing frustration and/or anxiety	Assess patient's ability to use nonverbal communication	A. Provide nonverbal means of communication 1. Writing equipment 2. Communication board 3. Artificial larynx 4. Generalized list of questions/answers B. Reassure patient that the inability to speak is a temporary effect of the ET tube passing the vocal cords	Patient will have nonverbal means to express needs and concerns
Anxiety, potential Etiology Inability to maintain adequate gas exchange and fear of the unknown outcome	Restlessness Afraid to sleep at night Uncooperative behavior Withdrawal Indifference Watches equipment vigilantly	Assess for signs of anxiety	If anxiety is present, see SCP in Ch. 1: Anxiety/fear	Anxiety level will decrease

Mechanical Ventilation—cont'd

NURSING DIAGNOSIS/ PATIENT PROBLEM	DEFINING CHARACTERISTICS	NURSING ORDERS		EXPECTED OUTCOMES
		ASSESSMENT	INTERVENTIONS	
Injury, potential for **Etiology** Mechanical ventilation	Improper ventilator settings Improper alarm settings Faulty disconnection of ventilator	Observe ventilator settings every ____ to see if patient is receiving the correct intermittent mandatory ventilation, (IMV), tidal volume, continuous positive airway pressure, and FIO$_2$ as ordered by physician. Notify respiratory therapist immediately of any discrepancy in ventilator settings	A. Listen for alarms, know the range in which the ventilator will sound off, and respond to alarms as they occur 1. High peak pressure alarm a. If patient is agitated, give sedation as ordered per physician b. Auscultate breath sounds, and institute suctioning as needed c. Notify respiratory therapist and physician if high pressure alarm continues 2. Low pressure alarm indicates possible disconnection or mechanical ventilatory malfunction a. If disconnected: reconnect patient to mechanical ventilator b. If malfunctioning: remove patient from mechanical ventilator, and use Ambu bag. Notify respiratory therapist to correct malfunction 3. Low exhale volume indicates that the patient is not returning delivered tidal volume, i.e., a leak or disconnection a. Reconnect patient to ventilator if disconnected, or reconnect exhale tubing and notify respiratory therapist if disconnected b. Check cuff volume by assessing if patient is able to talk or make sounds around the tube. Reinflate cuff with air slowly until no leak is detected. Notify anesthesiologist if leak persists 4. *Apnea alarm* is indicative of disconnection or absence of spontaneous respirations a. If disconnected, reconnect patient to ventilator b. Monitor ABGs, vital signs, and changes in mental status to make sure patient is receiving adequate IMV. If apnea persists with an inadequate IMV, use Ambu ventilation, and notify physician	Injury will be prevented

Continued.

Mechanical Ventilation—cont'd

NURSING DIAGNOSIS/ PATIENT PROBLEM	DEFINING CHARACTERISTICS	NURSING ORDERS		EXPECTED OUTCOMES
		ASSESSMENT	INTERVENTIONS	
Skin integrity, impairment of: potential **Etiology** Prolonged intubation	"Crusting" of secretions around ET tube Redness or irritation around ET tube and/ or beneath securing tape Skin breakdown under or around ET tube and/or tape	Observe skin for buildup of secretions, redness, or breakdown	A. If patient is nasally intubated, notify physician if skin is red, irritated, or breakdown is noted B. If patient is orally intubated, the tube should be repositioned from side to side q.24-48h. C. Change tape as needed when loosened or soiled D. Provide mouth care every ____ (e.g., may use 1:1 H_2O_2 and H_2O, and mouthwash afterwards)	Skin integrity will be maintained
Nutrition, alteration in: less than body requirements (potential) **Etiology** Intubation	Loss of weight with or without caloric intake $\geq$10%-20% under ideal body weight Documented inadequate caloric intake Caloric intake inadequate to keep pace with abnormal disease/metabolic state	A. Document patient's weight on admission and every day B. Obtain nutritional history C. Assess for bowel sounds D. Check for abdominal distention and tenderness	Give enteral or parenteral feedings as ordered per physician. Refer to appropriate SCP: Ch. 1: Nutrition, alteration in: less than body requirements; Ch. 5: Enteral tube feeding	Nutritional deficit will be minimized or prevented
Injury, potential for: infection **Etiology** Pulmonary invasive technique	Increased temperature Increased WBC Changes in tracheal secretions, color, consistency, and amount	A. Monitor temperature every ____, and notify physician if temperature is above ____ Core ____ Rectal ____ Oral ____ Axillary B. Monitor WBC and notify physician of elevation	A. Institute suctioning of airway every ____, and send sputum for culture and sensitivity per order of physician B. Administer antibiotics as ordered per physician C. Maintain aseptic suctioning techniques	Risk of infection will be minimized
Knowledge deficit **Etiology** Unfamiliarity with intubation and mechanical ventilation	Multiple questions Lack of concern Anxiety	Assess patient's perception and understanding of mechanical ventilation	A. Allow patient to express feelings and ask questions B. Explain that patient will not be able to eat or drink while intubated but assure him/her that alternative measures will be taken to provide nourishment, i.e., gastric feedings or hyperalimentation C. Explain to patient/significant others the necessity for procedures, e.g., obtaining ABGs D. Explain to patient the inability to talk while intubated E. Explain that the alarms may periodically sound off, which may be normal and the staff will be in close proximity F. Explain the need for frequent assessments, i.e., vital signs, ausculating breath sounds G. Explain the probable need for restraints H. Explain to patient the need for suctioning as needed	

Thoracotomy: postoperative care

NURSING DIAGNOSIS/ PATIENT PROBLEM	DEFINING CHARACTERISTICS	NURSING ORDERS		EXPECTED OUTCOMES
		ASSESSMENT	INTERVENTIONS	

Breathing pattern, ineffective: potential
Etiology
Malfunctioning chest tube drainage system
Positive pressure in the pleural space secondary to surgical incision
Collapse of lung on affected side (partial or complete)
	Dyspnea
	Shortness of breath
	Tachypnea
	Altered chest excursion
		A. Immediately perform complete respiratory assessment, and repeat at least every ____ hours
		B. Obtain vital signs every ____ hours, noting early signs of respiratory insufficiency; document and report abnormal parameters to physician
			A. Perform complete respiratory assessment
			B. Immediately perform complete assessment of the closed chest drainage system, and repeat at least every ____ hours
			  1. Check the H_2O seal for
			    a. Correct fluid level
			    b. Presence/absence of fluctuation. Absence of fluctuation indicates obstruction or lung reexpansion and must always be investigated
			    c. Presence of air leaks; document and report to physician
			  2. Check the suction control chamber for correct fluid level as specified in physician's order. The amount of suction (negative pressure) being applied to the pleural space is regulated by the amount of fluid in the *suction control chamber*, not the amount dialed on the Emerson/wall suction
			  3. Measure the output every ____ hours
			    a. Report drainage of bright red blood of 100 ml/hour for 2 consecutive hours to physician
			    b. Document color, amount, and characteristics of output every ____ hours
			  4. Position the chest drainage system below the patient's chest level
			  5. Make sure the tubing is free of kinks and clots. Milk the tubing from the insertion site downward
			  6. Set the Emerson suction machine correctly (if the system is connected to vacuum suction); 30 mm Hg = 20 L/air is recommended. If the system is disconnected from vacuum suction, it merely functions as a large drain with H_2O seal preventing air from entering the pleural space
			  7. Do not clamp chest tubes unless
			    a. A physician's order is present
				Optimal pulmonary function will be maintained

Originated by **Dorothy Lewis, RN,C BSN**
Resource person: **Carol Burkhart, RN, BSN, CCRN**

Continued.

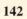

Thoracotomy: postoperative care—cont'd

NURSING DIAGNOSIS/ PATIENT PROBLEM	DEFINING CHARACTERISTICS	NURSING ORDERS		EXPECTED OUTCOMES
		ASSESSMENT	INTERVENTIONS	
			b. The closed chest drainage system is being changed to a new system c. The system becomes disconnected or the H_2O seal is disrupted NOTE: Clamping chest tubes is a dangerous practice. If chest tubes are clamped, you must be prepared to treat tension pneumothorax	
Airway clearance, ineffective **Etiology** Incisional pain Surgery	Subjective complaint of pain Refusal to cough Diminished breath sounds Splinting of respirations	A. Assess patient for any subjective complaints of discomfort or pain B. Perform respiratory assessment, noting signs of hypoventilation every _____	A. Instruct patient in 1. The use of pillow or hand splints when coughing 2. The use of "huff" or stair step ventilations and/or spirometry 3. The importance of early ambulation and/or frequent position changes B. Administer medication as ordered, offering pain medication *before* patient asks for it to avoid peak periods of pain C. Assist patient with ambulation/ position changes NOTE: The patient with a pneumonectomy should *never* be positioned with the remaining lung in a dependent position D. Assist patient in performing coughing and breathing maneuvers every _____	Airway will be free of secretions
Mobility, impaired physical (arm on affected side) **Etiology** Incisional pain and/or edema Decreased strength	Limited ROM Reluctance to attempt movement	Ask patient to raise arm on affected side laterally, documenting the degree of ROM present	A. Instruct patient to perform arm circles, with arm moving in a 360 degree arc every _____ B. Document progress	The patient will regain full ROM of the affected extremity before discharge
Knowledge deficit **Etiology** Unfamiliarity with discharge activity	Patient/significant others unable to restate appropriate discharge activity Patient/significant others verbalize questions/concerns regarding discharge activities	Assess knowledge base and readiness for learning	A. Instruct patient/significant others to 1. Have patient resume normal activities gradually as approved by physician, e.g., begin with short walks rather than stair climbing 2. Avoid inhaling noxious or harmful respiratory irritants, especially cigarette smoke 3. Keep follow-up appointments with physician 4. Report any complaint of shortness of breath or dyspnea at once B. Ask the patient/significant others verbally to reiterate activity plan C. Give written discharge information	The patient will be able to resume activities based on the limits of his/her existent pulmonary disease, avoid further damage from respiratory irritants, and recognize signs and symptoms of respiratory distress

Tracheostomy

NURSING DIAGNOSIS/ PATIENT PROBLEM	DEFINING CHARACTERISTICS	NURSING ORDERS		EXPECTED OUTCOMES
		ASSESSMENT	INTERVENTIONS	

Airway clearance, in-effective
Etiology
Tracheostomy
Fatigue
Thick secretions
Uncooperative patient
Confused patient
	Increasing restlessness
	Change in mental status
	Pallor, cyanosis
	Diaphoresis
	Nasal flaring
	Tachypnea
	Decreased breath sounds
		A. Assess for evidence of respiratory distress (tachypnea, nasal flaring, and increased use of accessory muscles of respiration)
		B. Assess vital signs every ____ and notify physician if out of prescribed range
		BP: ____ to ____
		Heart rate: ____ to ____
		Respiratory rate: ____ to ____
		Temperature ____ to ____
		C. Auscultate breath sounds, and inform physician of changes
			A. Keep suction equipment and Ambu at bedside
			B. Provide humidified air
			C. Administer O_2 as needed
			D. Encourage the patient to cough out secretions
			E. Institute suctioning of airway as needed to clear secretions
			  1. Irrigate with sterile saline if secretions are thick
			  2. Assess the color, consistency, etc., of secretions
			F. Maintain tracheostomy care
			G. Secure tracheostomy tube in position with umbilical tape
			  1. Use square knots, allowing one small finger breadth between tape and patient's neck
			  2. Do not remove old ties until new ties are secure
			H. Obtain a spare tracheostomy tube of the same size and keep at the bedside (note size: ____)
			I. Tape tracheal obturator at head of bed
				Patent airway will be maintained as evidenced by regular and unlabored breathing

Breathing pattern, in-effective
Etiology
Pneumonia
Copious tracheal secretions
Tracheostomy leak
	Hyperventilation
	Decreased breath sounds
	Adventitious breath sounds
	Increased respiratory effort (retractions)
	Tachypnea
	Increased heart rate
	Audible tracheostomy cuff leak
	Behavior changes
		A. Monitor respirations for rate and rhythm every ____ hours
		B. Assess changes in orientation and behavior pattern
		C. Assess changes in serial vital signs (including temperature)
		D. Auscultate breath sounds every ____ hours
			A. Position patient with proper body alignment for optimal breathing pattern
			B. Note presence of sputum; assess quality, color, consistency
			C. If abnormal breath sounds are present, use tracheal suction every ____ as needed
			D. Use humidified O_2 therapy
			E. Maintain adequate airway
			F. Maintain ABGs, and note changes in
			  1. pH: ____ to ____
			  2. Pao_2: ____ to ____
			  3. $Paco_2$: ____ to ____
			G. Check tracheostomy cuff for inflation (if patient is receiving mechanical ventilation). If leak is present, notify physician
			H. Decrease anxiety by staying with patient during episodes of respiratory distress
				Adequate ventilation will be evidenced by
				A. Regular respiratory rate
				B. Normal breath sounds
				C. Normal temperature

Originated by **Pam Harston, RN**
Resource person: **Susan Galanes, RN, MS, TNS, CCRN**

Continued.

Tracheostomy—cont'd

NURSING DIAGNOSIS/ PATIENT PROBLEM	DEFINING CHARACTERISTICS	NURSING ORDERS		EXPECTED OUTCOMES
		ASSESSMENT	INTERVENTIONS	
Gas exchange, impaired: potential **Etiology** Pneumothorax	Recent tracheostomy Respiratory distress Shortness of breath Apnea Tachypnea Anxiety Diaphoresis, pallor, vertigo	A. Assess patient for evidence of respiratory distress B. Assess vital signs every ___ hours C. Auscultate breath sounds D. Inform physician of change	A. Stay with patient, and notify physician if signs of respiratory distress are present B. Place patient in semi- to high Fowler's position C. Administer O_2 as needed D. When portable chest x-ray film is needed, check position of plate so that the patient's entire lung field can be x-rayed and optimal lung expansion can occur E. Set up for chest tube placement, as appropriate	Full lung expansion with adequate oxygenation and ventilation will be maintained
Nutrition, alteration in: less than body requirements (potential) **Etiology** Possible dysphagia secondary to tracheostomy Depression Anorexia Fatigue	Loss of weight with or without adequate caloric intake $\geq 10\%\text{-}20\%$ under ideal body weight Caloric intake inadequate to keep pace with abnormal disease/metabolic state	A. Document patient's actual weight on admission B. Obtain nutritional history as appropriate C. Assess patient's present nutritional intake: oral feeding vs enteral vs parenteral	If signs of altered nutrition are present, see SCP in Ch. 1: Nutrition, alteration in: less than body requirements	Patient will receive food/diet that will promote A. Adequate caloric intake B. Adequate wound healing C. Good skin turgor

Injury, potential for: stomal infection
 Etiology
 Alteration in skin integrity secondary to surgical incision
	Inability of wound to heal
	 Abnormal appearance of wound drainage
	 Purulent drainage from wound
	 Elevated temperature
	 Left shift in differential WBC count (including polymorphonucleus cells, bands)
	 Stoma red and warm to touch
		A. Observe stoma for erythema, exudates, odor, and crusting lesions
		 B. Assess vital signs every ___, and document abnormalities
		 C. Assess laboratory values of WBC differential
			A. Provide routine tracheostomy care every ___ and as needed
			 B. Do not allow secretions to pool around stoma. Suction area or wipe area with aseptic technique to keep stoma dry as possible
			 C. Keep skin under tracheostomy ties clean and dry as possible
			 D. If abnormal drainage and redness is present
			    1. Culture stoma and notify physician
			    2. Apply topical antifungal or antibiotic agent as ordered per physician
				Absence of stomal infection will be evidenced by
				 A. Normal temperature
				 B. Clean stoma
				 C. Lack of inflammation
				 D. Lack of discharge

Tracheostomy—cont'd

NURSING DIAGNOSIS/ PATIENT PROBLEM	DEFINING CHARACTERISTICS	NURSING ORDERS		EXPECTED OUTCOMES
		ASSESSMENT	INTERVENTIONS	
Communication, impaired: verbal **Etiology** Tracheostomy	Difficulty in making self understood Withdrawal Restlessness Frustration	A. Assess patient's ability to understand spoken word B. Assess patient's ability to express ideas	A. Provide call light within easy reach at all times B. Provide for easy observation of patient by nursing staff C. Provide patient with pad and pencil. Use communication or alphabet board if patient is unable to write D. Provide patient with reassurance and patience E. Use speech therapy for possible artificial larynx	Alternative methods of communication will be facilitated
Knowledge deficit of tracheostomy **Etiology** New procedure/intervention	Anxiety Lack of questioning Increased questioning Expressed need for more information	A. Assess knowledge of patient/significant others concerning tracheostomy B. Assess ability of patient/significant others to provide adequate home health care of patient C. Assess readiness to learn D. Assess ability to respond to emergency situations	A. Discuss the need for the patient to have a tracheostomy and its particular purpose B. Begin teaching skills early, and reinforce them daily C. Instruct need for sterile tracheostomy care and suctioning; include step-by-step care guidelines D. Reinforce knowledge of emergency techniques (who, when, why to contact physician and importance of follow-up appointments) E. Make appropriate referral to community health and visiting nurses	Patient/significant others will demonstrate skills appropriate for tracheostomy

CHAPTER FIVE

Gastrointestinal/Digestive

DISORDERS

Ascites

NURSING DIAGNOSIS/ PATIENT PROBLEM	DEFINING CHARACTERISTICS	NURSING ORDERS		EXPECTED OUTCOMES
		ASSESSMENT	INTERVENTIONS	
Fluid volume, alteration in: excess (extravascular) **Etiology** Liver disease Severe nutritional deficiency Hepatic malignancy Ovarian malignancy	Increased abdominal girth Fluid wave (ballottement) on abdominal examination Taut abdomen; dull to percussion	A. Assess for presence of ascites in patients at high risk (alcoholic liver disease, hepatic tumors, ovarian malignancies) by 1. Measuring abdominal girth on admission and every ____; document 2. Checking for ballottement on admission; document B. Monitor laboratory values 1. Serum protein and albumin levels every _____ 2. Serum electrolyte levels every _____	A. Record accurate I & O B. Restrict fluids (as ordered) to ____ml (days); ____ ml (evenings); ____ml (nights) C. Maintain sodium restriction as indicated D. Weigh patient daily E. Administer diuretics as ordered; monitor for side effects; document appropriately F. Evaluate complication of massive ascites 1. Decreased mobility, ability to perform ADL 2. Decreased appetite, nutrition 3. Decreased respiratory function 4. Body image alteration 5. Decreased skin integrity NOTE: In presence of complication, institute care plan G. If paracentesis is indicated 1. Instruct patient to void 2. Place patient in high Fowler's position 3. Prepare patient's abdomen with antiseptic 4. Remain with patient during entire procedure 5. Record vital signs every 15 min 6. Watch for signs of impending shock (increased pulse, decrease in BP, and diaphoresis) 7. Record color, amount, and consistency of fluid 8. Send specimens to appropriate laboratory 9. Monitor patient's vital signs, and check dressing for drainage as ordered	A. Worsening of ascites will be prevented B. Physical and psychologic complications will be minimized

Originated by **Denise Myles, RN,C**
Resource person: **Audrey Klopp, RN, MS, CCRN, CS, ET**

Ascites—cont'd

NURSING DIAGNOSIS/ PATIENT PROBLEM	DEFINING CHARACTERISTICS	NURSING ORDERS		EXPECTED OUTCOMES
		ASSESSMENT	INTERVENTIONS	

			H. If peritoneal-venous shunting is indicated
			  1. Preoperative
			    a. Teach patient how to use blow bottle (inspire against resistance)
			    b. Administer prophylactic antibiotics as ordered
			    c. Send appropriate blood specimens to laboratory
			    d. Witness consent
			  2. Postoperative
			    a. After patient returns from OR, place in low or semi-Fowler's position
			    b. Remind patient to use blow bottle four times a day, 15 min each time
			    c. Keep accurate hourly urine output records
			    d. Monitor Hct
			    e. Monitor for possible complications such as ascitic fluid leakage, infection at incision site, subcutaneous bleeding, disseminated intravascular coagulation, gastrointestinal bleeding, septicemia, shunt occlusion, and congestive heart failure	

Breathing pattern, ineffective: potential **Etiology** Upward pressure of ascitic fluid on diaphragm Decreased respiratory excursion	Labored, shallow respirations Dyspnea	Assess use of accessory muscles; rate, depth, and rhythm of respiration every _____	A. Place patient in high Fowler's position B. Administer and monitor O_2 therapy, if ordered C. See SCP in Ch. 1: Breathing pattern, ineffective	Optimal breathing pattern will be maintained
Knowledge deficit **Etiology** Cognitive limitation Lack of recall Lack of interest in learning	Erroneous perceptions Noncompliance with medical regimen Decreased mental status	Assess patient's general understanding of disease entity and management	A. Explain dietary restrictions in terms the patient understands. Have dietitian discuss restrictions in detail B. Explain rationale for monitoring weight C. Stress importance of weighing self at same time each day using same scale D. Explain importance of taking medications as prescribed. Discuss medication regimen thoroughly (name of medication, dosage, time schedule, and side effects) E. Assess readiness for alcoholic counseling. Refer to Alcoholics Anonymous. Arrange for social services to see patient	Patient will be able to verbalize basic understanding of the disease process and the steps he/she must follow to prevent recurrent hospitalizations

Crohn's Disease

NURSING DIAGNOSIS/ PATIENT PROBLEM	DEFINING CHARACTERISTICS	NURSING ORDERS		EXPECTED OUTCOMES
		ASSESSMENT	INTERVENTIONS	

Comfort, alteration in: abdominal pain
 Etiology
 Bowel inflammation and contractions of diseased bowel or colon
	Patient reports episodes of intermittent colicky abdominal pain associated with diarrhea and chronic joint pain
	 Abdominal rebound tenderness
	 Chronic pain in the joints
	 Hyperactive bowel sounds
	 Pallor
	 Diaphoresis
	 Anxiety
	 Restlessness
	 Fatigue
	 Malaise
	 Abdominal distention
	 Pain and cramps associated with eating
		A. Solicit patient's description of pain, documenting in patient's own words
		 B. Assess for presence of pain
		   1. Duration
		   2. Location
		   3. Frequency
		   4. Occurrence/ onset
		   5. Severity (scale 1-10, 10 most severe)
		 C. Solicit patient's perception of relief measures used to control pain
			A. Auscultate for bowel sounds every _____ and document
			 B. Check for rebound tenderness or distention every _____, and document
			 C. Provide adequate rest periods to facilitate sleep, comfort, and relaxation
			 D. Administer medications as ordered; evaluate and document effectiveness, and observe for signs of untoward effects
			 E. Institute use of diversional activities, hobbies, relaxation techniques, and psychosocial support systems to facilitate comfort and relaxation
			 F. Use techniques patient believes/ has found to be helpful if applicable
				Minimization or relief of pain will be evidenced by
				 A. Verbalization by patient
				 B. Calm, relaxed appearance of patient
				 C. Absence/decrease of abdominal distention/rebound tenderness

Nutrition, alteration in: less than body requirements **Etiology** Malabsorption Zinc deficiency Increased nitrogen loss with diarrhea Decreased intake	Nausea Diarrhea ≥10%-20% under ideal body weight Decreased/normal serum calcium, K^+, vitamins K and B_{12}, folic acid, and zinc Muscle wasting Pedal edema Skin lesions Poor wound healing	A. Document patient's *actual* weight on admission (*do not estimate*) B. Obtain nutritional history C. Assess for skin lesions, skin breaks, tears, decreased skin integrity, and edema of the extremities D. Assess serum electrolytes, Ca^+, vitamins K and B_{12}, folic acid, and zinc levels to determine actual or potential deficiencies E. Assess patterns of elimination: color, amount, consistency, frequency, odor, and for presence of steatorrhea F. Monitor laboratory analysis of serums as ordered; notify physician of abnormal results	A. Consult dietitian to review nutritional history, monitor calorie count, and assist patient with menu selection B. Weigh patient every _____, and document C. Document accurate I & O D. Encourage active/passive ROM to patient's tolerance E. Keep room as odor free as possible	Optimal nutritional state will be maintained

Originated by **Vivian Jones, RN**
Resource persons: **Susan Smalheiser, RN, MSN**
        Nola D. Johnson, RN

Crohn's Disease—cont'd

NURSING DIAGNOSIS/ PATIENT PROBLEM	DEFINING CHARACTERISTICS	NURSING ORDERS		EXPECTED OUTCOMES
		ASSESSMENT	INTERVENTIONS	
Fluid volume deficit: potential *Etiology* Presence of excessive diarrhea/nausea/ vomiting	Weight loss Decreased skin turgor Hypotension Concentrated urine	Assess hydration status: skin turgor, mucous membranes, I & O, weight, and vital signs every _____	A. Administer medications as ordered, noting possible reactions B. See SCP in Ch. 1: Fluid volume deficit (if problems exist)	Minimization of fluid volume deficit will be evidenced by A. Normal hydration status B. Weight stability or gain C. Adequate I & O balance D. Vital signs within normal range
Skin integrity, impairment of: potential *Etiology* Decreased nutritional status Frequent loose stools	Reddened or irritated areas over bony prominences Excoriated perianal skin	A. Assess skin integrity, noting color, texture, moisture, and temperature every _____ B. Assess psychologic conditions contributing to potential breakdowns, e.g., depression C. Assess perianal skin every _____	A. Use prophylactic pressure-relieving devices B. Encourage sitz baths every _____ and as needed to relieve pain from diarrhea C. Refer to SCP in Ch. 1: Skin integrity, impairment of: actual and potential (if problem exists)	Absence or healing of skin breakdown areas will be evidenced
Injury, potential for: infection *Etiology* Decreased nutrient absorption secondary to diseased bowel/ steroid therapy	Decreased total lymphocyte count Poor/diminished antigen response	A. Assess for poor wound healing, sore throat, fever B. Observe for fluid retention and cushingoid appearance ("moon-face") C. Monitor and record every _____: rectal temperature, heart rate, and respiratory rate. Notify physician if Heart rate: >_____ or <_____ Temperature: > _____or <_____ Respiratory rate: >_____ or <_____ D. If applicable 1. Monitor I & O every _____ 2. Check urine for sugar/acetone every _____. Notify physician if _____	A. Maintain good handwashing techniques B. Administer steroids as ordered, and notify physician of untoward effect	Risk of infection will be minimized

Continued.

Crohn's Disease—cont'd

NURSING DIAGNOSIS/ PATIENT PROBLEM	DEFINING CHARACTERISTICS	NURSING ORDERS		EXPECTED OUTCOMES
		ASSESSMENT	INTERVENTIONS	
Knowledge deficit of chronic disease process: potential **Etiology** Need for continuous and long-term management	Multiple questions by patient/significant others related to disease process and management Noncompliance with earlier therapy Anxiousness Depression	A. Assess understanding by patient/significant other of disease process and management B. Observe level of anxiety and learning capabilities	A. Set aside a specific uninterrupted time to spend with patient 1. Discuss disease process and management 2. Encourage patient/significant others to verbalize the disease process, management, concern, fears, and feelings. Document patient's understanding B. Make appropriate referrals 1. Dietary 2. Psychiatric counseling 3. Ostomy association C. Refer to SCP in Ch. 12: Grief over long-term illness/disability	Patient/significant others will be able to verbalize with understanding in a calm, relaxed manner A. Disease process and management B. Potential for complication C. Importance of follow-up care D. Medications and potential side effects

Enterocutaneous Fistula

NURSING DIAGNOSIS/ PATIENT PROBLEM	DEFINING CHARACTERISTICS	NURSING ORDERS		EXPECTED OUTCOMES
		ASSESSMENT	INTERVENTIONS	
Skin integrity, impairment of: actual/potential **Etiology** Continuous contact of bowel secretions with skin Altered nutritional/ metabolic state	Patient complains of burning, itching Skin is red, tender to touch Skin is excoriated	A. Assess condition of skin 1. Redness 2. Excoriation 3. Tenderness B. Assess amount, quality, and pH of secretions	A. Refer to SCP in Ch. 1: Skin integrity, impairment of B. Maintain intact perifistulous skin by 1. Dressing method a. Protect wound edges with Duoderm or Stomahesive barriers b. Change dressing every ____ to prevent secretion-soaked dressing from touching skin c. Use alternate methods (net panties, Montgomery straps) to hold dressing in place 2. Pouch method a. Choose appropriate pouch by evaluating (1) Skin condition (2) Size and shape of abdomen (3) Presence of current or recent sutures (4) Fistula site (5) Characteristics of fistula drainage b. Clean and prepare perifistulous skin c. Prepare pattern, and apply Stomahesive or Duoderm d. Fashion pouch; apply over skin barrier	Potential for altered skin integrity will be minimized

Originated by **Florencia Isidro-Sanchez, RN, BSN**
Resource person: **Audrey Klopp, RN, MS, CCRN, CS, ET**

Enterocutaneous Fistula—cont'd

NURSING DIAGNOSIS/ PATIENT PROBLEM	DEFINING CHARACTERISTICS	NURSING ORDERS		EXPECTED OUTCOMES
		ASSESSMENT	INTERVENTIONS	

			e. Attach to gravity drainage if indicated
			f. Keep pouch emptied routinely
			g. Change as necessary when leakage occurs
			3. Suction method (if neither pouch nor dressings maintain dryness)
			  a. Obtain permission from physician to place soft, fenestrated catheter near fistula site
			  b. Position and anchor catheter
			  c. Connect to low, intermittent suction device	

Fluid volume deficit: potential
Etiology
Loss of fluid via fistula
NPO status
	Decreased urine output
	Concentrated urine
	Dry mucous membranes
	Decreased venous filling
	Weight loss
	Increased heart rate
	Decreased skin turgor
	Abnormal electrolyte profile
	Complaints of thirst
	Complaints of weakness, dizziness
	Change in mental status
		A. Assess hydration status every ____
		  1. Skin turgor
		  2. Mucous membranes
		  3. I & O
		  4. Weight
		  5. Laboratory values
		  6. Vital signs
		  7. Subjective indicators
		B. Monitor serum and urine osmolality and specific gravity
			A. Document and report to physician signs/symptoms of electrolyte imbalance and/dehydration
			B. Administer parenteral fluids as ordered
			C. Offer ice chips and fluids as ordered/tolerated by patient
				Adequate fluid volume and electrolyte balance will be maintained as evidenced by
				A. Normal serum electrolytes
				B. Normal urine specific gravity
				C. Urine output of at least 30 ml/hour
				D. Moist mucous membranes

Nutrition, alteration in: less than body requirements
Etiology
Nutritional loss from fistula(s)
Decreased or bypassed absorptive surface
Prolonged therapeutic withholding of nutrients
	Complaints of weakness
	Weight loss
	Negative nitrogen balance
	Low serum albumin
	Low total iron-binding capacity (TIBC)
		A. See SCP in Ch. 1: Nutrition, alteration in: less than body requirements
		B. Assess nitrogen balance every ____
		C. Assess serum TIBC and serum albumin ____
		D. Inspect insertion site for redness, swelling, oozing, tenderness
		E. Weigh patient every ____
		F. Check electrolytes every ____
			A. Administer hyperalimentation per order; monitor response
			  1. Check vital signs every ____
			  2. Measure urine glucose every ____
			  3. Maintain flow rate (if administration is to be stopped or resumed for any reason, change flow rate to 50% of normal rate for at least 1 hour)
			  4. Change occlusive dressing and tubing q.48h. or as situation dictates
				Patient will be kept in anabolic state despite fistula

Continued.

Enterocutaneous Fistula—cont'd

NURSING DIAGNOSIS/ PATIENT PROBLEM	DEFINING CHARACTERISTICS	NURSING ORDERS		EXPECTED OUTCOMES
		ASSESSMENT	INTERVENTIONS	
Self-concept, disturbance in body image **Etiology** Continuous fecal drainage Fecal odor Necessity of pouch, dressings, and/or suction catheter	Verbalized concern of altered pattern of excretion Resistance to environmental change Reluctance to look at or touch pouch Altered socialization	A. Note verbal indications of altered self-concept/body image B. Note patient's willingness to socialize with family, friends, staff, other patients C. Note patient's involvement in self-care D. Note defensive behaviors regarding appearance	A. Encourage verbalization B. Provide adequate site care so that odor is minimized or eliminated	Patient will verbalize feelings about altered body image and understand the normal nature of his/her feelings
Anxiety/fear: potential **Etiology** Prolonged hospitalization Appearance of fistula/ pouch Painful/uncomfortable pouch/dressing changes Prolonged nutritional support Prolonged isolation from family, friends, work Possible need for surgery	Increased questioning Facial tension Verbalized anxiety Constant demands Restlessness Lack of participation in self-care Inability to accept care from others Derogatory comments about self	A. See SCP in Ch. 1: Anxiety/fear B. Assess for defining characteristics	A. Discuss present status/anticipated therapy B. Explain usual course of therapy C. Provide simple explanations and reassurance D. Take time to listen to fears, concerns E. Point out progress, however slight (e.g., decrease in drainage) F. Assist patient in using usual coping behaviors a. Express the normalcy of such feelings about oneself under the circumstances b. Verbalize for the nonverbal patient c. Reinforce that once the fistula is healed, elimination will return to normal d. Institute appropriate odor-control measures e. Initiate consultation with occupational/physical therapist to provide opportunity for exercise and activity f. Encourage use of distractors (television, radio, newspapers)	Anxiety/fear will be minimized as evidenced by appearance/behavior of patient and/or verbal report

Hemorrhoids/Hemorrhoidectomy

NURSING DIAGNOSIS/ PATIENT PROBLEM	DEFINING CHARACTERISTICS	NURSING ORDERS		EXPECTED OUTCOMES
		ASSESSMENT	INTERVENTIONS	
Fluid volume, excess in the superior (internal) and/or inferior (external) hemorrhoidal plexus (actual) **Etiology** Increased intravenous pressure in the hemorrhoidal plexus	Large, firm lumps protruding from rectum Presence of large, firm lumps on rectal examination Anal itching Painless, intermittent bleeding Constant discomfort and bleeding	A. Solicit patient's history of signs and symptoms of hemorrhoids. Severe bleeding and/or pain may be indications for proctoscopy to diagnose internal hemorrhoids vs rectal polyps B. Examine rectal area for external hemorrhoids 1. Covered by skin 2. Protruding from rectum 3. Likely to thrombose	A. Encourage patient to avoid prolonged standing or sitting B. Treat diarrhea/constipation (see SCP in Ch. 1: Bowel elimination, alteration in) C. Discuss patient's life-style and predisposing factors to development of hemorrhoids 1. Occupational standing or sitting for prolonged periods 2. Straining caused by diarrhea, constipation, vomiting, sneezing and coughing 3. Heart failure 4. Hepatic disease (abscess, hepatitis, cirrhosis) 5. Loss of muscle tone (old age, rectal surgery, pregnancy, episiotomy, anal intercourse) 6. Alcoholism 7. Anorectal infections D. Discuss self-care issues 1. Bowel elimination 2. Manual reduction of hemorrhoidal prolapse 3. Dietary habits (provide dietary consultation if necessary)	Complications/progression will be minimized
Comfort, alteration in: pain **Etiology** Thrombosis of external hemorrhoids or hemorrhoidal prolapse	Sudden rectal pain Large, firm lumps protruding from rectum Postoperative pain	A. Assess onset, duration, type of pain B. Elicit comfort factors used in past C. Examine rectal area	A. Provide local anesthetic as ordered B. Provide cold compresses C. Encourage warm sitz baths D. Administer analgesics as ordered for intractable pain (see SCP in Ch. 1: Comfort, alteration in: pain)	Pain/discomfort will be relieved or minimized
Fluid volume deficit: potential **Etiology** Bleeding hemorrhoids Preoperative or postoperative hemorrhoidal bleeding	Sudden, severe rectal bleeding Frequent, recurrent rectal bleeding (preoperative) Postoperative bleeding Pallor Weakness Fatigue	A. Assess onset and cause of bleeding B. Obtain history of past bleeding, frequency C. Assess vital signs every _____ D. Examine rectal area, assess amount of bleeding 1. Small, moderate, or profuse 2. Number of pads soaked	A. Notify physician of large amounts of blood loss and changes in vital signs B. Anticipate need for type and cross-match C. Prepare the patient for surgery if indicated D. If significant amount of bleeding occurs, see SCP in this chapter on acute GI bleeding **Postoperative care** A. Administer medications as ordered (Metamucil to increase stool bulk)	Rectal bleeding will be avoided or minimized

Originated by **Michele Knoll-Puzas, RN,C BS**

Continued.

Hemorrhoids/Hemorrhoidectomy—cont'd

NURSING DIAGNOSIS/ PATIENT PROBLEM	DEFINING CHARACTERISTICS	NURSING ORDERS		EXPECTED OUTCOMES
		ASSESSMENT	**INTERVENTIONS**	

			B. Keep wound site clean (sitz baths)
			 C. Instruct patient of importance of regular bowel habits
			 D. Discuss good anal hygiene
			   1. Suggest the use of plain, nonscented white toilet paper
			   2. Encourage the use of medicated astringent pads for cleansing
			   3. Discuss the avoidance of hand soaps and vigorous washing with hand towels
			 E. Provide patient with follow-up appointment and important telephone numbers	

Hepatic Encephalopathy

NURSING DIAGNOSIS/ PATIENT PROBLEM	DEFINING CHARACTERISTICS	NURSING ORDERS		EXPECTED OUTCOMES
		ASSESSMENT	**INTERVENTIONS**	

Cerebral metabolism, alteration in
 Etiology
 Liver failure
 Portal hypertension
 Ammonia intoxication
	Stage I
	 Minor mental aberrations
	 Confusion
	
	 Stage II
	 Asterixis
	 Apraxia
	
	 Stage III
	 Lethargy alternating with combativeness
	 Stupor
	 EEG slowing
	
	 Stage IV
	 Coma
	 Further EEG slowing
	 Fetor hepaticus
		A. Assess patient every ___ for signs and symptoms of
		   1. Stage I encephalopathy
		   2. Stage II encephalopathy
		   3. Stage III encephalopathy
		   4. Stage IV encephalopathy
		 B. Document improvement/deterioration in level of encephalopathy
		 C. Monitor vital signs (temperature, pulse, respiration, BP) every ___. Report heart rate greater than ___ or less than ___ to physician
			A. Stage I
			   1. Orient patient every ___ to time, place, and person
			     a. Place calendar and clock in room
			     b. Provide environmental stimulation (television, radio, newspaper, visitors)
			   2. Provide emotional support by reassuring patient that there is a physiologic cause of his/her confusion
			 B. Stages II and III
			   1. Evaluate and document presence of asterixis (flapping tremors) and apraxia every ___; notify physician of changes
			   2. Decrease intestinal bacteria content
			     a. Administer nonabsorbable antibiotics (neomycin, kanamycin) as or-
				Optimal stage of encephalopathy will be maintained

Originated by **Urakay Campbell, RN**
Resource person: **Audrey Klopp, RN, MS, CCRN, CS, ET**

Hepatic Encephalopathy—cont'd

NURSING DIAGNOSIS/ PATIENT PROBLEM	DEFINING CHARACTERISTICS	NURSING ORDERS		EXPECTED OUTCOMES
		ASSESSMENT	INTERVENTIONS	

		D. Monitor urine output every ___; report urine output less than ___ ml/hour to physician
		E. Monitor laboratory values reflecting hepatic function: serum transaminase, arterial serum ammonia level, bilirubin, coagulation profile, serum albumin, and protein every ___; report abnormalities to physician
		F. Monitor fluid and electrolyte balance, I and O every ___; serum electrolytes every ___; report imbalances to physician
			dered
			  b. Administer lactulose as ordered to alter colonic pH and stimulate evacuation
			3. Decrease ammonigenic potential
			  a. Order low-protein diet (20-40 g/daily)
			  b. Check drugs for ammonia content
			  c. Clean intestines of any old blood (lavage, suction, enemas)
			4. Evaluate factors that may increase cerebral sensitivity to ammonia (infections, acid-base imbalances)
			5. Protect patient from physical harm
			  a. Pad side rails
			  b. Keep bed in low position
			  c. Restrain, if necessary
			  d. Administer sedatives (nonhepatic metabolism) as ordered; document effectiveness; notify physician if dosage needs adjustment
			  e. Avoid oversedation that may precipitate coma
			C. Stage IV. See SCP in Ch. 3: Consciousness, alteration in level of	

Knowledge deficit **Etiology** Unfamiliarity with cause of encephalopathy	Inability to cope with illness Avoidance by significant others of patient's condition Inability to become involved in own care	A. Evaluate level of understanding by patient and significant others of patient's overall condition B. Evaluate patient's and family's ability and willingness to learn	A. Teach patient/significant others the cause of the encephalopathic event (noncompliance with drug or diet regime, alcohol abuse, infectious process) to minimize chance of recurrence B. Teach patient/significant others early signs of Stage I encephalopathy C. Teach patient/significant others purpose, dosage schedule, and expected action of medications D. Explain importance and rationale of low-protein diet, if prescribed for home use	Patient/significant others will verbalize understanding of precipitated event and will understand those measures prescribed to minimize recurrence

Hiatal Hernia: newly diagnosed

NURSING DIAGNOSIS/ PATIENT PROBLEM	DEFINING CHARACTERISTICS	NURSING ORDERS		EXPECTED OUTCOMES
		ASSESSMENT	INTERVENTIONS	
Comfort, alteration in Etiology Reflux of gastric contents secondary to Age (incidence higher in older individuals) Sex (incidence higher in females) Weakening of esophageal muscles Cancer of esophagus Kyphoscoliosis Diaphragm malformation Ascites Pregnancy Any increase in intraabdominal pressure (tumors)	Heart burn Chest pain Regurgitation Facial mask of pain Decreased physical activity Guarding behavior Moaning Alteration in sleep pattern Irritability Diaphoresis Change in pulse rate Change in BP	A. Assess for complaints of 1. Heartburn 2. Chest pain 3. Regurgitation B. Assess pain characteristics 1. Quality 2. Severity 3. Location 4. Onset 5. Duration 6. Precipitating factors 7. Relieving factors	A. Elevate head of bed at least 15 degrees B. Apply shock blocks to head of bed C. Use pillows behind back for support D. Respond quickly to complaints of pain or other discomfort E. Provide a quiet and restful environment F. Structure the patient's activities so that time is provided for rest periods G. Instruct the patient to avoid 1. Straining during a bowel movement 2. Wearing restricting clothes 3. Bending forward 4. Coughing H. Administer laxatives or stool softeners as ordered I. Discourage smoking (stimulates acid production and decreases bicarbonate secretions) J. Administer antacids as ordered	Discomfort because of gastric reflux will be minimized
Nutrition, alteration in: less than body requirement (potential) Etiology Gastric reflux Pain	Weight below body ideal for height and frame Documented, inadequate caloric intake Recent weight loss	A. Document patient's actual weight on admission B. Obtain a nutritional history C. Assess dental status D. Document foods that are known to cause symptoms	A. Order a bland diet B. Instruct patient 1. To eat frequent, small meals 2. To avoid eating for a minimum of 2 hours before lying down 3. To eat slowly C. Instruct patient to avoid spicy foods, fruit juices, alcohol, bedtime snacks, coffee, any other foods that bring on symptoms D. Encourage a reducing diet if patient is overweight (decreases abdominal pressure) E. Consult with dietitian for patient teaching 1. Foods to avoid 2. Foods high in spices 3. Caloric requirements needed to reduce weight F. Assist patient with meals when needed. G. Monitor blood and urine (electrolytes, BUN, creatinine, CBC, glucose) H. Maintain strict I & O I. Monitor caloric count if initiated by dietitian J. Obtain daily weights	Patient's optimal weight will be maintained

Originated by **Carolyn Bolton, RN**
Resource persons: **Sue A. Conneighton, RN, MSN**
    Audrey Klopp, RN, MS, CCRN, CS, ET

Hiatal Hernia: newly diagnosed—cont'd

NURSING DIAGNOSIS/ PATIENT PROBLEM	DEFINING CHARACTERISTICS	NURSING ORDERS		EXPECTED OUTCOMES
		ASSESSMENT	INTERVENTIONS	

Knowledge deficit
Etiology
Unfamiliarity with
  Diagnostic workup
  Disease process
  Treatment
	Lack of questions
	Multiple questions
	Verbalization of mis-information
		Evaluate patient's level of understanding about
		A. Diagnostic workup
		B. Disease process
		C. Treatment
			A. Explain the following to patient/significant others
			  1. Pathophysiology of hernia
			  2. Use of medications, including: purpose, proper administration, side effects
			  3. Diagnostic test, including purpose and special instructions
			    a. Chest x-ray film shows air behind heart
			    b. Barium study detects out-pouching, which will contain barium
			    c. Endoscopy and biopsy reveal perforation
			    d. Esophogeal motility detects esophageal abnormalities
			    e. pH studies detect gastric reflux
			    f. Guaiac stools detect blood in stool
			    g. CBC to determine possible blood loss
				Patient will verbalize an understanding of the diagnostic work-up

Activity intolerance
Etiology
Pain
Dyspnea
	Discomfort on exertion
	Dyspnea on exertion
	Patient's report of fatigue
	Abnormal heart rate
	Abnormal pulse rate
		A. Assess respiration before and after activities: quality and quantity
		B. Assess cardiac function before and after activity: pulse rate, BP, and skin color
		C. Assess mobility level
		D. Assess skin integrity; check for redness, tissue ischemia
		E. Assess potential physical injury with activity
		F. Assess need for assistance with ambulation
		G. Assess knowledge of family/significant others about immobility: what they know, need to know, misconceptions
		H. See SCP in Ch. 1: Activity intolerance
			A. Observe and document response to activity
			B. Report and document
			  1. Increased pulse
			  2. Palpitations
			  3. Decreased BP
			  4. Increased BP
			  5. Dyspnea
			  6. Fatigue
			  7. Chest pain
			C. Encourage rest periods between activities
			D. Gradually increase patient's responsibility for ADL
			E. Reassure patient that activity intolerance will improve as treatment progresses
				Optimal activity level will be maintained

Pancreatitis: acute

NURSING DIAGNOSIS/ PATIENT PROBLEM	DEFINING CHARACTERISTICS	NURSING ORDERS		EXPECTED OUTCOMES
		ASSESSMENT	INTERVENTIONS	
Comfort, alteration in **Etiology** Biliary tract disease (spasm of Vater's ampulla) Common channel involving biliary/pancreatic duct Reflux of duodenal contents Excessive alcohol intake Abdominal trauma/ surgery Infectious process Drugs	Epigastric pain or umbilical pain that radiates to the back/ shoulders Pain not relieved or made worse by certain narcotics Increasing pain when patient is in supine position Pain aggravated by food Abdominal distention with rebound tenderness Increased heart rate Splinted respirations Extreme restlessness Decreased or absent bowel sounds	A. Assess, document and report to physician pain characteristics 1. Quality 2. Location 3. Onset 4. Duration 5. History of previous attack B. Assess precipitating and relieving factors C. Observe for increased abdominal distention 1. Auscultate abdomen for bowel sounds every ____ 2. Report decrease or absence of bowel sounds D. Observe sclera and skin for jaundice E. Observe stool for fat, absence of bile, and odor	A. Reduce pancreatic stimulus by maintaining patient NPO or with a nasogastric tube to low suction as ordered B. Anticipate need for pain medication of ____ every _____ C. Respond immediately to complaints of pain D. Administer medication, such as anticholinergic drugs, as indicated: ____ every _____ E. Keep patient's environment conducive to rest F. Use repositioning and soothing back rubs G. Maintain bed rest H. Administer oral hygiene I. Use other measures for controlling discomfort 1. Provide quiet reassurance 2. Explain all procedures 3. Encourage communication with significant others 4. Remain with patient when extremely anxious or confused	Pain will be relieved or minimized
Fluid volume deficit **Etiology** Vomiting Decreased intake	Nausea and vomiting Abdominal distention Fever Hypotension Tachycardia Ileus	A. Assess hydration status 1. Skin turgor every _____ 2. BP every ____ 3. Weight every _____ 4. I & O every _____ 5. CVP every _____ B. Observe for complications of dehydration	A. Monitor vital signs, and report to physician 1. Heart rate > ____ or < ____ 2. Respiratory rate > ____ or < ____ 3. Systolic BP > ____ or < ____ 4. Diastolic BP > ____ or < ____ 5. CVP > ____ or < ____ 6. Temperature > ____ B. Maintain circulatory volume; replace fluid and electrolyte losses 1. Administer IV fluid of ____ at ____ ml/hour as ordered by physician 2. Administer volume expanders or blood transfusion as ordered by physician C. Keep the body metabolism of patient low 1. Maintain bed rest 2. Maintain body temperature in desired range	Maintenance of fluid volume and electrolyte balance will be evidenced by A. Absence of nausea and vomiting B. Absence of abdominal distention C. Normal body temperature D. Well-hydrated status E. Normotensive F. Heart rate within normal range G. Presence of bowel sounds

Originated by **Malu N. Viloria, RN, BSN**
Resource persons: **Audrey Klopp, RN, MS, CCRN, CS, ET**
Susan Galanes, RN, MS, TNS, CCRN

Pancreatitis: acute—cont'd

NURSING DIAGNOSIS/ PATIENT PROBLEM	DEFINING CHARACTERISTICS	NURSING ORDERS		EXPECTED OUTCOMES
		ASSESSMENT	INTERVENTIONS	
Breathing pattern, in-effective: potential **Etiology** Pain Abdominal distention or ascites Abdominal trauma or surgery Extravasation of pan-creatic enzymes	Dyspnea Shortness of breath Splinted respirations Tachypnea Cyanosis	A. Assess, document, and report to phy-sician 1. Respiratory rate every ____ 2. Breath sounds every ____ B. Note use of acces-sory muscles for breathing C. Assess position patient assumes for normal/easy breathing D. Assess for dys-pnea E. Note retractions and flaring nostrils F. Assess for changes in level of orientation	See SCP in Ch. 1: Breathing pat-tern, ineffective	Adequate airway and tissue oxygenation will be maintained
Skin integrity, alter-ation in: potential **Etiology** Dehydration Restricted/limited ac-tivity	Poor skin turgor Evidence of Stage I pressure areas	A. Assess skin integ-rity 1. Note color, moisture, and temperature 2. Ask patient about burning or itching B. Note patient's ac-tivity as ordered by physician 1. Bed rest 2. Turning from side to side C. Assess nutritional status 1. Diet as ordered 2. Daily weight	See SCP in Ch. 1: Skin integrity, impairment of	Absence of skin breakdown will be noted
Knowledge deficit **Etiology** Disease process of acute pancreatitis Strange environment	Multiple questions re-garding causes of pain, being NPO/or on a special diet, prognosis Questions indicating lack of information regarding hospital policies and proce-dures	A. Assess how much the patient and significant others understand about the disease process B. Assess knowledge of patient and sig-nificant others concerning such facts as hospital/ unit policy visiting hours, where to ask for patient's condition report, and relevant knowledge about hospital proce-dures	A. Explain hospital policies/proce-dures to patient and significant others 1. Visiting hours 2. Number of visitors 3. Telephone number to call to inquire about patient's con-dition B. Orient patient to bedside envi-ronment C. Explain any procedures that need to be done D. Instruct patient and significant others of the importance of calm and comfortable environ-ment	Patient and family will verbalize an under-standing of proce-dures and the envi-ronment

Peptic Ulcer

NURSING DIAGNOSIS/ PATIENT PROBLEM	DEFINING CHARACTERISTICS	NURSING ORDERS		EXPECTED OUTCOMES
		ASSESSMENT	INTERVENTIONS	
Alteration in mucosal barrier, erosion of gastric/duodenal mucosa by acidic gastric secretions **Etiology** Decreased mucosal resistance Defective mucus Inadequate mucosal blood flow Overproduction of gastric secretions Chronic gastritis Gastric irritants: aspirin, alcohol, caffeine, tobacco Dysfunctional pylorus (usually in elderly)	Pain (midepigastric) Indigestion or heartburn GI bleeding Diagnosis or history of peptic ulcer	Assess for signs and symptoms of ulcerations A. Events surrounding exacerbations and remission of symptoms B. Pain (see nursing diagnosis: Comfort, alteration in: pain) C. Nutrition (see nursing diagnosis: Nutrition, alteration in) D. Bleeding (see nursing diagnosis: Injury, potential for hemorrhage)	A. Assist with diagnostic evaluations as appropriate 1. Upper GI x-ray examinations 2. Gastric secretory studies 3. Upper GI endoscopy 4. Stools for occult blood 5. Esophagogastroduodenoscopy B. Administer medications as ordered 1. Antacids 2. Cimetidine (gastric secretions) 3. Anticholinergics (duodenal ulcers, gastric production) 4. Sedatives/tranquilizers (gastric ulcers only) C. Provide quiet, restful environment	Minimal mucosal erosion will be evidenced by a decrease in signs and symptoms and number of exacerbations
Comfort, alteration in: pain **Etiology** Lesion in gastric mucosa exposed to gastric secretions (hydrochloric acid, pepsin)	Patient reports or verbalizes pain (see Assessment)	A. Assess for site and type of pain 1. Heartburn 2. Indigestion 3. Back pain (pancreatic involvement) 4. Burning in throat 5. Localized midepigastric pain B. Assess for onset and duration of pain C. Assess for predisposing factors 1. Eating large meals 2. Ingestion of aspirin, alcohol, coffee, orange juice 3. Psychogenic factors D. Solicit techniques for relief of pain 1. Eating 2. Antacids 3. Analgesics	A. Provide medications as ordered 1. Antacids 2. Sedatives 3. Analgesics B. Maintain quiet, nonstressful environment C. Provide small frequent meals (4 to 6 per day) D. Encourage fluids (nonacidic) between meals E. Encourage patient to lie down after meals (see SCP in Ch. 1: Comfort, alteration in: pain)	Discomfort will be relieved or decreased

Originated by **Michele Knoll-Puzas, RN,C BS**

Peptic Ulcer—cont'd

NURSING DIAGNOSIS/ PATIENT PROBLEM	DEFINING CHARACTERISTICS	NURSING ORDERS		EXPECTED OUTCOMES
		ASSESSMENT	INTERVENTIONS	
Nutrition, alteration in: **Etiology** *Less than body requirements:* decreased intake caused by pain (gastric ulcers) *More than body requirements:* increased intake to relieve discomfort (duodenal ulcers)	**Less than body requirements** Loss of weight Inadequate caloric intake Pain upon eating **More than body requirements** Weight gain Reported dysfunctional eating pattern	A. Perform nutritional assessment B. Document weight on admission C. Obtain nutritional history	A. Consult dietitian when appropriate B. Document I & O, appetite C. Provide small meals, 4 to 6 times per day (see SCP in Ch. 1: Nutrition, alteration in: less than/more than body requirements)	Patient will practice good nutritional habits as evidenced by adequate, appropriate dietary intake
Injury, potential for: hemorrhage **Etiology** Perforation of gastric mucosal membrane	Frank, continual loss of bright, red blood in emesis Evidence of blood in stool (black, tarry, bright maroon)	A. Assess vital signs every ____ hours B. Assess emesis and stool for presence and amount of blood C. Maintain strict I & O D. Monitor electrolytes, CBC, and bleeding times	A. If bleeding occurs, see SCP in this chapter on acute GI bleeding	Potential effects of gastric perforation and hemorrhage will be minimized

Knowledge deficit related to cause and prevention of peptic ulcers
Etiology
New conditions
Unfamiliarity with treatment regime
	Frequent exacerbations
	Inability to verbalize causative and preventive factors
	Maintenance of dysfunctional destructive habits
		A. Assess level of understanding and ability to learn
		B. Assess current habits: dietary, smoking, drinking, medications
			A. Discuss ulceration site and common causative factors
			B. Discuss pain control, eating habits, and use of antacids and analgesics
			  1. Discuss avoidance of aspirin and all products containing aspirin
			  2. Provide rationale for use of antacids (cardiac and renal patients should use low-sodium antacids)
			  3. Warn patients of change in bowel habits caused by magnesium (diarrhea) or aluminum (constipation) in antacids
			  4. Discuss the use and side effects of anticholinergics (if appropriate)
			  5. Discuss avoidance of caffeine and alcohol, especially during an exacerbation
			  6. Encourage patients to stop smoking (increases secretion of gastric acids, decreases pancreatic bicarbonate secretions)
			C. Discuss signs and symptoms of perforation and hemorrhage
			D. Discuss availability of emergency care
			E. Discuss follow-up care and provide appropriate names and phone numbers if questions arise
				Patient will verbalize causative and preventive health care factors

Upper Gastrointestinal (UGI) Bleeding: acute

NURSING DIAGNOSIS/ PATIENT PROBLEM	DEFINING CHARACTERISTICS	NURSING ORDERS		EXPECTED OUTCOMES
		ASSESSMENT	INTERVENTIONS	
Fluid volume deficit **Etiology** Portal hypertension Altered mucosal barrier Retching Coagulopathy	Hematemesis Melena Cramping Signs/symptoms of hypovolemia: skin pallid and cool, altered mental status, oliguria, tachycardia, ischemic changes on ECG, dry mucous membranes, hypotension, thirst	A. Monitor amount, color, consistency of hematemesis, melena, or rectal bleeding B. Monitor BP for orthostatic changes (from patient lying prone to high Fowler's) *Note* orthostatic hypotension 1. >10 mm Hg drop; circulating blood volume decreased by 20% 2. >20-30 mm Hg drop; circulating blood volume decreased by 40% C. Assess for signs and symptoms of hypovolemia D. Monitor vital signs every ____ hours for evidence of hemorrhage. Notify physician of 1. Heart rate < ____ or > ____ 2. BP < ____ or > ____ 3. Respiratory rate < ____ or > ____ 4. CVP < ____, or > ____ 5. Urine output < ____ or > ____ E. Monitor patient's blood values. Notify physician of 1. Elevated PT/PTT 2. Elevation in liver function test 3. Prolonged bleeding time 4. Decrease in Hb/Hct	A. Insert a large-bore (no. 14, 16, 18 gauge) IV needle for fluid and blood B. Set up and assist with insertion of a central line C. Provide volume resuscitation as ordered by the physician 1. Give IV fluid at ____ ml/hour 2. Administer blood products a. Document number of units given b. Consider amount of citrate given D. Prepare for insertion of nasogastric Ewald evacuator or Sengstaken-Blakemore tube E. Lavage gastric tube with normal saline until clear F. Provide before and after procedures care 1. *Endoscopy* a. Explain purpose, and monitor vital signs before and during examination b. Administer topical anesthetic or sedatives c. Instruct the patient to remain NPO following the examination, until the gag reflex returns or until otherwise ordered 2. *Angiography* a. Explain procedure to patient and possibility of experiencing mild burning sensation during injection of contrast b. Position patient, and monitor vital signs throughout procedure c. Assess the insertion site every ____ following the procedure d. Turn the patient, and maintain skin integrity as permitted by hemodynamic status	Optimal fluid balance will be maintained The patient will verbalize understanding of the purpose and necessity of the procedure and of postprocedure care

Originated by **Marion C. Wallis, RN, CCRN**
Resource persons: **Susan Galanes, RN, MS, TNS, CCRN**
       Audrey Klopp, RN, MS, CCRN, CS, ET

Upper Gastrointestinal (UGI) Bleeding: acute—cont'd

NURSING DIAGNOSIS/ PATIENT PROBLEM	DEFINING CHARACTERISTICS	NURSING ORDERS		EXPECTED OUTCOMES
		ASSESSMENT	INTERVENTIONS	
		F. Assess venipuncture and incision sites for prolonged bleeding G. Assess patient for hematomas or petechiae		

Injury, potential for: complications of vasopressin (Pitressin) therapy
Etiology
Vasoconstriction
Antidiuretic effect
	Anginal pain
	ST segment changes on ECG
	Sinus bradycardia
	Side effects: tremors, sweating, vertigo, pounding in head, abdominal cramps, circumoral pallor, nausea/vomiting, flatus, urticaria, fluid retention
		A. Assess for side effects of vasopressin
		B. Monitor vital signs every ____ hours
		C. Assess peripheral pulses (rate, regularity) and capillary refill
		D. Assess for abdominal distention, and record abdominal girth
			A. Administer vasopressin per physician's orders
			B. If side effects occur
			  1. Stop infusion of vasopressin drip
			  2. Notify physician immediately
			  3. Have atropine on hand for decreased heart rate
			  4. Provide comfort and assurance for the patient
				Side effects from vasopressin therapy will be minimized

Anxiety/fear: potential **Etiology** Acute care setting Fear of the unknown Pain or discomfort	Restlessness Labile moods Depression Diaphoresis Nausea Anorexia Palpitations	Assess patient for signs and symptoms of anxiety, and if present, see SCP in Ch. 1: Anxiety/fear		Anxiety will be relieved or minimized
Knowledge deficit **Etiology** Unfamiliarity with disease process and treatment	Questioning Repeated admissions to the hospital for GI bleeding Verbalized misconceptions	Assess knowledge base and readiness to learn	A. Explain to patient the need to avoid large consumptions of alcohol or salicylates over a long period of time B. Inform patient of the signs and symptoms associated with the etiology of the disease and what interventions to take	The patient will verbalize an understanding of the cause of the ongoing disease process and be aware of signs and symptoms that it may precipitate

THERAPEUTIC INTERVENTIONS

Appendectomy

NURSING DIAGNOSIS/ PATIENT PROBLEM	DEFINING CHARACTERISTICS	NURSING ORDERS		EXPECTED OUTCOMES
		ASSESSMENT	INTERVENTIONS	

Injury, potential for: infection
 Etiology
 Appendectomy incision
	Febrile
	 Increased WBC
	 From incision site
	   Redness
	   Swelling
	   Drainage
	   Tenderness
	   Foul odor
		A. Assess incision site q.8h. for
		   1. Redness
		   2. Swelling
		   3. Drainage (note color and amount)
		   4. Tenderness
		   5. Foul odor
		 B. Assess vital signs q.4h., especially temperature
			A. Notify physician for any symptoms of infection
			 B. Keep incision clean and dry after initial dressing change
			 C. Administer antibiotics as ordered by physician
			 D. Administer antipyretic as ordered by physician
			 E. Instruct patient how to prevent tension on suture line by
			   1. Splinting
			   2. Bending of legs
			 F. Instruct patient in the following before discharge
			   1. Cleansing of incision
			   2. Bathing
			   3. Exercise
			   4. Proper diet
			   5. When to notify physician
				A. Patient will not develop a postoperative infection as evidenced by
				   1. Intact, clean incision site
				   2. Normal temperature
				 B. Patient will correctly verbalize home care instructions before discharge

Comfort, alteration in: pain
 Etiology
 Incision
	Subjective
	 Verbal complaints of pain and discomfort
	
	 Objective
	 Tachycardia
	 Tachypnea
	 Elevated BP
	 Facial grimacing
	 Little or no movement
	 Guarding of abdomen
	 Withdrawal
	 Diaphoresis
		A. Solicit patient's description of pain
		 B. Assess pain characteristics
		   1. Quality
		   2. Severity
		   3. Location
		   4. Duration
		 C. Assess relief obtained from analgesics
			A. Anticipate need for analgesics or additional methods of pain relief
			 B. Maintain a quiet, relaxed atmosphere
			 C. Alternate rest periods with activity
			 D. Refer to SCP in Ch. 1: Comfort, alteration in: pain
				Pain will be relieved or minimized

Originated by **Ruth E. Novitt, RN, MSN**

Appendectomy—cont'd

NURSING DIAGNOSIS/ PATIENT PROBLEM	DEFINING CHARACTERISTICS	NURSING ORDERS		EXPECTED OUTCOMES
		ASSESSMENT	INTERVENTIONS	
Airway clearance, in-effective: potential **Etiology** Anesthesia Pain	Abnormal breath sounds Frequent, congested cough Tachypnea Dyspnea	A. Assess respirations q.4h. or ____ for 1. Rate 2. Quality 3. Depth 4. Pattern 5. Use of accessory muscles B. Assess cough for 1. Frequency 2. Type C. Assess any sputum for 1. Color 2. Consistency 3. Amount D. Auscultate lungs q.4h. to assess air exchange E. See SCP in Ch. 1: Airway clearance, ineffective	A. Encourage patient to change position in bed frequently B. Elevate head of bed 30-45 degrees C. Encourage patient to deep breathe and cough at least q.2h. D. Instruct patient on how to splint abdominal incision E. Provide humidity if needed	Airway will be freed of secretions
Fluid volume deficit: potential **Etiology** NPO Increased metabolic requirements Bleeding from operative site	Dry mucous membranes Concentrated urine Decreased urine output Increased sodium level Frequent emesis Tachycardia Hypotension Hemoconcentration Thirst Restlessness Excessive bleeding from incision site	A. Assess fluid volume status (see Defining Characteristics) B. Assess incision site for bleeding C. Monitor electrolytes D. Refer to SCP in Ch. 1: Fluid volume deficit	A. Maintain adequate hydration B. Maintain strict I & O C. Monitor daily weights D. Monitor vital signs E. Report urine output <30 ml/ hour for 2 consecutive hours F. Report significant bleeding to physician	Adequate fluid and electrolyte balance will be maintained as evidenced by A. Electrolytes within normal limits B. Urine output ≥30 ml/hour C. Moist mucous membranes and good skin turgor
Fear/anxiety **Etiology** Emergency surgery Hospitalization	Frequent questions or calling of nurse Withdrawal Anger/hostility Restlessness Tension Tachypnea Elevated BP Tachycardia	A. Assess patient's level of anxiety B. Assess patient's pattern of coping C. Assess involvement of family or significant other D. See SCP in Ch. 1: Anxiety/fear	A. Establish rapport with patient and his/her family or significant other B. Encourage ventilation of feelings and concern C. Approach patient in a calm and relaxed manner D. Reassure patient that someone is here at all times if he needs something E. Medicate for pain as needed	Patient will exhibit a decreased level of anxiety as evidenced by A. Calm, relaxed appearance B. Verbalization of fears and feelings

Cholecystectomy

NURSING DIAGNOSIS/ PATIENT PROBLEM	DEFINING CHARACTERISTICS	NURSING ORDERS		EXPECTED OUTCOMES
		ASSESSMENT	INTERVENTIONS	

Fluid volume deficit, intravascular: potential
Etiology
Excessive wound/T tube loss
Excessive nasogastric (NG) tube output
Excessive third-space fluid losses
	Signs/symptoms of dehydration and shock
	Abnormal serum electrolyte profile
	Nausea, vomiting
	Tachycardia
	Fever, diaphoresis
	Apprehension
	Dark, tea-colored urine
		A. Monitor vital signs; note trends denoting dehydration or shocklike states
		B. Assess level of consciousness every ____, noting increase in apprehension or other changes
		C. Assess fluid balance every ____, documenting and reporting urine output < ____ ml
		D. Assess surgical dressings for amount and character of drainage every ____
		E. Assess T tube for patency every ____
		F. Assess drainage from T tube for amount and color every ____
		G. Assess patency of NG tube; note amount and color of output
			A. Maintain strict I & O and daily weight for ____ days
			B. Document any change in condition as related to assessments
			C. Inform service immediately if
			  1. Signs/symptoms of dehydration or shock occur
			  2. T tube is dislodged or not patent
			  3. Excessive drainage is noted on dressings
			D. Irrigate NG tube p.r.n. and at least every shift
			E. Check function of drains every ____; clamp T tube only if physician orders
			F. Administer IV fluids (____) at rate of ____ /hour as ordered
				Optimal fluid balance will be maintained

Injury, potential for infection: systemic **Etiology** Dislodgement of T tube with bacterial ingression Kinking, clotting off of tube with resultant increase in biliary pressure and possible leak of bile into peritoneum	Obviously displaced T tube Absence of bile flow Complaints of abdominal pain Elevated WBC count Jaundice	A. Monitor temperature and WBC counts every ____ B. Assess patency of T tube every ____ C. Observe and record color of urine and stool daily D. Monitor and record bile drainage every hour for 24 hours, then every ____ NOTE: Bile drainage should be bright yellow to dark green and have an acrid odor. Daily drainage should be <500 ml	A. If T tube is partially displaced, *do not remove it any further;* notify physician immediately B. Report any pus or other exudate from T tube site C. Position the drainage bag to promote gravity (below the level of the insertion site) D. Send stool/urine for bile pigment analysis as ordered E. When patient ambulates, place T tube in robe pocket or fasten below waist F. Change dressing to T tube site every ____, using aseptic technique	Risk of systemic infection will be minimized

Originated by: **Dorothy Lewis, RN,C BSN**
Resource person: **Carol Burkhart, RN, BSN, CCRN**

Cholecystectomy—cont'd

NURSING DIAGNOSIS/ PATIENT PROBLEM	DEFINING CHARACTERISTICS	NURSING ORDERS		EXPECTED OUTCOMES
		ASSESSMENT	INTERVENTIONS	
Breathing pattern, in-effective **Etiology** Painful surgical inci-sion Anxiety Decreased compliance secondary to general anesthesia Decreased diaphrag-matic movement	Shallow respirations Poor coughing efforts Adventitious breath sounds Guarded respirations with splinting	A. Perform respirato-ry assessment every ___; report any changes to physician B. See SCP in Ch. 1: Breathing pattern, ineffective	A. Explain importance of turning, coughing, and deep-breathing to patient B. Assist patient in use of incen-tive spirometer every ___ while awake C. Assist patient to change posi-tion every ___ while in bed; assist with ambulation D. Administer pain medications and other relieving measures as needed E. Teach patient to splint own in-cision while deep-breathing and coughing	Effects of altered breathing pattern will be minimized and complications prevented through aggressive attention to movement, coughing, and deep-breathing
Knowledge deficit re-lated to nutrition after cholecystectomy **Etiology** Unfamiliarity with postoperative nutri-tion plan	Patient/significant others unaware of need to alter diet following surgery Patient/significant others observed se-lecting fatty foods from menu	A. Take diet history regarding intake of fatty foods B. Note type of food selected from menu	A. Advise patient to avoid exces-sive fatty food intake B. Advise patient/significant others that no special food preparation is required. C. Encourage patient to maintain a well-balanced diet, avoiding extremes D. Consult dietitian if necessary	Patient/significant others will verbalize understanding of importance of eating a well-balanced diet, low in fat in-take following cho-lecystectomy
Knowledge deficit **Etiology** Unfamiliarity with T tube care after dis-charge	Multiple questions from patient/signifi-cant others Observed inability of patient/significant others to care for T tube	A. Assess ability of patient/significant others to under-stand care of T tube and site B. Assess willingness of patient/signifi-cant others to care for T tube and site	A. Explain purpose and location of T tube at a level patient/signifi-cant others can understand B. Inform patient/significant others to observe for jaundice, tea-colored urine, clay-colored stools, and signs/symptoms of peritonitis, and to notify physi-cian if any of these occur C. Teach patient/significant others to change dressing at site, using clean technique D. Teach patient/significant others proper tube clamping if indi-cated E. Stress importance of follow-up care	Patient/significant others will verbalize basic understanding of purpose for dis-charge with T tube in place, and will demonstrate safe care of tube and site

Enteral Tube Feeding

NURSING DIAGNOSIS/ PATIENT PROBLEM	DEFINING CHARACTERISTICS	NURSING ORDERS		EXPECTED OUTCOMES
		ASSESSMENT	INTERVENTIONS	
Airway clearance, ineffective: potential **Etiology** Aspiration as a result of Lack of gag reflex Poor positioning Overfeeding	Abnormal breath sounds Shortness of breath Coughing Diaphoresis Anxiety Restlessness Poor skin color	A. Assess correct position of tube before initiation of feeding B. Assess presence of gag reflex every ____ C. Assess level of consciousness before administration of feeding D. See SCP in Ch. 1: Airway clearance, ineffective	A. Position of patient 1. Elevate head of bed to 30 degrees for 30 min following feeding unless contraindicated 2. Document patient's baseline respiratory status 3. Monitor patient's respiratory status throughout feeding B. Placement of tube 1. Check tube placement before feeding by injecting air and listening over stomach 2. Check for residual feeding every ____ 3. Document correct tube placement and amount of residual feeding obtained C. In case of aspiration 1. Stop tube feeding 2. Monitor vital signs 3. Assess respiratory status 4. Notify physician 5. Keep head of bed elevated 6. Suction as necessary 7. Document time feeding was stopped, patient's appearance, and changes in respiratory status NOTE: a. High-risk patients are those who are comatose, who have decreased gag reflex, or who are unable to tolerate elevated head of bed b. Nasoduodenal or gastroduodenal feedings are preferred for high-risk patients	Potential for aspiration will be minimized
Nutrition, alteration in: less than body requirements **Etiology** Mechanical problems during administration of feedings such as Clogging of tube Inaccurate flow rate Incorrect tube administration set for pump Defective tube administration set	Continued weight loss Persistent anergy	A. Monitor equipment for proper functioning B. Assess tubing for passage of formula C. Assess nitrogen balance every ____ D. See SCP in Ch. 1: Nutrition, alteration in: less than body requirements	A. Care of tube 1. Flush tubing with ____ ml water following feedings or every ____ hours 2. Crush medications and dilute with water; use elixir form when possible 3. Flush tube following administration of medications 4. Check tubing connections B. Care of pump 1. Keep alarms on 2. Attach to outlet unless patient is walking	Nutritional support will be maximized

Originated by **Mary Martinat, RN, BSN**
Resource person: **Susan Smalheiser, RN, MSN**

Enteral Tube Feeding—cont'd

NURSING DIAGNOSIS/ PATIENT PROBLEM	DEFINING CHARACTERISTICS	NURSING ORDERS		EXPECTED OUTCOMES
		ASSESSMENT	INTERVENTIONS	
Bowel elimination, alteration in: diarrhea (potential) **Etiology** Intolerance to tube feeding because of Hyperosmolarity Temperature of feeding Rate of delivery Anxiety Bacterial contamination of feeding	Abdominal cramps Abdominal pain Frequency of stools Loose, liquid stools Urgency Hyperactive bowel sounds	A. Assess bowel sounds every ____ B. Assess number and character of stools C. See SCP in Ch. 1: Bowel elimination, alteration in: diarrhea	A. Delivery of formula 1. Begin feedings at ____ strength and at ____ ml/ hour 2. Increase rate and strength to prescribed amount but not at the same time 3. Administer feedings at room temperature 4. Monitor I & O 5. Change formula every ____ hours 6. Change setup daily 7. Administer feedings in a calm, relaxed atmosphere 8. Notify physician of any intolerance B. Patient activity 1. Encourage light activity following feeding 2. Document activity tolerance C. Bowel activity 1. Record frequency and consistency of all stools 2. When recording intake, differentiate tube feedings	Intolerance to feeding will be minimized
Fluid volume deficit: potential **Etiology** Osmolarity of feeding formula	Dry mucous membrane Poor skin turgor Elevated temperature Changes in mental status Azotemia	A. Assess patient for change in mental status every ____ B. See SCP in Ch. 1: Fluid volume deficit	A. Provide free water to patient: ____ ml as prescribed B. Document baseline mental status C. Document changes in mental status; notify physician	Fluid volume will be maintained as evidenced by A. Adequate urine output B. Good skin turgor C. Moist mucous membranes D. Normal urine specific gravity
Glucose and fat metabolism, alteration in **Etiology** Continuous feeding, rather than a physiologic intermittent bolus schedule	Glucose >120, flushed skin, headache, nausea, vomiting, fatigue, fruity breath Glucose <70, hunger, sweating, pallor, cold skin, tremor, blurry vision, fatigue, dizziness Foul-smelling, greasy stools	A. Review laboratory values B. Assess patient for mental status changes and other defining characteristics C. Assess stool for odor and greasiness	A. Glucose 1. Monitor blood glucose level by chemstick every ____ 2. Monitor urine sugar/acetone q.i.d., and notify physician if ____ 3. Administer hyperglycemic/ antihyperglycemic agents as ordered 4. Notify physician if feeding is stopped for any reason B. Fat 1. Monitor bowel sounds every ____ hours 2. Monitor number and characteristics of stools 3. Notify physician of any change in stools	Potential alteration in glucose and fat metabolism will be minimized

Continued.

Enteral Tube Feeding—cont'd

NURSING DIAGNOSIS/ PATIENT PROBLEM	DEFINING CHARACTERISTICS	NURSING ORDERS		EXPECTED OUTCOMES
		ASSESSMENT	INTERVENTIONS	
Comfort, alteration in: pain **Etiology** Dry mucous membranes and tape irritation	Dry, cracked lips Soiled tape Reddened area where tube is positioned Difficulty swallowing Verbalized discomfort	A. Assess mucous membranes B. Assess for reddened areas C. See SCP in Ch. 1: Comfort, alteration in: pain	A. Provide skin/mucous membrane care. Change position of tube at nares, and retape q.12h. B. Provide mouth care every q.4h C. Allow hard candy or gum if permissible	Pain will be minimized or relieved
Social isolation **Etiology** Change in body image	Patient stays in room and resists environmental changes Patient refuses visitors	Assess patient's behavior pattern during contact with significant others or staff	A. Allow time for verbalization B. Arrange privacy for visitation C. Encourage patient and significant others to participate in daily care D. Encourage activity outside of room if allowable	Antisocial behavior will be minimal as evidenced by patient interacting with significant others and staff
Self-concept, disturbance in **Etiology** Change in body image: feeding tube extending from nose	Patient verbalizes feelings of not being able to eat normally Patient will not look at tube Patient will not participate in daily hygiene	A. Assess patient's use of defense mechanisms in past crises B. Assess patient's support systems	A. Explain reason for tube feeding B. Allow patient time to express feelings and ask questions C. Allow patient/significant others to help with feedings D. Allow self-care to the extent possible	Patient will verbalize need for enteral feedings
Knowledge deficit regarding need for nutritional support **Etiology** New procedure and treatment	Patient verbalizes inaccurate information Patient exhibits inappropriate behavior Patient asks questions regarding tube feeding	A. Assess for prior experience with tube feeding B. Assess patient's knowledge regarding tube feeding	A. Demonstrate feedings and tube care B. Allow return demonstration C. Document progress	Patient will verbalize reasons for tube feedings and begin to participate in self-care

Fecal Ostomy (Ileostomy/Colostomy)

NURSING DIAGNOSIS/ PATIENT PROBLEM	DEFINING CHARACTERISTICS	NURSING ORDERS		EXPECTED OUTCOMES
		ASSESSMENT	INTERVENTIONS	

Preoperative knowledge deficit
 Etiology
 Lack of previous similar experience
 Need for additional information
	Verbalized need for information
	 Verbalized misinformation/misconceptions
		A. Assess previous surgical experience
		 B. Inquire as to information given by surgeon regarding formation of ostomy (i.e., purpose, site)
		 C. Ascertain (from chart, physician) whether stoma will be permanent or temporary
			A. Reinforce and reexplain proposed procedure
			 B. Answer questions directly and honestly
			 C. Use diagrams, pictures, and AV equipment to explain
			   1. Anatomy, physiology of GI tract
			   2. Pathophysiology necessitating ostomy
			   3. Proposed location of stoma
			 D. Explain need for pouch in terms of loss of sphincter
			 E. Show patient actual pouch or one similar to one he/she will have postoperatively
			 F. Allow patient to wear pouch preoperatively, if desired
				A. Patient will understand alteration in normal GI anatomy or physiology requiring the surgical creation of the ostomy
				 B. Patient will recognize that surgical loss of sphincter (or loss of function) will necessitate wearing a pouch

Originated by **Audrey Klopp, RN, MS, CCRN, CS, ET**
 Nola D. Johnson, RN

Fecal Ostomy (Ileostomy/Colostomy)—cont'd

NURSING DIAGNOSIS/ PATIENT PROBLEM	DEFINING CHARACTERISTICS	NURSING ORDERS		EXPECTED OUTCOMES
		ASSESSMENT	INTERVENTIONS	
Fear/anxiety **Etiology** Proposed creation of ostomy Previous contact with poorly rehabilitated ostomate	Verbally expresses concern/anxiety Tense facial expression Restlessness Multiple questions Lack of questions	A. Assess patient's level of anxiety; note nonverbal signs B. Elicit from patient (or other source) normal coping strategies	A. Ask patient to describe in detail what it is that is causing fear/anxiety B. Correct misconceptions, fill in knowledge gaps C. Offer a visit from rehabilitated ostomate D. See SCP in Ch. 1: Anxiety/fear	Level of anxiety will be decreased or manageable
Grief, anticipatory **Etiology** Proposed loss of fecal continence Anticipated loss of function, love, job, body image	Crying Rage Questioning Bargaining with self, God, health care professionals Withdrawal from usual relationships	A. Recognize the signs of anticipatory grief (see Defining Characteristics) B. Assess perceived loss of 1. Life 2. Function 3. Social status 4. Love 5. Control 6. Other	A. Encourage patient to verbalize feelings B. Assure patient that such grief is real, expected, and appropriate	Anticipatory grief will be recognized and facilitated
Bowel elimination, alteration in **Etiology** Preoperative preparation for surgery	Orders for dietary restriction, cathartics, cleansing enemas	Assess preparedness of bowel for surgery: clear/near clear returns on enemas	A. Explain necessity of bowel preparation B. Provide privacy during evacuation C. Allow for rest periods between enemas D. Observe for weakness, bradycardia, perianal discomfort	Bowel will be sufficiently prepared for surgical procedure
Self-care deficit, toileting: potential **Etiology** Need for preoperative stoma site marking	Presence of old abdominal scars Presence of bony prominences on anterior abdominal surface Presence of skin folds over abdomen Extreme obesity Pendulous breasts	Assess abdominal surface for presence of A. Old scars B. Bony prominences C. Skin folds D. Contour E. Visibility to patient	A. Indelibly mark proposed stoma site in area where 1. Patient can easily see 2. Patient can easily reach 3. Scars, bony prominences, skin folds are avoided 4. Hip flexion does not change contour B. Note usual sites for stoma 1. *Ileostomy:* lower right quadrant 2. *Ascending colostomy:* right upper or lower quadrant 3. *Transverse colostomy:* mid-waist or just below mid-waist 4. *Descending and sigmoid colostomies:* lower left quadrant C. If possible, have patient wear pouch over proposed site; evaluate effectiveness 12 to 24 hours after applying pouch	Potential for self-care deficit will be minimized by careful, individualized selection of appropriate stoma site

Continued.

Fecal Ostomy (Ileostomy/Colostomy)—cont'd

NURSING DIAGNOSIS/ PATIENT PROBLEM	DEFINING CHARACTERISTICS	NURSING ORDERS		EXPECTED OUTCOMES
		ASSESSMENT	INTERVENTIONS	

Postoperative bowel elimination, alteration in
Etiology
Surgical diversion of fecal stream
	Structural or functional absence of anal sphincter
	Presence of stoma
		A. Assess stoma every _____ postoperatively
		  1. Color
		  2. Shape
		  3. Size
		  4. Presence of supportive device (rod, catheter)
		  5. Function (flatus, stool)
		  6. Drainage that is not stool
		B. Assess bowel activity every _____
		  1. Stool (amount, consistency color, odor, frequency)
		  2. Bowel sounds
		  3. Flatus
		C. Note typical fecal output from newly created stomas
		  1. *Ileostomy:* mucoid, dark green or yellow liquid within 6 to 8 hours postoperatively
		  2. *Colostomies:* thin, brownish-mushy stool within 1 to 4 days postoperatively
		NOTE: A small amount of serosanguinous drainage in the first 24 to 48 hours is normal
			A. Apply pouch to stoma as soon as possible postoperatively to protect other surgical sites from fecal contamination and to protect peristomal skin
			B. Notify physician if stoma appears dusky or blue
				Bowel function via the stoma will return within 8 hours (ileostomy) or 1 to 4 days (colostomy)

Comfort, alteration in: pain **Etiology** Surgical incision(s)	Facial mask of pain Verbal complaints of pain Inability to turn; cough, deep breathe, get out of bed Decreased concentration	A. Assess level of comfort B. Elicit from patient possible sources of discomfort/recommendations for relief	A. Institute pain relief measures, incorporating patient's suggestions when possible B. See SCP in Ch. 1: Comfort, alteration in: pain	Patient will express relief from pain

Fecal Ostomy (Ileostomy/Colostomy)—cont'd

NURSING DIAGNOSIS/ PATIENT PROBLEM	DEFINING CHARACTERISTICS	NURSING ORDERS		EXPECTED OUTCOMES
		ASSESSMENT	INTERVENTIONS	
Self-concept, disturbance in: body image Etiology Presence of stoma; loss of fecal continence	Verbalized feelings about stoma and altered bowel elimination Refusal to discuss, acknowledge, touch, or care for stoma, pouch	A. Assess perception of change in body structure and function B. Assess perceived impact of change C. Note verbal references to stoma, altered bowel elimination	A. Acknowledge appropriateness of emotional response to perceived change in body structure and function B. Assist patient in looking at, touching, and caring for stoma when ready C. Reoffer a visit from a rehabilitated ostomate D. See SCP in Ch. 1: Body image: disturbance in	Patient will begin to acknowledge feelings about altered bowel function, stoma, and begin incorporating changes into self-concept
Knowledge deficit regarding self-ostomy care Etiology Presence of new stoma Lack of similar experience	Demonstrated inability to empty and change pouch Verbalize need for information regarding diet, odor, activity, hygiene, clothing, interpersonal relationships, equipment purchase, financial concerns	A. Assess 1. Ability to empty and change pouch 2. Ability to care for peristomal skin and identify problems, potential problems 3. Appropriateness in seeking assistance 4. Knowledge regarding a. Diet b. Activity c. Hygiene d. Clothing e. Interpersonal relationships f. Equipment purchase g. Financial reimbursement for ostomy equipment	A. Build on information given preoperatively B. Plan and share teaching plan with patient C. Begin psychomotor teaching during first and subsequent applications of pouch D. Gradually transfer responsibility for pouch emptying and changing to patient E. Allow at least one opportunity for supervised return demonstration of pouch change before discharge F. Instruct patient on the following 1. Diet a. *For ileostomy:* balanced diet; special care in chewing high-fiber foods (popcorn, peanuts, coconut, vegetables, string beans, olives); increased fluid intake during hot weather, vigorous exercise b. *For colostomy:* balanced diet; no foods are specifically contraindicated, although certain foods (eggs, fish, green leafy vegetables, carbonated beverages) may increase flatus and fecal odor 2. Odor control is best achieved by eliminating odor-causing foods from diet; oral agents and deodorant are available 3. Activity should not be restricted because of stoma or pouch; direct forceful blows to the stoma should be avoided	Patient will be capable of self-ostomy care on discharge

Continued.

Fecal Ostomy (Ileostomy/Colostomy)—cont'd

NURSING DIAGNOSIS/ PATIENT PROBLEM	DEFINING CHARACTERISTICS	NURSING ORDERS		EXPECTED OUTCOMES
		ASSESSMENT	INTERVENTIONS	
			4. *Hygiene.* Showers or baths may be taken with pouch on or off (spillage of stool may occur if pouch is removed, but this is no consequence, except aesthetically)	
			5. *Clothing.* There is no need for special clothing. Rigid metal strap in undergarments should be avoided	
			6. *Interpersonal relationships.* It is not necessary to tell everyone about stoma, although most patients find it less of a burden if shared with loved ones	
			7. *Sexual relationships.* The stoma will not be harmed during sexual intercourse. Extra measures toward hygiene or use of lingerie may lessen anxiety for both partners	
			8. Equipment should be purchased from a reputable dealer who carries a wide selection and can offer consultation (send a written list of needed equipment and supplies home with patient)	
			9. Because equipment required for stoma care is considered by law as prostheses, most public or private insurances reimburse all or part of the cost of equipment	
			10. *Need for follow-up.* Follow-up care with surgeon or enterostomal therapist is recommended every 1-2 months for 6-12 months postoperatively	
			11. *Support groups.* Give patient phone numbers to local ostomy support groups	

Gastrostomy Tube

NURSING DIAGNOSIS/ PATIENT PROBLEM	DEFINING CHARACTERISTICS	NURSING ORDERS		EXPECTED OUTCOMES
		ASSESSMENT	INTERVENTIONS	

Nutrition, alteration in: less than body requirements
Etiology
Complete obstruction of the esophagus
Obstruction resulting from scar tissue (lye burn)
Carcinomatous growth
Unconscious or debilitated patient
	Loss of weight with or without adequate caloric intake ≥10%-20% under ideal body weight
	Dehydration
	Anorexia
	Negative nitrogen balance
	Inability to swallow
		A. Check gastrostomy tube placement before each feeding by aspirating any gastric residual feeding
		B. Check for the presence or absence of bowel sounds before tube feeding is initiated
		C. Assess tube placement q.4h. during continuous gastrostomy feeding
		D. Document patient's base-line respiratory status
			A. Explain feeding procedure to patient
			B. Place patient in high Fowler's position (unless contraindicated)
			C. Assess patient's respiratory status during feeding and at two 1-hour intervals after completion of feeding
			D. Irrigate tube with _____ ml room-temperature tap water, and clamp after each feeding
			E. Administration of oral medications
			  1. Use medications in elixir form
			  2. If elixir form is not available, crush tablets and mix with _____ ml room-temperature tap water
			  3. Flush tube with _____ ml room-temperature tap water after medication is administered
				Adequate nutritional support will be maintained

Fluid volume deficit: potential Etiology Osmolarity of the feeding formula	Changes in mental status <20 ml urine output per hour Highly concentrated urine Daily fluid intake of <800 ml Increased serum Na Decreased venous filling Hypotension Dry mucous membranes Poor skin turgor Increased pulse rate Weakness Edema	Assess A. Hydration status: skin turgor and mucous membranes B. I & O C. Daily weights D. Mental status changes E. Defining characteristics	A. Document base-line mental status, and recheck q.4h. B. Maintain strict I & O every _____ hours C. Use the same scale to measure daily weight D. Monitor serum electrolytes/urine osmolarity E. Document specific gravity of urine every _____ hours F. Administer parenteral fluids as ordered, with accurate titration of flow G. Document gastric residual before each feeding H. Instill ≥60 ml gastric residual to prevent electrolyte loss I. Record vital signs every _____ hours J. Notify physician of any significant change in condition	Potential fluid volume deficit will be minimized

Continued.

Gastrostomy Tube—cont'd

NURSING DIAGNOSIS/ PATIENT PROBLEM	DEFINING CHARACTERISTICS	NURSING ORDERS		EXPECTED OUTCOMES
		ASSESSMENT	INTERVENTIONS	

Elimination, alteration in: diarrhea (potential)
 Etiology
 Mechanical, chemical, or bacterial irritation of intestinal mucosa
	Frequent, loose stools
	 Abdominal pain and cramping
	 Hyperactive bowel sounds
		A. Monitor frequency and consistency of stools
		 B. Assess q.4h. for feeding intolerance
		   1. Check for abdominal bloating and flatulence
		   2. Monitor for complaints of abdominal pain and cramping
		 C. See SCP in Ch. 1: Bowel elimination, alteration in: diarrhea
			A. Begin feeding at a low infusion rate: _____ ml/hour and at _____ strength
			 B. Gradually increase the rate to _____ ml/hour and _____ strength
			 C. Increase the rate and strength of feeding at different times to prevent intolerance
			 D. Administer feeding at room temperature
			 E. Prevent bacterial contamination of feeding and equipment
			   1. Change formula q.4h. (during a continuous feeding)
			   2. Rinse administration set with warm water
			   3. Change administration set q.24h. or as needed
			 F. Record frequency and consistency of stools
			 G. Maintain accurate I & O, with tube feeding recorded on a separate sheet
			 H. Notify physician of feeding intolerance
				Feeding intolerance will be minimized

Skin integrity, impairment of: potential
 Etiology
 Drainage from gastrostomy tube insertion site
	Redness and tenderness at insertion site
	 Area moist from gastric secretions
		Assess tube insertion site q.8h. for
		 A. Changes in skin color
		 B. Pus and/or drainage
		 C. Odor of drainage
		 D. Tenderness
			A. Provide skin care
			   1. Keep skin free of gastric secretions
			   2. Dress wound as appropriate
			   3. Obtain culture and sensitivity of drainage as ordered
			   4. Use hypoallergenic tape during dressing changes
			   5. Tape tube securely to the abdomen, avoiding tension on the tube
			 B. Consult with surgical clinical specialist as needed
				Skin breakdown will be avoided

Glucose and fat metabolism, alteration in: potential
 Etiology
 Continuous feeding
	Glucose >120
	 Glucose <70
	 Greasy, foul-smelling stools
		A. Monitor serum glucose levels
		 B. Assess for signs of hyper-hypoglycemia
		   1. Hyperglycemia: flushed skin, headache, nausea, vomiting, fatigue, fruity breath
		   2. Hypoglycemia: hunger, sweating, pallor, cold and clammy skin, fatigue, tremors, dizziness
		 C. Monitor for mental status changes
		 D. Assess odor and consistency of stool
			A. Monitor glucose
			   1. Check urine sugar/acetone four times a day; notify physician if _____
			   2. Monitor blood glucose by chemstick every _____
			   3. Administer hyperglycemic agents as ordered
			   4. Notify physician if feeding is stopped for any reason
			 B. Monitor fat
			   1. Check number and characteristic of stool
			   2. Notify physician of any changes
				Potential for alteration in fat and in glucose metabolism will be minimized

Gastrostomy Tube—cont'd

NURSING DIAGNOSIS/ PATIENT PROBLEM	DEFINING CHARACTERISTICS	NURSING ORDERS		EXPECTED OUTCOMES
		ASSESSMENT	INTERVENTIONS	
Knowledge deficit **Etiology** New procedure	Multiple questions Lack of questions Verbalization of inaccurate information Improperly demonstrated technique	Evaluate level of understanding by patient/significant others A. Purpose of feeding B. Necessary equipment C. Preparation and storage of formula D. Correct feeding procedure E. Schedule of feeding F. Administration of oral medications G. Signs and symptoms of aspiration H. Signs and symptoms of feeding intolerance	A. Explain to patient/significant others the purpose of the feeding B. Inform patient/significant others of equipment necessary for feeding 1. For bolus feeding: 50 ml syringe, ____ ml tap water at room temperature, Hoffman clamp 2. For continuous feeding: administration bag, ____ ml tap water at room temperature, Flexi-flow infusion pump (optional) C. Assemble all necessary equipment before initiating feeding D. Instruct patient/significant others in the proper preparation and storage of formula 1. Preparation: use _____ strength formula; dilute full strength formula with _____ ml tap water 2. Store unopened cans of formula at room temperature 3. Administer formula at room temperature 4. Store unused portion of formula in an airtight container in the refrigerator 5. Discard unused portion (of continuous feeding) formula after 4 hours E. Instruct patient/significant others in the proper feeding procedure 1. Place patient in an upright position during and for 30 min after feeding 2. Aspirate stomach contents before each feeding 3. Postpone feeding for 2 hours if the residual feeding is ≥60 ml 4. Reinstill residual feeding to prevent electrolyte imbalance 5. Discontinue feeding immediately if patient experiences respiratory difficulty, nausea, or vomiting 6. Instill ____ ml/feeding (for bolus feeding) 7. Administer ____ ml over a 4-hour period (for continuous feeding) 8. Flush tube with ____ ml room-temperature tap water after each feeding	Patient/significant others will verbalize and demonstrate an understanding of the tube feeding

Continued.

Gastrostomy Tube—cont'd

NURSING DIAGNOSIS/ PATIENT PROBLEM	DEFINING CHARACTERISTICS	NURSING ORDERS		EXPECTED OUTCOMES
		ASSESSMENT	INTERVENTIONS	
			9. Review feeding technique if patient complains of nausea, vomiting, fullness, cramping, or diarrhea 10. Notify visiting nurse and physician if any problems arise F. Have patient/significant others demonstrate correct feeding procedure ____ times before discharge G. Set up feeding schedule with patient/significant others (consider patient's life-style; keep as normal as possible) 1. Bolus feeding schedule: ____ ml every ____ hours 2. Continuous feeding schedule: ____ ml to run over ____ hours H. Administration of oral medications 1. Use elixir form if available; administer with a syringe, and flush with ____ ml room temperature tap water 2. Crush tablet(s) and mix with ____ ml room-temperature tap water; flush with _____ ml water I. Explain signs/symptoms of aspiration: coughing, choking, audible respirations, difficulty in breathing J. Explain signs/symptoms of feeding intolerance: cramping, diarrhea, excessive flatulence, vomiting	
Coping, ineffective individual: potential **Etiology** Altered body function	Repeated hospitalizations for weight loss and dehydration Withdrawal from social systems Verbalization of inability to cope	A. Assess patient's 1. Appearance 2. Behavior 3. Cognitive function (concentration, orientation) 4. Emotional status B. Identify patient's support systems (family, significant others) C. Identify previous ways of coping under stress	A. Provide consistency in care 1. The same nurse(s) should care for the patient (as much as possible) 2. Alter the patient's routine as little as possible B. Provide an atmosphere that will allow the patient to discuss his/ her feelings 1. Provide privacy 2. Approach patient in an unhurried manner 3. Listen carefully to the patient's attempts to verbalize C. Encourage the use of coping mechanisms that have worked in the past D. Encourage the family/significant others to participate in the patient's care E. Use other resources: psychiatric liaison, nutritional support service, social work, clergy	Patient will begin to A. Verbalize emotions B. Identify constructive coping behaviors

Herniorrhaphy: pediatric

NURSING DIAGNOSIS/ PATIENT PROBLEM	DEFINING CHARACTERISTICS	NURSING ORDERS		EXPECTED OUTCOMES
		ASSESSMENT	INTERVENTIONS	

Injury, potential for: infection
 Etiology
 Incision and break in skin integrity
	Elevated temperature, pulse, and respiratory rate
	 Presence of drainage, odor, redness and/or swelling to incision
		A. Assess incision line and/or dressing every ___ for cleanliness, approximation, swelling, hematoma, redness, drainage, and odor
		 B. Assess vital signs, especially temperature every ___
			A. Keep operative site clean and dry by changing
			   1. Dressing every day and when soiled
			   2. Diapers frequently to prevent contamination by urine and stool
			 B. Avoid pressure on operative site by lifting buttocks with support
			 C. Administer antipyretics for temperature >38.5° (rectal) per physician's order
			 D. Administer antibiotics as ordered
			 E. Obtain culture if there is any drainage from incision
				Risk of infection will be minimized as evidenced by a clean, dry, intact surgical incision

Airway clearance, ineffective **Etiology** Medications, anesthesia, and pain	Presence of rales, rhonchi and wheezes Tachypnea Dyspnea and apnea Cyanosis Ineffective cough Inability to voluntarily cough	A. Assess respiratory rate every ___ for quality, rate, and depth B. Auscultate breath sounds every ___ C. Assess for any symptoms of respiratory distress: retractions; rales, rhonchi, and wheezing; cyanosis; decreased/increased respiratory rate D. See SCP in Ch. 1: Airway clearance, ineffective	A. Provide humidity at bedside through use of humidifier/humidified O_2 B. Suction nasopharynx every ___ and as needed C. Reposition infant every ___ D. Stimulate infant every ___ to cry and/or cough	Airway will be free of secretions

Comfort, alteration in
 Etiology
 Surgery
	Crying
	 Restless
	 Listless
	 Irritable
	 Poor appetite
	 Altered sleep pattern
	 Difficult to soothe
		A. Observe for
		   1. Vocalizations, especially groaning, grunting, screaming, prolonged crying
		   2. Behavioral changes, irritability, restlessness, fretfulness, inability to soothe
		 B. Assess effectiveness of analgesics administered
		 C. See SCP in Ch. 1: Comfort, alteration in
			A. Assist in minimizing pain by
			   1. Gently lifting child and supporting buttocks
			   2. Avoiding direct pressure on incision
			 B. Provide comfort measures
			   1. Relaxed and quiet atmosphere
			   2. Warm baths
			 C. Satisfy physical needs
			   1. Hunger
			   2. Change diapers as needed
			 D. Administer analgesics as ordered
			 E. Provide diversional activities: toys, stimulation
			 F. Refer to foster grandmother program/child life department
				Pain will be minimized as evidenced by a decrease in undesirable verbal and nonverbal behaviors

Originated by **Andrea So, RN, BSN**
Resource person: **Ruth E. Novitt, RN, MSN**

Continued.

Herniorrhaphy: pediatric—cont'd

NURSING DIAGNOSIS/ PATIENT PROBLEM	DEFINING CHARACTERISTICS	NURSING ORDERS		EXPECTED OUTCOMES
		ASSESSMENT	INTERVENTIONS	
Fluid volume deficit: potential **Etiology** NPO preoperatively Discomfort postoperatively	Irritability Skin turgor poor to fair Sunken fontanel Crying Dry mucous membranes Decreased urine output (<30 ml/hour) Loss of weight Poor sucking/appetite	Assess child for defining characteristics (see SCP in Ch. 1: Fluid volume deficit)	A. Administer analgesics before feeding B. Provide well-balanced diet and adequate fluid based on weight and age (formula, food) C. Encourage parents to participate at meal time	Potential for dehydration will be minimized
Urinary elimination, alteration in patterns (retention): potential **Etiology** Retention related to surgery and anesthesia	Irritability Crying Abdominal/bladder distention Restlessness Absence of urine Inadequate I & O	A. Assess diaper for evidence of urine B. Assess urine for appearance, color, volume, specific gravity C. See SCP in Ch. 1: Urinary elimination, alteration in patterns	A. Obtain accurate I & O q.4h. B. Initiate measures to facilitate voiding 1. Encourage fluids as tolerated 2. Use warmth to relax sphincter (warm compress) 3. Credé's method 4. Administer analgesics as ordered C. Notify physician of urine output <____ ml/hour	Normal pattern of urine elimination will be maintained
Parental knowledge deficit **Etiology** Hospitalization of infant	Withdrawal Depression and silence Helplessness Crying Anxious and tense Demanding Asking questions frequently/repeatedly	A. Assess family's 1. Previous experience with surgery and hospitalization 2. Current understanding of surgery B. Assess previous coping mechanisms C. Assess support system 1. Family members 2. Relatives and friends 3. Clergy 4. Nursing staff 5. Social worker	A. Encourage communication and expression B. Encourage parental involvement in infant's care C. Explain home care of the operative site 1. Wash only with warm water 2. Change diaper frequently to prevent contamination of incision 3. Do not remove Steri-strips D. Explain possible postoperative complications 1. Check for increased bleeding and drainage from operative area 2. Check for symptoms of infection: elevated temperature, increased drainage, foul odor	Parents' fear and anxiety will be decreased Parents will verbalize understanding of: treatment plan, home care responsibilities, complications

CHAPTER SIX

Genitourinary

DISORDERS

Urinary Tract Infection (UTI)

NURSING DIAGNOSIS/ PATIENT PROBLEM	DEFINING CHARACTERISTICS	NURSING ORDERS		EXPECTED OUTCOMES
		ASSESSMENT	INTERVENTIONS	
Injury, potential for: infection Etiology Invading pathogens	Low back pain Suprapubic tenderness Urinary urgency and frequency Body malaise Nausea Low-grade fever Nocturia Incontinence	A. Assess signs and symptoms of UTI (see defining characteristics). Note that patient may be asymptomatic, especially with recurrent infections B. Assess laboratory data for the following 1. Urinalysis: hematuria, pyuria, bacteruria 2. Urine culture: causative organism 3. CBC: polymorphonuclear leukocytosis >11,000/ml C. Assess for prior history of UTI D. Assess for underlying conditions: pregnancy, sickle cell trait, hypertension, or diabetes mellitus	A. Attempt to enhance body's normal defense mechanisms 1. Encourage patient to drink liberal amounts of fluid to promote renal blood flow and to flush out bacteria in urinary tract 2. Instruct patient to void frequently (q.2-3h. during the day) and to empty bladder completely. This enhances bacterial clearance, reduces urine stasis, and prevents reinfection 3. Suggest drinking cranberry or prune juice to acidify urine B. Give prescribed antibiotic, and note its effectiveness	Patient will experience return of normal voiding pattern, with resolution of UTI
Comfort, alteration in Etiology Infection	**Subjective** Patient reports pain, cramps, or spasm in lower back and bladder area; dysuria; body malaise **Objective** Facial mask of pain Guarding behavior Protective decreased physical activity	A. Solicit patient's description of pain B. Assess pain characteristics, including quality, severity, location, onset, and duration	A. Apply heating pad to lower back for back pain B. Instruct patient in use of sitz bath for perineal pain C. Encourage adequate rest D. Administer analgesics and antispasmodics as ordered, and note their effectiveness E. Use distractions and relaxation techniques whenever appropriate	Patient will report relief or decrease of pain

Originated by **Caroline Sarmiento, RN, BSN**
Resource person: **Jackie Suprenant, RN, BSN**

Urinary Tract Infection (UTI)—cont'd

NURSING DIAGNOSIS/ PATIENT PROBLEM	DEFINING CHARACTERISTICS	NURSING ORDERS		EXPECTED OUTCOMES
		ASSESSMENT	INTERVENTIONS	
Knowledge deficit **Etiology** Unfamiliarity with nature and treatment of urinary tract infection	Lack of questions Apparent confusion over events Expressed need for more information	A. Assess patient's knowledge base regarding the nature of UTI B. Assess preventive measures patient may currently be using to minimize UTI	A. Provide information on UTI based on assessment data B. Provide health teaching and discharge planning to prevent recurrence of infection. Instruct patient in 1. Having follow-up urine studies to determine if asymptomatic infection is present (thus a marked tendency for infection to recur) 2. Following hygienic measures to decrease introital concentration of pathogens by washing in shower or while standing in tub and washing perineum with soap and water from front to back after each bowel movement 3. Voiding immediately after each sexual intercourse 4. Voiding at the first urge to avoid urinary distention 5. Changing underpants daily and wearing a well-ventilating material such as cotton. Cotton-crotched pantyhose should also be worn 6. Taking medication for long-term antimicrobial therapy just before bedtime to ensure concentration of drug during overnight period	Patient will verbalize understanding of the nature of UTI

THERAPEUTIC INTERVENTIONS

Transurethral Resection of Prostate

NURSING DIAGNOSIS/ PATIENT PROBLEM	DEFINING CHARACTERISTICS	NURSING ORDERS		EXPECTED OUTCOMES
		ASSESSMENT	INTERVENTIONS	
Knowledge deficit **Etiology** Scheduled for new procedure	Asks information Verbalizes misconceptions No previous surgical experience	A. Assess the patient's level of understanding about 1. Surgical plan 2. Previous surgical experience B. Assess his level of anxiety related to knowledge deficit	A. Visit patient preoperatively and discuss perioperative plan B. Allow patient to verbalize questions, misconceptions C. Teach and practice postoperative exercises such as deep breathing and coughing D. Explain procedures before and as they are done E. Explain reason for retention catheter and continuous bladder irrigation F. Encourage the patient to discuss with his physician specific postoperative activities	Patient will verbalize understanding of necessity of procedure and associated postoperative treatment
Anxiety/fear **Etiology** Possibility of postoperative impotence	Appears very anxious Expresses fear of postoperative impotence Repeats misconceptions Asks questions about other patients who have undergone the same surgery with resultant impotence	Assess the patient's mental state and emotional maturity	A. Use visual aids while teaching B. Ask the patient to repeat in his own words the location and functions of the prostate gland C. Refer questions you cannot address to the physician D. Clarify misunderstandings or relate them to the surgeon	Patient will discuss his symptoms and communicate feelings verbally and nonverbally
Comfort, alteration in **Etiology** Pain during and after resection	Verbalizes hypogastric pain Experiences fullness of bladder Becomes restless and starts to move around	Assess level of pain during and after procedure	A. Minimize movement of patient B. Keep external stimuli to a minimum C. Instruct patient to breathe slowly and deeply at onset of pain D. Keep catheter in place and patent	Patient will verbalize minimal discomfort
Comfort, alteration in **Etiology** Spinal anesthesia	Headache Nausea Vomiting Low BP	Assess vital signs every _____	A. Provide emesis basin in case of vomiting B. Keep the patient in a flat position, and instruct him not to raise his head C. Minimize movement during procedure	Patient's discomfort will be minimized

Originated by **Encarnacion Mendoza, RN, BSN**
Resource person: **Katie Wyatt, RN**

Transurethral Resection of Prostate—cont'd

NURSING DIAGNOSIS/ PATIENT PROBLEM	DEFINING CHARACTERISTICS	NURSING ORDERS		EXPECTED OUTCOMES
		ASSESSMENT	INTERVENTIONS	
Anxiety/fear Etiology Planned anesthesia	Appears anxious Verbalizes misconceptions Relates previous negative experience Expresses need for more explanations about anesthesia	A. Assess level of anxiety B. Assess level of understanding about proposed anesthesia	A. Provide emotional support to the patient B. Reinforce that he will be monitored continuously by the anesthesiologist C. Explain that the anesthesiologist will give him some medications to keep him relaxed	Patient will accept explanations and realize the importance of anesthesia
Injury, potential for Etiology Position during procedure	Soreness of body parts Body not properly aligned Tingling, pinching sensation Numbness	Assess patient's body alignment throughout procedure	A. Move and position patient gently to prevent pathologic fractures and dislocations B. Apply soft pads or folded sheets on stirrup to relieve pressure under popliteal region C. Extend arm on a padded arm board D. Provide head support E. Provide soft pads under bony prominences F. Keep heavy sheets away from chest	Potential for injury related to position will be minimized
Injury, potential for: infection Etiology Instrumentation Manipulation	Past history of recurrent UTI Increased WBC Cloudy urine Purulent postoperative discharge from catheter	A. Check length of time instruments are soaked in disinfecting/sterilizing agents B. Observe aseptic technique used by urologist and assistants throughout procedure	A. Soak instruments in disinfecting/sterilizing agent for at least 10 min for effectiveness against microorganisms B. Rinse instruments thoroughly in sterile water to eliminate all traces of chemicals C. Administer antibiotics as ordered D. Use aseptic technique when catheterizing patient E. Lubricate catheter before insertion F. Use bacteriocidal soap in cleaning the genitalia to suppress or reduce microbial population G. Connect all tubing aseptically	Risk of infection will be minimized
Fluid volume deficit: potential Etiology Blood loss	Blood drainage from catheter Gradually decreasing BP Decreasing Hb and Hct	Assess for signs of fluid volume deficit	A. Document signs and symptoms of shock. Use nonhemolysing irrigation, solutions B. Check for blood type and cross-match C. Have blood available in OR	Optimal fluid volume will be maintained
Body temperature, alteration in: potential Etiology Cool OR environment Prolonged exposure of genitalia	Decreased body temperature from preoperative baseline temperature Skin cold to touch Patient states that he feels cold	A. Observe change of body temperature every _____ B. Note room temperature	A. Keep room temperature at an optimal level B. Cover the patient with warm blankets C. Use warm irrigating solution during resection D. Prevent pooling of solution beneath patient	Patient's body temperature will be maintained with minimal variations

CHAPTER SEVEN

Renal

DISORDERS

Hypocalcemia and Bone Disease in End-Stage Renal Disease

NURSING DIAGNOSIS/ PATIENT PROBLEM	DEFINING CHARACTERISTICS	NURSING ORDERS		EXPECTED OUTCOMES
		ASSESSMENT	INTERVENTIONS	
Fluid composition, alteration in: hypocalcemia **Etiology** Increased phosphorus level Renal failure	Tingling sensations at the end of fingers Muscle cramps Tetany Convulsion	A. Assess for signs and symptoms of hypocalcemia 1. Tingling sensations at the ends of fingers 2. Muscle cramps and carpopedal spasms 3. Tetany 4. Convulsion B. Observe for signs and symptoms of calcium-phosphorus imbalance 1. Pruritus 2. Blurred vision 3. Cardiac arrhythmias	A. Monitor calcium and phosphorus levels every ____, and report values to physician B. Administer phosphate-binding medications as ordered C. Apply lotion for itchiness, and recommend use of scratcher rather than fingernails	Normal calcium levels will be maintained
Bone injury: potential for **Etiology** Decreased blood calcium level (demineralization of the bones makes bones brittle, porous, and thinner)	Change in bone structure History of bones breaking easily Severe pain	A. Assess for signs and symptoms of extreme pain and joint swelling B. Observe patient's gait C. Assess patient's history for a tendency to fracture easily D. Observe ambulation and movement of extremities	A. Provide safety measures such as 1. Side rails 2. Uncluttered room 3. Orientation to surroundings 4. Proper lighting B. Refer to rehabilitation medicine department as indicated for 1. Use of crutches 2. Transport from wheelchair to chair or vice versa	Patient will demonstrate use of appropriate ambulation and safety measures

Originated by **Ofelia Zafra, RN, BSN**
Resource person: **Lumie Perez, RN, BSN, CCRN**
        Susan Galanes, RN, MS, TNS, CCRN

Hypocalcemia and Bone Disease in End-Stage Renal Disease—cont'd

NURSING DIAGNOSIS/ PATIENT PROBLEM	DEFINING CHARACTERISTICS	NURSING ORDERS		EXPECTED OUTCOMES
		ASSESSMENT	INTERVENTIONS	
Self-concept, disturbance in: body image **Etiology** Stunted growth Disfigured face, body, extremities Waddling gait	Verbalizes about appearance Verbalizes feeling of isolation Refuses to participate in any social activities	A. Assess patient's perception of his/her body image B. Assess patient's readiness for help C. Assess patient's coping mechanisms	A. Establish a continuing one-to-one patient-nurse relationship B. Allow patient opportunity to verbalize his/her feelings C. Accept patient's feelings, as appropriate D. Encourage patient to maintain ADL E. Include significant others in planning activities F. Use health team members from related disciplines for support: psychiatric liaison, social worker, etc.	Minimized alteration in body image will be evidenced by A. Verbalization of feelings B. Participation in activities that patient enjoys C. Expressed desire to resume activities i.e.: going back to work, sports, traveling, etc.
Knowledge deficit **Etiology** Unfamiliarity with disease process	Multiple questions Noncompliance with medications and diet	A. Assess patient's knowledge of condition, readiness to learn, and ability to learn B. Assess patient's knowledge of medication and diet	A. Discuss the causes and complications of hypocalcemia and bone disease B. Teach patient/significant others to observe for signs and symptoms of hypocalcemia. Provide a list of symptoms on discharge C. Discuss the importance of taking prescribed medications D. Discuss thoroughly, before discharge, patient's medications, dosages, and side effects E. Explain the need for a special diet and the need for adhering to it. Use resources as appropriate: list, pamphlet, dietitian F. Encourage significant others to verbalize their feelings, insecurities, and other concerns before discharge G. Refer to other health team members as indicated	The patient will A. Verbalize a general understanding of the disease and prevention of complications B. State signs and symptoms of hypocalcemia C. Verbalize knowledge of dosage, side effects, administration, and contraindications of medications

Nephrotic Syndrome: pediatric

NURSING DIAGNOSIS/ PATIENT PROBLEM	DEFINING CHARACTERISTICS	NURSING ORDERS		EXPECTED OUTCOMES
		ASSESSMENT	INTERVENTIONS	

Fluid/electrolyte balance, alteration in
 Etiology
 Decreased filtering
 Fluid loss into interstitial spaces
	Total body edema
	 Low BP
	 Puffy eyelids
	 Elevated BUN and creatinine levels
	 Abnormal electrolytes
	 Decreased Hb and Hct
		A. Check vital signs every ____ (especially pulse and BP)
		 B. Assess postural BP every _____
		 C. Maintain accurate I & O
		 D. Weigh patient every _____
		 E. Check urine every ____ for
		   1. Specific gravity
		   2. Dipstick
		 F. Measure abdominal girth every
		 _____
		 G. Assess for edema every _____
		 H. Monitor daily laboratory work as ordered
		   1. Hb
		   2. Hct
		   3. Electrolytes
		   4. BUN/creatinine
		 I. Assess for signs of anemia
		   1. Stools for blood
		   2. Pallor
			A. Administer diuretics as ordered. Assess for signs of shock
			 B. Administer salt-poor albumin as ordered
			 C. Administer electrolytes as ordered
				A. Vital signs will remain stable for child
				 B. Optimal fluid/ electrolyte balance will be maintained

Skin integrity, impairment of: potential **Etiology** Tissue edema	Poor skin turgor Skin taut over bony areas Redness to bony areas	A. Assess dependent areas for skin breakdown every _____ B. Assess child for pitting edema C. Observe open wounds for proper healing	A. Change child's position every 2 hours B. Use pillows to support child when positioning to relieve pressure areas C. Keep skin clean and dry D. Apply baby powder between skin folds E. Check temperature every _____ F. Avoid having the child wear tight clothing G. Refer to SCP in Ch. 1: Skin integrity, impairment of	Optimal skin integrity will be maintained
Nutrition, alteration in: less than body requirements **Etiology** Impaired renal function	Low serum protein Proteinuria Muscle wasting	A. Monitor child's intake daily, both liquids and solids B. Monitor protein loss in urine every _____	A. Provide a high-protein, high-calorie diet B. Restrict sodium intake C. Offer small, frequent meals D. Provide foods high in K + E. Provide vitamin supplements as ordered	Adequate dietary requirements will be provided through diet

Originated by **Kathy Alexander, RN**
Resource persons: **Janice L. Miller, RN,C MSN**
        Ruth E. Novitt, RN, MSN

Nephrotic Syndrome: pediatric—cont'd

NURSING DIAGNOSIS/ PATIENT PROBLEM	DEFINING CHARACTERISTICS	NURSING ORDERS		EXPECTED OUTCOMES
		ASSESSMENT	INTERVENTIONS	
Injury, potential for infections **Etiology** Immunosuppression of steroid therapy	Elevated temperature Elevated WBC Malaise	A. Assess child for signs of infection B. Assess vital signs, especially temperature, every _____ C. Observe visitors for any obvious symptoms of infection	A. Keep visitors with infectious symptoms away from child B. Do not put child in a room with other children who have infectious diseases	Exposure to potential infectious agents will be minimized

Knowledge deficit
 Etiology
 Chronicity of disease
 Long-term medical management
	Asking no questions
	 Overly anxious
	 Inability to talk about present status
		Assess knowledge base and readiness for learning of parents/child	A. Explain nephrotic syndrome to parents/child
			 B. Instruct parents to observe for increased edema by
			   1. Daily weights
			   2. Periorbital edema
			   3. Abdominal distention
			   4. Ankle edema
			 C. Instruct parents/child in the proper use of dipsticks for protein (provide with dipstick and sheet to record results of urine protein)
			 D. Instruct parents to inform physician of signs of infection or relapse: fever, lethargy, oliguria, weight gain
			 E. Instruct parents/child in the need to
			   1. Restrict sodium in the diet
			   2. Keep a list of low sodium foods and those high in potassium, protein, and carbohydrates
			   3. Provide small frequent meals if child has nausea and vomiting
			 F. Inform parents of the importance of proper medication administration
			   1. Types of medications, dosage, and side effects
			   2. Importance of antacid/foods administered along with steroids to prevent GI disturbances (ulcers)
			 G. Inform parents not to discontinue steroids or to alter times and doses without physician's guidance
			 H. Inform parents/child that patient should wear identification denoting the need for supplemental systemic glucocorticoids during stress (trauma, OR, dental work, or injury)
				A. Parents/child will verbalize an understanding of
				   1. Nephrotic syndrome
				   2. Treatments/ procedures
				   3. Complications
				   4. Diet
				   5. Medication
				     a. Dosage
				     b. Side effects
				     c. When to notify physician
				 B. Parents/child will demonstrate proper use of urine dipstick testing

End-Stage Renal Disease: outpatient on dialysis with fluid volume excess

NURSING DIAGNOSIS/ PATIENT PROBLEM	DEFINING CHARACTERISTICS	NURSING ORDERS		EXPECTED OUTCOMES
		ASSESSMENT	INTERVENTIONS	
Fluid volume, alteration in: excess **Etiology** Excess fluid intake Excess sodium intake Compromised regulatory mechanisms	Edema Elevated BP before dialysis (elevated from patient's normal BP) Weight gain	A. Assess patient's vital signs every _____ B. Assess amount of edema by palpating area over tibia, at ankles, sacrum, back, and assessing appearance of face C. Assess patient's compliance to dietary and fluid restrictions at home	A. Weigh at every visit before and after dialysis (weight gain not to exceed 1 kg between visits) B. Restrict fluid intake to ____ / ____ C. Restrict dietary sodium intake to ____ /____ D. Advise patient to elevate feet when sitting down E. Instruct patient of necessity to follow prescribed fluid/dietary restriction F. Give antihypertensive medications if prescribed G. At initiation of treatment, run off normal saline in the lines, and use patient's own blood as a prime	The effects of the fluid volume excess will be minimized, as evidenced by A. Verbalization of fluid and dietary restrictions B. Normalizing trends in BP
Gas exchange, impaired: potential **Etiology** Altered blood flow Alveolar-capillary membrane changes	Shortness of breath Tachypnea Orthopnea Chest pain Tachycardia Restlessness Confusion	A. Assess vital signs every _____ B. Auscultate for moist rales C. Check for distended neck veins D. Assess for cyanosis E. Assess breathing pattern. If abnormal, see SCP in Ch. 1: Breathing pattern, ineffective	A. Maintain optimal positioning for air exchange. Have patient sit up if he/she complains of shortness of breath B. Notify physician if signs of impaired gas exchange are present C. Perform ultrafiltration as ordered per physician	Optimal gas exchange will be maintained
Skin integrity, impairment of: potential **Etiology** End-stage renal disease	Pitting of extremities on manipulation Low Hct Puffy eyelids Demarcation of clothing and shoes on patient's body	Assess skin integrity. See SCP in Ch. 1: Skin integrity, impairment of	A. Instruct the patient to wear loose-fitting clothing when edema is present B. Teach patient factors important to skin integrity 1. Nutrition 2. Mobility 3. Hygiene 4. Early recognition of skin breakdown	Optimal skin integrity will be maintained
Self-concept, disturbance in: potential **Etiology** Prolonged outpatient dialysis Loss of body function	Depression Expressed anger Withdrawal	Assess for disturbed self-concept	A. Talk with patient, significant others, and friends, if possible, regarding chronic outpatient dialysis B. Discuss problems and possible solutions with patient C. Explore strengths and resources with patient D. Have social worker see patients on a regular basis as a preventive measure E. Refer to psychiatric consultant as necessary	Patient will demonstrate some acceptance of altered body image

Originated by **Laura Watanabe, RN**
Resource person: **Susan Galanes, RN, MS, TNS, CCRN**

End-Stage Renal Disease: outpatient on dialysis with fluid volume excess—cont'd

NURSING DIAGNOSIS/ PATIENT PROBLEM	DEFINING CHARACTERISTICS	NURSING ORDERS		EXPECTED OUTCOMES
		ASSESSMENT	INTERVENTIONS	

Knowledge deficit
Etiology
 	
Lack of interest in learning
Unfamiliarity with disease process
Information misinterpretation
	Verbalization of misconceptions
	Questioning
	Noncompliance
	Signs to look for: fluid volume excess, edema, respiratory signs
		A. Assess patient's understanding of end-stage renal disease
		B. Observe for dietary deviations and noncompliance when patient is on unit
			A. Instruct the patient in various methods to relieve a dry mouth and maintain fluid restriction
			  1. Allow ice chips as needed
			  2. Suggest keeping hard candy on hand to alleviate dry mouth
			  3. Suggest frequent mouth rinses with ½ cup mouth wash mixed with ½ cup ice water
			B. Instruct patient in dietary restrictions: _____
			C. Use available resources to aid the instruction as necessary: dietitian, pamphlets, books, dietary list
			D. Involve significant others in instruction sessions on special diets and fluid restrictions
			E. Instruct patient in recognition of signs of fluid volume excess
				Patient will verbalize an understanding of necessary dietary restrictions

Renal Failure, Acute

NURSING DIAGNOSIS/ PATIENT PROBLEM	DEFINING CHARACTERISTICS	NURSING ORDERS		EXPECTED OUTCOMES
		ASSESSMENT	INTERVENTIONS	
Urinary elimination, alteration in patterns **Etiology** Severe renal ischemia secondary to sepsis, shock, or severe hypovolemia with hypotension (usually after surgery or trauma) Nephrotoxic drugs or antibiotics such as amphotericin and gentamycin Renal vascular occlusion Hemolytic blood transfusion reaction	Increased BUN and creatinine Urine specific gravity fixed at or near 1.010 Hematuria, proteinuria Urine output <400 ml/24 hours (in the absence of inadequate fluid intake or fluid losses by another route)	A. Assess patient for any alteration in urinary elimination B. Monitor and record I & O every _____. Include all fluid losses such as stool, emesis, and wound drainage C. Monitor urine specific gravity, and check for protein and blood every _____ D. Palpate bladder for distention E. Assess for patency of Foley catheter (if present) F. Notify physician of urine output <____ ml/hour	A. Monitor vital signs every ____ hours B. Maintain strict I & O C. Administer fluids and diuretics as ordered, and document patient's response D. Maintain patency of Foley catheter E. Obtain daily weights F. When administering medications metabolized by the kidneys (such as antibiotics), remember that the excretion of these drugs may be altered. The dosages may require adjustment	Optimal urine elimination will be maintained

Originated by **Deborah Lazzara, RN, CCRN**
Resource person: **Susan Galanes, RN, MS, TNS, CCRN**

Continued.

Renal Failure, Acute—cont'd

NURSING DIAGNOSIS/ PATIENT PROBLEM	DEFINING CHARACTERISTICS	NURSING ORDERS		EXPECTED OUTCOMES
		ASSESSMENT	INTERVENTIONS	

		G. Monitor blood and urine chemistries as ordered
		    Electrolytes (Na, K, Cl, Ca, phosphorus, magnesium)
		    BUN, creatinine
		    Urinalysis, urine electrolytes
		    (Notify physician of abnormalities		

Fluid volume, alteration in: excess **Etiology** Inability of the body to properly excrete fluid and electrolytes Excessive administration of oral/IV fluids during periods of decreased renal function	Increased central venous pressure and BP Acute weight gain, edema Signs/symptoms of congestive heart failure: jugular vein distention, rales Shortness of breath, dyspnea Pericarditis, friction rub	A. Assess patient for signs of circulatory overload, congestive heart failure, and pulmonary congestion B. Monitor heart rate, BP, CVP, and respiratory rate every _____ C. Monitor and record I & O every _____. Include all stools, emesis, and drainage	A. Maintain strict I & O B. Weight patient daily (before and after dialysis), and record C. Auscultate breath sounds and heart sounds every ____. Notify physician of any abnormalities D. Administer oral and IV fluids per physician's orders to replace sensible and insensible losses E. Administer medications (such as diuretics) per physician's orders, and document patient's response F. Monitor laboratory work (such as serum electrolytes and osmolality) as ordered G. Prepare patient for hemodialysis, ultrafiltration, or peritoneal dialysis if indicated	Optimal fluid balance will be maintained

Cardiac output, alteration in: decreased (potential)
Etiology
Arrhythmias caused by electrolyte imbalance from acute renal failure
A. Primary hyperkalemia
  1. Decreased renal elimination of electrolytes: K, phosphorus, magnesium, Na)
	A. Decreased cardiac output
	  1. Change in BP, heart rate, CVP, peripheral pulses
	  2. Decreased urine output
	  3. Abnormal heart sounds and cardiac enzymes
	  4. Arrhythmias
	  5. Anxiety/restlessness
		A. Assess patient for signs of decreased cardiac output and electrolyte disturbances
		B. Monitor vital signs every ____ hours. Notify physician of abnormalities
		C. Monitor serum electrolytes as ordered
			A. Administer oral and IV fluids as ordered to maintain optimal fluid balance. Note the effects
			B. Monitor cardiac rhythm, and notify physician of abnormalities. Determine patient's hemodynamic response to arrhythmias
			C. Administer medications (such as sodium bicarbonate [NaHCO₃], calcium salts, glucose/insulin, K exchange resins) per order in an attempt to equilibrate the electrolyte disturbances temporarily. Note patient's response
				Optimal cardiac output will be maintained

Renal Failure, Acute—cont'd

NURSING DIAGNOSIS/ PATIENT PROBLEM	DEFINING CHARACTERISTICS	NURSING ORDERS		EXPECTED OUTCOMES
		ASSESSMENT	INTERVENTIONS	
2. Metabolic acidosis (present with acute renal failure) exacerbates hyperkalemia by causing the cellular shift of H and K. Excess H ions are traded intracellularly with K ions, causing increased extracellular K B. Hyponatremia results from excessive extracellular fluid (dilutional effect), edema, and restricted IV or dietary intake C. Hypocalcemia can also occur, although exact cause is unknown	B. Hyperkalemia (K > 5.5) 1. ECG changes such as a. Widened QRS segment, increased T waves b. Prolonged PR interval c. Bradycardia, arrhythmias, cardiac arrest C. Hyponatremia (Na <115 mEq/L) 1. Nausea/vomiting 2. Lethargy, weakness 3. Seizures (with severe deficit) D. Hypocalcemia (Ca <6.0) 1. Perioral paresthesias 2. Twitching, tetany, seizures 3. Cardiac arrhythmias		D. Maintain hemodynamic parameters as indicated; notify physician of variations Heart rate: _____ BP: _____ CVP: _____ Urine output: _____ Pulmonary capillary wedge pressure/pulmonary artery diastolic pressure: _____ E. Assist in providing optimal tissue perfusion 1. Administer O_2 as needed 2. Provide calm environment with minimal stressors 3. Restrict activity to conserve O_2 F. Prepare patient for dialysis or ultrafiltration when indicated G. For additional interventions/assessment, see SCPs in Ch. 1: Activity intolerance and Cardiac output, alteration in: decreased	
Breathing pattern, ineffective **Etiology** Volume overload leading to congestive heart failure/left ventricular failure Metabolic acidosis (caused by the kidney's inability to properly excrete hydrogen ions) leading to hyperventilation as a compensatory mechanism	Shortness of breath Rales, wheezes Dyspnea Hyperventilation Orthopnea	A. Assess rate and depth of respirations every ____ hours B. Auscultate breath sounds every ____ hours, and document findings. Notify physician if adventitious sounds are present C. Monitor ABGs as ordered and as needed. Notify physician of abnormal results D. Monitor results of chest radiographs	A. Encourage pulmonary toilet, turning, coughing, and deep breathing exercises every ____ hours B. Use tracheal suction as needed C. Maintain head of bed at an angle of at least 30 degrees D. Administer O_2 as ordered E. Administer medications such as diuretics/bronchodilators as ordered F. For further interventions/assessment see SCPs in Ch. 1: Airway clearance, ineffective and Breathing pattern, ineffective	Pulmonary complications will be minimized

Continued.

Renal Failure, Acute—cont'd

NURSING DIAGNOSIS/ PATIENT PROBLEM	DEFINING CHARACTERISTICS	NURSING ORDERS		EXPECTED OUTCOMES
		ASSESSMENT	INTERVENTIONS	
Nutrition, alteration in: less than body requirements **Etiology** Acute renal failure causes an accumulation of urea and other metabolic wastes The stress of acute illness can lead to GI hemorrhage and decreased appetite	Stomatitis Anorexia, decreased appetite Nausea, vomiting Diarrhea Constipation Melena, hematemesis	A. Assess for possible etiology of patient's decreased appetite or GI discomfort B. Assess patient's actual oral intake; obtain calorie counts as necessary C. Monitor serum laboratory values such as electrolytes and albumin level D. Record output of emesis and stools. Observe appearance, and notify physician of abnormalities E. Assess weight gain pattern F. See SCP in Ch. 1: Nutrition, alteration in: less than body requirements	A. Administer small frequent feedings as tolerated B. Consult dietitian to assist in providing patient with a low K, high carbohydrate diet as indicated C. Administer enteral/parental feedings as ordered D. Provide frequent oral hygiene E. Offer ice chips/hard candy if not contraindicated F. Offer antiemetics such as diphenhydramine (Benadryl) or dimenhydrinate (Dramamine) as ordered per physician G. Observe all stools/emesis for gross blood, and test for occult blood (guaiac/Hematest). Report results to physician	Nutritional state will be maximized
Tissue perfusion, alteration in: potential **Etiology** Anemia Bone marrow suppression secondary to insufficient renal production of erythropoietic factor Increased hemolysis leading to decreased life span of red blood cells secondary to abnormal chemical environment in plasma Decreased platelets and defective cohesion of platelets Inhibition of certain clotting factors Blood loss in GI tract	Fatigue Pallor Dyspnea Hct <30% Prolonged PT/PTT Bleeding tendencies, especially from GI tract	A. Observe patient for signs of fatigue, pallor, bleeding from puncture sites and incisions, and bruising tendencies. Document accordingly B. Monitor laboratory work as ordered and report results to physician: Hb and Hct, platelets, and coagulation studies	A. Check for guaiac in all stools and emesis. Report results to physician B. Administer O_2 as ordered C. Administer blood transfusions as ordered 1. Observe for signs of fluid overload and adverse reactions during transfusion 2. Administer diuretics, e.g., furosemide (Lasix), as ordered after transfusion D. Prepare patient for dialysis	Complications of anemia and decreased platelets will be minimized

Renal Failure, Acute—cont'd

NURSING DIAGNOSIS/ PATIENT PROBLEM	DEFINING CHARACTERISTICS	NURSING ORDERS		EXPECTED OUTCOMES
		ASSESSMENT	INTERVENTIONS	

Consciousness, altered levels of: actual or potential
Etiology
Accumulation of toxic waste products of metabolism
Electrolyte imbalances
Hypoxia
	Decreased concentration
	Apathy
	Confusion
	Lethargy leading to coma
	Convulsions
	Neuromuscular irritability
	Asterixis
		A. Assess for alteration in level of consciousness, muscular weakness, and irritability every _____
		B. Document patient's neurologic status
		C. Check electrolyte/ ABG results for abnormalities to determine actual or potential cause of change in level of consciousness
			A. Notify physician of any changes in patient's level of consciousness
			B. Reorient patient to environment as needed
			C. Maintain bed in low position with side rails up at all times
			D. Keep call light within easy reach of patient
			E. Use seizure precautions for patient with decreased level of consciousness
			  1. Keep side rails padded
			  2. Keep oral airway and padded tongue blades at bedside at all times
			F. See SCP in Ch. 3: Consciousness, altered levels of
				Optimal state of consciousness will be maintained

Injury, potential for systemic or local infection **Etiology** Debilitated state with poor nutrition Poor skin integrity and wound healing Use of indwelling catheters, subclavian lines, Foley catheters, ET tubes, etc.	Increased temperature Increased white blood cell count Local inflammation, redness or abnormal drainage Positive culture results (blood, wound, sputum, or urine)	A. Assess for potential sites of infection: urinary, pulmonary, wound, or IV line B. Monitor temperature every ____. Notify physician of temperature >38° C. Monitor WBC count D. Note and report promptly any signs of localized or systemic infection	A. Provide scrupulous perineal and catheter care every _____ B. Provide meticulous skin care to avoid skin breakdown over pressure areas C. Use strict aseptic technique when performing dressing changes, wound irrigations, catheter care, and suctioning D. Avoid the use of indwelling catheters or IV lines whenever possible E. If the use of indwelling catheters or IV lines are mandatory, change them per unit/hospital policy F. Protect patient from exposure to other patients with infection G. If infection is suspected, obtain specimens of blood, urine, sputum, etc., for culture and sensitivity as ordered H. If infection is present, administer antibiotics as ordered	Potential for systemic/ local infection will be minimized

Continued.

Renal Failure, Acute—cont'd

NURSING DIAGNOSIS/ PATIENT PROBLEM	DEFINING CHARACTERISTICS	NURSING ORDERS		EXPECTED OUTCOMES
		ASSESSMENT	INTERVENTIONS	
Knowledge deficit **Etiology** Change in body function secondary to acute renal failure (usually occurring secondary to an injury or illness)	Patient/significant others will verbalize questions and concerns regarding patient's condition and associated procedures and treatments	A. Assess current knowledge and understanding of illness by patient/ significant others B. Encourage patient to verbalize feelings and questions	A. Discuss need for monitoring equipment and frequent assessments B. Explain all tests and procedures *before* they occur. Use terms the patient is capable of understanding; be clear and direct C. Explain purpose of fluid and dietary restrictions D. Explain the need for dialysis and what the patient should expect during the procedure E. Instruct the patient to perform deep breathing and coughing exercises F. Involve the patient's family in caring for him/her as much as possible (when appropriate) G. Encourage family conferences with members of patient's health care team (e.g., physicians, nurses, rehabilitation personnel, social workers) as necessary H. Consult appropriate resource persons such as rehabilitation personnel, physicians, social workers, psychologists, clergy, occupational therapists, and clinical specialists as needed	Patient/significant others will verbalize understanding of the disease process and associated treatments

THERAPEUTIC INTERVENTIONS

Arteriovenous Shunt for Dialysis Purposes

NURSING DIAGNOSIS/ PATIENT PROBLEM	DEFINING CHARACTERISTICS	NURSING ORDERS		EXPECTED OUTCOMES
		ASSESSMENT	INTERVENTIONS	
Circulation, impairment of: potential **Etiology** Interruption in arteriovenous (A-V) shunt blood flow	Pain over access area Absence of pulse above the venous exit site Absence of thrill over the shunt area Absence of bruit over the arterial site Decreased temperature of the affected limb	A. Assess A-V shunt for signs and symptoms of inadequate blood flow every _____ B. Analyze and interpret available blood work results, particularly PT, PTT, Hb and Hct	A. Maintain proper positioning of cannulated arm; has to be elevated B. Administer anticoagulants as ordered C. Promote the following preventive measures to ensure adequate blood flow 1. Do not take BP in the cannulated limb 2. Do not draw blood specimens from the cannulated limb D. Instruct patient/significant others to *avoid* the following 1. Sleeping on the shunt limb 2. Wearing tight clothing over the limb with shunt 3. Carrying handbags or packages over the shunt arm 4. Participating in activities or sports that involve active use of cannulated limb E. Teach patient/significant others to check for adequate blood flow 1. Arrange teaching sessions when participants are ready 2. Demonstrate how to feel for pulses and thrill 3. Designate specific areas to feel for pulses and thrill 4. Allow adequate time for return demonstration F. Provide list of available printed materials on cannula care: pamphlets, booklets	A. Patency of the A-V shunt will be maintained as evidenced by 1. Absence of pain over the access area 2. Presence of thrill 3. Presence of bruit 4. Presence of pulse in the venous exit area B. Patient/significant others will state the restrictions for the cannulated limb C. Patient/significant others will be able to do a return demonstration on pulse taking

Originated by **Ofelia Mallari, RN**
Resource person: **Lumie Perez, RN, BSN, CCRN**

Continued.

Arteriovenous Shunt for Dialysis Purposes—cont'd

NURSING DIAGNOSIS/ PATIENT PROBLEM	DEFINING CHARACTERISTICS	NURSING ORDERS		EXPECTED OUTCOMES
		ASSESSMENT	INTERVENTIONS	

Injury, potential for infection
 Etiology
 A-V shunt access
	Pain over access site
	 Fever
	 Red, swollen, warm area around access site
	 Drainage from access site
		Assess the A-V shunt for signs and symptoms of infection	A. Maintain asepsis with the A-V shunt during dialysis
			   1. Clean the area daily with antiseptics. Povidone-iodine (Betadine) solution is the recommended agent
			   2. Apply povidone-iodine or neomycin sulfate ointment to the exit site
			   3. Dress the arm with sterile gauze, then wrap with Kerlix dressing
			   4. Obtain specimen for culture when infection is suspected
			   5. Administer antibiotics as needed, per physician's order
			 B. Explain to patient/significant others the importance of maintaining asepsis with the A-V shunt
			 C. Demonstrate to patient/significant others ways to maintain asepsis
			   1. Cleaning the area with antiseptics
			   2. Applying the povidone-iodine or neomycin sulfate (Neosporin) ointment to the exit site
			   3. Dressing the site with sterile gauze
			   4. Wrapping the cannulated limb with Kerlix dressing
			 D. Instruct the patient/significant others to keep the dressing clean and dry at all times
			 E. Instruct patient/significant others to inform the physician or to call the dialysis unit *immediately* for any signs and symptoms of infection
			   1. Pain over the access site
			   2. Fever
			   3. Red, swollen, and warm access site
			   4. Drainage from access site
				Potential for infection will be minimized
				
				Patient/significant others will be able to state signs and symptoms of infection

Anxiety/fear
 Etiology
 Fear of changes in way of life and living
 Fear of losing job
 Fear of financial burden
 Fear of altered body image
	Verbalizes fear
	 Increased questioning
	 Withdrawn or talks excessively
		Assess patient for
		 A. Anxiety
		 B. Available support systems
		 C. Coping mechanisms
			A. Establish rapport with patient
			 B. Encourage patient to ventilate concerns, questions, and feelings
			 C. Refer to other support groups as appropriate
			   1. Psychologist/psychiatrist
			   2. Social worker
			   3. Psychiatric liaison nurse
			   4. Refer to appropriate groups for peer support
				Fear/anxiety will be minimized as evidenced by patient
				 A. Appearing more calm and relaxed
				 B. Asking appropriate questions

Peritoneal Dialysis: pediatric

NURSING DIAGNOSIS/ PATIENT PROBLEM	DEFINING CHARACTERISTICS	NURSING ORDERS		EXPECTED OUTCOMES
		ASSESSMENT	INTERVENTIONS	
Fluid volume/electrolyte balance, alteration in: potential **Etiology** Renal insufficiency Peritoneal dialysis not functioning properly	Abdominal pain Complaints of fullness Shortness of breath Nausea Decreased urinary output Increased abdominal girth Weight gain Weight loss beyond dry weight Diarrhea	A. Obtain baseline vital signs and dry weight B. Monitor patient's BP q.4h. during dialysis C. Record fluid I & O D. Weigh patient b.i.d. (once before dialysis is begun) E. Measure abdominal girth daily at the end of the drain time F. Monitor patient for tachypnea, retractions, nasal flaring G. Auscultate breath sounds q.4h. H. Monitor patient's electrolytes, especially K+ I. Observe for nausea, vomiting, edema, or disorientation	A. Monitor each exchange, checking to see that outflow is equal to or greater than inflow B. Change child's position at least q.2h. to maximize drainage. Put head of bed at 45 degrees, and turn patient on side C. Check catheter for kinks D. Check catheter for fibrin or clots E. Discontinue dialysis if signs of hypokalemia are present F. Notify physician, and change dialysate concentrate when patient reaches dry weight	Electrolytes and hydration will remain stable during dialysis
Injury, potential for infection **Etiology** Contamination to entry site of peritoneal catheter	Patient complaints of abdominal pain, tenderness, feeling warm, and having chills Rigid abdominal wall Pericatheter site reddened with discharge Fever Cloudy returned dialysate Positive culture and sensitivity	A. Assess peritoneal drainage with each exchange (normal is clear) B. Assess area around catheter site. Catheter site should be clean with no signs of inflammation C. Assess patient for complaint of abdominal tenderness D. Assess vital signs q.4h. unless patient is febrile, then q.2h.	A. Use strict aseptic technique when setting up dialysis and hooking up patient B. Maintain drainage receptacle below the level of the peritoneum to avoid backflow of dialysate C. Notify physician for any signs of infection	Potential for infection will be minimized

Originated by **Agnes Jones, RN**
Resource persons: **Janice L. Miller, RN,C MSN**
            Michele Knoll-Puzas, RN,C BS

Continued.

Peritoneal Dialysis: pediatric—cont'd

NURSING DIAGNOSIS/ PATIENT PROBLEM	DEFINING CHARACTERISTICS	NURSING ORDERS		EXPECTED OUTCOMES
		ASSESSMENT	INTERVENTIONS	
Comfort, alteration in **Etiology** Length of procedure Actual infusing of dialysate Distended abdomen	Patient complains of abdominal pain during procedure Tossing about in bed Complaints of feeling full Patient crying Patient is restless and irritable	Assess patient continually for signs of discomfort	A. Remain at bedside during initiation of dialysis B. Allow/encourage parental involvement during dialysis C. Change patient position to relieve discomfort during inflow D. Allow patient to ambulate if permitted E. Provide diversional play and school activities F. Refer to SCP in Ch. 1: Comfort, alteration in	Relief or minimization of pain will be evidenced by verbalization and appearance of improved comfort
Knowledge deficit, parent/child **Etiology** New procedure	Anxious Restless Withdrawn Regressed Frequent questions Frequent complaints Vague physical complaints	A. Assess knowledge levels of parent and child B. Assess child's developmental stage C. Assess parent-child interactions	A. Review patient diagnosis B. Review peritoneal dialysis and rationale C. Discuss dietary/fluid requirements and restrictions: low sodium, low potassium, adequate protein, high calories, free fluids D. Arrange dietary consultation if necessary E. Discuss medications and their use F. Demonstrate and request return demonstration of peritoneal catheter care G. Discuss return appointments, follow-up care, emergency numbers H. Arrange social service consultation if necessary	A. The parents (and child, if applicable) will verbalize purpose and potential outcomes of peritoneal dialysis B. The parents/child will be able to verbalize and demonstrate appropriate home care measures

CHAPTER EIGHT

Endocrine/Metabolic

DISORDERS

Adrenocortical Insufficiency: Addison's disease

NURSING DIAGNOSIS/ PATIENT PROBLEM	DEFINING CHARACTERISTICS	NURSING ORDERS		EXPECTED OUTCOMES
		ASSESSMENT	INTERVENTIONS	
Tissue perfusion, alteration in **Etiology** Any situation requiring an increased need for corticosteroids (e.g., stress, infection, GI upsets) may lead to shock or vascular collapse	Headache Listlessness and lethargy Physical weakness Nausea and vomiting Intractable abdominal pain Decreased BP Weak, thready pulse Decreased blood sugar Increased potassium Orthostatic hypotension Decreased sodium Increased temperature	A. Assess and record any changes in mentation B. Monitor and record vital signs every _____ C. Assess for orthostatic hypotension by taking postural BP D. Assess for alteration in nervous system: weakness, paresthesia or paresis, and possible paralysis E. Assess patient's muscle strength and ability to ambulate F. Assess GI functioning	A. Minimize stressful situations 1. Promote a quiet environment 2. Provide rest periods 3. Explain all procedures and answer all questions B. Assist patient with activities as needed C. Monitor and record I & O D. Monitor electrolytes E. Monitor ABGs F. Observe for signs of infection G. Closely monitor if patient complains of headache H. Refer to SCP in Ch. 1: Cardiac output, alteration in: decreased (as appropriate)	Optimal tissue perfusion will be maintained
Nutrition, alteration in: less than body requirements **Etiology** Decreased GI enzymes, which result in loss of appetite and decreased tolerance for oral intake Decreased gastric acid production Decreased urinary nitrogen excretion	Recent weight loss Decreased blood sugar Nausea and vomiting Diarrhea Abdominal cramps Anorexia General malaise	A. Assess patient's general appearance B. Assess GI function C. Assess patient's appetite D. Monitor and record weight daily E. Assess which foods patient is able to tolerate	A. Provide foods patient is able to tolerate B. Avoid fasting C. Offer frequent small meals D. Create an environment conducive to eating E. Encourage rest periods F. Encourage patient to follow a diet high in protein, low in carbohydrates, and high in sodium G. Explain need for diet supplements	Adequate nutritional status will be evidenced by A. Maintained weight B. Increased oral intake C. Normal blood sugar D. Decreased GI disturbances E. Increased appetite F. Increased energy level

Originated by **Cathy Croke, RN, MSN**
Resource person: **Susan Galanes, RN, MS, TNS, CCRN**

Adrenocortical Insufficiency: Addison's disease—cont'd

NURSING DIAGNOSIS/ PATIENT PROBLEM	DEFINING CHARACTERISTICS	NURSING ORDERS		EXPECTED OUTCOMES
		ASSESSMENT	INTERVENTIONS	
Knowledge deficit about long-term steroid therapy **Etiology** No past experience with adrenocortical insufficiency	Verbalizes frustrations Expresses need for further information Denial of disease Lack of compliance	A. Assess patient's feelings about disease B. Assess patient's feelings about need for life-long medication C. Assess support systems that are available D. Assess patient's ability to comply with treatment	A. Instruct patient in self-administration of steroids, including expected effects, side effects, and dosage B. Offer information about the need to adjust dosage when under stress C. Emphasize need for a morning or an evening dose D. Discuss the signs and symptoms that require consultation with physician E. Stress the importance of regular physician visits F. Explain how to obtain a medication identification tag and the importance of wearing it G. Inform patient that an injectable form of cortisol with a sterile syringe is available	Patient will verbalize understanding of disease process and guidelines for replacement therapy

Diabetes: insulin-dependent

NURSING DIAGNOSIS/ PATIENT PROBLEM	DEFINING CHARACTERISTICS	NURSING ORDERS		EXPECTED OUTCOMES
		ASSESSMENT	INTERVENTIONS	
Altered metabolic status **Etiology** Reduction of islet of Langerhans cells of pancreas (decreased insulin) Glucose unable to enter cells and blood concentration increased Renal tubular capacity is exceeded, leading to glycosuria	Polydipsia Polyphagia Polyuria Weight loss Increased blood glucose/abnormal glucose tolerance test	Assess for signs and symptoms of hyperglycemia or diabetic ketoacidosis A. Assess vital signs q.4h. B. Monitor blood glucose chemistry every _____ for _____ hours and then q.4h. C. Monitor strict I & O D. Check laboratory results; glucose, electrolytes, acetone levels	A. Administer insulin as ordered (progressively) 1. Insulin drip (if condition warrants) 2. Regular insulin subcutaneously preprandially 3. Regular/NPH AM and PM split-mixed dose when indicated B. Rotate injection sites; document site with each injection (for optimal absorption) C. Provide appropriate diet 1. Obtain dietary consultation 2. Reinforce need for patient to consume all foods on tray and not save for later use 3. Check for proper identification on each meal tray 4. Reinforce dietary instructions	Insulin will be adequate to maintain blood glucose within normal range Nutritional requirements will be adequate for growth and development while *controlling* diabetic state

Originated by **Linda Rosen-Walsh, RN, BSN**
Resource person: **Michele Knoll-Puzas, RN,C BS**
Margaret A. Cunningham, RN, MS

Continued.

Diabetes: insulin-dependent—cont'd

NURSING DIAGNOSIS/ PATIENT PROBLEM	DEFINING CHARACTERISTICS	NURSING ORDERS		EXPECTED OUTCOMES
		ASSESSMENT	INTERVENTIONS	
Fear Etiology Diagnostic and treatment course	Regressive behavior in patient Anger/noncompliance with regimen Refusal to attempt procedures independently	A. Assess coping mechanisms of patient/parents regarding diagnosis and treatment B. Assess for noncompliance, anger, regressive behavior in patient C. Assess overall patient/parent relationship	A. Explain *all* procedures, using a calm and unhurried manner B. Encourage verbalization of feelings regarding diagnosis and chronicity C. Reinforce fact that anger and "mourning" over loss of freedom is a normal coping mechanism D. Support and reinforce progress made toward independence E. Answer any and all questions patient/parents may have	Child/parent will begin to demonstrate coping behaviors with diabetic condition
Knowledge deficit Etiology Initial diagnosis of chronic disease Multifaceted treatment involved in controlling diabetics	Anxiety Fear Anger regarding chronicity Asking many questions Asking no questions Noncompliance with dietary restrictions Failure to attempt own insulin injections or blood glucose chemistry	A. Assess parental/ child willingness to learn B. Assess developmental level of child C. Assess physical ability of child to listen and learn D. Assess parental/ child level of anxiety	A. Contact diabetic teaching service B. Reinforce and encourage progress made toward independence at blood glucose chemistry and insulin techniques C. Reassess level of learning daily D. Allow patient/parent to ask questions E. Explain definition of diabetes, including signs and symptoms F. Reinforce fact that diabetes is a chronic condition for which there is no cure G. Explain that diabetes is controlled through diet, insulin, and exercise H. Define insulin, and discuss different types, action, and duration, especially split-mixed insulin regimen I. Demonstrate accurate method of drawing up and administering insulin. Explain rationale for rotating injection sites J. Explain need for diet-controlled exchange system and importance of strict adherence K. Explain that daily exercise is important for lowering blood sugar and also allowing child to socialize normally with peers. Reinforce that diabetes does *not* restrict physical activity L. Explain that blood glucose monitoring is necessary in diabetic control and that normal glucose levels are 70-110 mg/dl M. Demonstrate accurate use of autolet and interpretation of blood glucose Chemstrips N. Define hypoglycemia (blood glucose <40 mg/dl) and possible causes	A. Readiness and ability of parent/ child to learn about diabetes and its management will be accurately assessed B. Parent/child will verbalize accurate definition of diabetes C. Parent/child will verbalize understanding of types of insulin and will accurately demonstrate drawing up and administering insulin D. Parent/child will verbalize dietary exchange system and specific number-of-calories diet child is on E. Parent/child will verbalize rationale of urine testing and will demonstrate accurate technique F. Parent/child will verbalize knowledge of normal blood glucose levels and will accurately demonstrate blood glucose chemistry procedure

Diabetes: insulin-dependent—cont'd

NURSING DIAGNOSIS/ PATIENT PROBLEM	DEFINING CHARACTERISTICS	NURSING ORDERS		EXPECTED OUTCOMES
		ASSESSMENT	INTERVENTIONS	

			O. Discuss signs and symptoms of hypoglycemia
			  1. Mild: cool, sweaty, shaky, irritable, tired, weak, headache, hungry, personality changes
			  2. Moderate: nausea, sleepiness, disorientation, fainting, decreased level of consciousness
			  3. Severe: coma or convulsion
			P. Instruct child/parents in treatment for symptoms of hypoglycemia (e.g., 4 oz orange juice, hard candy, sugar, candy bar). Discuss use of glucagon for hypoglycemic coma
			Q. Define hyperglycemia (serum glucose >140 mg/dl) and possible causes. Instruct on signs and symptoms: glycosuria, polyuria (bed-wetting), polydipsia, polyphagia, acetone breath
			R. Discuss/define diabetic ketoacidosis and the need to seek immediate medical attention
			S. Discuss need for careful monitoring of blood sugar during illness as it may require an insulin adjustment
			T. Reinforce need to wear Medic-Alert identification
			U. Reinforce need for regular follow-up care, including eye and dental care
			V. Refer to outside agencies and support groups (e.g., American Diabetic Association)
				G. Parent/child will verbalize definition of hypoglycemia and hyperglycemia and necessary steps when these conditions are recognized
				H. Parent/child will verbalize need for proper identification
				I. Parent/child will verbalize need for routine follow-up care
				J. Parent/child will verbalize knowledge of available outside referral and support groups

Diabetic Patient with Recurrent Hypoglycemia/Hyperglycemia

NURSING DIAGNOSIS/ PATIENT PROBLEM	DEFINING CHARACTERISTICS	NURSING ORDERS		EXPECTED OUTCOMES
		ASSESSMENT	INTERVENTIONS	
Health maintenance, alteration in **Etiology** Altered or impaired communication Inability to make deliberate or thoughtful judgments Perceptual/cognitive impairments Complete/partial lack of necessary motor skills Ineffective coping Lack of interest or motivation Unfamiliarity with resources	Demonstrated lack of knowledge regarding basic health practices Demonstrated lack of adaptive behaviors to internal/external environmental change Reported or observed inability to take responsibility to meet health needs History of lack of help-seeking behavior Reported or observed lack of equipment, financial, or other resources Reported or observed impairment of personal support system	A. Assess patient's past pattern of health maintenance and health concept 1. Body/self-image 2. Coping style 3. Compliance with recommendations 4. Use of resources B. Assess patient's health perception and health management pattern specific to diabetes mellitus, including 1. Medications 2. Patterns of monitoring and controlling symptoms of acute/chronic complications and management 3. Use/availability of resources 4. Refer to diabetic assessment checklist for additional information C. Assess ability and willingness to learn or change present pattern(s)	A. Facilitate patient's review of past/present health status via nursing history B. Encourage verbalization of feelings C. Offer guidance and support in realistic problem identification and problem-solving process D. Assist patient in identification of aspects of care for which he/she may be unable to be responsible (temporarily or permanently) E. Assume appropriate responsibility for those aspects of patient's care identified and agreed to in nurse-patient contract F. Assist in identification of available resources and facilitate referrals as appropriate: e.g., financial counselor, social worker, diabetes teaching service, visiting nurse, speech and audiology, psychiatric liaison G. Provide appropriate guidelines for future health maintenance	Patient/significant others will demonstrate progress toward assumption of adequate health maintenance program
Knowledge deficit **Etiology** Intellectual limitations Impairment of memory Impairments to learning, e.g., anxiety, language difficulties, visual, auditory, or tactile difficulties Lack of interest or motivation Lack of information or inadequate resources	Misinterpretation of information Inability to perform return demonstration(s) of skills Inaccurate demonstration or absence of follow-through on previous instruction Inadequate recall or understanding of information Inappropriate behavior (e.g., anger, hostility, withdrawal, apathy)	A. Assess patient's knowledge base regarding diabetes mellitus and specifically hypoglycemia and hyperglycemia. Use diabetic assessment checklist B. Review patient history regarding 1. Medical problems 2. Dietary habits 3. Exercise patterns 4. Medication(s) 5. Frequency and nature of acute complications and treatment	A. Assist patient in monitoring of blood glucose level Fasting blood sugar: ____/____ Urine fractional every _____ Ketones _____ Types of test(s) used B. Observe and assist patient in recognition of signs and symptoms of altered glucose metabolism 1. *Hypoglycemia:* hunger, sweating, pallor, tremor, feelings of nervousness or anxiety, lethargy, irritability, tingling or numbness in lips or tongue (early). Blurred or double vision, mental dullness, change in behavior, fatigue, confusion, dizziness, slurred speech, slow or uncoordi-	Patient/significant others will verbalize A. Signs/symptoms of hypoglycemia and hyperglycemia B. Possible causes of hypoglycemia and hyperglycemia

Originated by **Eileen Raebig, RN,C**
Resource person: **Verda Abernathy, RN, MA**

Diabetic Patient with Recurrent Hypoglycemia/Hyperglycemia—cont'd

NURSING DIAGNOSIS/ PATIENT PROBLEM	DEFINING CHARACTERISTICS	NURSING ORDERS		EXPECTED OUTCOMES
		ASSESSMENT	INTERVENTIONS	

		6. Evidence of chronic complications
		7. Monitoring methods
		C. Observe patient behavior for evidence of altered mental status and or other impairments to learning
			nated movement (gradual)
			2. *Hyperglycemia:* polydipsia, polyphagia, polyuria, nocturia, nausea, vomiting, dim or blurred vision, cephalgia (early). Abdominal pain, GI cramps, constipation, drowsiness, headache, weakness, flushed/dry skin, rapid labored or deep breathing, weak rapid pulse, temperature, acetone breath odor, hypotension, coma (gradual)
			C. Institute prompt treatment for altered glucose states in conjunction with physician
			  1. Hypoglycemia
			    a. Provide approximately 10 g carbohydrate source (4 oz fruit juice, 2 teaspoons honey, 5 Life savers, or 1 glass soft drink)
			    b. Inform physician
			    c. Observe for response
			    d. Administer IV glucose source as ordered
			  2. Hyperglycemia
			    a. Keep patient flat and warm
			    b. If patient is conscious, administer sugar-free fluids
			    c. Notify physician
			    d. Obtain blood/urine specimens
			    e. Prepare to administer parenteral fluids and/or insulin as ordered
			D. Provide information to patient/significant others as immediately as practical regarding possible causes, signs and symptoms observed by nurse and patient, and possible future prevention
			E. Record nursing measures taken and response of patient/significant others
			F. Use a variety of approaches to patient teaching, considering specialized needs identified in assessment area	

Continued.

Diabetic Patient with Recurrent Hypoglycemia/Hyperglycemia—cont'd

NURSING DIAGNOSIS/ PATIENT PROBLEM	DEFINING CHARACTERISTICS	NURSING ORDERS		EXPECTED OUTCOMES
		ASSESSMENT	INTERVENTIONS	
			G. Use principles of adult education in formulating teaching plan, e.g., 1. Progress from simple to complex 2. Build on present accurate knowledge base 3. Information related to patient's unique situation and learning interests may best be received first H. Use a variety of resources in educational efforts as appropriate, e.g., written pamphlets, diabetic teaching service personnel/classes, films, equipment demonstration, dietitian I. Reinforce information provided by diabetic teaching service/ physician/other nursing staff J. Educate patient as to management of altered glucose states such as 1. Carrying carbohydrate source in event of hypoglycemic reaction 2. Carrying identification card or alert bracelet (American Diabetic Association or Medic-Alert Foundation) 3. Promptly seeking attention for anticipated/actual problems K. Educate patient as to means of avoiding alterations in glucose levels 1. Importance of uniformity in diet, exercise, and hypoglycemic agent administration 2. Distribution of carbohydrate load in diet over period of maximum insulin effect (if insulin dependent) 3. Accurate, regular monitoring of serum blood glucose and urine testing 4. Anticipation of change in needs with illness, unusual stress/activity, etc. 5. Importance of regular health supervision L. Provide patient with copy of discharge instruction sheet covering medications, treatments, activity level, and dietary instruction	

Diabetic Ketoacidosis: acute

NURSING DIAGNOSIS/ PATIENT PROBLEM	DEFINING CHARACTERISTICS	NURSING ORDERS		EXPECTED OUTCOMES
		ASSESSMENT	INTERVENTIONS	

Fluid composition, alteration in: diabetic ketoacidosis
Etiology
Omission/reduction of insulin
Initial onset of diabetes
Infection/intercurrent illness
Acute pancreatitis
Stress
	Clinical
	Polydipsia, polyuria
	Weakness, anorexia
	Abdominal pain
	Kussmaul's respirations
	Acetone breath
	Blurred vision
	Nausea, vomiting
	Pallor, diaphoresis
	
	Laboratory
	Serum glucose >300 mg/dl and <900 mg/dl
	Serum ketones ≤ 4:1
	Decreased serum pH, phosphate, bicarbonate
	Normal/low/elevated serum potassium
	Urine glucose: 2%
	Urine acetone: strong
		A. Assess for significant alterations in
		  1. Respiratory rate, depth, type and presence of acetone breath
		  2. I & O
		  3. Serum laboratory values: glucose, ketones, electrolytes, phosphate, and ABGs
		  4. Urine sugar/ acetone
		  5. Bowel sounds, presence of acute abdomen
		B. Assess for underlying cause of ketoacidosis: history of diabetes in family, stress, infection, etc.
			A. Monitor and record respiratory rate, depth, and presence of Kussmaul's respirations every ____ , and notify physician of respiratory rate <____ or >____
			B. Monitor ABGs as ordered. Notify physician if abnormal, and maintain O_2 as ordered
			C. Monitor serum laboratory values as ordered, and notify physician of abnormality. Use blood glucose Chemstrips to monitor serum glucose as necessary
			D. Monitor and record urine sugar/ acetone every ____; notify physician if >____
			E. Administer and record IV fluids and additives as ordered
			F. Administer and record insulin/ insulin drip as ordered. Follow hospital/unit procedure for preparation of insulin drip
			G. Monitor for hypoglycemia. Signs and symptoms include confusion, tremors, pallor, weakness, diaphoresis, serum glucose <60 mg/dl. If signs are present, administer sugar under tongue if NPO or orange juice if patient is tolerating oral fluids. Document and notify physician
			H. Be prepared to administer D5W if serum glucose is <300 mg/dl
			I. Document consistency and amount of emesis; notify physician if present, elevate head of bed 30 degrees, and prepare for possible nasogastric tube placement
			J. Auscultate for bowel sounds every ____. Assess for abdominal pain, checking intensity of pain and location every ____; document and notify physician of any changes
			K. Administer medications, e.g., trimethobenzamide (Tigan) and prochlorperazine (Compazine) as ordered, evaluating for signs and symptoms of any untoward effects
			L. Maintain patient on complete bed rest, and instruct patient as activity level changes occur
				Alteration in fluid composition will be minimized as evidenced by early resolution of diabetic ketoacidosis

Originated by **Nola D. Johnson, RN**
Resource persons: **Susan Galanes, RN, MS, TNS, CCRN**
    Margaret A. Cunningham, RN, MS

Continued.

Diabetic Ketoacidosis: acute—cont'd

NURSING DIAGNOSIS/ PATIENT PROBLEM	DEFINING CHARACTERISTICS	NURSING ORDERS		EXPECTED OUTCOMES
		ASSESSMENT	INTERVENTIONS	
Fluid volume deficit **Etiology** Osmotic diuresis from hyperglycemia	Decreased skin turgor Hypotension, tachycardia Dilute urine Output greater than intake Increased serum values: WBC, Hb, Hct, glucose, BUN Increased sodium, creatinine	A. Monitor and record vital signs every ____; notify physician of any abnormalities: heart rate <____ or >____; BP systolic: <____ or >____; BP diastolic: <____ or >_____ B. Check and record skin turgor every ____ C. Monitor and record I & O every ____ ; notify physician if urine output is <30 ml for 2 consecutive hours D. Monitor and record urine specific gravity every ____ E. Weigh patient daily, and record F. Monitor serum and urine laboratory values, and notify physician of results as indicated	A. Allow fluids that are sugar free for complaints of thirst if patient is not NPO B. Administer IV fluids as ordered to maintain fluid balance	Fluid volume deficit will be minimized as evidenced by A. Normal skin turgor B. Normal vital signs C. Normal serum and urine laboratory values, and normal specific gravity D. Normal I & O
Cardiac rhythm, alteration in: potential **Etiology** Electrolyte imbalance	Irregular pulse Elevated cardiac enzymes Serum K+ abnormalities Arrhythmias per ECG or cardiac monitor	A. Assess laboratory data frequently associated with the development or perpetuation of arrhythmias B. Maintain continuous cardiac monitoring for prompt recognition of changes in rhythm, and document rhythm strip q.12h. C. Check pulses for presence, equality, and quality every ____ D. Assess for any associated chest pain or discomfort, palpitations, or alterations in BP	A. Obtain 12-lead ECG, as necessary, for any consistent arrhythmias, and notify physician B. Correct fluid and electrolyte imbalances as ordered per physician C. Document patient's complaints of chest pain, and notify physician for treatment	Alteration in cardiac rhythm will be minimized as evidenced by A. Regular pulse B. Normal serum K+ levels C. Absence of ectopics on ECG

Diabetic Ketoacidosis: acute—cont'd

NURSING DIAGNOSIS/ PATIENT PROBLEM	DEFINING CHARACTERISTICS	NURSING ORDERS		EXPECTED OUTCOMES
		ASSESSMENT	INTERVENTIONS	
Consciousness, altered levels of: potential **Etiology** Electrolyte imbalance or dehydration	Change in alertness, orientation, verbal response; motor response, pupillary reaction (on neurologic flow sheet) Seizure activity Agitation Impaired judgment	Assess level of consciousness every ____ or as indicated, using coma scale on neurologic flow sheet	A. Maintain serial documentation on neurologic flow sheet B. Keep oral airway at bedside; be prepared to protect patient if seizures occur C. Keep side rails up at all times, bed in low position, and a functional call light within patient's reach D. Reorient patient, as necessary, to environment and procedures E. If alteration in level of consciousness is present, see SCP in Ch. 3: Consciousness, altered levels of	Alteration in level of consciousness will be minimized as evidenced by A. Appropriate verbal and motor response B. Alert patient C. Absence of seizure activity
Knowledge deficit **Etiology** Unfamiliarity with disease process and treatment	Noncompliance: medications; testing urine and blood; follow-up care Unawareness of factors leading to ketoacidosis Signs and symptoms of hypoglycemia Verbalization of lack of knowledge; questions about ketoacidosis Initial diagnosis of diabetes	Seek understanding of disease process by patient/significant others and how it affects patient's lifestyle	Explain to patient and significant others A. Symptoms of early acute diabetic ketoacidosis (drowsiness, nausea, vomiting, flushed skin, thirst, excessive urination, glycosuria, ketonuria) B. Factors that predispose to diabetic ketoacidosis (illness, stress, infection, insufficient insulin, decreased activity and exercise) C. Importance of balanced diet, routine exercise, weight control, accurate medication administration, regular urine and blood testing, and follow-up care D. "Sick day" management: importance of taking insulin even if feeling ill and not eating and supplementing with small amounts of carbonated noncola beverages through the day; frequent testing of urine and blood; keeping physician informed	Patient/significant others will demonstrate or verbalize A. Knowledge of disease process B. Importance of medications and urine and blood testing C. Signs and symptoms of hypoglycemia D. "Sick day" management

Excessive Glucocorticoids: Cushing's syndrome

NURSING DIAGNOSIS/ PATIENT PROBLEM	DEFINING CHARACTERISTICS	NURSING ORDERS		EXPECTED OUTCOMES
		ASSESSMENT	INTERVENTIONS	
Fluid volume excess: potential Etiology Retention of sodium and water resulting from water miner-alocorticoid excess Depletion of potassium because of mineralocorticoid excess	Hypertension Hypokalemia Cardiac arrhythmias Signs and symptoms of congestive heart failure (CHF): rales, jugular vein disten-tion Elevated plasma corti-sol levels in the morning with no normal decline as the day proceeds Hypernatremia Impaired renal con-centrating capacity	A. Assess patient for signs of circulato-ry overload, CHF, and pulmonary congestion B. Monitor and re-cord heart rate, BP, CVP, and re-spiratory rate every _____ C. Assess pulse for regularity every _____ D. Monitor and re-cord I & O every _____ E. Assess patient for signs of muscle weakness F. Assess ECG for appearance of U wave	A. Maintain strict I & O _____ ml/24 hours B. Weigh patient daily and record C. Ausculate lungs and heart. No-tify physician of any abnormal-ities D. Monitor laboratory work (espe-cially potassium and sodium) E. Encourage a diet low in calo-ries, carbohydrates, and so-dium but that has ample protein and potassium content	Fluid volume balance will be maintained as evidenced by A. Normal BP B. Normal potassium and sodium levels C. No muscle weak-ness D. Normal diurnal pattern of cortisol level with a grad-ual decrease until evening
Fluid volume deficit: potential Etiology Glycosuria-induced diuresis, leading to intravascular deple-tion secondary to excessive secretion of glucocorticoids	Decreased urine out-put Increased specific gravity of urine Output greater than in-put Sudden weight loss Hemoconcentration Increased serum so-dium Decreased skin turgor Hypotension Dry mucous mem-branes	Assess for presence of defining characteris-tics	See SCP in Ch. 1: Fluid volume deficit	Adequate fluid vol-ume and electrolyte balance will be maintained as evi-denced by A. Normal urine spe-cific gravity B. Urine output at least 30 ml/hour C. Normal potassium and sodium levels D. Normal skin tugor E. Moist mucous membranes
Potential for injury: infection Etiology Increased cortisol se-cretion keeps the body in a chronic stress state Increased cortisol sup-presses leukocyte adherence to the en-dothelial surface Increased cortisol de-creases leukocyte accumulation at the injury site	Increased temperature Increased white blood cells Local inflammation, redness, or abnor-mal drainage Positive culture results (blood, wound, spu-tum, or urine) Thin skin	A. Assess potential sites of infection: urinary, pulmo-nary, wound, or IV line B. Monitor and re-cord temperature every _____ C. Monitor WBC count D. Note and report promptly any signs of localized or systemic infec-tion	A. Use strict aseptic technique when performing dressing changes, wound irrigations, catheter care, or suctioning B. Avoid the use of indwelling catheters or IV lines whenever possible C. Protect patient from exposure to other patients with infections D. Obtain specimens of blood, urine, serum, etc., for culture and sensitivity if infection is suspected E. Administer antibiotics as or-dered when infection is present	Potential for systemic/ local infection as evidenced by A. Normal WBC count B. Normal tempera-ture C. Prompt detection and treatment of actual infection

Originated by **Cathy Croke, RN, MSN**
Resource person: **Susan Galanes, RN, MS, TNS, CCRN**

Excessive Glucocorticoids: Cushing's syndrome—cont'd

NURSING DIAGNOSIS/ PATIENT PROBLEM	DEFINING CHARACTERISTICS	NURSING ORDERS		EXPECTED OUTCOMES
		ASSESSMENT	INTERVENTIONS	
Increased cortisol impairs WBC migration, antibody formation, and lymphocyte proliferation Increased cortisol increases protein breakdown		E. Assess for signs of skin breakdown	F. Protect patient from bumping and bruising G. Change patient's position every _____ H. Pad bony prominences I. Keep skin clean and dry J. If needed, see SCP in Ch. 1: Skin integrity, impairment of	
Potential for injury: fracture **Etiology** As protein catabolism increases, protein synthesis decreases, leading to osteoporosis from wasting of the bone matrix. In children it can lead to retarded linear growth Chronic cortisol hypersecretion redistributes body fat	Awkward, poorly coordinated movements Abnormal fat distribution; fat from arms and legs deposited on the face, shoulder, trunk, and abdomen Kyphosis or height loss	A. Assess patient's ability to ambulate, and observe gait B. Observe for loss of muscle mass and osteoporosis after minor trauma C. Assess patient for signs of kyphosis or height loss D. Assess fat distribution	A. Keep floor in patient's room clean, dry, and uncluttered B. Encourage the use of a cane or walker if patient's gait is unsteady C. Encourage the patient to wear properly fitted low-heeled shoes D. Notify physician of even minor trauma E. Measure actual height at time of admission, and compare with past medical records	Potential for fractures will be minimized as evidenced by A. Steady gait alone or with use of assistive device B. Prompt detection and early treatment of actual fracture
Self-concept, disturbance in: body image **Etiology** Increased production of androgens may occur, giving rise to virilism in women; hirsutism (abnormal growth of hair) Disturbed protein metabolism results in muscle wasting, capillary fragility, and wasting of bone matrix: ecchymosis, osteoporosis, slender limbs, striae, usually purple Abnormal fat distribution along with edema resulting in moon face, cervicodorsal fat (buffalo hump), obesity of trunk	Verbal identification of feeling about altered body structure Verbal preoccupation with changed body Refusal to discuss or acknowledge change Actual change in body structure Refusal to look at, touch, or care for altered body part Focusing behavior on changed body part Change in social behavior (withdrawal, isolation, flamboyancy) Compensatory use of concealing clothing, other devices	Assess for presence of defining characteristics	See SCP in Ch. 1: Body image: disturbance in	Patient will begin to acknowledge feelings about altered structure
Knowledge deficit about disease process **Etiology** No past experience with excessive glucocorticoids	Questioning, especially if repetitive Silence Anxiety Repeated admission to the hospital for complications Verbalized misconceptions	A. Assess level of knowledge regarding Cushing's syndrome B. Assess patient's 1. Resources 2. Strengths and weaknesses C. Assess for defining characteristics	A. Explain all tests to patient B. Answer all questions honestly C. Explain the methods, rationale, and expected effects of appropriate treatment 1. Surgery 2. Radiation 3. Drug therapy 4. Diet restrictions	Patient will discuss treatment options and ask appropriate questions

Hepatitis

NURSING DIAGNOSIS/ PATIENT PROBLEM	DEFINING CHARACTERISTICS	NURSING ORDERS		EXPECTED OUTCOMES
		ASSESSMENT	INTERVENTIONS	
Activity intolerance Etiology Decreased fat, carbohydrate, and protein metabolism and utilization	Abnormal cardiac response to activity Patient reports of fatigue and weakness Abnormal respiratory response to activity	A. Assess respiratory status before activity 1. Respiratory rate 2. Use of accessory muscles 3. Need for supplemental O$_2$ B. Assess cardiac status before activity 1. Pulse rate 2. Cardiac rhythm 3. BP 4. Skin color and perfusion C. Assess need for ambulation aids D. Assess understanding by patient/significant others of change in activity level and tolerance	A. Maintain bed rest with bathroom privileges B. Provide quiet environment C. Limit visitors as needed D. Help patient learn relaxation E. Plan nursing care to provide long periods of rest F. Medicate with sedatives or tranquilizers as ordered G. Increase activity levels as tolerated by patient H. Monitor patient for signs of relapse precipitated by increased activity that is too rapid or premature 1. Increasing serum/enzymes 2. Increasing anorexia 3. Increasing liver tenderness	Patient will increase activity levels as tolerated without recurrence of hepatitis
Nutrition, alteration in: less than body requirements Etiology Alteration in absorption of nutrients Alteration in metabolism of nutrients Decreased intake of nutrients	Loss of weight with or without adequate calorie intake Documented inadequate calorie intake Increased metabolic state that is not met by calorie intake Anorexia Nausea/vomiting	A. Document patient's actual weight B. Obtain nutritional history C. Obtain baseline laboratory values 1. Serum protein 2. Serum albumin 3. Vitamin assays (as appropriate) 4. Mineral and trace element levels (as appropriate) 5. Serum osmolarity	A. Maintain bed rest to decrease metabolic needs B. Increase activity as patient tolerates C. Provide diet with 1. High carbohydrates; low fats; protein modified as patient tolerates 2. Small meals 3. Largest meal at breakfast D. Give antiemetics before meals E. Encourage patient to take fruit juice, carbonated beverages F. Avoid alcoholic beverages G. Administer vitamin supplements H. Administer enteral supplements or parenteral nutrition as ordered I. See SCP in Ch. 1: Nutrition, alteration in: less than body requirements	Optimal nutritional status will be maintained
Fluid volume deficit: potential Etiology Vomiting Diarrhea Decreased dietary intake	Decreased urine output Concentrated urine Hemoconcentration Increased serum sodium Thirst Edema Dry mucous membranes Decreased pulse pressure Increased heart rate	A. Monitor I & O every shift B. Check patient's weight every _____ C. Monitor 1. Serum sodium 2. Serum osmolarity 3. Total protein 4. Serum albumin D. Check for formation of edema	A. Encourage oral intake of fluids B. Administer enteral and parenteral fluids as ordered C. Note enteric losses of fluid, e.g., vomiting, diarrhea D. Monitor patient for signs and symptoms of dehydration E. See SCP in Ch. 1: Fluid volume deficit	Patient will maintain adequate hydration status

Originated by **Martha Dickerson, RN, MS, CCRN**

Hepatitis—cont'd

NURSING DIAGNOSIS/ PATIENT PROBLEM	DEFINING CHARACTERISTICS	NURSING ORDERS		EXPECTED OUTCOMES
		ASSESSMENT	INTERVENTIONS	
Bowel elimination, alteration in: constipation/diarrhea (potential) **Etiology** Alteration in dietary intake Alteration in digestive processes Decreased activity level	**Constipation** Straining at stool Passage of liquid feces around impaction Abdominal distention Nausea/vomiting Fecal incontinence **Diarrhea** Frequency of stool Loose/liquid stool Urgency Abdominal pain Hyperactive bowel sounds	A. Establish patient's history of elimination B. Determine whether patient uses medications to provide regular elimination	A. Observe stool for color, consistency, frequency, amount B. Provide adequate dietary and fluid intake C. Administer medications for diarrhea or constipation as ordered (SCPs in Ch. 1: Bowel elimination, alteration in)	Patient will have normal bowel function

Skin integrity, impairment of
 Etiology
 Accumulation of bile salts in skin
 Prolonged bed rest
 Mechanical forces associated with bed rest: pressure, shearing
 Frequent diarrhea
 Poor nutritional status
	Itching
	 Disruption of skin surface
		A. Check patient's skin for any signs of breakdown or presence of lesions
		 B. Assess nutritional status: diet, laboratory data, weight
			A. Position patient at least q.2h. to prevent development of pressure lesions
			 B. Use pressure-relieving devices as necessary (see SCP in Ch. 1: Skin integrity, impairment of)
			 C. For itching
			    1. Encourage cool shower or bath with baking soda
			    2. Use calamine lotion
			    3. Administer antihistamines as ordered
			    4. Keep fingernails short
			    5. Provide patient with gloves to wear
				A. Itching will be relieved
				 B. Trauma to skin will be minimized

Diversional activity, deficit: potential **Etiology** Isolation	Verbal complaints of boredom Verbal reports of "feeling isolated" Pacing Daydreaming Excessive napping	A. Assess tolerated activity level (see first assessment) B. Solicit from patient desire for activities/social contact	A. Encourage expression of feelings regarding isolation B. Encourage use of radio, television, newspapers, telephone, calendar, photographs C. Plan nursing intervention to space contact throughout the day D. Encourage family members/ friends to visit as tolerated	Potential for boredom and feelings of isolation will be minimized
Knowledge deficit **Etiology** New condition Unfamiliarity with treatment and disease course	Lack of questions Many questions Noncompliance with isolation procedure	A. Determine understanding by patient/significant others of disease process, complications, and treatment B. Determine understanding of disease transmission C. See SCP in Ch. 1: Knowledge deficit	A. Provide information to patient/ significant others regarding disease and isolation procedures in patient teaching sessions B. Encourage patient/significant others to ask questions C. Assess understanding of information following teaching session D. Observe compliance with treatment regimen E. Observe compliance with isolation procedures F. Observe development of complications	Patient and significant others will demonstrate knowledge of and compliance with treatment regimen and isolation procedures

Hypercalcemia

NURSING DIAGNOSIS/ PATIENT PROBLEM	DEFINING CHARACTERISTICS	NURSING ORDERS		EXPECTED OUTCOMES
		ASSESSMENT	INTERVENTIONS	
Body fluid composition, alteration in **Etiology** Excess calcium in blood secondary to A. Loss from bones because of immobilization, as in cancer with bone metastasis and multiple myeloma B. Excess calcium intake in the diet C. Increase in factors causing mobilization from bones, as in increased parathyroid hormone, increased vitamin D, steroid therapy, thiazide diuretics	**Central nervous system** Depressed or absent deep tendon reflexes, drowsiness, lethargy, confusion, blurred vision, coma **Muscular system** Fatigue, hypotonia, weakness, GI atony, anorexia, nausea, vomiting, abdominal pain **Skeletal system** Bone pain, osteoporosis, pathologic fractures **Cardiovascular system** Arrhythmias, bradycardia, shortened Q-T intervals, cardiac arrest	A. Monitor laboratory values: calcium and other electrolytes (e.g., sodium, potassium and magnesium, which are excreted along with calcium) every _____ B. Monitor renal status: BUN and creatinine levels every _____ C. Assess general appearance 1. Level of consciousness 2. Skin turgor 3. Activity and mobility levels 4. Appetite D. Check patient's medical history related to cancer and drug therapy	A. Reduce calcium intake and restore calcium level to normal 1. Promote renal calcium excretion by a. Saline hydration with use of normal saline infusion as ordered b. Administration of loop diuretics such as furosemide c. Use of acidic juices (e.g., cranberry and prune juices, which dissolve calcium salts) 2. Decrease calcium absorption a. Inhibition of bone resorption through administration of glucocorticoids, cytotoxic antibiotics (e.g., plicamycin), calcitonin, decreased vitamin D intake 3. Decrease intestinal absorption a. Through diets low or absent in calcium, as ordered b. By giving phosphate supplements B. Minimize side effects from these interventions 1. Administer the right IV fluids and drugs as ordered (i.e., the correct amount, route, rate) 2. Monitor for side effects of drug therapy 3. Maintain accurate I & O 4. Obtain daily weights 5. Check vital signs every _____ , with neurologic checks as needed 6. For calcitonin therapy, keep epinephrine at bedside in case of anaphylactic reaction	Calcium balance will return to within normal limits

Originated by **Bella Biag, RN, BSN**
Resource person: **Audrey Klopp, RN, MS, CCRN, CS, ET**
         Dawnetta Collins, RN,C

Hypercalcemia—cont'd

NURSING DIAGNOSIS/ PATIENT PROBLEM	DEFINING CHARACTERISTICS	NURSING ORDERS		EXPECTED OUTCOMES
		ASSESSMENT	INTERVENTIONS	
Fluid volume excess/ deficit: potential **Etiology** Fluid therapy Diuretic therapy	**Excess** Acute weight gain Edema Moist rales on lung auscultation Shortness of breath Puffy eyelids Decreased level of consciousness with confusion **Deficit** Acute weight loss Decreased body temperature Dry skin and mucous membranes Longitudinal wrinkles Furrows of tongue Oliguria Anuria	**General appearance** A. Check skin turgor by observation and palpation for dryness, swelling, or flushing B. Check eyes for puffiness or dryness C. Auscultate lungs for presence of rales. Observe character of respirations: rate, rhythm, depth, and use of accessory muscles D. Palpate bladder for any distention or retention. Also observe for incontinence, pain, or increasing tenderness **Parameters** A. Monitor CVP, and notify physician if <____ cm or >____ cm B. Monitor output; insert Foley catheter if needed as ordered per physician C. Check weight every _____ D. Monitor electrolyte levels, especially potassium, every _____	A. Refer to physician any abnormal findings B. Check vital signs every ____ with neurologic checks and CVP readings C. Regulate IV fluids as ordered; use mechanical pumps or regulators as needed D. Increase fluid intake or restrict fluids as needed: _____ E. Record accurate I & O F. Maintain routine Foley care, including perineal area G. Obtain daily weight with same scale H. Observe signs and symptoms of potassium deficit/excess such as anorexia, ileus, weakness, diarrhea, colic, intestinal irritability, and nausea I. See SCP in Ch. 1: Fluid volume deficit	Hazards of fluid/electrolyte imbalance will be minimized
Consciousness, altered levels of: potential **Etiology** Hypercalcemia Fluid/electrolyte imbalance	Lethargy Restlessness Coma	A. Assess level of consciousness, and check for orientation/disorientation every ____ B. Check pupils for size and reaction to light every ____	See SCP in Ch. 3: Consciousness, altered levels of	Optimal level of consciousness will be maintained

Continued.

Hypercalcemia—cont'd

NURSING DIAGNOSIS/ PATIENT PROBLEM	DEFINING CHARACTERISTICS	NURSING ORDERS		EXPECTED OUTCOMES
		ASSESSMENT	INTERVENTIONS	
Mobility, impaired physical: potential **Etiology** Decreased level of consciousness Bone pain	Presence of pain on movement Stiffness of joints Inability to do active movements with or without assistance Decreased intake of fluid and foods	A. Assess character, nature, and location of pain B. Assess skin, joint, and muscle integrity 1. Check pressure areas for any skin breakdown 2. Check joints for ROM 3. Check muscle tone for loss of muscle mass 4. Check patient's level of activity	A. Decrease bone pain 1. Medicate with analgesics as needed, and record patient's response to medication 2. Provide assistance and support if pain is present on movement B. Promote safety by preventing contractures and decubitus ulcers 1. Provide assistance with ADL, ROM exercises, turning, ambulation 2. Use assistive devices such as pillows, footboards, air mattress or water mattress, Stryker boots 3. Keep all side rails up, especially at night, with small light left on 4. Use restraints as needed 5. Avoid back rubs to prevent pathologic fractures	Hazards of immobility will be minimized
Airway clearance, ineffective: potential **Etiology** Mucous plug or mucous stasis	Decreased level of consciousness Impaired mobility	Auscultate lungs for presence of diminished breath sounds. Observe and record character of respiratory rate/rhythm with complaint of shortness of breath	A. Prevent mucous stasis 1. Encourage increased fluid intake 2. Provide respiratory therapy (e.g., postural drainage, percussion, and vibration) as ordered 3. Help and supervise patient with regularly scheduled breathing exercises (e.g., diaphragmatic breathing and use of incentive spirometer) 4. Establish and maintain regular turning schedule B. See SCP in Ch. 1: Airway clearance, ineffective	Airway will be free of secretions

Hypercalcemia—cont'd

NURSING DIAGNOSIS/ PATIENT PROBLEM	DEFINING CHARACTERISTICS	NURSING ORDERS		EXPECTED OUTCOMES
		ASSESSMENT	INTERVENTIONS	
Knowledge deficit **Etiology** Unfamiliarity with cause of hypercalcemia	Questions from patient/significant others Demanding/manipulative behavior Inability of patient/ significant others to describe diet therapy or drug therapy	A. Assess patient's socioeconomic background B. Assess level of understanding of disease entity by patient/significant others C. Assess level of understanding and knowledge of therapy D. Assess patient's support systems	A. Encourage patient/significant others to verbalize feelings/ needs or problems 1. Establish trusting relationship 2. Create privacy during discussions 3. Show interest and willingness to listen B. Provide health teaching and counseling 1. Provide information to patient/significant others based on identified needs or problems 2. Stress importance of following strict diet therapy, exercise, increased fluid intake, and drug therapy, as well as potential complications 3. Stress importance of regular follow-up to monitor serum calcium levels 4. Provide information as to the various health and governmental agencies that can be used for assistance 5. Encourage maximum participation of patient/significant others in total care, e.g., eating, mobility, ROM exercises, and performing ADL C. Refer patient/significant others to social service and occupational therapy personnel for follow-up	Patient and family will understand the importance of adhering to medical regimen to prevent recurrence of hypercalcemia

THERAPEUTIC INTERVENTIONS

Thyroidectomy

NURSING DIAGNOSIS/ PATIENT PROBLEM	DEFINING CHARACTERISTICS	NURSING ORDERS		EXPECTED OUTCOMES
		ASSESSMENT	INTERVENTIONS	

Airway clearance, in-effective
Etiology
Hematoma
Laryngeal edema
Vocal cord paralysis
Tracheal collapse
 	
Indications for thyroidectomy
 	
Benign or malignant tumor
Graves' disease (hyperthyroidism, thyrotoxicosis)
Hashimoto's thyroiditis
	Neck swelling, tightness
	Stridor, dyspnea, cyanosis
	Intercostal rib retraction during inspiration
	Voice normal, hoarse, or absent
	Immobility of vocal cord as visualized by laryngoscopy
		A. Observe respiratory rate, rhythm every _____
		B. Note quality of voice every _____
		C. Observe neck for swelling, tightness every _____
		D. Examine wound for evidence of hematoma, oozing every _____
		E. Observe for presence of stridor
			A. Keep tracheostomy tray at bedside
			B. Keep head of bed elevated to 45 degrees
			C. Notify physician of any change in
			  1. Respiratory pattern
			  2. Quality of voice
				Airway will be free of secretions

Body fluid constituents, alteration in: hypocalcemia (potential)
Etiology
Inadvertent surgical removal of parathyroid glands (hypoparathyroidism)
Blood supply to parathyroids is damaged (usually temporary but may be permanent)
	A. Paresthesia of circumoral region, fingers, toes
	B. Total serum calcium level <7.7 mg/100 ml indicative of impending tetany (normal: 8.8-10.8 mg/100 ml)
	C. Increased excitability of nervous tissue
	  1. Tetanic spasms
	  2. Positive (+) Chvostek's sign
	  3. Positive (+) Trousseau's sign
	  4. Laryngeal stridor
	  5. Seizure
	  6. Lethargy
	  7. Headache
		A. Note circumoral and peripheral paresthesia every _____
		B. Observe for tremors in extremities every _____
		C. Check for presence of Chvostek's and Trousseau's sign every _____
		D. Monitor serum calcium level. Draw blood specimens as ordered
			A. Notify physician if $Ca^{++} < 8.0$ mg/100 ml
			B. Keep calcium gluconate and syringe at bedside
			C. Maintain IV access
			D. Administer/monitor IV infusions of calcium gluconate. Also, administer oral calcium, vitamin D, as ordered
				Serum calcium level will remain within normal limits

Injury: potential for wound dehiscence (low transverse anterior neck incision) **Etiology** Hematoma Excessive strain on suture line Improper positioning, movement	Wound edges not approximated	Assess neck incision for approximated edges, redness, swelling, drainage, presence of staples/ sutures every _____	A. Notify physician if wound edges are not approximated B. Elevate head of bed 45 degrees C. Avoid flexion of neck D. Avoid rapid movements of head E. Support head with hands when rising	A. Incisional line will be intact B. Stress on suture line will be prevented

Originated by **Laura Vieceli-Brooks, RN, BSN**
Resource person: **Audrey Klopp, RN, MS, CCRN, CS, ET**

Thyroidectomy—cont'd

NURSING DIAGNOSIS/ PATIENT PROBLEM	DEFINING CHARACTERISTICS	NURSING ORDERS		EXPECTED OUTCOMES
		ASSESSMENT	INTERVENTIONS	
Alteration in metabolism, thyroid storm: hyperthyroidism (potential) **Etiology** Inadequate preoperative preparation (euthyroid state not achieved) Increased production of thyroid hormone leads to sensitivity to sympathetic nervous system	Increased pulse (up to 200 BPM) Elevated temperature Increased BP Diaphoresis Nausea, vomiting, diarrhea, abdominal pain Tremor Restlessness, possibly delirium Arrhythmias	A. Assess environment for excessive stimulation B. Assess anxiety level C. Assess for presence of defining characteristics as appropriate	A. Monitor vital signs every _____, and notify physician of abnormalities B. Provide quiet environment (control noise level) C. Reduce anxiety (see SCP in Ch. 1: Anxiety/fear) D. Lower temperature by keeping covers off, use of hypothermia blanket, antipyretic agents, sponge bath E. Promote rest, and administer sedatives as ordered; assist with ADL F. Maintain IV infusion (for hydration, nutrition, electrolyte balance) G. Maintain adequate nutritional intake, especially protein, carbohydrates, vitamins; avoid caffeine H. Administer antithyroid drug (iodine), beta-receptor blocking agent (propranolol), adrenal corticosteroid as ordered	Complications of altered metabolism will be minimized
Knowledge deficit related to home care **Etiology** Lack of previous experience	Increased (or lack of) questioning Verbalized anxiety	A. Assess ability and readiness to learn B. Assess knowledge level regarding postoperative care	A. Instruct patient to inform physician if the following develop 1. Circumoral, peripheral paresthesia; tremors 2. Difficulty breathing 3. Any alteration in voice 4. Sensation of pressure, tightness, fullness in neck 5. Excessive or continual drainage from incision line 6. Incision open and/or red 7. Signs/symptoms of thyroid storm B. Instruct patient to avoid abrupt head, neck movements C. Instruct patient to keep wound dry. May shower when approved by physician	

CHAPTER NINE

Integumentary/Musculoskeletal

DISORDERS

Arthritis, Rheumatoid

NURSING DIAGNOSIS/ PATIENT PROBLEM	DEFINING CHARACTERISTICS	NURSING ORDERS		EXPECTED OUTCOMES
		ASSESSMENT	INTERVENTIONS	

Comfort, alteration in: joint pain
Etiology
Inflammation associated with increased disease activity
Degenerative changes secondary to long-standing inflammation
	Subjective
	Patient/significant other reports pain
	
	Objective
	Guarding on motion of affected joints
	Facial mask of pain
	Moaning or other sounds associated with pain
		A. Solicit patient's description of pain
		  1. Quality
		  2. Severity
		  3. Location
		  4. Onset
		  5. Duration
		  6. Aggravating and alleviating factors
		B. Assess for signs of joint inflammation (redness, warmth, swelling, decreased motion)
		C. Determine past measures used to alleviate pain
		D. Assess interference with lifestyle
			A. Administer antiinflammatory medication as prescribed. The first dose of the day should be given early in the morning with a small snack. Antiinflammatory drugs should not be given on an empty stomach
			B. Use nonnarcotic analgesic as necessary
			C. Encourage patient to assume an anatomically correct position. Do not use the knee gatch or pillows to prop knees. Use a small flat pillow under head
			D. Use hot (e.g., heating pad) or cold packs on painful, inflamed joints. Consult the clinical specialist or physical or occupational therapist for suggestions
			E. Encourage the use of ambulation aid(s) when pain is related to weight bearing
			F. Apply bed cradle to keep the pressure of bed covers off inflamed lower extremities
			G. Consult occupational therapist for the proper splinting of affected joints
			H. See SCP in Ch. 1: Comfort, alteration in: pain
				Patient will verbalize decrease or relief of pain

Comfort, alteration in: stiffness
Etiology
Inflammation associated with increased disease activity
Degenerative changes secondary to long-standing inflammation
	Subjective
	Patient/significant other verbalizes complaint of joint stiffness
	
	Objective
	Guarding on motion of affected joints
	Refusal to participate in usual self-care activities
	Decreased functional ability
		A. Solicit patient's description of the stiffness
		  1. Location: generalized or localized
		  2. Timing: morning, night, all day
		  3. Length of stiffness. Ask patient: "How long does it take you to loosen up after you get out of bed?" Record in hours or fraction of hour
			A. Encourage patient to take a 15-min warm shower or bath on rising. Localized heat (hand soaking) is also useful
			B. Encourage patient to perform ROM exercises after taking a shower or bath. Each joint should be put through two repetitions
			C. Allow sufficient time for patient to carry out all activities
			D. Avoid scheduling tests or treatments when stiffness is present
			E. Administer antiinflammatory medication as prescribed. The first dose of the day should be given early in the morning with a small snack. Antiinflammatory drugs should not be given on an empty stomach
				Patient will verbalize decrease or relief of stiffness

Originated by **Sue A. Conneighton, RN, MSN**

Arthritis, Rheumatoid—cont'd

NURSING DIAGNOSIS/ PATIENT PROBLEM	DEFINING CHARACTERISTICS	NURSING ORDERS		EXPECTED OUTCOMES
		ASSESSMENT	INTERVENTIONS	
		4. Relationship to activities 5. Aggravating/ alleviating factors B. Determine past measures used to alleviate stiffness C. Assess interference with lifestyle	F. Suggest the use of elastic gloves (e.g., Isotoner) at night to decrease hand stiffness G. Remind patient to avoid prolonged periods of inactivity	

Comfort, alteration in: fatigue
Etiology
Increased disease activity
	Subjective
	Patient/significant other describes lack of energy, exhaustion, listlessness
	
	Objective
	Excessive sleeping
	Decreased attention span
	Facial expressions: yawning, sadness
	Decreased functional capacity
		A. Solicit patient's description of fatigue
		  1. Timing (afternoon or all day)
		  2. Relationship to activities
		  3. Aggravating and alleviating factors
		B. Determine nighttime sleep pattern (see Sleep pattern disturbance in this section)
		C. Assess interference with lifestyle
		D. Determine if fatigue is related to psychologic factors (stress, depression)
		E. Determine past measures used to alleviate fatigue
			A. Provide for periods of uninterrupted rest throughout the day (30 min 3-4 times/day)
			B. Reinforce principles of energy conservation as taught by occupational therapist
			  1. Pacing activities (alternating activity with rest)
			  2. Adequate periods of rest (throughout the day and at night)
			  3. Organization of activities and environment
			  4. Proper use of assistive/ adaptive devices
			C. If fatigue is related to interrupted sleep, see the following nursing diagnosis: Sleep pattern disturbance
			D. Consult clinical specialist if fatigue may be related to psychologic factors (see nursing diagnosis on p. 232: Psychosocial adaptation, ineffective)
				Patient will verbalize decrease or relief of fatigue

Sleep pattern disturbance: potential
Etiology
Pain
Stiffness
Psychosocial factors
	Subjective
	Patient/significant other reports inability to fall asleep or frequent awakening through the night
	
	Objective
	Interrupted sleep pattern on several nights
		A. Solicit patient's description of the sleep pattern disturbance
		  1. Difficulty falling asleep
		  2. Frequent awakening throughout the night
		  3. Inhibition of sleep because of pain/stiffness
		  4. Aggravating and alleviating factors
			A. Encourage patient to take a warm shower or bath immediately before bedtime
			B. Encourage gentle ROM exercises (after shower/bath) to help relieve pain and stiffness
			C. Encourage patient to sleep in an anatomically correct position (do not prop knees or head). Change positions frequently through the night
			D. Suggest the use of an electric blanket (set on low temperature)
			E. Provide a quiet and restful environment. Avoid wakening the
				Patient will verbalize an increase in undisturbed sleep

Continued.

Arthritis, Rheumatoid—cont'd

NURSING DIAGNOSIS/ PATIENT PROBLEM	DEFINING CHARACTERISTICS	NURSING ORDERS		EXPECTED OUTCOMES
		ASSESSMENT	**INTERVENTIONS**	
		B. Determine patient's nighttime rituals C. Assess the need for special sleep devices (e.g., bed board, special pillow) D. Determine if sleep pattern disturbance is related to psychologic factors (stress, depression)	patient for unnecessary reasons (routine vital signs) F. Encourage patient to carry out normal nighttime rituals G. Provide special sleep devices or ask family to bring them from home H. Avoid stimulating foods (caffeine) and activities before bedtime I. Encourage the use of relaxation techniques J. Administer a nighttime analgesic and/or long-acting antiinflammatory drug as ordered K. Administer sleeping medication as ordered if requested by patient L. Consult clinical specialist if sleep pattern disturbance may be related to psychologic factors	

Mobility, impaired physical
Etiology
Pain
Stiffness
Fatigue
Psychosocial factors
Altered joint function
Muscle weakness
	Subjective
	Patient/significant other verbalizes difficulty with purposeful movement
	
	Objective
	Decreased ability to transfer and ambulate
	Reluctance to attempt movement
	Decreased muscle strength
	Decreased ROM
		A. Observe patient's ability to
		  1. Ambulate
		  2. Move all joints in a functional manner
		B. Solicit patient's description of
		  1. Aggravating and alleviating factors
		  2. Joint pain and stiffness
		  3. Interference with life-style
			A. Allow patient adequate time to carry out all activities
			B. Provide adaptive equipment (e.g., cane, walker) as necessary, or ask significant other to bring them from home
			C. Reinforce the proper use of ambulation devices as taught by physical therapy
			D. Encourage patient to wear proper footwear (well-fitting, good support) when ambulating
			E. Assist with ambulation as necessary
			F. Reinforce the techniques of therapeutic exercise (ROM and muscle strengthening) as taught by physical therapist
			G. Reinforce principles of joint protection as taught by occupational therapist
				Patient will verbalize/demonstrate increased ability to move purposefully

Self-care deficit
Etiology
Pain
Stiffness
Fatigue
Psychosocial factors
Altered joint functions
Muscle weakness
	Subjective
	Patient/significant other verbalizes difficulty with self-care activities
	
	Objective
	Decreased functional ability of upper and/or lower extremities
		A. Observe patient's ability to
		  1. Bathe
		  2. Carry out personal hygiene
		  3. Dress
		  4. Toilet
		  5. Eat
		B. Assess interference with life-style
			A. Encourage independence
			  1. Assist as necessary
			  2. Provide necessary adaptive equipment (raised toilet seat, dressing aids, eating aids), or ask significant other to bring them from home
			  3. Refer to occupational therapy for specialized needs
			B. Allow patient adequate time to carry out self-care activities
				Patient will verbalize/demonstrate an increased ability with self-care activities

Arthritis, Rheumatoid—cont'd

NURSING DIAGNOSIS/ PATIENT PROBLEM	DEFINING CHARACTERISTICS	NURSING ORDERS		EXPECTED OUTCOMES
		ASSESSMENT	INTERVENTIONS	
		C. Determine assistive/adaptive devices used in self-care activities	C. Encourage patient to take a shower or bath rather than a bed bath D. Refrain from scheduling tests/activities during self-care time E. Offer guidance to patient in pacing activities F. Reinforce the self-care techniques taught by the occupational therapist	

Knowledge deficit
Etiology
New disease/procedures
Unfamiliarity with treatment regime
	Multiple questions
	Lack of questions
	Verbalization of misconceptions
	Verbalized lack of knowledge
		A. Assess patient's level of knowledge about rheumatoid arthritis and its treatment
		B. Identify priorities for patient education
		C. Assess patient's cognitive style of learning (visual, verbal)
		D. Assess the degree to which discomfort will interfere with learning
			A. Provide a private, quiet environment for patient education
			B. Schedule educational sessions when patient is most comfortable
			C. Keep duration of sessions appropriate to patient's attention span and ability to integrate the information
			D. Teach patient according to cognitive style
			E. Introduce/reinforce disease process information
			  1. Unknown etiology
			  2. Chronicity of rheumatoid arthritis
			  3. Process of inflammation
			  4. Joint and other organ involvement
			  5. Remissions and exacerbations
			  6. Control vs cure
			F. Introduce/reinforce information on drug therapy
			  1. Name of drug
			  2. Purpose
			  3. Use of drug
			  4. Directions for administrations
			  5. Potential side effects
			  6. Any other pertinent information
			G. Introduce/reinforce self-management techniques
			  1. ROM exercises
			  2. Muscle strengthening exercises
			  3. Pain management
			  4. Joint protection
			  5. Pacing activities
			  6. Adequate rest
			  7. Splinting
			H. Stress the importance of long-term follow-up
			I. Introduce/reinforce the concept of quackery
				Patient will verbalize an increased awareness about the disease and treatment

Continued.

Arthritis, Rheumatoid—cont'd

NURSING DIAGNOSIS/ PATIENT PROBLEM	DEFINING CHARACTERISTICS	NURSING ORDERS		EXPECTED OUTCOMES
		ASSESSMENT	INTERVENTIONS	
Psychosocial adaptation, ineffective **Etiology** Altered body structure and function Biophysical Psychosocial Inadequate coping mechanism Inadequate support	Patient/significant other verbalizes ineffective psychosocial adaptation to rheumatoid arthritis *Grieving:* anger, depression, withdrawal *Diminished self-concept:* refusal to discuss limitations/altered body function, disparaging remarks about self, withdrawal from role responsibilities *Diminished coping:* expressed hopelessness, prolonged denial of health status, verbalized inability to cope, altered behavior toward self or others *Sexual dysfunction:* verbalization of problem, expressing dissatisfaction, change in sexual relationship	A. Identify behaviors that are suggestive of grieving B. Assess behavioral patterns suggesting an altered self-concept C. Identify behavioral cues suggestive of ineffective individual coping D. Assess cues suggesting sexual dysfunction E. Identify behavioral cues suggestive of ineffective family coping	See SCP in Ch. 12: Grief over long-term illness/disability: psychosocial aspects	Patient/significant other will explore adaptive alternatives

Fracture: extremity

NURSING DIAGNOSIS/ PATIENT PROBLEM	DEFINING CHARACTERISTICS	NURSING ORDERS		EXPECTED OUTCOMES
		ASSESSMENT	INTERVENTIONS	
Comfort, alteration in **Etiology** Injury	**Subjective** Patient/significant others verbalize complaint of pain or discomfort **Objective** Guarding behavior Altered muscle tone (rigid or flaccid) Diaphoresis Increased pulse rate Increased BP Increased or decreased respirations Pallor Crying, moaning Grimacing Anxiety Restlessness Withdrawal Irritability	A. Assess for subjective or objective symptoms of pain or discomfort B. Assess pain characteristics 　Location 　Quality 　Severity 　Onset 　Duration 　Precipitating factors 　Relieving factors C. Determine patient's past experience with pain and pain-relief measures	A. Maintain immobilization and support of affected part B. Reposition and support unaffected parts as permitted C. Elevate affected part D. Apply cold to decrease swelling (for the first 24 hours) E. Anticipate patient's need for analgesia F. Respond immediately to patient's request for analgesia if appropriate to give G. Medicate 30 min before wound/pin care or physical therapy H. See SCP in Ch. 1: Comfort, alteration in	Patient will verbalize and/or demonstrate relief or decrease in pain

Originated by **Marilyn Magafas, RN,C BSN**
　　　　　　Joanne Shearer, RN, MSN
Resource person: **Helen Snow-Jackson, RN, BSN, TNS, CEN**

Fracture: extremity—cont'd

NURSING DIAGNOSIS/ PATIENT PROBLEM	DEFINING CHARACTERISTICS	NURSING ORDERS		EXPECTED OUTCOMES
		ASSESSMENT	INTERVENTIONS	
Fluid volume deficit, potential **Etiology** Multiple fractures Femur fracture Blood vessel damage with bleeding or large areas of ecchymosis and/or third spacing of fluids	Weak, rapid pulse Cool, clammy skin Rapid, shallow respirations Decreased BP Slow capillary refill Decreased urinary output Anxiety Altered level of consciousness	A. Assess for symptoms of hypovolemia (see Defining Characteristics) B. Assess amount of bleeding from external wounds or internal bleeding C. Assess for third spacing or bleeding around fracture site	A. Apply pressure to bleeding wounds B. Administer O$_2$ as ordered C. Use antishock trousers (MAST) as ordered D. Administer IV fluids and blood products as ordered E. Monitor baseline Hct or CBC every _____ hours F. Maintain/restore proper alignment of fracture site. Exception: Splint joints of elbows and knees where found. Do not attempt realignment G. Obtain a circumference measurement of injured area every _____ to assess for further bleeding/third space fluid loss	Occurrence of fluid volume deficit will be minimized

Tissue perfusion, alteration in: peripheral (potential)
 Etiology
 Edema
 Hemmorhage
 Immobilization of fracture site
	Distal to fracture site
	   Skin cool, cyanotic
	   Diminished or absent pulse
	   Slow/absent capillary refill
	   Edema
	   Hematoma
	   Paralysis of muscle groups
	   Altered sensation
	   Numbness, tingling
	   Pain
		A. Assess distal to fracture site every _____ hours
		   Color
		   Sensation
		   Movement
		   Capillary refill
		   Swelling
		   Pulses (presence and quality)
		   Pain
		 B. Compare to opposite extremity
			A. Remove restrictive clothing and/or jewelry from affected part
			 B. Elevate affected part on pillows or by suspension traction if ordered
			 C. Encourage exercise of unaffected parts distal to site as allowed
			 D. Report immediately any neurovascular compromise to physician
			 E. Document all findings completely
				Neurovascular compromise will be minimized

Infection, potential for **Etiology** Open fracture External fixation pins	**Local** Pain/tenderness Redness Swelling Excess warmth Purulent drainage Delayed healing Loosening of pins **Systemic** Increased pulse rate Fever Change in level of consciousness Decreased urinary output Increased WBC	A. Assess wound and/or pin site for 1. Local signs of infection 2. Signs of developing gangrene vesicles filled with red watery fluid and gas bubbles coming from tissue 3. Odors or drainage through immobilization devices that are not removed, i.e., casts	A. Maintain adequate hydration and nutritional status B. Use sterile technique if changing wound dressings C. Keep dressing dry and intact. Give wound care as ordered every _____ D. Observe wound precautions if purulent drainage is present E. Document appearance of wound F. Administer antibiotics as ordered G. Administer tetanus toxoid as indicated	Occurrence of infection will be minimized

Continued.

Fracture: extremity—cont'd

NURSING DIAGNOSIS/ PATIENT PROBLEM	DEFINING CHARACTERISTICS	NURSING ORDERS		EXPECTED OUTCOMES
		ASSESSMENT	INTERVENTIONS	

		B. Inspect wound and/or pin site every _____
		 C. Assess for systemic signs of infection
		 D. Monitor vital signs every _____
		 E. Monitor laboratory values
			H. Pin site care
			 1. Provide care to all pin sites every _____
			 2. Adhere to strict schedule (staff or patient)
			 3. Use aseptic technique in pin care
			   a. Cleanse each pin site with hydrogen peroxide, using sterile applicator, and rinse with normal saline to remove crusting from pin site
			   b. Apply sterile dressing/ ointment as ordered
			   c. Wipe fixator off daily with alcohol
			   d. Document observations	

Nutrition, alteration in: less than body requirements **Etiology** Increased nutritional needs for wound and fracture healing	Poor dietary selection Poor wound and fracture healing Delayed bone repair Decreased total protein/albumin levels	A. Monitor dietary intake and calorie count if indicated B. Assess patient preferences C. Assess laboratory values	A. Encourage and teach importance of diet with adequate amounts of protein, calcium, vitamin C, iron, and calories B. Refer to clinical dietitian as needed C. Provide adequate rest periods	Wound/fracture healing will be maximized by selection and consumption of balanced diet
Mobility, impaired physical **Etiology** Immobilization device (cast, sling pins) Pain	Reluctance to attempt movement Limited ROM Mechanical restriction of movement Decreased muscle strength and/or control Impaired coordination Inability to purposefully move within physical environment, including bed mobility, transfer, ambulation	A. Assess ROM of unaffected parts proximal and distal to immobilization device B. Assess patient's ability to perform basic ADL C. Assess patient's ability to ambulate D. Assess present and preinjury level of mobility E. Assess muscle strength to all extremities	A. Encourage isometric and active ROM, and perform resistive ROM exercises to all unaffected joints q.i.d. and as tolerated B. Splint to support foot in neutral position applied to lower extremity frames (occupational therapy referral for splint) C. Perform flexion and extension exercises to proximal and distal joints of affected extremity, when indicated D. Assist to chair or wheel chair when ordered. Teach transfer technique E. Lift extremity by frame/immobilizer if stable; avoid handling of soft tissue F. Reinforce crutch ambulation taught by physical therapist; assist with gait belt until gait becomes stable G. Use SCP in Ch. 1: Injury: potential for high-risk fall status (as appropriate) H. If patient is bedridden because of immobilization device, see SCP in Ch. 1: Mobility, impaired physical	Limitations related to physical mobility will be minimized

Fracture: extremity—cont'd

NURSING DIAGNOSIS/ PATIENT PROBLEM	DEFINING CHARACTERISTICS	NURSING ORDERS		EXPECTED OUTCOMES
		ASSESSMENT	INTERVENTIONS	
Breathing patterns, ineffective: potential **Etiology** Fat embolism Pulmonary embolus Type of immobilization device/site of fracture	Tachycardia Tachypnea Precordial chest pain Rales, wheezing Cough Dyspnea Shortness of breath Cyanosis Petechiae Altered level of consciousness	Assess for symptoms of breathing pattern abnormality (see Defining Characteristics)	A. Administer O₂ as ordered B. Report symptoms to physician immediately C. See SCP in Ch. 1: Breathing pattern, ineffective D. See SCP in Ch. 4: Pulmonary embolism	Occurrence of altered breathing pattern will be minimized
Knowledge deficit **Etiology** New procedures/treatment New condition	Patient/significant other verbalizes lack of adequate knowledge regarding care/ use of immobilization device, mobility limitations, complications, and follow-up care Confusion; asking multitude of questions Lack of questions Inaccurate follow-through of instruction Improper performance Inappropriate or exaggerated behaviors, e.g., hostile, agitated, hysterical, apathetic	A. Encourage patient to verbalize questions B. Solicit patient's current understanding of his/her diagnosis, treatment, follow-up, etc. C. Assess readiness and ability of patient/significant others to assume responsibility for care	A. Instruct patient (and significant others as needed) regarding 1. Signs of possible complications and appropriate actions to take if they occur (see Potential for infection and Potential alteration in peripheral tissue perfusion in this section) 2. Mobility restrictions 3. Exercises (ROM and isometric) as allowed 4. Pain relief measures (see Alteration in comfort in this section) 5. Nutritional and rest needs 6. Proper use of ambulatory devices (e.g., crutches, canes) if needed 7. Proper use/care of immobilization devices (e.g., casts, slings, pin care) 8. Follow-up care after discharge B. Involve patient/significant others in procedures from beginning, e.g., opening packages, pouring solutions C. Supervise patient/significant others performing the procedure D. Provide patient with own supplies as appropriate	A. Patient and significant other will verbalize understanding of treatment modalities, possible complications, and follow-up care B. Patient/significant others properly perform care as appropriate
Skin integrity, impairment of: potential **Etiology** Presence of immobilization device Improper immobilization device	Pain/tenderness Redness Swelling Delayed wound/fracture site healing Spasm	A. Assess immobilized extremity for redness/breakdown B. If patient has cast, check edges of cast for roughness; check structural integrity of cast for cracks	A. Maintain padding under immobilization device to prevent rubbing B. Use antipressure devices (i.e., flotation devices, air mattress) as appropriate C. Maintain proper immobilization of affected part D. Maintain adequate hydration status E. See SCP in Ch. 1: Skin integrity, impairment of	Impairment of skin integrity will be minimized as a result of proper care of immobilization device

Continued.

Fracture: extremity—cont'd

NURSING DIAGNOSIS/ PATIENT PROBLEM	DEFINING CHARACTERISTICS	NURSING ORDERS		EXPECTED OUTCOMES
		ASSESSMENT	INTERVENTIONS	
Body image, disturbance in **Etiology** Change or loss of body part	Refusal to participate in care Unrealistic perception of course of treatment	Assess feelings of patient/significant others and level of acceptance about injury and method of treatment	A. Perform preoperative teaching if time permits; use pictures of device B. Explain procedures and treatment modalities (show x-ray studies to aid teaching) C. Encourage and give permission to verbalize feelings D. Encourage/support a realistic assessment of the situation E. Avoid false reassurances F. Consult with occupational therapist for modification of clothing G. See SCP in Ch. 1: Body image, disturbance in	Injury and method of treatment will be accepted
Self-esteem, disturbance in **Etiology** Loss of body function Inability to perform role responsibilities Loss of control	Withdrawal behavior Demanding behavior Inability to problem solve Anger Denial Hostility Noncompliance	Assess coping mechanism used by patient/significant others	A. Help patient identify previous stress situations and ways of dealing with them B. Identify and reinforce patient's strengths C. Support continued meaningful roles with significant others and friends: provide for visits, telephone calls, written work, etc., as tolerated D. Encourage patient to plan and participate in activities of care. Adapt care to patient's routines and needs E. Provide opportunities for independent activities F. Continually teach and inform patient and significant others about physical status, treatment plan, etc. G. Make Social Service referral early in hospitalization for financial and resource counseling as needed	Patient will achieve positive expressions, feelings, and reactions about self and situation

Shingles (Herpes Zoster)

NURSING DIAGNOSIS/ PATIENT PROBLEM	DEFINING CHARACTERISTICS	NURSING ORDERS		EXPECTED OUTCOMES
		ASSESSMENT	INTERVENTIONS	
Injury, potential for: secondary infection **Etiology** Skin lesions: papules, vesicules, pustules, and crusting	Itching of lesions Redness and discharge from lesions	A. Assess for presence of skin lesions, defining type, description, and location B. Assess for itching or irritation from lesions C. Assess for signs of localized infection: redness and discharge	A. Discourage scratching of lesions 1. Remind patient not to scratch 2. Trim fingernails B. Use gauze to separate lesions in the skin folds (e.g., breasts, axilla, fingers, toes) C. Implement appropriate isolation precautions 1. Wound and skin precautions for localized infection 2. Strict isolation for disseminated infection D. Do not use topical steroids if a secondary infection is suspected E. Obtain culture and sensitivity of suspected secondary infected lesions as ordered per physician to indicate appropriate antibiotic treatment	Secondary infection will be prevented
Comfort, alteration in **Etiology** Nerve pain, which most commonly affects Thoracic (55%) Cervical (20%) Lumbar and sacral (15%) and the ophthalmic division of the trigeminal nerve	Complaints of pain localized to affected nerve Complaints of sharp, burning, or dull pain Facial mask of pain Alteration in muscle tone	A. Solicit patient's description of pain/discomfort including the characteristics Quality Severity Location Onset Duration Precipitating factors and/or relieving factors B. Assess for nonverbal signs of pain/ discomfort	A. Apply cool wet dressing to pruritic lesions B. Use appropriate pharmaceuticals per physician's order 1. Corticosteroids (antiinflammatory effect) 2. Topical steroid ointment such as triamcinolone acetonide (Kenalog) 3. Vidarabine (Vira-A) which halts new vesicle formation; provides rapid pain relief 4. Antihistamines: relief of itching C. Prevent irritation of lesions 1. Avoid rubbing of the skin or lesion 2. Avoid extreme temperatures 3. Avoid pressure against the skin; use loose, nonrestrictive clothing	Patient's discomfort will be relieved

Originated by **Susan Galanes, RN, MS, TNS, CCRN**

Continued.

Shingles (Herpes Zoster)—cont'd

NURSING DIAGNOSIS/ PATIENT PROBLEM	DEFINING CHARACTERISTICS	NURSING ORDERS		EXPECTED OUTCOMES
		ASSESSMENT	INTERVENTIONS	
Anxiety/fear: potential **Etiology** Isolation Possibility of underlying disease in those past middle age	Restlessness Insomnia Facial tension Overexcited/jittery Expressed concern	A. Assess for signs of anxiety or expressed fear B. Assess patient's coping patterns	A. Allay fears regarding isolation by describing 1. Necessity for isolation 2. Isolation techniques 3. Possible duration of isolation B. Support the patient undergoing diagnostic studies to investigate the presence of internal disease (Hodgkin's disease, lymphosarcoma, malignancy) 1. Display a confident, calm manner and an understanding attitude 2. Establish rapport with the patient 3. Encourage ventilation of feelings C. Refer to the SCP in Ch. 1: Anxiety/fear	Patient will display a calm, relaxed appearance
Consciousness, altered levels of: potential **Etiology** CNS inflammation	Change in alertness Change in orientation Memory impairment Impaired judgment Irritability	A. Assess level of consciousness every ____ or as indicated B. Determine contributing factors to any change in level of consciousness 1. Medications 2. Awakening from a sound sleep 3. Not understanding the question	Refer to SCP in Ch. 3: Consciousness, alteration in level of	Alteration in level of consciousness will be minimized
Breathing pattern, ineffective: potential **Etiology** Varicella pneumonia (present in 15% of adults with herpes zoster)	Dyspnea Shortness of breath Cough Tachypnea	A. Assess respiratory rate and depth every ____ B. Assess breath sounds every ____	Refer to SCP in Ch. 4: Pneumonia	Regular and unlabored breathing pattern will be maintained
Body image, disturbance in: potential **Etiology** Skin lesions	Verbal preoccupation with lesions Focusing behavior on the lesion Refusal to look at or to take part in caring for the skin lesions	A. Assess perception of change in appearance B. Note verbal references to skin lesions	Refer to SCP in Ch. 1: Body image, disturbance in	Patient will begin to acknowledge feelings about the skin lesions

Shingles (Herpes Zoster)—cont'd

NURSING DIAGNOSIS/ PATIENT PROBLEM	DEFINING CHARACTERISTICS	NURSING ORDERS		EXPECTED OUTCOMES
		ASSESSMENT	INTERVENTIONS	

Knowledge deficit
 Etiology
 New condition and procedures
	Questions
	 Confusion about treatment
	 Inability to comply with treatment regimen
	 Lack of questions
		Determine understanding by patient and significant others of disease process, complications, and treatment regimen	A. Encourage patient/significant others to ask questions
			 B. Provide necessary information to patient/significant others
			   1. Description of herpes zoster, including spread of disease
			   2. Explanation of need for isolation, including correct isolation procedures to follow
			   3. The need to prevent scratching or irritation of the lesions
			   4. The need to notify health professionals if any signs of CNS inflammation or signs of pneumonia develop
			 C. Evaluate understanding of information following teaching sessions
			 D. Observe for compliance with treatment regimen
				Patient/significant other will verbalize needed information regarding the disease, treatment, and complications of herpes zoster

Skin Loss, Full-Thickness: comparable to burn injury

NURSING DIAGNOSIS/ PATIENT PROBLEM	DEFINING CHARACTERISTICS	NURSING ORDERS		EXPECTED OUTCOMES
		ASSESSMENT	INTERVENTIONS	
Skin integrity, impairment of **Etiology** Destruction of structures underneath the skin, along with the thickness of skin (potential destruction/damage of epithelium, fat, muscles, bone, and blood vessels) Burns Crushing injuries Thrombocytopenia purpura	Blanching of the skin Redness Leathery appearance Color changes of the skin: brown to black Blistering, weeping skin Pain or absence of pain	Examine skin surface immediately to determine classification A. Check color, texture, turgor, and depth of wound B. Check for blisters, large open wounds, blanching C. Assess degree of pain D. Assess for any odors E. Assess for adherent debris/hair	A. Maintain aseptic technique: wear mask and sterile gloves with physical contact B. Use burn pack or nonadherent sheeting (to prevent sticking) C. Use hydrotherapy tub as ordered per physician to aid in cleansing and loosening slough, exudate, eschar D. Apply topical bacteriostatic substances as directed by physician. Use extreme care when removing topical ointments during dressing change to prevent the removal of granulating skin E. Elevate extremities, if possible	Optimal skin integrity will be maintained

Originated by **Linda Marie St. Julien, RN, BSN**
 Resource persons: **Susan Galanes, RN, MS, TNS, CCRN**
   Audrey Klopp, RN, MS, CCRN, CS, ET

Continued.

Skin Loss, Full-Thickness: comparable to burn injury—cont'd

NURSING DIAGNOSIS/ PATIENT PROBLEM	DEFINING CHARACTERISTICS	NURSING ORDERS		EXPECTED OUTCOMES
		ASSESSMENT	INTERVENTIONS	

Injury, potential for infection
Etiology
Altered skin integrity
	Elevated WBCs
	Elevated temperature
	Presence of positive cultures
	Wound sepsis: abdominal distention, ileus, disorientation
		A. Review laboratory data for any abrupt changes
		B. Monitor and record vital signs every ____, and notify physician if out of range
		BP: ____ to ____
		Respiratory rate: ____ to ____
		Pulse: ____ to ____
		Temperature: ____ to ____
		C. Observe potential sites of infection
		  1. Assess odor and wound appearance at each dressing change
		  2. Routinely assess IV line sites, Foley catheter, and any other invasive sites for infection
			A. Use rigid aseptic technique when wound is exposed
			B. Keep area clean
			C. Promote personal hygiene
			D. Monitor topical agent's effectiveness via wound cultures as ordered per physician
			E. Administer antibiotics on schedule as ordered per physician
				The risk for infection will be minimized

Fluid volume, deficit: potential NOTE: Fluid volume deficit is directly proportional to extent and depth of "burn" injury **Etiology** Massive fluid shifting and loss of circulating volume results in fluid accumulation in the tissues with blister formation; increased capillary permeability Hemorrhage: stress ulcer (curling ulcer)	Altered mental status Tachycardia Hypotension Thirst Skin pale and cool, dusty-looking in dark skinned person Oliguria Restlessness Hypoxia Alteration in electrolytes, especially hyperkalemia Alteration in the acid-base balance Catabolism (outpouring of $K+$ and nitrogen) Coffee-ground emesis Bright-red blood emesis via nasogastric tube Melena stools	A. Assess for signs and symptoms of fluid volume deficit (see Defining Characteristics) B. Monitor vital signs and hemodynamic status, and report to physician if out of range BP: ____ to ____ Heart rate: ____ to ____ Respiratory rate: ____ to ____ CVP: ____ to ____ Pulmonary wedge pressure: ____ to ____ C. Monitor urine specific gravity ____ D. Monitor I & O every ____, and report to physician if urine output is <____ ml/hour E. Obtain daily weight	A. Administer IV and oral fluids as ordered: ____ at ____ ml/hour B. See SCP in Ch. 1: Fluid volume deficit C. Administer antacids and other medications as ordered by physician D. See SCP in Ch. 5: Upper gastrointestinal bleeding, acute (as needed)	Fluid volume deficit will be minimized

Skin Loss, Full-Thickness: comparable to burn injury—cont'd

NURSING DIAGNOSIS/ PATIENT PROBLEM	DEFINING CHARACTERISTICS	NURSING ORDERS		EXPECTED OUTCOMES
		ASSESSMENT	INTERVENTIONS	
		F. Observe for cardiac arrhythmias associated with hyperkalemia, ectopy G. Observe for coffee-ground emesis, bloody emesis, melena stools, abdominal distention, and epigastric pain		
Altered breathing pattern/impaired gas exchange: potential **Etiology** Metabolic acidosis	Tachycardia Decreased breath sounds Alterations in ABGs Tachypnea Cheyne-Stokes respiration	A. Monitor ABGs every _____ B. Monitor respiratory status	A. Administer O₂ as ordered B. See SCP in Ch. 1: Breathing pattern, ineffective	Altered breathing pattern/impaired gas exchange will be minimized
Tissue perfusion, alteration in: peripheral (potential) **Etiology** Blockage of the microcirculation Blood loss Compartment syndrome	Weak thready pulses Edema and swelling Pallor, extremities cool to touch Pain Numbness Decreased platelets Prolonged PT/PTT	A. Check pulses of all extremities every _____ B. Monitor vital signs every ___: BP, heart rate, and respiratory rate for any abrupt changes C. Assess the color and temperature of extremities D. Check for any pain, numbness, or swelling of extremities E. Monitor laboratory data, and report findings to physician (e.g., platelets, PT/PTT)	A. Maintain good alignment of extremities to allow for adequate blood flow without compression on arteries B. Notify physician immediately of any noted alterations in perfusion C. Administer blood products as ordered	Optimal tissue perfusion will be maintained
Nutrition, alteration in: less than body requirements (potential) **Etiology** Excessive metabolic demands resulting from prolonged interference of patient's ability to ingest or digest food Increased basal metabolic rate	Increased ketones Decreased albumin Generalized weakness Negative nitrogen balance (hypoproteinemia) Increased BUN Alterations in fluid and electrolyte status	A. Closely monitor caloric intake B. Monitor urine, serum glucose and ketone levels C. Assess for muscle weakness D. Monitor serum and urine electrolytes and BUN E. Check for bowel sounds F. Monitor gastric pH	A. See SCP in Ch. 1: Nutrition, alteration in: less than body requirements B. Consult dietitian	Alteration in nutritional status will be corrected with minimal catabolism

Continued.

Skin Loss, Full-Thickness: comparable to burn injury—cont'd

NURSING DIAGNOSIS/ PATIENT PROBLEM	DEFINING CHARACTERISTICS	NURSING ORDERS		EXPECTED OUTCOMES
		ASSESSMENT	INTERVENTIONS	
Comfort, alteration in Etiology Pain of injury	**Subjective** Patient or family member verbalizes pain **Objective** Increased restlessness Alterations in sleep pattern Irritability Facial grimaces Guarding	Assess pain characteristics A. Quality B. Severity C. Location D. Onset E. Duration F. Precipitating factor	A. Administer sedatives and analgesics prescribed for pain (via IV while patient is critical) as ordered per physician B. Administer medications on time C. Position patient to promote comfort D. Alleviate all unnecessary stressors or sources of discomfort E. Allay fears and anxiety F. Turn patient to aid in alleviating any pressure points G. Use distraction/relaxation techniques as indicated	Relief of pain or reduction of pain will be evidenced by verbal or nonverbal cues
Anxiety Etiology Change in health status	Restlessness Combativeness Tachypnea Tachycardia	A. Observe patient for signs of anxiety B. Identify normal baseline level of coping	A. See SCP in Ch. 1: Anxiety/fear	Anxiety will be eliminated or reduced
Knowledge deficit Etiology New injury New treatment	Multiple questions Noncommunication Staring Change in behavior Guarding	Assess patient's baseline knowledge of injury and treatment	A. Explain all procedures and tests B. Explain need for sterile techniques with dressing changes C. Explain the reason for frequent assessment/orientation to environment D. Explain the reason for frequent turning and repositioning E. To alleviate fears, explain reason for gloves and mask during sterile procedures	Patient will verbalize knowledge and understanding of injury and treatment

THERAPEUTIC INTERVENTIONS

Arthroscopy of Knee

NURSING DIAGNOSIS/ PATIENT PROBLEM	DEFINING CHARACTERISTICS	NURSING ORDERS		EXPECTED OUTCOMES
		ASSESSMENT	INTERVENTIONS	
Mobility, impaired physical **Etiology** Torn segment of meniscus Loose body in knee joint Degenerated or osteochondritic areas of knee Internal derangement of knee Acute injuries of knee Ligamentous knee injuries Patellar dislocation	Patient/significant others complain of pain, "locked knee," subsequent or intermittent giving-away Swelling Ability to feel loose body Loss of limited motion Positive McMurray test ("click" heard with possible pain on flexion with rotation)	A. Evaluate patient history/onset of injury 1. Mechanism of injury 2. Date of onset 3. Pertinent medical problems (i.e., osteoarthritis, hemophilia, vascular disease) B. Assess physical findings preoperatively and postoperatively (see Defining Characteristics)	A. Stage mobilization from lying to partial sitting, to sitting in a chair, standing, then ambulation B. Demonstrate immediate postoperative exercises, such as quadricep and hamstring strengthening, straight-leg raising, and ambulation with supportive devices such as a walker or crutches C. Monitor 1. Motor strength every ___ hours as necessary 2. Patient's tolerance to the rehabilitation exercises 3. Patient for possible hazards of immobility D. Assist with ambulation when initiated by physical therapy and with weight-bearing as ordered per physician E. Document outcome of interventions	Rapid rehabilitation will be promoted with minimal or no impaired physical mobility
Tissue perfusion, alteration in **Etiology** Altered neurovascular function	Complaints of pain, feelings of severe numbness or coolness of affected extremity Swelling Sluggish/absent capillary refill Coldness Pallor Pulselessness Abnormal calf edema Unusual postoperative bleeding	Assess and compare neurovascular status of both lower extremities preoperatively and postoperatively every ___ as needed. Include color, warmth, circulation, movement, sensation, pulses, and capillary refill	A. Elevate the affected extremity B. Apply ice packs to decrease swelling C. Monitor lower extremities every ___ hour, as needed, for any signs or symptoms of neurovascular insufficiency (see Defining Characteristics) D. Maintain a clean, snug-fitting but comfortable dressing that will absorb leakage of blood or fluid E. Document all signs and symptoms of neurovascular deficit, and notify physician immediately	Adequate tissue perfusion (neurovascular function) will be maintained throughout the postoperative course

Originated by **Lori Luke, RN**
Resource person: **Marilyn Magafas, RN,C BSN**

Continued.

Arthroscopy of Knee—cont'd

NURSING DIAGNOSIS/ PATIENT PROBLEM	DEFINING CHARACTERISTICS	NURSING ORDERS		EXPECTED OUTCOMES
		ASSESSMENT	INTERVENTIONS	
Comfort, alteration in: pain **Etiology** Surgical pain and rehabilitation program	Patient/significant others complain of pain Facial grimacing Moaning or crying Guarding behavior Limited movement Reluctance to move Irritability Restlessness Altered vital signs	A. Determine the source of pain B. Assess the degree and character of pain C. Determine patient's expectations of pain relief	A. Foresee the need for and offer the prescribed analgesics every _____ hour as needed B. Encourage diversional activities C. Instruct that overactivity may portray itself as pain D. If pain persists after taking the prescribed analgesics, rest, and elevation of the affected leg, the physician should be notified E. Document any presence of pain, what was done for it, and what, if any, relief patient expressed	Patient will verbalize and demonstrate relief or decrease of pain
Injury, potential for: infection **Etiology** Incision	Complaint of pain, chills, lethargy Increased warmth of tissue surrounding wound Temperature >37° C (100° F) Erythema around the wound Purulent/foul-smelling drainage Induration Positive wound culture	Perform assessment of A. Skin color and temperature (in general and around the wound) B. Absence/presence of fever C. Character of any drainage present D. Laboratory results	A. Deliver antipyretics and/or antibiotics as prescribed B. Change bandage with sterile-to-clean technique as often as necessary C. Provide and maintain clean and dry linens D. Encourage increased amounts of liquids E. Document subjective and objective findings, and notify physician	Risk of postoperative infection will be minimized
Knowledge deficit: potential **Etiology** New conditions New procedures	Patient verbalizes misconceptions/lack of knowledge concerning hospitalization, the surgical procedure, and the rehabilitation program Patient demonstrates lack of or abundance of questions and increased anxiety	A. Assess patient's previous hospitalization/injury experience B. Assess previous use of crutches or other supportive devices C. Assess expectations of the surgical outcome D. Assess willingness to learn	A. Maintain relaxed and comfortable environment B. Document stress response and action taken C. Teach patient that exercise is essential to strengthen the structures that support and stabilize the knee and *must* be routinely performed D. Increase activity as tolerated. Until the first postoperative visit with physician, the leg should be elevated whenever patient is sitting or lying down E. Keep dressing clean and dry until the first postoperative visit; showers can be taken within 48 hours if the dressing is kept dry F. Instruct that "splashing" or "squishing" inside the knee is normal (this residual liquid left from surgery will be absorbed) G. Instruct that bruises at the puncture site will eventually disappear and that no creams or lotions should be applied to the incision	Patient will verbalize and demonstrate adequate knowledge of procedure and rehabilitation program prescribed before discharge

Arthroscopy of Knee—cont'd

NURSING DIAGNOSIS/ PATIENT PROBLEM	DEFINING CHARACTERISTICS	NURSING ORDERS		EXPECTED OUTCOMES
		ASSESSMENT	INTERVENTIONS	
			H. Instruct on safe use of crutches 1. Patient should wear flat-heeled, well-fitting shoes 2. Crutches should be 1-1½ inches below axillae with the arms slightly flexed 3. Patient should look ahead when walking, not down 4. Tingling or numbness in upper torso may indicate incorrect use of crutches or the wrong size of crutches 5. Crutches should have rubber tips and pads to prevent slipping 6. Crutches used for support may be discontinued when patient is able to walk without a limp (generally after the first 48 hours) I. The follow-up appointment should occur within 7 days of the procedure J. Inform patient that physician will give permission for return to work, sports, activities, etc. (generally 4-6 weeks for running, jogging, or "stop-and-go" sports)	

Bryant's Traction: pediatric

NURSING DIAGNOSIS/ PATIENT PROBLEM	DEFINING CHARACTERISTICS	NURSING ORDERS		EXPECTED OUTCOMES
		ASSESSMENT	INTERVENTIONS	
Tissue perfusion, alteration in **Etiology** Restricted movement and diminished functional use of affected limb(s) Presence of traction with both hips flexed at 90-degree extension and legs suspended by pulleys and weights Posey restraint to maintain child's position in bed (to prevent moving side to side)	Cool extremities Edema, swelling of affected limb Pain, tingling, numbness Pallor Limited movement Decreased or absent pulse	A. Assess neurovascular status q.2h. for color, temperature, capillary refill, edema, peripheral pulses, sensation, movement B. Check proper functioning of traction equipment every ___ hours for 1. Ropes: taut and in center of tract, knots tied securely 2. Pulleys: wheels move freely; secured to attachment bar 3. Weights: correct amount (___ pounds), hanging freely C. Observe for proper body alignment 1. Child in center of bed 2. Buttocks slightly elevated off the bed 3. Legs extended at right angles 4. Traction pull in line with the long axis of bone	A. Maintain proper body alignment by 1. Positioning 2. Restraining 3. Diversional activity B. Maintain traction equipment C. Rewrap Ace bandages as ordered D. Notify physician of any changes	Neurovascular compromise will be minimized
Skin integrity, impairment of: potential **Etiology** Adhesive strips and Ace bandages used in application of Bryant's traction	Redness Blanching Irritation Excoriation Cyanosis	A. Assess skin condition before application of traction/bandages for integrity, color, temperature, dryness, blistering B. Assess pressure areas over bony prominences (heels, back/buttocks, top and dorsum of feet) for redness, dryness, excoriation, blistering, blanching	A. Provide daily skin care to exposed areas B. Gently massage around pressure areas every ___ hours C. Keep bed linen smooth and dry D. See SCP in Ch. 1: Skin integrity, impairment of: actual and potential	Skin integrity will be maintained

Originated by **Lillian Navarrete, RN**
Resource person: **Ruth E. Novitt, RN, MSN**

Bryant's Traction: pediatric—cont'd

NURSING DIAGNOSIS/ PATIENT PROBLEM	DEFINING CHARACTERISTICS	NURSING ORDERS		EXPECTED OUTCOMES
		ASSESSMENT	INTERVENTIONS	
Bowel elimination, alteration in: potential **Etiology** Immobilization	Irritability Crying Abdominal distention Decreased stools (dark, hard, dry, pellet-formed stools)	A. Question parents regarding child's normal stool pattern B. Assess stool for appearance, consistency, frequency, color C. Auscultate bowel sounds every ____ hours D. Assess fluid/food intake E. See SCP in Ch. 1: Bowel elimination, alteration in: constipation	A. Encourage regular meals with child's favorite foods B. Provide diet with increased roughage C. Limit milk intake to meals only D. Supplement with fruit juices and water E. Provide ____ ml/24 hours F. Refer to dietitian G. Record fluid/food intake	Child will maintain normal pattern of bowel elimination
Urinary elimination, alteration in: retention **Etiology** Immobility	Irritability Bladder distention Decreased urinary output Absence of urine Restlessness	A. Assess diapers for evidence of voiding every ____ hours B. Assess urine for appearance, color, volume, frequency C. Assess for bladder distention D. See SCP in Ch. 1: Urinary elimination, alteration in patterns: retention	A. Record I & O B. Notify physician of significant changes in output C. Encourage fluids: ____ ml/hour	Urinary retention will be prevented

Diversional activity, deficit
 Etiology
 Immobility imposed by traction
	Continuous/intermittent crying
	 Attention seeking
	 Child always searching for parent or caregiver
	 Apathy
	 Inactive
	 Withdrawn
	 Irritability
		A. Assess activity limitations imposed by traction
		 B. Assess developmental level of child
		 C. Assess for unusual behavior
		   1. Increased crying
		   2. Irritability
		   3. Boredom
		   4. Withdrawn/inactive
		   5. Attention seeking
			A. Provide age-appropriate stimulation and activities that child can do in bed
			 B. Encourage ROM exercises of uninvolved joints/limb(s)
			 C. Refer to occupational/physical therapist and child life therapist
			 D. Assign a foster grandmother to child during the day
			 E. Encourage frequent parental visits and involvement in child's care
			 F. Pull child's bed into the playroom when possible or place his/her bed close to other children
				Adequate age-appropriate stimulation will be provided while child is in traction

Continued.

Bryant's Traction: pediatric—cont'd

NURSING DIAGNOSIS/PATIENT PROBLEM	DEFINING CHARACTERISTICS	NURSING ORDERS		EXPECTED OUTCOMES
		ASSESSMENT	INTERVENTIONS	
Nutrition, alteration in, less than body requirements: potential **Etiology** Increased needs for bone growth and repair Poor appetite Difficult/uncomfortable positioning for feedings	Weight loss Inadequate fluid/calorie intake for weight/age	A. Assess child's 1. Appetite 2. Likes and dislikes 3. Food/fluid intake B. Assess child's weight C. See SCP in Ch. 1: Nutrition, alteration in: less than body requirements	A. Weigh child before application of traction and before applying cast B. Provide well-balanced diet and adequate fluids based on child's weight and age 1. Formula (____ ml/day) 2. Solid foods/baby foods a. Amount _____ b. Type _____ c. Frequency _____ C. Record fluid/food intake D. Provide fluids/foods that child loves to eat and drink E. Encourage parent to be present during meal times F. Refer to dietitian	Altered nutrition will be minimized as evidenced by bone repair and normal growth
Comfort, alteration in **Etiology** Pain and immobilization	Irritable Crying Poor appetite Altered sleep patterns Poor sucking Difficult to soothe	A. Observe for any of the following pain characteristics 1. Altered facial expressions 2. Vocalizations: groaning, crying, screaming 3. Behavioral changes: irritability, restlessness, fretfulness, interrupted sleep B. Assess for presence of pressure or friction from traction bandages C. Assess for proper body and traction alignment D. Assess effectiveness of any analgesics administered	A. Provide comfort measures 1. Relaxed, quiet environment 2. Proper body alignment 3. Daily hygiene 4. Toys B. Satisfy daily needs 1. Hunger 2. Comfort 3. Soiled diapers C. Administer analgesics as ordered D. Provide emotional support through personal contact, use of toys, and adequate stimuli E. See SCP in Ch. 1: Comfort, alteration in: pain	Pain will be minimized as evidenced by a decrease in verbal and nonverbal pain behaviors
Parental knowledge deficit **Etiology** Hospitalization of child and implementation of Bryant's traction	Anxious Asking questions Silent Inconsistent visiting No physical interaction	A. Assess parent's level of knowledge related to hospitalization and implementation of traction B. Observe parent-child interaction	A. Review and reinforce the following 1. Type of traction and its importance 2. Traction principles to obtain effectiveness 3. Restrictions and limitations of movement 4. How to perform neurovascular checks B. Prepare parents for surgical correction and application of cast (if applicable) C. Encourage parental participation in child's care	Parents will verbalize an understanding of the child's hospitalization and implementation of Bryant's traction

Clubfoot Repair: pediatric

NURSING DIAGNOSIS/ PATIENT PROBLEM	DEFINING CHARACTERISTICS	NURSING ORDERS		EXPECTED OUTCOMES
		ASSESSMENT	INTERVENTIONS	
Comfort, alteration in **Etiology** Postoperative pain	Irritable Crying Restless Difficult to soothe Altered sleep patterns Moaning Tachypnea Tachycardia	A. Assess pain characteristics 1. Quality 2. Location 3. Onset 4. Duration B. Assess for behavioral characteristics (see Defining Characteristics) C. Evaluate effectiveness of pain medication and non-medication measures to relieve pain D. Refer to SCP in Ch. 1: Comfort, alteration in	A. Provide comfort measures 1. Quiet, relaxed environment 2. Reduced noise and light 3. Adequate rest and sleep B. Satisfy physical needs 1. Offer food on a regular basis 2. Provide for sucking if patient is small child or infant 3. Lift child carefully and as a whole unit (do not lift by legs) C. Administer pain medication as ordered by physician	Pain will be relieved or minimized
Airway clearance, in-effective: potential **Etiology** Anesthesia Limited activity Pain medication	Coarse breath sounds Rales and rhonchi Wheezing Shortness of breath Cyanosis Congested cough Weak cough Tachypnea	A. Assess respiratory status q.4h. 1. Auscultate breath sounds 2. Check respiratory rate, depth, and quality 3. Check for presence of rales, rhonchi, wheezing, nasal flaring, and retractions 4. Check skin color B. Evaluate effects/ side effects of medications given	A. Encourage fluids B. Elevate head of bed at 45-degree angle C. Encourage deep breathing and coughing D. Suction nasopharyngeal secretions as needed E. Evaluate effectiveness of respiratory treatments prescribed F. Maintain O_2 and humidity as ordered 1. Bed-side humidifier 2. Mist tent 3. Face mask	Child's airway will remain clear
Tissue perfusion, alteration in: potential **Etiology** Surgery; cast application to lower extremities	Impaired movement of legs Peripheral edema Cyanosis of toes Loss of sensation to toes Mottling of extremities Decreased capillary refill Extremities are cool to touch Restlessness	A. Assess neurovascular status of lower extremities every ____ for 1. Color 2. Sensation 3. Edema and/or swelling 4. Presence/absence of pulses 5. Movement of toes B. Assess cast for any bleeding	A. Elevate casted legs on pillow when patient is in bed B. Encourage deep breathing and coughing C. Perform passive stretching exercises for 10-15 min four times a day D. Maintain functional body alignment E. Keep small objects away from child to avoid objects from being put down cast F. Notify physician(s) if a decrease in perfusion is present	Adequate circulation to lower extremities will be maintained

Originated by **Andrea So, RN, BSN**
Resource person: **Ruth E. Novitt, RN, MSN**

Continued.

Clubfoot Repair: pediatric—cont'd

NURSING DIAGNOSIS/ PATIENT PROBLEM	DEFINING CHARACTERISTICS	NURSING ORDERS		EXPECTED OUTCOMES
		ASSESSMENT	INTERVENTIONS	
Anxiety and fear of parent(s) and child **Etiology** Surgery and hospitalization	Depression Withdrawal Crying Hostility Demanding Restless Tense Overexcited/anxious Tachycardia Tachypnea Elevated BP	A. Assess parent's knowledge and comprehension of hospitalization and surgery B. Assess parent-child relationship C. Assess support system of parents and child: family members, friends, clergy	A. Orient parent(s) and child to hospital environment B. Establish rapport with patient and family C. Encourage expression of feelings and fears D. Explain all tests, procedures, surgery, etc. E. Provide a quiet, relaxed, and private environment F. Encourage participation and involvement of parent(s) in child's care G. Use support staff (e.g., social worker, clergy) H. See SCP in Ch. 1: Anxiety/fear	Parent(s) and child will have a decrease in anxiety level
Skin integrity, impairment of: potential **Etiology** Cast application	Dryness and peeling of skin around cast Decreased circulation to extremity Discoloration of skin around cast	A. Assess skin around cast q.4h. for 1. Color 2. Drainage 3. Sensation 4. Texture 5. Intactness 6. Dryness 7. Breakdowns 8. Rashes B. Assess for signs of tissue impairment 1. Redness or cyanosis 2. Verbal/nonverbal pain behaviors C. Refer to SCP in Ch. 1: Skin integrity, impairment of	A. Massage skin under cast edges with alcohol B. Keep skin around and under cast clean and dry C. Relieve itching by 1. Blowing cool air down cast using an Asepto syringe 2. Inserting a strip of gauze through the cast to massage skin gently D. Petal edges of cast E. Prevent cast from contamination with feces and urine by 1. Changing diaper when soiled 2. Offering bedpan frequently 3. Placing a sheet of plastic under the front and back edges of cast openings 4. Elevating head of bed slightly F. Encourage increased fluid and protein intake	Child's skin integrity will remain intact
Injury, potential for: infection **Etiology** Surgical incision	Odors from cast Drainage on cast near incision site Elevated temperature, pulse, and respiratory rate Elevated WBC Complaints of pain at incision site	A. Assess cast q.4h. for intactness, color, odor, drainage B. Monitor temperature q.4h.	Notify physician if any symptoms of infection are present (see Defining Characteristics)	Risk of infection will be minimized

Clubfoot Repair: pediatric—cont'd

NURSING DIAGNOSIS/ PATIENT PROBLEM	DEFINING CHARACTERISTICS	NURSING ORDERS		EXPECTED OUTCOMES
		ASSESSMENT	INTERVENTIONS	
Knowledge deficit **Etiology** New condition; unfamiliarity with treatment regime	Anxiety Crying Asking frequent questions Demanding Failure to comply with instructions	A. Assess parents' knowledge of clubfoot and surgery B. Assess parents' behaviors and relationship C. Assess parents' ability to learn	A. Establish rapport with parents B. Instruct parents on frequency and method of skin care C. Instruct in signs of complications 1. Discoloration or cyanosis 2. Loss of sensation to toes 3. Edema 4. Pain D. Instruct in methods to prevent complications 1. Elevate cast on pillows 2. Keep skin clean and dry 3. Avoid pressure on chest 4. Maintain high fluid intake 5. Provide age-appropriate activities E. Instruct parents on follow-up care and cast changes	Parents will verbalize A. Signs and symptoms of infection and appropriate interventions if infection occurs B. Necessity of follow-up care

Harrington Rod for Scoliosis

NURSING DIAGNOSIS/ PATIENT PROBLEM	DEFINING CHARACTERISTICS	NURSING ORDERS		EXPECTED OUTCOMES
		ASSESSMENT	INTERVENTIONS	
Anxiety/fear **Etiology** Anticipation of physical harm or psychologic threat (e.g., impending surgery) Forced adaptation to change in health status	**Mild** Restlessness Increased awareness Increased questioning **Moderate-severe** Avoids looking at equipment Moves very little in bed Withdrawal Tense/anxious appearance	A. Recognize child's level of anxiety (mild, severe). Note any signs/ symptoms, especially nonverbal communication B. Assess child's normal coping patterns (by interview with patient/family/significant others/physician) C. Assess knowledge levels of parent/ child: reason for hospitalization, scoliosis, body image, anatomy involved, Harrington rod placement, and postoperative expectations (i.e., ICU, Stryker frame) D. See SCP in Ch. 1: Anxiety/fear	A. Orient child to environment B. Display confident, calm manner and understanding attitude C. Establish rapport with child through continuity of care D. Explain preoperative and postoperative procedures/routines through parent/child teaching E. Encourage ventilation of feelings F. Place child in quiet environment; reduce distracting stimuli G. Adapt care, if possible, to child's routines H. Encourage child to ask questions to clear up misconceptions I. Encourage family to visit J. Use other supportive measures (e.g., medications and psychiatric liaison) K. Provide diversional measures L. Monitor changes in anxiety level M. Introduce child/parent to a nurse from ICU N. Have child practice aspects of anticipated therapy such as deep breathing, spirometer, leg exercises, use of Stryker frame, fracture bedpan	Decreased level of anxiety will be evidenced by A. Calmer, relaxed appearance B. Verbalization of fears/feelings C. Restful night

Originated by **Denise Birkner, RN, BSN**
Resource person: **Michele Knoll-Puzas, RN,C BS**

Continued.

Harrington Rod for Scoliosis—cont'd

NURSING DIAGNOSIS/ PATIENT PROBLEM	DEFINING CHARACTERISTICS	NURSING ORDERS		EXPECTED OUTCOMES
		ASSESSMENT	INTERVENTIONS	
Circulation, alteration in: peripheral (potential) **Etiology** Immobility with venous stasis (preventing normal blood flow and facilitating clot formation) Reactions to anesthesia and medications Blood loss	Distention or decreased pulsation of neck veins and lower extremities Ischemic pain Increased coldness, numbness, loss of hair, trophic skin changes, pallor, or rubor Swelling of lower extremities Delayed healing of lesions Changes in BP **Pulmonary embolism** Dyspnea Tachycardia Chest pain Fever Neck vein distention Cyanosis Restlessness Hypoxemia Hemoptysis	A. Inspect neck (jugular vein) for pulsation and/or distention B. Observe skin over extremities for color, pallor, rubor, hair distribution C. Inspect for distention of any superficial vessels of lower extremities and along IV site D. Assess vital signs every ___ hours E. Assess circulation, mobility, and sensation of all extremities F. Assess peripheral pulses G. Assess for development of thrombophlebitis: leg swelling, redness, pain on dorsiflexion H. Assess for pulmonary embolism (see Defining Characteristics)	A. Compare temperature of extremities; palpate pulses (radial, femoral, pedal), and compare symmetry. Palpate extremities for edema B. Measure calves and thighs if symptoms of deep vein thrombosis are present C. Maintain body alignment D. Apply TED hose E. Turn patient on Stryker frame as ordered F. Encourage coughing and deep breathing q.2h. G. Demonstrate and encourage leg exercises H. Question child for chest pain, shortness of breath, or hemoptysis	Circulatory complications will be prevented or at least minimized
Gas exchange, impaired: potential **Etiology** Hypostatic pneumonia related to Prolonged anesthesia Immobilization in OR and on Stryker frame	Sudden onset of shaking chills Fever Flushed skin Productive cough (pink-tinged) Sharp chest pain, increased on inspiration Headache Rales/rhonchi Tachypnea Decreased breath sounds over affected lung area Hypoxemia	A. Assess respiratory rate, rhythm, amplitude every ___ hours B. Auscultate breath sounds every ___ hours C. Assess vital signs every ___ hours	A. Turn child on Stryker frame as scheduled B. Encourage coughing and deep breathing exercises every ___ hours and suction as needed C. Note chest pain, shortness of breath, or hemoptysis D. Demonstrate breathing exercises and use of spirometer (blow bottles, glove) to prevent hypostatic pneumonia E. Monitor ABGs F. Evaluate symptoms of hypoxia G. Obtain sputum for culture and sensitivity H. Encourage child to avoid dehydration by drinking plenty of fluids I. Administer antibiotics, if ordered J. Perform chest percussion and postural drainage as necessary K. Administer humidified air or O_2 as ordered	Prevention of hypostatic pneumonia will be evidenced by A. Breath sounds that are clear on auscultation B. Respiratory rate within normal limits

Harrington Rod for Scoliosis—cont'd

NURSING DIAGNOSIS/ PATIENT PROBLEM	DEFINING CHARACTERISTICS	NURSING ORDERS		EXPECTED OUTCOMES
		ASSESSMENT	INTERVENTIONS	
Fluid volume deficit **Etiology** Rapid blood loss or excess fluid loss (through fever, diarrhea, nasogastric drainage, diaphoresis, and inadequate fluid intake)	Specific gravity >1.025 Output greater than intake Decreased urine output Sudden weight loss Hypotension Thirst Tachycardia Decreased skin turgor Dry mucous membranes Weakness	A. Assess hydrational status and nutritional needs: skin turgor, mucous membranes, I & O B. Observe for signs of dehydration, and report to physician C. Evaluate nutritional value of diet	A. Monitor strict I & O every ____ hours B. Report urine output <30 ml/ hour for 2 consecutive hours C. Administer parenteral fluids as ordered D. Monitor electrolytes E. Monitor urine specific gravity F. Monitor and document child's vital signs every ____ hours; report abnormalities G. Encourage liquid intake of 2000-3000 ml/day unless contraindicated H. Provide appropriate dietary supplements I. See SCP in Ch. 1: Fluid volume deficit	Fluid volume and electrolyte balance will be maintained as evidenced by A. Normal electrolytes B. Urine output of at least 30 ml/hour C. Balanced I & O D. Normal skin turgor E. Moist mucous membranes F. Normal urine specific gravity
Injury: potential for infection **Etiology** Harrington rod insertion	Surgical incision Swelling Hematoma Redness Odor Burning/itching Pain Numbness Fever Increased WBC	A. Assess skin integrity 1. Note color, moisture, texture, and temperature 2. Assess incision line and dressing for drainage every ____ hours 3. Check incision for cleanliness, approximation, swelling, hematoma, redness, odor, every ____ hours 4. Ask child about burning or itching B. Assess nutritional status C. See SCP in Ch. 1: Skin integrity, impairment of	A. Keep dressing dry and intact B. Maintain Steri-strips to back incision until removed with alcohol ____ days postoperatively before casting C. Prevent skin breakdown by meticulous skin care with each turning D. Report any changes (i.e., redness, swelling, drainage, or heat) at incisional area E. Prevent pressure on incisional area by 1. Turning patient as scheduled on Stryker frame 2. Using prophylactic antipressure devices 3. Maintaining proper body alignment F. Encourage adequate nutrition and hydration	Risk of skin breakdown will be minimized, and tissue integrity will be maintained

Continued.

Harrington Rod for Scoliosis—cont'd

NURSING DIAGNOSIS/ PATIENT PROBLEM	DEFINING CHARACTERISTICS	NURSING ORDERS		EXPECTED OUTCOMES
		ASSESSMENT	INTERVENTIONS	
Alteration in neurologic function (potential) **Etiology** Surgery proximal to spinal cord and nerve roots Increased potential for neurologic injury at surgical site Prolonged immobilization Development of edema, infection, hematoma at surgical site with nerve root/ cord compression	Increased back pain Radiating pain in distal nerve root (thigh, calf, foot) Paresthesia (numbness, tingling of extremities) Urinary retention Ileus, constipation Weakness in leg, foot, or toes Absent or decreased reflexes (nerve root) or increased reflexes (spinal cord) Asymmetric lower extremity reflexes Change in sensory function Pain in extremities Signs and symptoms of infection	Assess for neurologic deficits every _____ hours (see Defining Characteristics)	A. Use verbal commands: ask child to do simple tasks (e.g., wiggle toes and dorsiflex feet) to assess motor function B. Use light touch and pain to check sensations C. Check child's GI activity and fluid/electrolyte balance D. Check bowel/bladder control E. Document and communicate findings of neurologic assessment	Optimal neurologic function will be maintained
Urinary elimination, alteration in: urinary retention (potential) **Etiology** Neurogenic bladder Obstructive uropathy Recent anesthesia Medications Obstructed catheter	**Subjective** Complaints of lower abdominal pain or discomfort Desire but inability to urinate **Objective** Decreased (<30 ml/ hour) or absent urinary output for 2 consecutive hours Frequency Hesitancy Urgency Lower abdomen distention Restlessness	Assess for symptoms of urinary retention	See SCP in Ch. 1: Urinary elimination, alteration in patterns: retention	Child will not retain urine
Bowel elimination, alteration in: constipation/impaction (potential) **Etiology** Anesthesia Inadequate fluid or food intake Decreased mobility Emotional tension Analgesics	**Subjective** Feeling of fullness Cramping pain Tender abdomen Headache Nausea Anorexia **Objective** Abdominal distention Gurgling, decreased or absent bowel sounds Hard masses of stool on examination or expelled Flatulence Dehydration Vomiting	Assess for signs and symptoms of constipation/impaction	See SCP in Ch. 1: Bowel elimination, alteration in: constipation/ impaction	Child will return to normal preoperative bowel habits

Harrington Rod for Scoliosis—cont'd

NURSING DIAGNOSIS/ PATIENT PROBLEM	DEFINING CHARACTERISTICS	NURSING ORDERS		EXPECTED OUTCOMES
		ASSESSMENT	INTERVENTIONS	
Comfort, alteration in: pain **Etiology** Surgical procedure	**Subjective** Child/significant other reports discomfort **Objective** Guarding behavior Self-focus, withdrawal Crying Moaning Restlessness Irritability Facial mask of pain Altered muscle tone Changes in vital signs, respiration, color Altered sleep pattern	Assess for signs and symptoms of discomfort	See SCP in Ch. 1: Comfort, alteration in: pain	Pain will be relieved or minimized
Mobility, impaired physical **Etiology** Immobilization on Stryker frame, by cast or brace	Inability to purposefully move within the physical environment Reluctance to attempt mobility, limited ROM, decreased muscle strength and control Imposed restrictions of movement, including mechanical devices, medical protocol, impaired coordination	A. Assess for impaired mobility B. See SCP in Ch. 1: Mobility, impaired physical	A. Encourage early ADL when possible B. Turn patient on Stryker frame as scheduled C. Encourage appropriate use of assistive devices D. Maintain patient's body in good alignment E. Use antipressure devices prophylactically as ordered/indicated F. Perform meticulous skin care (use moisturizer) every _____ hours G. Encourage breathing exercises and coughing every _____ hours H. Maintain I & O I. Encourage fluid intake of 2000-3000 ml/day J. Monitor and record daily bowel activity K. Explain progressive physical activity L. Instruct child and family on importance of ROM and breathing exercises M. Encourage verbalization of feelings N. Explain to child length of time he/she will be on Stryker frame and unable to get up and walk	Normal physiologic function will be promoted and complications minimized
Injury, potential for **Etiology** Postoperative placement on Foster or Stryker frame Unstable condition of spine and Harrington rod	Trying to get up Brakes not on bed Improper lifting Improper turning	A. Assess environment for safety hazards B. Assess all equipment for proper working conditions, e.g., safety straps, brakes, screws in place	A. Provide safe environment for child B. Avoid jolting frame and child, especially in turning C. Ensure equipment is in good working condition D. Maintain safety straps on child at all times E. Prevent displacement of Harrington rod; do not lift child under axillae, and instruct child not to lift hands over head	Injury will be prevented

Continued.

Harrington Rod for Scoliosis—cont'd

NURSING DIAGNOSIS/ PATIENT PROBLEM	DEFINING CHARACTERISTICS	NURSING ORDERS		EXPECTED OUTCOMES
		ASSESSMENT	INTERVENTIONS	
Self-concept, disturbance in **Etiology** Body image changes Body cast Lack of privacy Separation from family/significant others and peers	**Subjective** Dependence Depression Denial/grief Withdrawal Restlessness Regression Anger Sadness **Objective** Frequent questions Frequent complaints Negative attitude Crying/irritability Distorted self-image Expressions of self-doubt Verbalizes discontent with body	A. Assess child's normal coping mechanisms (by interviews) B. Assess knowledge levels of child/family C. Assess child's intellectual skills and provide him/her with necessary information to use in problem solving D. Assess the impact of scoliosis, surgery, and limitations on child	A. Allow child to continue as many normal activities as possible (e.g., ADL, schooling) B. Provide diversionary activities (e.g., telephone, television, friends), and establish schedules C. Be sensitive to child's concerns about body image, and intervene appropriately D. Provide as much privacy as possible, especially during bathing and toileting E. Allow child/family to verbalize concerns F. See SCP in Ch. 1: Self-concept: disturbance in	Parent/child will verbalize understanding of temporary changes in body image

Parent/child knowledge deficit
Etiology
Changes in postoperative self-care activities
	Subjective
	Anxious
	Restless
	Withdrawn
	Regressed
	
	Objective
	Frequent questions
	Frequent complaints
	Vague physical complaints
		A. Assess knowledge levels of parent/child concerning necessity, duration, care, and application of body cast
		B. Assess child's developmental stage as applicable
		C. Assess parent/child interactions
			A. Teach child/parent necessity of body cast
			B. Teach factors important to skin integrity and recognition of skin breakdown
			  1. Signs and symptoms
			  2. What to report
			  3. Nutrition
			  4. Mobility
			  5. Hygiene
			C. Explain and assist child in home exercise program
			D. Demonstrate observations for circulation checks: change in color, sensation, temperature, respiration difficulty, and abdominal discomfort
			E. Explain home medications, dosages, and times
			F. Discuss return appointments
			G. Discuss restrictions/limitations placed on child
			H. Instruct in home cast care
			I. Arrange for home equipment with available services for transportation
			J. Suggest appropriate community agencies as referral sources
				Parent/child will verbalize and demonstrate appropriate home care measures for cast and skin care

Laminectomy

NURSING DIAGNOSIS/ PATIENT PROBLEM	DEFINING CHARACTERISTICS	NURSING ORDERS		EXPECTED OUTCOMES
		ASSESSMENT	INTERVENTIONS	
Fear/anxiety (potential) of impending surgery **Etiology** Knowledge deficit Loss of control of activity Possible complications Lack of success	Withdrawn behavior Verbal cues: crying, hostility, negative expectations Avoiding subject of surgery Obsession with possible complications Obsession with idea of failure	A. Encourage patient to verbalize concerns B. Assess patient's knowledge regarding his/her surgery C. Assess patient's need for additional information 1. Patient exhibits anxiety with increased information 2. Patient avoids receiving information 3. Patient asks questions/seeks information D. Assess patient's understanding of information regarding surgery 1. Patient able to repeat information in own words 2. Patient able to explain instructions to significant other accurately 3. Patient able to perform return demonstrations correctly 4. Patient able to state rationale for each instruction	A. Encourage patient to verbalize his/her picture of the surgical procedure B. Review with patient the purpose and general procedure C. Instruct patient regarding postoperative therapy 1. Use of incentive spirometer _____ times, every _____ hours 2. Practice coughing and deep breathing 3. Practice log rolling from side to side 4. Practice log rolling onto bedpan 5. Request analgesic for discomfort 6. Familiarize patient with a pain scale: 0-5, with 5 most severe 0 ————— 5 3 No Moderate Severe pain pain 7. Instruct patient on sequential compression sleeves, their purpose, and duration 8. Introduce patient to TED hose: purpose and duration 9. Introduce patient to Foley catheter: purpose and duration 10. Introduce patient to Hemovac drains: purpose and duration 11. Inform patient that he/she will be checked frequently by nurses 12. Inform patient of probable length of bed rest: _____ days (varies with physician) 13. Point out to patient positive aspects of surgery 14. Educate significant other regarding postoperative therapy 15. Encourage significant other to support patient	Patient's fear will be eliminated or reduced

Originated by **Linda M. Jones, RN, BSN**
Resource person: **Marilyn Magafas, RN,C BSN**

Continued.

Laminectomy—cont'd

NURSING DIAGNOSIS/ PATIENT PROBLEM	DEFINING CHARACTERISTICS	NURSING ORDERS		EXPECTED OUTCOMES
		ASSESSMENT	INTERVENTIONS	
Comfort, alteration in: pain **Etiology** Surgical incision Limited mobility Stiffness/soreness Spasms	Restlessness Verbal cues Facial expressions Body rigidity Rings nurse's light frequently Requests frequent position changes	A. Assess patient for signs and symptoms of discomfort (see Defining Characteristics) B. Assess effect of repositioning C. Assess effect of analgesic 1. Patient sleeps 2. Patient appears restless 3. Patient exhibits signs and symptoms of side effects	A. Encourage patient to describe discomfort: character, location, intensity, radiation, precipitating factor B. Encourage patient to *rate discomfort* on pain scale C. Encourage patient to request analgesic or muscle relaxant at early sign of discomfort D. Maintain correct body alignment at all times E. Log roll patient side to side q.2h. F. Maintain pillows behind back, hips, between legs, and under upper arms G. Prevent strain on back muscles by 1. Maintaining head of bed flat unless otherwise indicated by physician 2. Flexing upper legs with pillows when patient is supine, or use knee gatch (avoid flexing knees with pillows directly under popliteal space) H. Gently massage back and extremities with lotion I. Encourage quiet environment J. Offer analgesic every _____ hours K. Instruct patient to evaluate *effect of analgesic* in relieving discomfort, using the pain scale 0 ——————— 5 3 Complete Moderate No relief relief relief L. Instruct patient to avoid soreness/stiffness by 1. ROM of ankles 2. Bending and extending knees 3. Flexion and extension exercises of arms _____ times every _____ hours	A. Patient will verbalize minimal/ tolerable discomfort or no discomfort B. Patient rating of discomfort on the pain scale will be <3

Laminectomy—cont'd

NURSING DIAGNOSIS/ PATIENT PROBLEM	DEFINING CHARACTERISTICS	NURSING ORDERS		EXPECTED OUTCOMES
		ASSESSMENT	INTERVENTIONS	

Tissue perfusion, alteration in: to lower extremities (neurovascular status)—potential
 Etiology
 Surgical procedure
 Immobility
	Numbness/tingling
	 Absent or diminished reflexes
	 Absent or faint pedal pulse
	 Absent or sluggish capillary refill
	 Pallor
	 Coolness
	 Edema
	 Unrelieved pain
		A. Assess patient's lower extremities for altered sensation
		   1. Sharp vs dull
		   2. Cool vs warm
		   3. Bilateral vs unilateral
		 B. Assess patient's mobility in lower extremities
		   1. Active ROM
		   2. Passive ROM
		   3. Strong vs weak
		   4. Bilateral or unilateral
		   5. Presence or absence of Babinski's reflex
		 C. Assess patient's vascular status in lower extremities
		   1. Color
		   2. Capillary refill
		   3. Temperature
		   4. Pulses
		   5. Homans' sign
		 D. Assess bowel and bladder status
		 E. Assess for deep vein thrombosis
			A. Encourage patient to perform ankle ROM exercises
			 B. Check sequential compression sleeves (if ordered) for
			   1. Correct position (space for knees)
			   2. Tightness
			   3. Looseness
			   4. Excessive warmth
			 C. Remove sequential compression sleeves every shift, and note circulatory status
			 D. Check TED hose (if applicable) for
			   1. Correct position
			   2. Constriction at thighs, ankles
			 E. Remove TED hose every shift, and note circulatory status
			 F. Reposition (log roll) q.2h. and as needed
				Neurovascular status of lower extremities will remain unchanged from preoperative condition

Breathing pattern, ineffective: potential **Etiology** Anesthesia Immobility Inability to adequately cough and deep breathe Atelectasis Embolism	Increased respiration >24/min Decreased respiration <10/min Patient complains of shortness of breath or dyspnea Decreased breath sounds Auscultation of wheezes, rhonchi, congestion Altered character of respiration: shallow, retractions	Assess respiratory status (see Defining Characteristics)	A. Encourage patient to use incentive spirometer _____ times, every _____ hours B. Encourage patient to cough and deep breathe C. Log roll patient from side to side q.2h. D. Monitor patient for temperature >38.5° C (101° F) E. Encourage patient to notify nurse or physician of shortness of breath or dyspnea	Optimal respiratory status will be maintained

Continued.

Laminectomy—cont'd

NURSING DIAGNOSIS/ PATIENT PROBLEM	DEFINING CHARACTERISTICS	NURSING ORDERS		EXPECTED OUTCOMES
		ASSESSMENT	INTERVENTIONS	

Mobility, impaired physical
Etiology
Surgical procedure
Bed rest activity
Discomfort
	Patient requesting assistance on movement
	Patient verbalizing difficulty in moving
	Patient requesting analgesic before movement
		A. Assess patient's ability to reposition self in bed
		  1. Independent
		  2. Requires assistance
		  3. Poor coordination
		  4. Poor use of body mechanics
		B. Assess patient's muscular strength
		  1. Strong
		  2. Weak/flaccid
		  3. Stiff
		C. Assess patient's ability to follow instructions
		D. Assess patient's tolerance to activity
		  1. No complaints
		  2. Tires easily
		  3. Verbalizes discomfort
		    a. Immediately
		    b. Within ___ minutes
		  4. Requests additional or progression of activity
		E. Assess patient's ability to perform ADL (see *A*)
			A. Offer analgesic before activity
			B. Encourage active ROM of extremities
			C. Encourage patient's independent repositioning in bed when tolerated
			D. Assist patient to dangle at side of bed (when approved by physician postoperative day ___)
			  1. Patient must be in side-lying position, near edge of bed, with knees bent
			  2. Elevate head of bed
			  3. Use hands (patient's) to push up upper torso and to pivot buttocks to sitting position with straight back
			E. Dangle for 3-5 min
			F. Ambulate patient as tolerated
			  1. Patient uses hands/arms to push up hips from bed
			  2. Patient stands for a few minutes
			  3. Patient uses assistance first time
			G. Progress ambulation as tolerated. Use cane as needed
			H. Instruct patient in sitting
			  1. Use straight-back chair
			  2. Place pillows in seat to reduce strain if seat is low
			  3. Bend knees
			  4. Support weight with arms
			  5. Elevate feet with one pillow on floor (relaxes back muscles)
			I. Instruct patient to ambulate or sit while wearing corset (if prescribed)
			J. Patient is not to sleep with corset on
			K. Patient is to sit for no longer than 10-15 min (first time) and progress as tolerated. No prolonged sitting at any time
				Patient will be independent or need minimal assistance with mobility

Laminectomy—cont'd

NURSING DIAGNOSIS/ PATIENT PROBLEM	DEFINING CHARACTERISTICS	NURSING ORDERS		EXPECTED OUTCOMES
		ASSESSMENT	INTERVENTIONS	
Nutrition, alteration in: less than body requirements (potential) **Etiology** Altered GI status	Nausea/vomiting Abdominal distention Absent bowel sounds Constipation	A. Assess bowel sounds 1. Absent 2. Hypoactive 3. Active B. Assess abdominal girth C. Assess patient's tolerance to fluids	A. Auscultate bowel sounds in all quadrants q.4h. B. Measure abdominal girth every morning C. Monitor patient tolerance to fluids D. Monitor I & O E. Encourage patient to verbalize nausea or flatulence F. If patient has nasogastric (NG) tube 1. Monitor output 2. Perform fluid challenge (if ordered) a. Instill hourly for 3 hours, and clamp after each instillation b. On the fourth hour, aspirate; if >150 ml, do not discontinue NG tube G. If NG tube remains 1. Monitor IV rate for adequate fluid intake 2. Monitor potassium level 3. Monitor NG pH every _____ hours 4. Notify physician of pH <5 H. If patient has no BM within 2 days of resuming regular diet 1. Notify physician 2. Administer laxatives (if ordered) 3. Push oral fluids 4. Encourage bulk in diet 5. Increase activity	Optimal nutritional status will be maintained
Injury, potential for infection to body **Etiology** Surgical procedure Poor aseptic technique during dressing changes Foley catheter	Elevated temperature ≥38.5° C (101° F) Purulent drainage from incision Elevated WBC Signs/symptoms of wound infection	A. Assess surgical incision every shift for appearance and drainage: color, odor, amount B. Assess urine for color, odor, specific gravity, consistency	A. Use aseptic technique during dressing changes B. Perform Foley care every day as needed C. Encourage patient to drink adequate amount of fluids D. Monitor WBC E. Obtain samples for urinalysis and culture and sensitivity after Foley catheter is discontinued and/or on signs/symptoms of urinary tract infection F. Notify physician of these interventions	Risk for infection will be minimized

Continued.

Laminectomy—cont'd

NURSING DIAGNOSIS/ PATIENT PROBLEM	DEFINING CHARACTERISTICS	NURSING ORDERS		EXPECTED OUTCOMES
		ASSESSMENT	INTERVENTIONS	
Knowledge deficit related to discharge **Etiology** New condition and procedures	Questions Lack of questions Confusion about treatment	Determine knowledge of postdischarge recovery guidelines	**Discharge instructions** **Car ride home** A. Lie on back seat of automobile with pillows or B. Sit with pillow behind back, with buttocks to back of seat and knees slightly elevated on book (reduce stress on back muscles) **Sleep** A. Maintain correct body alignment B. Use pillows as indicated while hospitalized. A firm mattress is recommended. Sleeping on the side, with knees and hips flexed, is preferable to sleeping on the back or abdomen **Activities** A. Ambulate as tolerated with or without corset (per physician's instructions) B. Perform exercises (if indicated) per physician's order and as instructed by physical therapist C. Sit for short periods; may increase as tolerated D. Avoid lifting or carrying heavy objects E. Avoid reaching/stretching to pick up an object. Raise yourself to the level required F. Sexual activity: recommended abstinence for about 3 weeks or as instructed by physician G. Resume driving _____ per physician H. Return to work _____ per physician **Complications** Notify physician of persistent lower back pain, leg pain, numbness, weakness; change in bowel and bladder status; or wound changes, fever; change in gait	Patient will verbalize understanding of discharge instructions

Le Fort I Osteotomy

NURSING DIAGNOSIS/ PATIENT PROBLEM	DEFINING CHARACTERISTICS	NURSING ORDERS		EXPECTED OUTCOMES
		ASSESSMENT	INTERVENTIONS	
Breathing patterns, altered **Etiology** Wired jaws Possible nasal or pharyngeal swelling Possible laryngeal edema caused by prolonged endotracheal intubation	Elevated respiratory rate Labored respirations Nasal breathing resulting from jaws being wired	A. Assess rate and rhythm of respirations every _____ B. Assess nasal airway for patency every _____ C. Auscultate breath sounds every _____	A. Keep head of bed elevated at all times B. Have wire cutters taped to wall at head of bed C. Have aspirator with Yankaeur suction at bedside D. Instruct patient on oral suctioning with Yankaeur suction tube E. Clean nasal airway with normal saline as appropriate F. Maintain humidified air per face tent G. Administer decongestants as ordered per physician	Complications of altered breathing pattern will be minimized
Nutrition, alteration in: less than body requirements **Etiology** Wired jaws Change in dietary habits	Weight loss Documented inadequate caloric intake	A. Monitor I & O every shift B. Determine patient's dietary preference C. Assess patient's weight every _____	A. Arrange for dietary consult for patient/significant other B. Keep head of bed elevated C. Instruct patient on proper use of feeding syringes D. Instruct patient not to attempt to open mouth E. Provide patient with antiemetics as ordered F. Instruct patient who feels about to vomit to sit up and turn head to the side and suction out secretions G. Reassure patient that emesis will be liquid in form, that it will pass between the teeth, and that it can be easily suctioned H. Provide patient with a diet that is high in calories, protein, and vitamin C I. Provide patient with liquids and soft and blenderized foods that require no chewing J. Have dietary supplements at bedside K. Maintain IV fluids as ordered L. Push oral fluids	Adequate nutritional and fluid balance will be maintained while jaws are wired

Originated by **Patricia A. Hannon, RN**
Resource person: **Audrey Klopp, RN, MS, CCRN, CS, ET**

Continued.

Le Fort I Osteotomy—cont'd

NURSING DIAGNOSIS/ PATIENT PROBLEM	DEFINING CHARACTERISTICS	NURSING ORDERS		EXPECTED OUTCOMES
		ASSESSMENT	INTERVENTIONS	

Injury, potential for: intraoral infection
 Etiology
 Improper oral hygiene
	Elevated temperature
	 Excessive oral secretions
	 Foul odor coming from mouth
	 Increased facial swelling
	 Excessive drainage on head and face dressing
		A. Check head and face dressing for excessive drainage, noting color, amount, and presence of foul odor
		 B. Check vital signs, noting any increase in temperature
		 C. Observe for increased facial swelling, and loosen dressing as needed
			A. Administer IV antibiotics as ordered
			 B. Administer corticosteroids as ordered
			 C. Apply ice packs to both sides of face
			 D. Instruct patient on proper mouth care
			   1. Normal saline rinses after each meal and at bedtime
			   2. Brushing teeth with a child-size, soft toothbrush after meals and at bedtime, beginning 48 hours after surgery
				Potential for intraoral infection will be minimized

Communication, impaired: verbal **Etiology** Wired jaws	Increased facial swelling Difficulty understanding patient verbally	A. Determine if patient can speak so he/she is understood by others B. Determine if patient can write	A. Have call light within patient reach B. Provide patient with paper and pen at bedside C. Instruct patient not to attempt to open his/her mouth D. Inform patient that the wires will usually be removed in 6-8 weeks E. Offer patient support and reassurance	Alternate means of communication will be enhanced
Knowledge deficit related to home care **Etiology** Lack of previous, similar experiences	Patient repeatedly asking same questions Lack of questions being asked by patient Patient unable to perform return demonstrations on proper use of feeding syringes and proper oral hygiene maintenance	A. Determine if patient has any questions B. Determine if patient can use feeding syringes and perform proper oral hygiene with ease	Teach patient/significant other the following A. Wire cutters are provided but should be used only in an emergency B. Correct way to cut wires C. Dietary instructions will be provided per dietitian, along with syringes and suction catheters for home use D. Proper cleaning of feeding syringes after each use E. Avoid alcohol because it causes loss of control of secretions F. Best position to assume for vomiting G. Importance of maintaining proper oral hygiene H. Facial swelling will usually be gone in 1 week	Patient will demonstrate and verbalize appropriate, safe self-care

Shoulder Arthroplasty, Total

NURSING DIAGNOSIS/ PATIENT PROBLEM	DEFINING CHARACTERISTICS	NURSING ORDERS		EXPECTED OUTCOMES
		ASSESSMENT	INTERVENTIONS	
Neurovascular status, alteration in: potential **Etiology** Altered circulation/ perfusion of affected arm	Cool, cyanotic, or pulseless extremity Altered sensation or movement of extremity Sluggish/absent capillary refill Edema	A. Assess color, peripheral pulses, sensation, and motor function postoperatively, and compare to patient's preoperative status B. Measure extremity to detect increase in circumference or presence of edema	A. Monitor and document neurovascular assessment every ____ hours 1. Recommended: q.4h. for 24 hours postoperatively, then q.8h. after that if neurovascular status is stable 2. Report any change to appropriate physician immediately B. Measure and record increase in circumference/presence of edema every ____ hours. Notify appropriate physician if increase in circumference is noted	Optimal neurovascular status will be maintained
Mobility, impaired physical **Etiology** Preoperative: adhesions/pain Postoperative: pain, spasm, other factors	Preoperative: may have limited ROM of affected extremity Postoperative: initially will have limitations in flexion, abduction, and extension	A. Assess full ROM of affected extremity preoperatively, and document B. Assess postoperative ROM, documenting improvement or failure to progress C. Assess/document the performance of ADL	A. Maintain arm in shoulder immobilizer for ____ days (as ordered) B. After immobilizer is removed (with physician's order), apply sling C. Begin ROM exercises of hand, elbow, and wrist in conjunction with physical therapy personnel: extension, abduction, flexion D. Reinforce/assist with shoulder exercises after initiation/demonstration in physical therapy department E. Encourage and assist patient in performance of basic ADL: self-feeding, brushing teeth, combing hair	Full ROM will be maintained
Comfort, alteration in **Etiology** Surgical pain and physical therapy treatment	**Subjective** Patient/significant others complain of pain or discomfort **Objective** Withdrawal, guarding behavior, crying, moaning, grimacing, anxiety, rigidity, tachycardia, diaphoresis	A. Assess patient/significant others for subjective complaints of pain or discomfort B. Assess patient for objective symptoms of pain or discomfort C. Document observations D. Assess effectiveness of intervention(s) in relieving pain/discomfort	A. Assess the vital signs every ____ hours; document tachycardia B. Give analgesics as ordered and as needed. Encourage patient to take medications *before* pain becomes severe 1. Evaluate the effectiveness of analgesia 2. Offer analgesia 30-45 min before physical therapy C. Try other measures to relieve pain/discomfort 1. Ice pack to shoulder after exercise as needed (with physician's order) 2. Reposition patient q.1-2h. Avoid positioning on operative side 3. Evaluate/document effectiveness of these pain-relief measures	Pain will be relieved or minimized

Originated by **Cynthia Gordon, RN, BSN**
Resource person: **Marilyn Magafas, RN,C BSN**
       Janet I. Linder, Registered Physical Therapist

Continued.

Shoulder Arthroplasty, Total—cont'd

NURSING DIAGNOSIS/ PATIENT PROBLEM	DEFINING CHARACTERISTICS	NURSING ORDERS		EXPECTED OUTCOMES
		ASSESSMENT	INTERVENTIONS	
Knowledge deficit **Etiology** Lack of information regarding surgical procedure	Patient expresses lack of familiarity with exact nature of procedure Apparent confusion over events Lack of questions	A. Question patient/ significant others regarding procedure and surgical events B. Assess patient/significant others for subjective response to questions/fears regarding surgery	A. Encourage/answer any questions before and after surgery B. Review procedure and perioperative events 1. Purpose of surgery 2. Actual procedure in terms suited to intellectual/cognitive level of patient 3. Postoperative events and care, with emphasis on exercise C. Inform patient about and encourage use of other teaching resources 1. Hospital television channel for movie on perioperative events and care 2. Ancillary departments such as physical therapy/occupational therapy D. Review information after patient teaching session E. Document questions/concerns of patient and instruction given	Patient will verbalize understanding of surgical procedure
Pulmonary function, alteration in: potential **Etiology** Surgery Immobility Pain Anesthesia Fat embolus	A. Abnormal breath sounds, respirations B. Abnormal ABGs C. Symptoms of early respiratory insufficiency/failure D. Abnormal sputum production because of inability to cough productively E. Signs/symptoms of fat embolus 1. Respiratory insufficiency/ failure 2. CNS manifestations a. Headache, irritability b. Delirium c. Progression to marked alteration in level of consciousness	Assess respiratory system at least every ____ hours, documenting and reporting any significant abnormalities	A. Encourage patient to use spirometer, to cough, and to turn to nonoperative side every ____ hour B. If respiratory abnormalities develop, send urine for fat analysis, and notify physician (fat embolus is most likely to develop on second postoperative day) C. Assist patient with ambulation per physician's order D. Monitor vital signs every ____ hour; document and report any abnormalities E. Document any signs/symptoms of systemic manifestation of fat emboli and report immediately to physician F. Administer pain medication to assist patient to cough, turn, and deep breathe more effectively	Optimal pulmonary function will be maintained

Shoulder Arthroplasty, Total—cont'd

NURSING DIAGNOSIS/ PATIENT PROBLEM	DEFINING CHARACTERISTICS	NURSING ORDERS		EXPECTED OUTCOMES
		ASSESSMENT	INTERVENTIONS	

	3. Cardiovascular
	  a. Early: tachycardia, mild drop in BP
	  b. Late: shock symptoms
	4. Renal: fat globules in urine
	5. Integument: petechial hemorrhages on torso, axillae, conjunctiva			

Injury, potential for infection **Etiology** Interruption of skin integrity secondary to surgical incision	Inability of wound to heal Abnormal appearance of wound, drainage Elevated temperature Left shift in differential WBC count (include polymorphonuclear cells, bands) Complaints of severe incisional pain Incision warm to touch	A. Monitor the appearance of incision for redness, pus, bulging, dehiscence B. Assess vital signs every ___ hours, taking the temperature q.4h. and notifying physician if temperature exceeds 38° C C. Assess laboratory values in regard to WBC differential, documenting and reporting abnormal left shift	A. Administer preoperative scrub to area per physician's order B. Use sterile/aseptic technique for dressing changes and during wound inspection C. Inspect wound at least every shift D. Administer appropriate antibiotics as ordered E. Obtain culture and sensitivity and Gram stain per physician's order if infection is suspected F. Notify appropriate personnel, and document if any signs/ symptoms of infection appear	Risk for infection will be minimized

Knowledge deficit
Etiology
Unfamiliarity with discharge activity
	Multiple questions
	Lack of questions
		A. Ask patient to verbalize questions related to activities/limitations after total shoulder arthroplasty
		B. If patient has limited or poor cognitive ability, involve significant others or guardian in discharge teaching
			Instruct the patient/significant others in discharge care
			A. Perform only passive ROM exercises for the first 25 days. Thereafter active exercises may be started
			B. Avoid activities such as heavy lifting, pulling, pushing
			C. Avoid activities that involve exaggerated external rotation and abduction
			  1. E.g., push-ups, golf, volleyball
			  2. Any activity in which the affected extremity is required to support the weight of the body
				Patient will verbalize those activities to avoid that may cause dislocation of the affected extremity

Skeletal Traction: pediatric

NURSING DIAGNOSIS/ PATIENT PROBLEM	DEFINING CHARACTERISTICS	NURSING ORDERS		EXPECTED OUTCOMES
		ASSESSMENT	INTERVENTIONS	

Mobility, impaired physical
Etiology
Fractured limb
Decreased strength
Imposed restrictions of movement
	Inability to move within the physical environment
	Limited active joint ROM
	Decreased muscle strength, control, mass
		A. Assess child's ability to move both unaffected and affected limb(s)
		B. Assess child's vital signs
		C. Auscultate breath sounds every ___ hours
		D. Assess cough (if present)
			A. Maintain child's body in functional alignment
			B. Use assistive devices for moving, especially with lower limb fractures (e.g., overhead trapeze, side rails)
			C. Assist child with repositioning every ___ hours
			D. Encourage coughing, turning, and deep breathing every ___ hours
			E. Encourage child to move unaffected limbs as much as possible
			F. Initiate use of antipressure devices
			G. Instruct family/child in
			  1. Complications of immobility
			  2. Measures to decrease occurrence of complications
			H. See SCPs in Ch. 1: Mobility, impaired physical; skin integrity, impairment of
				Family/child will demonstrate proper methods of movement and measures to prevent complications

Injury, potential for infection at insertion site of Steinmann pins
Etiology
Break in skin on each side of affected limb
Interruption of bone structure
	Redness
	Swelling
	Discharge
	Odor
	Increased temperature
	Pain
	Tenderness
		A. Assess area surrounding pins every ___ hours for
		  1. Condition
		  2. Odor, redness, swelling, discharge, and warmth
		  3. Excessive pain and tenderness
		B. Assess vital signs (especially temperature) every ___ hours
			A. Treat pin entry sites as surgical wounds
			B. Provide pin care every ___ hours as ordered
			C. Encourage foods high in protein and vitamin C
			D. Instruct family/child in
			  1. Potential for infection: signs and symptoms of infection
			  2. Prevention of infection: pin care and purpose
				Risk of infection will be minimized

Originated by **Mary P. Knoezer, RN, BSN**
Resource person: **Ruth E. Novitt, RN, MSN**

Skeletal Traction: pediatric—cont'd

NURSING DIAGNOSIS/ PATIENT PROBLEM	DEFINING CHARACTERISTICS	NURSING ORDERS		EXPECTED OUTCOMES
		ASSESSMENT	INTERVENTIONS	
Tissue perfusion, alteration in: potential **Etiology** Fractured limb and immobility imposed by traction	Complaints of numbness or tingling Pale and cool extremity Absence of pulse distal to injury Cyanosis	A. Assess neurovascular status every ____ hours for 1. Capillary refill 2. Pain 3. Change in sensation to extremity 4. Temperature 5. Mobility B. Assess circulatory status every ____ hours for 1. Pulse 2. Color 3. Homans' sign 4. Redness 5. Localized swelling	A. Encourage movement of all extremities B. Report any circulatory compromise to physician C. Instruct family/child in 1. Complications/warning signs of impaired circulation 2. Methods to prevent complications	A. Neurocirculatory compromise will be minimized B. Family/child will verbalize methods to prevent complications
Bowel elimination, alteration in: potential **Etiology** Immobility	Complaints of abdominal pain or fullness Absent or decreased BMs Decreased bowel sounds Oozing of stool Decreased appetite Small, very hard stools Crying on defecation Increased straining on defecation Grimacing	A. Assess child's normal pattern of bowel elimination B. Assess BMs for frequency, amount, color, consistency, straining, incontinence, presence of blood C. Auscultate bowel sounds every ____ hours D. Assess dietary/fluid intake E. Palpate abdomen for intestinal distention F. Assess presence of stool in rectum	A. Encourage fluids (water, fruit juices): ____ ml q.8h. B. Refer to dietitian to increase intake of fiber in diet C. Administer stool softeners as ordered D. Provide privacy while child is using bedpan E. Encourage position changes as child is able F. See SCP in Ch. 1: Bowel elimination, alteration in: constipation G. Instruct family in appropriate diet and fluid intake to prevent constipation H. Instruct child not to ignore the signs of defecation	A. Child's normal pattern of GI elimination will be maintained B. Family/child will verbalize measures to prevent constipation
Urinary elimination, alteration in patterns: retention (potential) **Etiology** Immobility	Inability to void Urgency Dribbling Bladder distention Restlessness Pain, discomfort Absence of urine	A. Assess patterns of urinary elimination B. Monitor I & O	A. Offer bedpan/urinal every ____ hours B. Place bedpan/urinal within easy reach C. Provide privacy when child is voiding D. Offer fluids of preference or foods with a high water content E. Encourage fluids ____ ml q.24h. F. Instruct family on measures to assist the child with voiding: privacy, positioning, fluid intake G. Explain to child (age permitting) importance of voiding frequently H. See SCP in Ch. 1: Urinary elimination, alteration in patterns: retention	A. Urinary retention will be prevented B. Family will demonstrate measures that will enhance voiding

Continued.

Skeletal Traction: pediatric—cont'd

NURSING DIAGNOSIS/ PATIENT PROBLEM	DEFINING CHARACTERISTICS	NURSING ORDERS		EXPECTED OUTCOMES
		ASSESSMENT	INTERVENTIONS	

Diversionary activity, deficit
Etiology
Immobility imposed by skeletal traction
	Complaints of boredom and loneliness
	Lack of expression
	Withdrawn, irritable, demanding behavior
	Regression
		Assess child's ability for play
		A. Pain
		B. Mood
		C. Behavior (both verbal and nonverbal)
		D. Previous experience with illness
		E. Family input
		F. Age
		G. Level of growth and development
			A. Plan a daily schedule that alternates rest with play
			B. Encourage family to call and visit frequently
			C. Provide age-appropriate activities: books, games, television/movies, painting, sewing, drawing
			D. Refer child to child life therapist
			E. Assign foster grandmother to visit at bedside
			F. Instruct parents on importance of maintaining contact with child by
			  1. Telephoning frequently
			  2. Visiting every day
			  3. Bringing favorite toys, books, foods from home
				A. Home and family interactions will be maintained
				B. Child will maintain usual level of growth and development

Comfort, alteration in
Etiology
Fractured limb
	Child (or family member) verbalizes complaint of discomfort or pain
	Withdrawal
	Irritability
	Crying
	Rigidity
	Unwilling to change position
	Tachycardia
	Tachypnea
		A. Observe child for behaviors associated with pain, especially
		  1. Increased crying/irritability
		  2. Unwilling to suck
		  3. No movement in bed
		  4. Increased muscle tension
		  5. Increased pulse and respirations
		  6. Inability to sleep
		  7. Inability to soothe child
		B. Assess pain characteristics (of any child who can verbalize)
		  1. Location
		  2. Onset
		  3. Duration
		  4. Intensity. Use color scale (blue, yellow, red) or number scale 1-3 (3 being most severe)
		C. Assess past experience with pain
		D. Assess past and present measures employed to relieve pain
			A. Anticipate need for pain relief
			B. Provide environment with decreased visual and auditory stimuli
			C. Administer pain medication per order
			D. Provide comfort measures
			  1. Distraction (e.g., mobiles, sucking, play, television)
			  2. Touch (hold, back rubs)
			  3. Breathing techniques
			  4. Reassurance (verbal and physical)
			  5. Position change
			E. Evaluate effectiveness of pain relief measures
			F. Instruct familiy/child on
			  1. Measures to relieve pain
			  2. How to administer pain medication
			  3. Side effects associated with pain medications
			G. See SCP in Ch. 1: Comfort, alteration in: pain
				A. Pain will be alleviated or relieved
				B. Family/child will verbalize and use appropriate measures to relieve pain

Total Hip Arthroplasty

NURSING DIAGNOSIS/ PATIENT PROBLEM	DEFINING CHARACTERISTICS	NURSING ORDERS		EXPECTED OUTCOMES
		ASSESSMENT	INTERVENTIONS	
Knowledge deficit, potential **Etiology** New procedures	Patient verbalizes lack of knowledge regarding hospitalization and surgical regime Increased anxiety level Lack of/multitude of questions	A. Assess patient's experience of past hospitalizations B. Assess patient's preexisting medical problems C. Assess patient's cognitive/intellectual level. Observe for confusion, forgetfulness, disorientation, etc. D. Assess patient's level of knowledge regarding present hospitalization, surgical procedures, etc. (include patient's desire for information)	A. Obtain complete nursing history on admission. Include past hospitalization and medical/surgical history B. Review/explain procedure and preoperative, perioperative, and postoperative events C. Encourage and answer any questions about information given D. Include family members/significant others in teaching program E. Instruct patient in preoperative routine; include 1. Surgical consent 2. Admission blood work, urinalysis, chest x-ray study, ECG 3. Anesthesia visit 4. NPO after midnight 5. Preoperative medications F. Instruct patient to watch educational television, if relevant program is available G. Instruct patient regarding total hip replacement (postoperative position protocol) 1. Maintain abduction of legs; avoid adduction 2. Maintain hip flexion <90-degree angle 3. Avoid internal rotation of affected extremity H. Instruct patient in leg exercises. Include quad sets, gluteal sets, active ankle ROM I. Instruct in immediate postoperative tubes, drains, assistive devices, routine care, etc. Include Hemovac (or surgical drain), IVs, Foley catheter, pain medication, diet, abduction splint, antiembolic devices, activity level J. Document all instructions given	Patient will demonstrate/recall instructions given preoperatively

Originated by **Hope Hlinka, RN**
Resource person: **Marilyn Magafas, RN,C BSN**

Continued.

Total Hip Arthroplasty—cont'd

NURSING DIAGNOSIS/ PATIENT PROBLEM	DEFINING CHARACTERISTICS	NURSING ORDERS		EXPECTED OUTCOMES
		ASSESSMENT	INTERVENTIONS	
Comfort, alteration in: pain **Etiology** Surgical pain Physical rehabilitation program	Patient and/or significant others complain of pain Facial grimaces, guarding behavior, crying, anxiety, withdrawal, restlessness, irritability, altered vital signs	A. Assess patient's previous experience with pain and analgesia B. Observe facial expressions and behavior C. Inquire as to patient's description of pain	A. Anticipate need for analgesics, and medicate as ordered B. Turn and position every _____ as needed C. Respond quickly to complaints of pain D. Eliminate additional stressors or sources of discomfort; provide diversional activity E. Once physiotherapy is initiated, encourage use of analgesia 30-45 min before therapy F. Provide egg crate mattress as needed G. Instruct patient that analgesics are not given routinely but as needed H. Instruct patient to request analgesic before pain becomes severe	Patient will experience pain relief as exhibited by behavior and verbalization of such relief
Injury, potential for: hip dislocation **Etiology** Improper positioning	Legs may be positioned in internal rotation or adduction Increased pain in affected hip X-ray film confirmation of dislocation	A. Assess patient's knowledge of proper position after total hip replacement B. Assess patient's position while in bed, out of bed, getting into a chair, and while ambulating	A. Maintain abduction of legs with abduction splint (in or out of bed) B. Turn patient side to side in bed with abduction splint between legs (may turn onto affected hip unless otherwise noted by physician) C. Maintain slouch position while in chair D. Use raised toilet seat E. Frequently instruct and/or remind patient regarding hip precautions (abduction of legs, flexion of hip <90 degrees, neutral or external rotation of affected leg) F. Review precautions as outlined in home instruction sheet	Patient will maintain proper positioning during all activities

Total Hip Arthroplasty—cont'd

NURSING DIAGNOSIS/ PATIENT PROBLEM	DEFINING CHARACTERISTICS	NURSING ORDERS		EXPECTED OUTCOMES
		ASSESSMENT	INTERVENTIONS	
Tissue perfusion, alteration in: potential (lower extremities) **Etiology** Surgical procedure	Pain Pallor Cyanosis Pulselessness Paresthesia Paralysis Edema Sluggish/absent capillary refill NOTE: May be present in either or both lower extremities	A. Assess and compare neurovascular status of both lower extremities preoperatively and postoperatively, including color, warmth, circulation, movement, sensation, pulses (dorsalis pedis and posterior tibial), and capillary refill B. Assess lower extremities for signs/symptoms of neurovascular damage (see Defining Characteristics) C. Assess for perineal nerve palsy secondary to improper positioning of abduction splint straps	A. Monitor and compare neurovascular status every _____ hours for 48 hours immediately after surgery, then every shift if neurovascular status is stable. Report any changes immediately B. Keep abduction splint straps from pressing against head of fibula at proximal lateral aspect of lower leg to prevent perineal nerve palsy	Tissue perfusion will remain adequate throughout postoperative course
Injury, potential for: infection **Etiology** Surgical procedures	Signs/symptoms of wound infection Redness at incision Elevated WBC Elevated temperature Drainage from incision Warmth on palpation Edema	A. Assess incisional area every _____ hour for signs/symptoms of infection (see Defining Characteristics) B. Assess temperature every _____ hour; notify physician of temperature over _____ C. Assess laboratory values, especially WBC D. Assess patient's bladder and bowel habits, especially incontinence	A. Inspect wound every _____ hour for signs/symptoms of infection B. Change incisional dressing daily (more frequently if increased drainage is noted), using aseptic technique C. Observe patient for incontinence, and clean immediately D. Document and immediately notify physician of any signs/symptoms of infection E. Administer appropriate antibiotics as ordered	Risk of infection will be minimized

Continued.

Total Hip Arthroplasty—cont'd

NURSING DIAGNOSIS/ PATIENT PROBLEM	DEFINING CHARACTERISTICS	NURSING ORDERS		EXPECTED OUTCOMES
		ASSESSMENT	INTERVENTIONS	
Tissue perfusion, alteration in: potential **Etiology** Deep vein thrombosis (DVT) Pulmonary embolism (PE) Fat embolism secondary to surgery and immobility	**Deep vein thrombosis** Homan's sign Swelling, tenderness, redness in calf Palpable cords Abnormal blood flow studies **Pulmonary embolism** Abnormal ABGs Abnormal ventilation-perfusion scan Tachypnea Signs/symptoms of DVT Chest pain Dyspnea Tachycardia Hemoptysis Cyanosis Anxiety **Fat embolism** (usually second day after surgery) A. *Pulmonary:* Dyspnea, tachypnea, cyanosis B. *Cerebral:* Headache, irritability, delirium, stupor, coma C. *Cardiac:* Tachycardia; decreased BP; petechial hemorrhage of upper chest, axillae, and conjunctivae; fat globules in urine	Assess for signs/ symptoms of DVT, PE, fat embolism every ____ hour (See Defining Characteristics)	A. Apply antiembolic devices as ordered (sequential compression devices or thigh-high hose). Remove every ____ hour. Inspect skin for signs/ symptoms of breakdown and impaired circulation, and reapply B. Turn q.2-4h. as needed, side to side while in bed. Encourage and assist with early ambulation when ordered C. Monitor respiratory status every ____ hour(s). Note dyspnea, tachypnea, productive hemoptysis, adventitious breath sounds. Report any abnormalities immediately D. Encourage use of incentive spirometry every ____ hour(s) while awake E. Encourage leg exercises, including quad sets, gluteal sets, ankle ROM	Risk of deep vein thrombosis, pulmonary embolus, and fat embolism will be minimized

Total Hip Arthroplasty—cont'd

NURSING DIAGNOSIS/ PATIENT PROBLEM	DEFINING CHARACTERISTICS	NURSING ORDERS		EXPECTED OUTCOMES
		ASSESSMENT	INTERVENTIONS	
Bowel elimination, alteration in: constipation **Etiology** Immobility	Passage of small, hard, dry stool or no stool Distended, hard abdomen Patient complains of feeling full, having "not moved bowels in days"	A. Assess patient's bowel habits before hospitalization B. Assess bowel sounds postoperatively C. Assess passage of flatus D. Assess dietary intake	A. Encourage fluids B. Increase roughage in diet C. Encourage ambulation when ordered D. Use laxatives/stool softeners as ordered E. Offer bedpan, or ambulate to bathroom on regular routine	Patient's regular bowel habits will be resumed postoperatively, and complications of constipation or impaction will be minimized
Skin integrity, impairment of: potential **Etiology** Prolonged bed rest in supine position Shearing forces Friction Maceration	**Actual skin breakdown** Stage I: redness, skin intact Stage II: blisters Stage III: necrosis Stage IV: necrosis involving bones and joints	A. Assess on admission patient's skin, especially over bony prominences. Note any break in skin or decubitus. Document all findings B. Assess patient's position postoperatively	A. Turn patient q.2h.; may turn to operative side unless otherwise indicated by physician. NOTE: Before turning, maintain abduction of legs with abduction splint B. Remove splints and antiembolic devices during morning care to inspect skin (but maintain abduction of legs) C. Massage bony prominences D. For actual skin breakdown, see SCP in Ch. 1: Skin integrity, impairment of	Optimal skin integrity will be maintained
Self-care deficit, potential/actual **Etiology** Surgical procedure	Patient verbalizes lack of knowledge regarding discharge from hospital and self-care following surgery Increased anxiety level Lack of/multitude of questions	A. Assess patient's home environment including family/ significant others/ support services B. Assess patient's level of knowledge regarding home care postoperatively	A. Coordinate interdisciplinary teams of physiotherapy/occupational therapy/social work early during hospitalization to provide adequate time for discharge planning B. Encourage and answer patient questions regarding discharge C. Reinforce all instructions given in physiotherapy/occupational therapy D. Reinforce instructions given regarding needed equipment (e.g., raised toilet seat, walker, reacher)	Adequate discharge planning and teaching will promote safety and allay fears concerning discharge from hospital

Total Knee Arthroplasty

NURSING DIAGNOSIS/ PATIENT PROBLEM	DEFINING CHARACTERISTICS	NURSING ORDERS		EXPECTED OUTCOMES
		ASSESSMENT	INTERVENTIONS	
Knowledge deficit: potential (regarding surgical procedure) **Etiology** New procedures Unfamiliarity with surgical routines	Many questions Lack of questions Increased anxiety level Verbalized misconceptions	A. Assess patient's previous hospital experiences B. Assess patient's cognitive/intellectual level C. Assess patient's existing medical problems D. Assess patient's knowledge of present hospitalization	A. Obtain complete nursing history B. Review surgical procedure C. Instruct patient to watch television channel for general preoperative, intraoperative and postoperative information D. Instruct patient in preoperative routine, including surgical consent, admission blood work, urinalysis, chest x-ray examination, ECG, anesthesia visit, NPO after midnight, preoperative medications, and immediate preoperative routine E. Instruct patient on immediate postoperative routine, including surgical Hemovac, IV infusion, diet, activity level, medications, Foley catheter F. Instruct patient on postoperative use of continuous passive motion (CPM) machine; inform of purpose and usage G. Instruct patient about leg exercises (quad sets, gluteal sets, and active ankle ROM), allowing patient to perform H. Instruct patient on cough and deep breathing exercises, allowing to perform I. Encourage questions, and answer with complete information J. Document all instructions given	Patient will demonstrate or verbalize understanding of preoperative instructions given
Comfort, alteration in: pain **Etiology** Surgical procedure Physical rehabilitation program	Patient/significant other reports pain Facial grimaces Moaning, crying Protective, guarded behavior Restlessness Withdrawal Irritability	A. Assess patient's description of pain B. Assess patient's behavior and facial expressions C. Assess patient's previous experiences with pain and pain relief D. Assess pain relief measures for their effectiveness	A. Give analgesics as ordered, and evaluate effectiveness B. Alter patient's position, i.e., turning, adjusting pillows C. Respond immediately to complaints of pain D. Encourage use of analgesics 30 min before physiotherapy E. Encourage appropriate rest periods F. Eliminate additional stressors, and encourage diversional activity G. Instruct patient to report pain so relief measures can be started H. See SCP in Ch. 1: Comfort, alteration in	Patient will verbalize relief of or decrease in pain

Originated by **Sandra Eungard, RN, BSN**
Resource person: **Marilyn Magafas, RN,C BSN**

Total Knee Arthroplasty—cont'd

NURSING DIAGNOSIS/ PATIENT PROBLEM	DEFINING CHARACTERISTICS	NURSING ORDERS		EXPECTED OUTCOMES
		ASSESSMENT	INTERVENTIONS	

Mobility, impaired physical
 Etiology
 Postoperative activity limitations
	Restrictive movement resulting from post-operative protocol
	 Decreased muscle strength and coordination
	 Reluctance to move
		A. Assess patient's ability to carry out ADL
		 B. Assess patient's ROM
		 C. Assess patient's knowledge of the use of continuous passive motion (CPM)
		 D. Assess patient's knowledge of early ambulation and physical therapy
		 E. Assess patient's previous experiences with use of crutches or walker
			A. If ordered by physician, apply CPM to affected leg at prescribed degrees
			 B. Maintain proper position of CPM
			   1. Apply egg-crate mattress to bed
			   2. Attach extension bar of CPM to traction bar at end of bed
			   3. Keep cords of CPM free
			 C. Instruct patient on proper positioning in CPM
			   1. Maintain leg in neutral position
			   2. Adjust CPM so that knee joint corresponds to bend in CPM machine
			   3. Adjust foot plate so that foot is in neutral position in boot
			   4. Instruct patient to keep opposite leg away from machine
			 D. Assist and encourage patient to perform quad sets, gluteal sets, and ankle ROM
			 E. Turn and position every ____ hours as needed
			 F. Encourage ambulation after initiated by physiotherapy; weight bearing as prescribed
			 G. Encourage and assist patient to sit in chair
			 H. Reinforce ROM (extension/flexion) and muscle strengthening exercises as taught by physical therapist
			 I. Encourage use of assistive devices provided by occupational therapist to carry out ADL
				A. Patient will achieve acceptable level of knee strength and ROM
				 B. Patient will achieve independence in ambulation and ADL

Tissue perfusion, alteration in: to lower extremities (arterial)—potential **Etiology** Surgical procedure Restricted movement Swelling	Coldness Pallor Pain Pulselessness Edema Sluggish or absent capillary refill	A. Assess lower extremities, and compare for temperature, color, sensation, movement, pulse, edema, and capillary refill B. Assess for increased pain in lower extremity	A. Use preoperative neurovascular assessment to establish baseline status for postoperative comparison B. Monitor neurovascular status every ____ hours C. Maintain functional alignment D. If signs of altered tissue perfusion are noted, see SCP in Ch. 1: Tissue perfusion, alteration in	Tissue perfusion will be maintained

Continued.

Total Knee Arthroplasty—cont'd

NURSING DIAGNOSIS/ PATIENT PROBLEM	DEFINING CHARACTERISTICS	NURSING ORDERS		EXPECTED OUTCOMES
		ASSESSMENT	INTERVENTIONS	
Tissue perfusion, alteration in: deep vein thrombosis (DVT) (potential) **Etiology** Restricted movement	Pain Swelling Redness Tenderness on palpation of calf Increased warmth Positive Homans' sign	Assess for signs/ symptoms of DVT (see Defining Characteristics)	A. Encourage ROM exercises B. Apply TED hose or sequential compression devices as prescribed by physician C. Remove antiembolic devices every ____ for inspection of skin, and reapply	Risk of DVT will be minimized
Injury, potential for infection **Etiology** Surgical procedure Incision	Increased warmth Redness Swelling Tenderness at incision site Increased WBC count Increased temperature	Assess patient for signs/symptoms of infection (see Defining Characteristics)	A. Administer antibiotics as ordered B. Encourage fluid intake C. Maintain strict aseptic technique for dressing changes D. Monitor vital signs, and notify physician of abnormalities	Risk of infection will be minimized
Skin integrity, impairment of: potential **Etiology** Physical immobility and/or contact with CPM	Stage I: redness, skin intact Stage II: blisters Stage III: necrosis Stage IV: necrosis involving bones and joints	A. Assess patient's skin preoperatively and postoperatively every ____ hours for breakdown B. Assess patient's position postoperatively in CPM	A. Turn q.2h. unless otherwise indicated B. Inspect skin every ____ hours, removing TED hose or sequential compression devices, and reapply C. Clean, dry, and moisturize skin every ____ hours or as indicated D. Massage and moisturize skin every ____ hours, especially over bony prominences E. Apply egg-crate mattress to bed F. Inspect leg in CPM for pressure points, especially the knee and thigh (medial, lateral, and posterior) area G. Pad any areas resting on hard parts of the CPM H. If skin breakdown occurs, see SCP in Ch. 1: Skin integrity, impairment of	Risk of skin breakdown will be minimized
Bowel elimination, alteration in: constipation (potential) **Etiology** Immobility Medications Altered nutrition	Hard stools Straining for stool Abdominal distention Frequent attempts to defecate Nausea/vomiting	A. Compare preoperative stool pattern with postoperative pattern B. Assess preoperative laxative use C. Assess dietary habits D. Assess activity level E. Assess current medications and their contributing factors to constipation	A. Encourage increased dietary bulk B. Encourage fluid intake C. Encourage ambulation, and assist as needed D. Give laxatives and stool softeners as prescribed per physician E. Provide privacy and comfort during elimination F. When possible, assist with ambulation to bathroom	Normal bowel patterns will be resumed

Total Knee Arthroplasty—cont'd

NURSING DIAGNOSIS/ PATIENT PROBLEM	DEFINING CHARACTERISTICS	NURSING ORDERS		EXPECTED OUTCOMES
		ASSESSMENT	INTERVENTIONS	
Urinary elimination, altered patterns: retention (potential) **Etiology** Restricted activity Surgical procedure	Decreased output Frequency Urgency Lower abdominal distention	A. Assess amount and frequency of urine B. Palpate over bladder for distention C. Evaluate time intervals between voids	A. Initiate methods to encourage voiding B. Provide privacy C. Place urinal or bedpan within reach D. Use straight catheter or insert Foley catheter per physician's orders E. Monitor I & O F. See SCP in Ch. 1: Urinary elimination, alteration in patterns: retention	Adequate urinary output will be maintained
Breathing pattern, ineffective: potential **Etiology** Immobility Fatigue	Increased temperature Adventitious breath sounds Chest pains Abnormal ABGs Increased anxiety Tachypnea Dyspnea Tachycardia Cyanosis	A. Assess respiratory rate and rhythm every ____ hours B. Auscultate breath sounds every ____ hours C. Assess signs/ symptoms of respiratory compromise/pulmonary embolus every ____ hours (see Defining Characteristics)	A. Instruct patient on incentive spirometer usage and cough and deep breathing exercises preoperatively B. Encourage patient to use incentive spirometer every 1-2 hours while awake C. Turn every ____ hours as tolerated	Risk of respiratory compromise will be minimized
Tissue perfusion, alteration in: pulmonary (potential) **Etiology** Obstruction in venous blood flow secondary to pulmonary embolus	Decreased breath sounds on affected side Tachypnea Tachycardia Abnormal ABGs Chest pain Dyspnea Febrile	A. Auscultate breath sounds every ____ B. Assess respiratory pattern (rate, rhythm, quality)	If signs of pulmonary embolus are noted, call physician and institute SCP in Ch. 4: Pulmonary embolism	Risk of pulmonary embolism will be minimized
Self-care deficit: potential/actual **Etiology** Postoperative condition/recovery process	Patient verbalizes knowledge deficit in home care Increased anxiety as discharge approaches	A. Assess patient's knowledge of care on discharge B. Assess patient's home situation regarding availability of family/significant others C. Assess patient's physical environment at home relating to mobility	A. Reinforce all instructions given to patient B. Coordinate social service, physiotherapy, and occupational therapy early to provide adequate discharge planning C. Encourage patient questions D. Instruct patient regarding discharge medications, exercises, and follow-up physician visits	Patient will verbalize readiness for discharge

CHAPTER TEN

Hematologic/Neoplastic

DISORDERS

Acquired Immune Deficiency Syndrome (AIDS)

NURSING DIAGNOSIS/ PATIENT PROBLEM	DEFINING CHARACTERISTICS	NURSING ORDERS		EXPECTED OUTCOMES
		ASSESSMENT	INTERVENTIONS	
Infection: potential for **Etiology** Alteration in immuno-logic function Decreased num- ber of T4 helper cells Altered T4 helper cell function Reversed T4:T8 ratio Altered cellular immune re- sponse Altered humoral immune re- sponse	Fatigue Fever Weight loss Persistent diarrhea Swollen lymph nodes Signs/symptoms of other opportunistic infections or neo- plasms	A. Assess for pres- ence of defining characteristics B. Check laboratory reports for T-lym- phocytes C. Assess response to cutaneous skin testing	A. Use frequent handwashing be- fore and after entering room B. Prevent patient's contact with other diseases 1. Use private room if possi- ble; if not possible do not allow exposure to anyone with a known infection 2. Advise staff and visitors to avoid contact with patient if they suspect cold or influ- enza 3. Use reverse isolation proce- dures as indicated C. Leave all equipment frequently used inside the room: e.g., thermometer, BP cuff, stetho- scope, tourniquet D. Use precautions to prevent the spread of acquired immune de- ficiency syndrome (AIDS) 1. Avoid exposure to blood or other body fluids a. Use gloves for all direct contact with blood and body fluid b. Always wear gloves when handling any spec- imens c. Label specimens with blood/body fluid precau- tion label d. Wear gown when soiling by secretions is antici- pated e. Keep a disposable Ambu bag and mask at bedside f. Clean blood spills imme- diately with sodium hy- pochlorite solution 2. Double bag all linens, and label with precautions 3. Prevent injury with a sharp instrument to caretakers or visitors a. Dispose of needle and syringe in puncture resis- tant container immedi- ately after use. NOTE: Do not place contaminated needles in sheath before disposal b. Keep the needle disposal receptacle in the room	The potential for in- fection will be mini- mized

Originated by **Dorothy Rhodes, RN**
Resource persons: **Martha Dickerson, RN, MS, CCRN**
            Susan Galanes, RN, MS, TNS, CCRN

Acquired Immune Deficiency Syndrome (AIDS)—cont'd

NURSING DIAGNOSIS/ PATIENT PROBLEM	DEFINING CHARACTERISTICS	NURSING ORDERS		EXPECTED OUTCOMES
		ASSESSMENT	INTERVENTIONS	
Temperature regulation: alteration in **Etiology** Infectious process	Increased body temperature Chills Flushing Perspiration Tachycardia Convulsions	A. Monitor temperature at least q.4h., and note pattern of temperature elevations. Report elevations B. Assess for associated symptoms (e.g., chills, flushing, tachycardia), and document	A. Administer antipyretics as ordered, and monitor effectiveness B. Use cold therapy to decrease temperature C. Encourage intake of oral fluids as permitted D. Administer parenteral fluids as ordered E. Monitor vital signs F. Obtain specimens for culture and sensitivity as ordered per physician, and monitor reports G. Maintain isolation procedures if deemed necessary following culture reports H. Administer appropriate antibiotics as ordered per physician	Patient will maintain body temperature within normal limits

Ineffective breathing pattern and ineffective airway clearance: potential for
 Etiology
 Pneumonia from opportunistic infection
 Fatigue
	Dyspnea
	 Tachypnea
	 Use of accessory muscles
	 Rhonchi
	 Wheezes
	 Cough
	 Decreased PaO_2
	 Cyanosis
		A. Assess respiratory rate and depth, noting breathing patterns
		 B. Note use of accessory muscles
		 C. Assess position assumed for breathing
		 D. Assess for changes in vital signs every _____
		 E. Auscultate breath sounds every _____
		 F. Assess for presence of cough, noting presence of sputum: quantity, color, and consistency. NOTE: Use gloves when handling secretions
		 G. Assess for signs of hypoxemia
		   1. Decreased PaO_2
		   2. Skin color changes
		   3. Changes in orientation (If appropriate, see SCP in Ch. 3: Consciousness, alteration in level of)
			See SCP in Ch. 4: Pneumonia	Patient's respiratory exchange will be optimized, and airway will be maintained free of secretions

Continued.

Acquired Immune Deficiency Syndrome (AIDS)—cont'd

NURSING DIAGNOSIS/ PATIENT PROBLEM	DEFINING CHARACTERISTICS	NURSING ORDERS		EXPECTED OUTCOMES
		ASSESSMENT	INTERVENTIONS	
Fluid volume deficit: potential **Etiology** Diarrhea Altered nutritional status Altered temperature regulation	Output greater than intake Sudden weight loss Decreased urine output Increased urine specific gravity Decreased skin tugor Increased serum sodium Dry mucous membranes Change in vital signs: increased heart rate, hypotension	Assess hydration status (see Defining Characteristics)	A. Monitor I & O every shift B. Record daily weight C. Encourage oral fluid intake D. Administer parenteral fluids as ordered E. Monitor electrolytes, serum and urine osmolarity, and specific gravity F. Monitor and document vital signs, and report abnormalities	Adequate fluid volume and electrolyte balance will be maintained

Skin integrity, impairment of: potential
 Etiology
 Prolonged unrelieved pressure
 Altered nutritional status
 Presence of excretion and secretions
	Reddened skin
	 Pain
	 Numbness
	 Blisters
		A. Check skin color, moisture, texture, and temperature
		 B. Assess for signs of ischemia, redness, pain, and numbness on admission and every _____ hours (at least q.2h.)
		 C. Assess nutritional status
			A. Turn patient according to established schedule
			 B. Provide prophylactic use of pressure relieving devices
			   1. Alternating pressure mattress
			   2. Egg crate mattress
			   3. Stryker boots
			   4. Elbow pads
			 C. Maintain functional body alignment
			 D. Increase tissue perfusion by massaging *around* affected areas
			 E. Keep skin clean and dry
			 F. Maintain adequate hydration and nutrition
			 G. See SCP in Ch. 1: Skin integrity, impairment of
				Skin breakdown will be prevented

Nutritional status, alteration in: less than body requirements **Etiology** Loss of appetite Fatigue	Weight loss (may be up to 20% of normal body weight) Calorie intake inadequate to meet metabolic requirements	A. Document patient's actual weight on admission B. Obtain nutritional history	A. Document dietary and fluid I & O B. Provide dietary planning to encourage intake of high caloric, protein foods C. Encourage patient participation in menu planning D. Assist patient with meals as needed E. Obtain weight every _____ (at least once a week) F. Monitor serum/urine electrolytes, albumin, CBC, glucose and acetone as necessary G. Encourage exercise as tolerated	Optimal nutritional support will be maintained

Acquired Immune Deficiency Syndrome (AIDS)—cont'd

NURSING DIAGNOSIS/ PATIENT PROBLEM	DEFINING CHARACTERISTICS	NURSING ORDERS		EXPECTED OUTCOMES
		ASSESSMENT	INTERVENTIONS	
Coping, ineffective: individual **Etiology** Stigma attached to disease	Depression Withdrawal from relationships with significant others Anger/hostility Alienation/isolation Inability to meet role expectations Inability to care for self	A. Assess patient's perception of self B. Determine patient's previous coping patterns	A. Maintain nonjudgmental approach when giving care B. Observe and document expressions of grief, anger, hostility, and powerlessness C. Monitor patient's ability to care for self and cope with environment D. Encourage patient to participate in own care E. Provide an opportunity for family to express feelings F. Provide opportunities for interaction among patient/family/ significant others G. Refer to psychiatric liaison or social worker as needed	A. Patient will verbalize fears and concerns B. Patient/family/significant others will have an avenue for relieving tensions and promoting psychologic well-being

Knowledge deficit regarding disease and transmission
 Etiology
 New condition
	Multiple questions
	 Lack of questions
	 Confusion regarding disease and complications
	 Noncompliance with prevention behavior, isolation techniques
	 Transmission of disease to another person
		Assess patient's knowledge of disease process, complications, and treatment modalities	A. Instruct patient in signs and symptoms of disease, opportunistic infections, and neoplasms, and to whom this information should be reported
			 B. Instruct patient in routes of disease transmission
			 C. Instruct patient in methods of preventing disease transmission
			   1. Information on sexual transmission
			   2. Use of "dirty" intravenous needles
			   3. Donation of blood, semen, or other organs
			   4. Do not share personal items
			 D. Allow patient to discuss feelings and reactions to the information
			 E. Help patient integrate information into daily life
				Patient will verbalize understanding of disease process, complications, and treatment modalities

Anemia

NURSING DIAGNOSIS/ PATIENT PROBLEM	DEFINING CHARACTERISTICS	NURSING ORDERS		EXPECTED OUTCOMES
		ASSESSMENT	INTERVENTIONS	
Activity intolerance **Etiology** Decreased O$_2$ supply to cells Decreased cellular ability to meet energy requirements	Weakness Fatigue Dyspnea on exertion Abnormal cardiac response to activity Abnormal respiratory response to activity	A. Assess respiratory status before activity 1. Respiratory rate 2. Use of accessory muscles 3. Need for supplemental O$_2$ B. Assess cardiac status before activity 1. Pulse rate 2. Cardiac rhythm 3. BP 4. Skin color and perfusion C. Assess patient's ability to perform ADL D. Assess potential for injury with activity E. Assess understanding of change in activity level and tolerance by patient/significant others	A. Plan nursing activities to provide patient with adequate rest periods B. Provide quiet atmosphere to allow patient to rest C. Provide assistance for activities that patient cannot perform independently D. Increase activity levels as tolerated by patient E. Monitor patient for cardiac or respiratory complications	Patient will perform ADL independently as tolerated Patient will increase activity levels as tolerated without occurrence of respiratory or cardiac complications
Breathing patterns, ineffective: potential **Etiology** Decreased Hb level resulting in decreased O$_2$ content of blood and decreased O$_2$ carrying capacity of blood	Dyspnea Shortness of breath Orthopnea Tachypnea Cyanosis Tachycardia Use of accessory muscles Nasal flaring Retractions	Assess respiratory status A. Respiratory rate B. Depth of respiration C. Use of accessory muscles D. Presence of flaring nostrils, retractions E. Dyspnea, shortness of breath F. Position for optimal breathing	A. Monitor vital signs B. Observe for changes in breathing patterns C. Pace activities to patient's tolerance D. Monitor ABGs E. Administer supplemental O$_2$ as ordered F. Elevate head of bed as needed G. See SCP in Ch. 1: Breathing pattern, ineffective	Patient's optimal breathing pattern will be maintained

Originated by **Martha Dickerson, RN, MS, CCRN**

Anemia—cont'd

NURSING DIAGNOSIS/ PATIENT PROBLEM	DEFINING CHARACTERISTICS	NURSING ORDERS		EXPECTED OUTCOMES
		ASSESSMENT	INTERVENTIONS	
Injury, potential for: cardiac complications of anemia (angina, myocardial infarction, congestive heart failure) **Etiology** High output state Tachycardia Tachypnea Increased metabolic needs Significantly decreased Hb levels	Shortness of breath Orthopnea Edema Palpitations Angina, chest pain Cold, clammy skin Changes in color of skin, mucous membranes Arrhythmias	A. Assess factors that affect the symptomatology of the anemic state 1. Speed with which anemia developed 2. Metabolic needs of the patient 3. Other physical disorders B. Assess cardiac status 1. Pulse rate 2. Cardiac rhythm 3. BP 4. Skin color and perfusion 5. Complaints of angina, chest pain	A. Monitor vital signs B. Observe for changes in cardiac status C. Pace activities to patient's tolerance D. Observe for angina and chest pain (see SCP in Ch. 2: Angina, unstable) E. Observe for conditions that increase metabolic needs of patient	Optimal cardiac status will be maintained
Skin integrity, impairment of: potential **Etiology** Decreased blood and O$_2$ supply to skin	Skin cool to touch Altered circulation Altered sensation Altered nutrition	A. Assess skin integrity: color, moisture, temperature, texture of skin; presence of existing skin lesions B. Assess nutritional status: diet, laboratory data, weight C. Assess physical impairments that may contribute to breakdown: altered circulation, altered sensation	A. Reposition patient frequently (at least q.2h.) B. Use pressure-relieving devices as necessary C. Provide extra blankets and clothing to keep patient warm D. Teach patient to avoid heating pads E. Provide adequate nutritional support (see next Nursing Diagnosis: Nutrition, alteration in)	Patient will maintain optimal skin integrity

Continued.

Anemia—cont'd

NURSING DIAGNOSIS/ PATIENT PROBLEM	DEFINING CHARACTERISTICS	NURSING ORDERS		EXPECTED OUTCOMES
		ASSESSMENT	INTERVENTIONS	
Nutrition, alteration in: less than body requirements **Etiology** Decreased intake of iron, protein Disease of GI tract, liver Deficiency in metabolism of nutrients Increased need for nutrients beyond normal intake Blood loss	Loss of weight Nausea/vomiting Anorexia	A. Document patient's weight B. Obtain nutritional history C. Determine presence of underlying disease process (iron, vitamin deficiency, etc.) D. Obtain baseline laboratory values Serum iron Total iron-binding capacity RBC Hb; Hb electrophoresis Reticulocyte count Red cell shape and size Bilirubin Bone marrow examination Bleeding/coagulation studies Occult blood in urine/stool	A. Assist patient in selecting meals B. Provide diet with high-protein, high-carbohydrate, iron-containing foods C. Encourage good oral hygiene D. Provide small, frequent meals E. Administer vitamin and mineral supplements as ordered F. Administer nutritional supplements as ordered G. Monitor laboratory values	Patient will have adequate nutrients to manufacture sufficient numbers of RBCs and Hb
Bowel elimination, alteration in: constipation and/or diarrhea **Etiology** Decreased dietary intake Decreased digestive processes Decreased activity level Drug therapy	**Constipation** Frequency less than usual pattern Straining at stool Hard-formed stool Passage of liquid feces around impaction Abdominal distention Nausea/vomiting Fecal incontinence Decreased bowel sounds **Diarrhea** Increased frequency of stool Loose/liquid stool Urgency Cramping Abdominal pain Hyperactive bowel sounds	A. Establish patient's history of elimination B. Determine whether patient uses medications to provide regular elimination	A. Observe stool for color, consistency, frequency, amount B. Provide adequate dietary and fluid intake C. Administer medications for diarrhea or constipation as ordered (see SCPs in Ch. 1: Bowel elimination, alteration in [constipation; diarrhea])	Patient will have normal bowel function

Anemia—cont'd

NURSING DIAGNOSIS/ PATIENT PROBLEM	DEFINING CHARACTERISTICS	NURSING ORDERS		EXPECTED OUTCOMES
		ASSESSMENT	INTERVENTIONS	
Consciousness, altered levels of: potential **Etiology** Decreased blood and O_2 supply to vital organs	Visual changes Dizziness Fainting Postural hypotension Change in alertness Memory impairment Impaired judgment Change in alertness	A. Assess level of consciousness and neurologic status B. Assess patient's ability to carry out ADL C. Assess potential for injury	A. Provide patient with assistance in completing ADL B. Teach patient to avoid sudden movements such as sitting up too quickly or getting out of bed rapidly C. Observe patient for changes in orientation, neurologic function, vision D. Place objects within patient's reach E. If signs of altered level of consciousness are noted, see SCP in Ch. 3: Consciousness, alteration in level of	Optimal state of consciousness will be maintained
Knowledge deficit **Etiology** Unfamiliarity with disease process, treatment plan, and complications	Multiple questions by patient/significant others Lack of questions Confusion about treatment Inability to comply with treatment regimen Development of complications	Determine understanding by patient/ significant others of disease process, treatment, and complications	A. Encourage patient/significant others to ask questions B. Provide information to patient/ significant others regarding disease process, treatment, and complications C. Evaluate understanding of information following teaching sessions D. Observe compliance with treatment program 1. Improved activity tolerance 2. Ability to manage ADL more effectively 3. Increased Hct and Hb 4. Selection of well-balanced diet 5. Compliance with medication regimen, e.g., vitamin, mineral, and nutritional supplements E. Observe for development of complications such as 1. Dyspnea 2. Angina, myocardial infarction 3. Skin breakdown 4. Constipation, diarrhea 5. Altered level of consciousness	Patient will demonstrate understanding of and compliance with treatment regimen

Disseminated Intravascular Coagulation (DIC)

NURSING DIAGNOSIS/ PATIENT PROBLEM	DEFINING CHARACTERISTICS	NURSING ORDERS		EXPECTED OUTCOMES
		ASSESSMENT	INTERVENTIONS	
Fluid volume deficit **Etiology** Blood loss. DIC always occurs secondary to some other pathology Infection Neoplastic disorders Obstetric complications Tissue damage Trauma Burns	**Laboratory data** PT >15 sec PTT >60-90 sec Hypofibrinogenemia Thrombocytopenia Elevated fibrin split products Prolonged bleeding time **Clinical symptoms** Oozing of blood from IV sites, drains, or wounds Petechiae, purpura, hematomas Bleeding from mucous membranes Hematuria, hemoptysis, occult positive stools Cardiovascular changes (hypotension, arrhythmias) CNS changes (decreased mental status, possible cerebral hemorrhage)	A. Examine skin surface for signs of bleeding; note 1. Petechiae, purpura, hematomas 2. Oozing of blood from IV sites, drains, and wounds 3. Bleeding from mucous membranes B. Observe for signs of bleeding from GI/GU tracts C. Note any hemoptysis or blood obtained during suctioning D. Observe for changes in mental status; institute neurologic checklist E. Monitor vital signs every _____ 1. Heart rate 2. BP 3. CVP, pulmonary capillary wedge pressure	A. Protect patient 1. Eliminate pressure by turning patient every _____ 2. If patient is confused/agitated, pad side rails to prevent bruising 3. Minimize IM/SC injections; apply pressure to injection site if puncture is unavoidable 4. Prevent stable clots from dislodging; if clot dislodges, apply pressure and cold compress 5. Apply pressure to any oozing site 6. Prevent trauma to catheters/ tubes by proper taping; minimize pulling 7. Minimize number of cuff BPs; maintain arterial line B. Document blood loss and report to physician 1. Document amount and character of drainage on dressings; note frequency of dressing changes 2. Do hemoccult test on all stools and guaiac test on aspirate from all GI tubes/ drains 3. Note hematuria; test urine for blood every _____ 4. Note hemoptysis; use gentle suctioning technique to prevent trauma to mucosa 5. Report all blood loss to physician C. Document changes in mental status 1. Check neurologic status every _____, using neurologic checklist 2. Note abnormal behavior, confusion, pupil changes, strength deficit D. Maintain fluid volume/balance 1. Notify physician of BP <_____ or of orthostasis 2. Notify physician of tachycardia >_____; note ST segment and T-wave changes or arrhythmias 3. Notify physician of CVP <_____; wedge pressure <_____ or >_____; cardiac output <_____; pulmonary artery diastolic pressure <_____ or >_____ 4. Notify physician of urine output <30 ml/hour	Optimal fluid balance will be maintained

Originated by **Gail L. Dykstra, RN**
Resource person: **Audrey Klopp, RN, MS, CCRN, CS, ET**

Disseminated Intravascular Coagulation (DIC)—cont'd

NURSING DIAGNOSIS/ PATIENT PROBLEM	DEFINING CHARACTERISTICS	NURSING ORDERS		EXPECTED OUTCOMES
		ASSESSMENT	INTERVENTIONS	

			E. Monitor coagulation profile every _____
			 F. Monitor Hct and Hb every _____
			 G. Institute medical management
			   1. Administer fluids as ordered
			   2. Administer blood products as ordered; monitor patient response (observe for transfusion reaction)
			   3. Administer heparin therapy as ordered to interrupt abnormal accelerated coagulation
			     a. Infuse continuous heparin drip on IVAC/IMED (usually 1000-1500 U/hour)
			     b. Maintain PTT at _____ × normal; monitor PTT every _____
			     c. Observe for any increase in bleeding after initiating heparin therapy. If bleeding increases, notify physician for possible need to decrease drip
			     d. Consider dosage alteration in patients with hepatic or renal failure	

Injury, potential for **Etiology** Possible complications of drug therapy related to too much or too little heparin. Note that heparin aborts the clotting process by blocking the production of thrombin	**Too much heparin** Bleeding from IV sites, drains, wounds Petechiae, purpura, hematomas Bleeding from mucous membranes GI, GU bleeding Bleeding from respiratory tract PTT > 2½ times normal **Too little heparin** Continued evidence of further clot formation (e.g., newly developed signs of pulmonary emboli or peripheral thromboemboli) Continued evidence of bleeding from DIC (abnormal clotting) PTT < twice normal	Note adverse effects of heparin therapy A. Any increase in bleeding from IV sites, GI/GU tracts, respiratory tract, wounds B. Development of new purpura, petechiae, or hematomas	**Too much heparin** A. Check PTT; notify physician B. Reevaluate heparin dosage **Too little heparin** A. Check to make sure infusion is not interrupted (infiltrated IV, malfunctioning infusion device) B. Check PTT; notify physician C. Reevaluate heparin dosage	Side effects of heparin therapy will be minimized

Continued.

Disseminated Intravascular Coagulation (DIC)—cont'd

NURSING DIAGNOSIS/ PATIENT PROBLEM	DEFINING CHARACTERISTICS	NURSING ORDERS		EXPECTED OUTCOMES
		ASSESSMENT	INTERVENTIONS	
Tissue perfusion, alteration in **Etiology** Microvascular clot formation Inappropriate coagulation Possible blood loss Decreased Hct and Hb Acidosis Decreased circulation Poor O_2 exchange at cellular level	**Laboratory data** Decreased PO_2 or decreased O_2 saturation Decreased Hb Increased PCO_2 Blood pH < 7.3 Bicarbonate < 22 Acidic urine, pH 4.6-5.02 **Clinical signs** Dyspnea Poor capillary refill Acral cyanosis Changes in mental status (confusion)	A. Observe for signs of dyspnea, respiratory distress, poor capillary refill, acral cyanosis B. Note changes in patient's mental function (confusion) C. Observe for changes in cardiac rhythm D. Note abnormal breath sounds E. Note Kussmaul's respiration	A. Monitor respirations, and notify physician of rate >30 min (adult) and/or abnormal breath sounds B. Maintain airway 1. Encourage coughing 2. Use suction as needed 3. Elevate head of bed >45 degrees for dyspnea C. Maintain O_2 therapy as ordered D. Monitor ABGs every ____, and notify physician if abnormal O_2 Sat <90% PO_2 <50 PCO_2 >45 pH <7.30 Bicarbonate <22 E. Monitor heart rate and vital signs every ____; notify physician of change in vital signs, cardiac arrhythmias, or heart rate <_____ or >____ F. Use neurologic checklist every ____ to monitor trends in mental status/loss of consciousness	O_2 sat of at least ____ % and blood pH between ____ and ____ will be maintained
Knowledge deficit **Etiology** Lack of familiarity with procedures	Increased questioning Lack of questions	Assess knowledge base and readiness for learning	A. Instruct patient to notify nurse of bleeding from wounds, IV sites, etc. B. Instruct patient to inform nurse of feelings of fatigue or dizziness C. Instruct patient to try to avoid any trauma D. Explain purpose of drug/transfusion therapy E. Explain rationale for therapy to significant others and encourage them and other visitors to remain calm while visiting	Patient will verbalize a basic understanding of what is happening and what nursing care procedures are being performed
Anxiety/fear **Etiology** Presenting symptoms of DIC and/or staff reaction to disease process	Restlessness Increased awareness Increased questioning	A. Assess level of anxiety B. Assess normal coping patterns	A. Inform significant others of patient's prognosis, and prepare them for patient's appearance B. Minimize staff conversations at the bedside C. Use calm approach with patient D. See SCP in Ch. 1: Anxiety/fear	Anxiety will be minimized

Granulocytopenia: risk for infection

NURSING DIAGNOSIS/ PATIENT PROBLEM	DEFINING CHARACTERISTICS	NURSING ORDERS		EXPECTED OUTCOMES
		ASSESSMENT	INTERVENTIONS	
Injury, potential for: infection **Etiology** Granulocytopenia, secondary to Radiation therapy Chemotherapy Hypersplenism Bone marrow depression/failure Autoimmune responses	Decrease in circulating granulocytes Total neutrophil level <1000 m	A. Monitor WBC (especially neutrophils/bands) every _____ B. Identify the source(s) leading to the low WBC C. Identify sites that pose a risk for infection (e.g., orifices, wounds, catheter sites) D. Note any abnormalities in the color/character of sputum/urine/stool E. Assess for local/ systemic signs/ symptoms of infection (such as fever, chills, diaphoresis, local redness, heat, pain, excessive malaise, sore throat, dysphagia, or cellulitis. Note that inflammation and exudate may be absent because of decrease or lack of neutrophils F. Identify medication patient may have taken that would mask signs/ symptoms of infection (e.g., steroids, antipyretics) G. Identify any nosocomial pathogens in the patient care area (e.g., respiratory bacteria, urine bacteria)	A. Wash hands before and after each contact with the patient B. Utilize sterile technique with dressing changes and catheter care. Patient has the following catheter sites: ____ care includes ____ ____ care includes ____ ____ care includes ____ C. Use isolation procedures as ordered or appropriate; isolation ordered: _____ D. Limit visitors. Discourage anyone with current or recent infection from visiting E. Encourage daily shower and perineal care (with soap and water) after urination and defecation F. Encourage patient to brush teeth with toothsponge and use lukewarm saline soaks after each meal and at bedtime G. Encourage oral fluids, ____ ml q.24h. H. Assist patient with selection of a high-protein, high-vitamin, high-calorie diet (refer to dietitian as needed) I. Avoid unnecessary invasive procedures J. Monitor temperature q.4h. around the clock K. Notify physician immediately of temperature >38.5° C, hypotension, or any other signs/ symptoms of acute systemic infection L. Send cultures as ordered for temperature >38.5° C M. Initiate measures for control of fever (e.g., cool sponge bath, blanket, light covers) for temperature of _____ N. Administer medications as ordered for infection (antibiotics), for prevention of mucosal damage (stool softeners) and to allay signs and symptoms of infections (antipyretics)	The risk of infection will be minimized

Originated by **Vanessa Randle, RN**
Resource person: **Christa M. Schroeder, RN, MSN**

Continued.

Granulocytopenia: risk for infection—cont'd

NURSING DIAGNOSIS/ PATIENT PROBLEM	DEFINING CHARACTERISTICS	NURSING ORDERS		EXPECTED OUTCOMES
		ASSESSMENT	INTERVENTIONS	

Knowledge deficit
Etiology
Unfamiliarity with nature, treatment of condition
	Multiple questions
	Lack of questions
	Misconceptions
	Request for information
		A. Assess readiness for teaching by patient/significant others
		B. Assess knowledge base regarding infection (recognition of, plan of care for, evaluation of care)
			A. Explain to patient/significant others that the low WBC leaves the patient highly susceptible to infection
			B. Explain factors that have contributed to the low WBC (e.g., chemotherapy, drug sensitivity, etc.)
			C. Explain signs/symptoms of infection to patient/significant others, and instruct them to contact appropriate health team member immediately if any should occur or are suspected
			D. Provide an explanation of the plan of care to patient/significant others (e.g., need for private room, isolation, etc.)
			E. Instruct patient/significant others about
			  1. Use of prescribed medications (indications, dosages, side effects)
			  2. Avoidance of activities that may result in bodily injury. Suggest alternatives where appropriate (e.g., oral/axillary temperatures instead of rectal; electric razor instead of razor blades; sanitary napkins instead of tampons; toothsponge instead of toothbrush)
			  3. Avoidance of crowds and persons with current or recent infection
			  4. Avoidance of sharing drinking and eating utensils
			  5. Avoidance of animal excreta
			F. Instruct patient to make routine dental visits
				Patient/significant others will demonstrate an understanding of
				A. Medical diagnosis
				B. Treatment plan
				C. Safety measures
				D. Follow-up care

Leukemia: acute

NURSING DIAGNOSIS/ PATIENT PROBLEM	DEFINING CHARACTERISTICS	NURSING ORDERS		EXPECTED OUTCOMES
		ASSESSMENT	INTERVENTIONS	
Coping, ineffective: potential **Etiology** Situational crisis Inadequate support system Inadequate coping methods	Patient verbalizes fear, anxiety, and feelings of hopelessness/meaninglessness Asks questions about illness, procedures, and therapy Noncompliance in diet, medications, precautionary measures	A. Assess patient's concept and knowledge of the disease B. Assess patient for 1. Events/illnesses preceding hospitalization 2. Awareness and comprehension of the illness; importance of procedures; importance of hospitalization 3. Coping mechanisms used in previous illnesses and hospitalization experiences 4. Level of understanding, modes of communication, and readiness to learn 5. Dynamics of relationship with significant others C. Assess patient's readiness and need for information	A. Establish open lines of communication 1. Initiate brief visits to patient 2. Define your role as a patient informant and advocate 3. Understand the grieving process, and respect your patient's feelings as they ensue a. Request a break when you have approached your emotional limit b. Introduce patient to the staff, and orient him/her to the unit's physical environment B. Meet with medical team to discuss plan of care to maintain consistency C. Assist patient/significant others in redefining hopes, the components of their individuality, e.g., roles, values, and attitudes D. Provide reading materials and resource persons as needed E. Introduce new information about disease treatment 1. Use simple terms 2. Add to current knowledge 3. Reinforce instructions/repeat information as necessary F. Use a calm approach with patient/significant others G. Refer to SCP in Ch. 12: Grief over long-term illness/disability: psychosocial aspects	A. Patient and nurse will have effective communication B. Patient will show signs of coping as evidenced by less apprehension, fear, and anxiety C. Patient will verbalize an understanding of 1. Illness and how it affects his/her body 2. Treatments/ procedures: states their importance, potential side effects; measures to minimize side effects

Originated by **Marlene T. de la Cruz, RN, BSN**
Resource person: **Christa M. Schroeder, RN, MSN**
           Ruth E. Novitt, RN, MSN

Continued.

Leukemia: acute—cont'd

NURSING DIAGNOSIS/ PATIENT PROBLEM	DEFINING CHARACTERISTICS	NURSING ORDERS		EXPECTED OUTCOMES
		ASSESSMENT	INTERVENTIONS	

Injury, potential for: infection
Etiology
Altered immunologic responses as related to
  The disease process
  Immunosuppression secondary to chemotherapy
	Rales
	Cyanosis
	Decreased breath sounds
	Rhonchi
	Cough
	Tachypnea
	Abnormal sputum
		A. Auscultate lung field every day or as necessary
		B. Observe patient for coughing spells and for nature and character of sputum
			Report any findings to physician, and initiate treatment as follows
			A. Place patient in protective isolation if laboratory results indicate neutropenia
			  1. Inform patient/significant others
			  2. Screen all visitors to minimize traffic in patient's room
			  3. Bathe patient with chlorhexidine (Hibiclens) before entering room and every day thereafter
			B. Initiate meticulous oral hygiene. Instruct patient
			  1. To brush teeth with soft toothbrush q.i.d. and as necessary
			  2. To remove dentures at night
			  3. To rinse mouth after each emesis or when expectorating phlegm
			C. Instruct patient to maintain personal hygiene
			  1. To wash hands well before eating and after using the bathroom
			  2. To wipe perineal area from front to back
			D. Observe aseptic technique for all invasive procedures
			E. Minimize risk of infection from central lines and arteriovenous punctures
			  1. Observe for evidence of infection and culture as ordered
			  2. Observe strict aseptic technique when changing dressings
			  3. Avoid wetting central catheter dressings
			F. Apply lotion to intact skin every morning and as needed
			G. Explain to patient the definition, etiology, and effects of leukopenia
			  1. Normal range of blood count
			  2. Functions of leukocytes and neutrophils
				A. The risk of local/ systemic infection will be minimized
				B. Patient will demonstrate an understanding of neutropenia/leukopenia by stating
				  1. Its definition
				  2. Function of leukocytes
				  3. Etiology of leukopenia
				  4. Importance of avoiding exposure to people with transmittable diseases
				C. Patient will participate in minimizing potential for infection by monitoring his/her own body responses

Leukemia: acute—cont'd

NURSING DIAGNOSIS/ PATIENT PROBLEM	DEFINING CHARACTERISTICS	NURSING ORDERS		EXPECTED OUTCOMES
		ASSESSMENT	INTERVENTIONS	

			H. Instruct patient to observe for fever spikes, flulike symptoms: malaise, weakness, and myalgia and to notify the nurse/physicians if they occur
			I. Instruct patient to avoid crowds or contact with persons with contagious illness
			J. Teach patient how to take oral and axillary temperature
			K. Encourage patient to observe good handwashing technique
			L. Teach patient how to monitor counts and report those not within normal limits
			M. Refer patient to a dietitian for instructions on maintenance of a well-balanced diet
			N. Explain to patient the importance of regular medical and dental checkups
			O. Teach patient how to inspect the oropharyngeal area daily for
			  1. White patches in the mouth
			  2. Coated/encrusted oral ulcerations
			  3. Swollen and erythematous tongue with white/brown coating
			  4. Infected throat and pain on deglutition
			  5. Note texture, color, and character of the oropharynx
			  6. Check for any debris on teeth
			  7. Note any ill-fitting dentures
			  8. Note amount and viscosity of saliva
			  9. Observe for any changes in vocal tone
			  10. Avoid mouthwashes that contain alcohol
			  11. Avoid irritating foods/acidic drinks
			  12. Teach patient how to use prescribed topical medications such as nystatin (Nilstat) and lidocaine (Xylocaine)
			  13. See preceding SCP: Granulocytopenia	

Continued.

Leukemia: acute—cont'd

NURSING DIAGNOSIS/ PATIENT PROBLEM	DEFINING CHARACTERISTICS	NURSING ORDERS		EXPECTED OUTCOMES
		ASSESSMENT	INTERVENTIONS	

Injury, potential for: bleeding
Etiology
Replacement of bone marrow with leukemic cells
Bone marrow depression secondary to chemotherapy
	Decrease in total circulating platelets <50,000
	Petechiae and bruising, especially venipuncture sites
	Headaches and changes in mental and visual acuity
	Hemoptysis
	Hematemesis
	Hematochezia
	Melena
	Vaginal bleeding
	Dizziness
	Orthostatic changes
	Decreased BP
	Increased pulse rate
		A. Monitor platelet count daily
		B. Observe for changes in the neurologic status q.4h.
		C. Monitor vital signs q.4h. and as needed
		D. Note any change in the color of emesis, urine, and stool
		E. Note any bleeding at puncture sites (e.g., venipuncture, bone marrow aspiration site)
			A. Institute bleeding precautions for platelet count <50,000 by
			  1. Avoiding use of toothpicks and dental floss
			  2. Avoiding rectal suppositories, thermometers, enemas, constipation, vaginal douches, and use of tampons
			  3. Avoiding IM/SC injections. If you must use small-bore needles for injections, apply pressure to site for 10 min. Observe for oozing from site
			  4. Avoid straight-edged razors
			  5. Avoid aspirin, alcohol, anticoagulants, or any products containing these
			  6. Avoid coarse foods/snacks
			  7. Administer antacids as ordered for patients taking steroids
			  8. Avoid urinary/rectal tenesmus by administering stool softeners as ordered
			  9. Prevent sneezing and coughing if possible
			  10. Inspect gums for any oozing
			  11. Count used sanitary pads during menstruation
			  12. Place a sign over patient's bed as a reminder to apply pressure after venipunctures
			  13. Use fingerstick if possible. Coordinate laboratory work so all tests can be drawn at one time
			  14. Apply pressure dressing/sandbag to bone marrow aspiration site
			  15. Inflate BP cuff as little as possible to get accurate reading
			  16. Check urine, emesis, and stool for blood
			B. Maintain a safe environment for patient, especially during episodes of chills, fever, confusion, and weakness. Assist patient during ambulation and shower/tub bath
			C. Encourage rest to decrease pulse rate, which will assist clot formation
			D. Apply ice or topical thrombin promptly as ordered if bleeding from mucous membranes occurs
				A. Patient will have minimal or no incidence of bleeding related to low platelet count
				B. Patient will demonstrate an understanding of thrombocytopenia by
				  1. Stating the function of platelets and effects on the body of a decreased count
				  2. Adhering to precautionary measures

Leukemia: acute—cont'd

NURSING DIAGNOSIS/ PATIENT PROBLEM	DEFINING CHARACTERISTICS	NURSING ORDERS		EXPECTED OUTCOMES
		ASSESSMENT	INTERVENTIONS	

			E. Ensure the availability and readiness of blood products
			F. Assess vital signs during and after blood transfusion(s)
			G. Explain to patient/significant others the definition, etiology, and symptoms of thrombocytopenia and functions of platelets
			  1. Normal range of platelet count
			  2. Effects of thrombocytopenia
			  3. Rationale of bleeding precautions
			H. Instruct patient to
			  1. Use electric razor
			  2. Avoid sharp objects such as scissors
			  3. Use emery boards
			  4. Avoid wearing tight/constrictive clothing
			  5. Lubricate nostrils with saline drops as necessary
			I. Protect self from injury/trauma, e.g., falls, bumps, strenuous exercises
			J. Report to physician any changes in menstrual cycle
			K. Advise patient to contact physician before any dental work
			L. Encourage patient to be gentle during intercourse, to use lubrication, and to avoid trauma	

Fluid volume deficit: potential **Etiology** Side effects of chemotherapy	Parched tongue Poor skin turgor Weight loss with output exceeding intake Thirst Weakness Lethargy Changes in pulse Change in BP Increased serum BUN and creatinine levels	Assess for presence of defining characteristics	Refer to SCP in Ch. 1: Fluid volume deficit; SCP in Ch. 10: Chemotherapy	Optimal fluid status will be maintained
Nutrition, alteration in: less than body requirements **Etiology** The disease process Side effects of chemotherapy (e.g., nausea, vomiting, stomatitis)	Nausea and vomiting Parched tongue Poor skin turgor Weight loss with output exceeding intake Thirst Weakness Lethargy Lethargy in pulse Increased serum BUN and creatinine levels	Assess for presence of defining characteristics	See SCP in Ch. 1: Nutrition, alteration in: less than body requirements	Patient will maintain present weight or will not lose more than 10% of original body weight

Continued.

Leukemia: acute—cont'd

NURSING DIAGNOSIS/ PATIENT PROBLEM	DEFINING CHARACTERISTICS	NURSING ORDERS		EXPECTED OUTCOMES
		ASSESSMENT	INTERVENTIONS	
Mobility, impaired physical: potential **Etiology** Fluid volume deficit secondary to side effects of chemotherapy Pain and discomfort Depression/severe anxiety	Weakness Lethargy Decreased attempt to move around Physical restrictions on movements (e.g., protective isolation) Requires help/assistance during meals/ ambulation Verbalizes inability to move freely without fear of falling Stays in bed most of the time	Assess for presence of defining characteristics	See SCP in Ch. 1: Mobility, impaired physical	Patient will maintain optimal level of independence
Social isolation: potential **Etiology** Protective isolation Impaired mobility secondary to disease entity	Verbalization of being isolated from ''the world''; ''I want to get out of here'' Reduced social acceptance and interactions Unrealistic expectations of self Outbursts Withdrawal Impaired ability to ambulate	A. Recognize early verbal/nonverbal communication cues reflecting need to socialize B. Monitor blood counts to determine duration of isolation C. Observe patient closely for any behavioral changes D. Assess level of activity	A. Allow patient to exert some control over environment 1. Remove unnecessary equipment to provide a space for patient 2. Open blinds during daytime 3. Dim lights at night 4. Ask significant others to bring in familiar objects, e.g., pictures and pillows 5. Muffle noises B. Visit and talk with patient at frequent intervals C. Avoid using intercom when responding to patient's call D. Provide normal aids for interaction (e.g., eyeglasses, hearing aids, writing materials) E. Encourage participation of significant others through visits and telephone calls F. Provide diversional therapy/activities (e.g., radio, television, magazines, occupational therapy) G. Assist patient in grooming when entertaining visitors 1. Encourage use of makeup 2. Encourage use of wig during daytime H. Encourage patient to ambulate during the course of protective isolation as permitted by physician and own physical limitations I. Leave patient's door open J. Acknowledge patient's efforts in maintaining a sense of wellbeing	Optimal state of socialization will be maintained

Multiple Myeloma

NURSING DIAGNOSIS/ PATIENT PROBLEM	DEFINING CHARACTERISTICS	NURSING ORDERS		EXPECTED OUTCOMES
		ASSESSMENT	INTERVENTIONS	

Comfort, alteration in
 Etiology
 Pain resulting from invasion of marrow and bone by plasma cells
	Constant, severe bone pain on movement
	 Low back pain
	 Swelling, tenderness
	 Guarding behavior
	 Decreased physical activity
	 Moaning, crying
	 Pacing, restlessness, irritability, alteration in sleep pattern
		Assess pain characteristics
		 A. Quality (sharp, dull, aching, shooting, stabbing, or burning)
		 B. Severity of pain (scale of 1-10; 10 most severe)
		 C. Location (where pain located)
		 D. What caused the pain
		 E. Duration of pain (intermittent or continuous)
			A. Anticipate need for pain medication
			 B. Reduce additional stress and discomfort
			 C. Give pain medication as ordered; observe for signs and symptoms of any untoward effects
			 D. Use additional measures for comfort
			   1. Decreased noise and excess activity
			   2. Relaxation techniques
			   3. Good body alignment
			   4. Clean comfortable bed
			 E. Additional rest and sleep periods
			 F. Notify physician if pain medications have not worked within certain time: _____
				Relief or decrease of pain will be evidenced by verbalization and appearance of comfort

Injury, potential for: infection
 Etiology
 Decrease in synthesis of immunoglobulin by plasma cells secondary to
   Bone marrow depression/failure
 Decrease in normal circulating antibodies
 Decreased autoimmune response
 Chemotherapy
	Temperature > 37.7° C (100° F)
	 Chills
	 Fever
	 Swelling localized
	 Soreness localized
	 Redness localized
	 Pain
		A. Check body for general skin appearance
		   1. Open wounds
		   2. Skin breakdown
		   3. Swelling
		   4. Redness
		 B. Monitor temperature q.4h.
		 C. Monitor urine output, color and odor, pain or burning on urination
		 D. Watch for signs and symptoms of bronchopneumonia, coughing (productive and nonproductive), and color and odor of sputum
		 E. Obtain urine, sputum, and blood for culture and sensitivity if temperature > 37.7° C, as ordered per physician
		 F. Check medications (patient taking steroids may not have overt symptoms of infection)
		 G. Notify physician of any of the above symptoms
			A. Use good hand-washing technique before and after each patient contact
			 B. Use sterile technique for dressing change and catheter care
			 C. Maintain reverse isolation as ordered
			 D. Discourage visitors with current or recent infection; e.g., if family member has upper respiratory infection but feels he/she must visit, have him/her wear a mask and limit the stay to 10 min
			 E. Avoid unnecessary invasive procedures
			 F. Maintain normal or near normal body temperature
			   1. Medications as ordered per physician
			   2. Alcohol bath
			   3. Cooling blanket
				Risk of nosocomial infection will be minimized

Originated by **Geraldine Rowden, RN**
Resource persons: **Christa M. Schroeder, RN, MSN,**
    Susan Galanes, RN, MS, TNS, CCRN
    Meg Gulanick, RN, MSN, CCRN

Continued.

Multiple Myeloma—cont'd

NURSING DIAGNOSIS/ PATIENT PROBLEM	DEFINING CHARACTERISTICS	NURSING ORDERS		EXPECTED OUTCOMES
		ASSESSMENT	INTERVENTIONS	
Injury, potential for bleeding **Possible causes** Bone marrow depression or failure Replacement or invasion of bone marrow by neoplastic plasma cells Abnormal hepatic or renal functions	Petechiae Purpura Hematomas Unexplained bruises or areas of ecchymoses Bleeding from any body orifice Prolonged oozing of blood from IM, IV, venipuncture, or bone marrow sites	A. Identify factors that lower platelet count or predispose patient to bleeding B. Check platelet count C. Check current chemotherapy regimens for potential myelosuppression D. Identify drugs interfering with platelet function E. Observe and report signs and symptoms of spontaneous or excessive bleeding	A. Draw all blood for laboratory work with one daily venipuncture (fingersticks when possible) B. Avoid IM injection; if necessary, use smallest needle possible C. Apply direct pressure for 3-5 min after IM injection, venipuncture, and bone marrow aspiration D. Avoid rectal temperatures and enemas E. Prevent constipation (straining causes breakage of small blood vessels around anus) by increased oral fluid intake and/or stool softeners as ordered per physician F. Use soft toothbrushes G. Use electric razor, not blades H. Avoid aspirin, aspirin compounds, and other drugs interfering with hemostatic platelet function I. Place sign near patient, informing other health team members of bleeding precautions J. Transfuse platelets as ordered per physician	Risk of bleeding will be minimized
Mobility, impaired physical **Etiology** Bone weakness caused by invasion of plasma cells	Inability to move purposefully within the physical environment Decrease in ADL Reluctance to attempt movement Limited ROM Decreased muscle strength or control Restricted movement and impaired coordination	A. Assess patient's ability to carry out ADL B. Assess patient's ROM and muscle strength	A. Assist patient with ADL B. Gather supportive aid, e.g., walker, cane C. Apply back brace as ordered per physician D. Ambulate patient at least q.i.d. E. Prevent contractions of upper and lower extremities by doing passive ROM every _____ F. Allow rest periods after ambulation G. Prevent unnecessary trauma to extremities	Optimal state of mobility will be maintained

Multiple Myeloma—cont'd

NURSING DIAGNOSIS/ PATIENT PROBLEM	DEFINING CHARACTERISTICS	NURSING ORDERS		EXPECTED OUTCOMES
		ASSESSMENT	INTERVENTIONS	

Urinary elimination, alteration in patterns: potential
 Etiology
 Renal insufficiency/ renal failure
	Decreased urine output
	 Increased BUN, creatinine, Ca, and uric acid level
	 Repeated UTI
	 Hypertension
	 Increase in weight
	 Pedal edema
	 Puffy eyes
	 Oliguria
	 Anuria
		A. Monitor serum laboratory values (BUN, creatinine, Ca, K, and uric acid)
		 B. Assess for edema
		 C. Check I & O
		 D. Check urine for specific gravity, color, and odor
		 E. Monitor weight daily
		 F. Check for dyspnea, tachycardia, pneumonia, pulmonary edema, distended neck veins, and peripheral edema
			For renal insufficiency
			 A. If hypercalcemia is present, push fluids 2500 ml-3000 ml or per day as ordered by the physician
			 B. Monitor dietary intake
			    1. Check that the patient is adhering to a renal diet
			    2. Restrict sodium intake as ordered per physician
			 C. Monitor indwelling catheter; check for infection, patency, or kinking
			 D. Notify physician of any decrease in urine output or increase in K, BUN, or creatinine
			 E. For acute renal failure see SCP in Ch. 7: Renal failure, acute
				Optimal renal function will be maintained

Nutrition, alteration in: less than body requirements (potential) **Etiology** Chemotherapy	Nausea Vomiting Anorexia Diarrhea Weight loss	A. Monitor food intake: obtain diet list B. Assess what food patient likes C. Assess for signs of nausea, vomiting, anorexia, diarrhea, weight loss	A. Increase diet when patient is able to tolerate it B. Obtain food patient likes and give supplements such as Ensure shakes C. Check food for protein, carbohydrate, and fat content. Consult dietitian as appropriate D. Give prochlorperazine (Compazine) for nausea and vomiting as ordered E. Maintain Hickman or Hyperal line fluid as ordered per physician	Patient's nutritional status will be improved

Acute grieving
 Etiology
 Terminal illness
	Fear
	 Denial
	 Regression
	 Depression
	 Anger
	 Shame
	 Guilt
	 Grief
	 "Why me" attitude
		A. Assess patient's awareness of disease
		 B. Monitor patient's mental state
		    1. Withdrawal
		    2. Anger
		    3. Crying
		    4. Disbelief
			A. Obtain literature for patient to read
			    1. Contact U.S. Department of Health and Human Services for information on multiple myeloma
			    2. Contact American Cancer Society
			 B. Contact local chapter of multiple myeloma support group (if available in area)
			 C. Work with patient during grieving stage
			    1. Give patient time to adjust to diagnosis
			    2. Have patient express feelings
			    3. Listen to patient's complaints
			    4. Channel some of patient's anger
				A. Patient will be able to vent some hostility and anger
				 B. Patient will begin to work through the grieving process to the best of his/her ability

Continued.

Multiple Myeloma—cont'd

NURSING DIAGNOSIS/ PATIENT PROBLEM	DEFINING CHARACTERISTICS	NURSING ORDERS		EXPECTED OUTCOMES
		ASSESSMENT	INTERVENTIONS	
Knowledge deficit **Etiology** Unfamiliarity with disease process	Asking questions Lack of question Confusion over disease and outcome	Assess knowledge of patient and significant others concerning A. Pain and medications B. Possible infection C. Bleeding disorders D. Mobility E. Dietary and fluid restriction	A. Instruct patient to report pain so that relief measure can be given B. Explain the need to know if pain medication works C. Explain to patient the side effects of medication being taken D. Explain to patient the side effects of chemotherapy E. Instruct patient to avoid crowded places and people with infections or colds F. Explain need to monitor skin, open sores, or wounds for redness, oozing, pus, or swelling G. Instruct patient to be aware of drugs that mask symptoms of infection, e.g., prednisone H. Explain to patient the need for good hand-washing techniques I. Explain relationship between platelets and bleeding, and between bone marrow function and platelet numbers J. Explain the rationale and measures to prevent bleeding K. Explain the need to observe and report to the nurse or physician any signs of spontaneous or excessive bleeding, petechiae, ecchymoses, or hematomas L. Explain to the patient the need to maintain adequate nutrition M. Instruct patient to increase fluid intake if dehydrated (e.g., signs of dry skin, feeling of thirst) or to decrease fluid if overloaded (e.g., signs of edema) N. Educate patient about need to know about I & O O. Caution patient about importance of decrease in or absence of urine P. Instruct patient about signs and symptoms of UTI, frequent urination, abdominal and/or low back pain Q. Explain the need for maintenance of physical mobility R. Explain to patient the need to voice anger and fear S. Use available handouts, pamphlets, books, or audiovisual material	Patient and significant others will be aware of the various components of the disease entity and treatments as evidenced by their ability to respond appropriately to questions

Sickle Cell Pain Crisis: pediatric

NURSING DIAGNOSIS/ PATIENT PROBLEM	DEFINING CHARACTERISTICS	NURSING ORDERS		EXPECTED OUTCOMES
		ASSESSMENT	INTERVENTIONS	
Comfort, alteration in Etiology Vasoocclusive crisis Hypoxia, which causes the cells to become rigid and elongated, thus forming a crescent shape Stasis of RBCs	Complaint of generalized or localized pain Tenderness on palpation Inability to move affected joint Swelling to area Deformity to joint Warmth, discoloration	A. Assess pain q.2-4h. 1. Precipitation 2. Quality 3. Radiation 4. Severity 5. Timing B. Check laboratory values, e.g., Hb electrophoresis for amount of sickling	A. Administer medications according to pediatric sickle cell pain protocol 1. Administer IM injections (meperidine [Demerol] or MSO₄) q.3h. for first 48 hours 2. Use antiinflammatory agent simultaneously with IM injections q.3h. (Ascriptin or aspirin: 2 tablets) 3. Start oral analgesic 48 hours after admission: Tylenol no. 3, Empirin, Percodan, Darvocet-N, or Darvon B. Apply warm compresses to swollen and painful areas C. Try positioning patient to promote comfort D. Use pillows to promote comfort E. Apply heating pads to affected extremities F. Respond immediately to complaints of pain G. Use any additional comfort measures 1. Alteration in environment 2. Distractional devices 3. Relaxation techniques H. Provide rest periods to facilitate comfort, sleep, and relaxation	Patient will verbalize that pain is decreased
Fluid volume deficit: potential Etiology Inability to take fluids by mouth	Decreased urine output Concentrated urine Output greater than intake Sudden weight loss Decreased skin turgor Increased thirst Dry mucous membranes Sunken fontanels Hypokalemia Hyponatremia	A. Assess hydrational status 1. Skin turgor 2. Mucous membranes 3. Daily weight B. Monitor strict I & O q.4-8h. C. Report urine output < 30 ml/hour for 2 consecutive hours D. Monitor serum/ urine electrolytes and specific gravity E. Monitor and document vital signs. Report any abnormal findings	A. Administer parenteral fluids as ordered 1. D5W.2NS at 1½-2 times maintenance 2. Maintain patent IV flow rate 3. Continue IV fluids for 24-48 hours after oral pain management has begun B. Push oral fluids as soon as possible C. Provide desired fluids such as ice, tea, Popsicles, milk	A. Fluid volume and electrolyte balance will be evidenced by 1. Normal electrolytes 2. Urine output at least 30 ml/ hour 3. Balanced I & O 4. Normal skin turgor 5. Moist mucous membranes 6. Normal urine specific gravity B. Dehydration and recurrence of pain crisis will be prevented

Originated by **Carol Boyd, RN**
Resource person: **Michele Knoll-Puzas, RN,C BS**

Continued.

Sickle Cell Pain Crisis: pediatric—cont'd

NURSING DIAGNOSIS/ PATIENT PROBLEM	DEFINING CHARACTERISTICS	NURSING ORDERS		EXPECTED OUTCOMES
		ASSESSMENT	INTERVENTIONS	
Nutrition, alteration in: less than body requirements (potential) **Etiology** The child with sickle cell may spend his/ her nutrient resources on responses to illness	Loss of weight with or without adequate caloric intake ≥10%-20% under ideal body weight Caloric intake inadequate to keep pace with abnormal disease/metabolic state	A. Document patient's actual weight on admission B. Obtain nutritional history as appropriate	A. Document appetite and I & O 1. Encourage patient participation (daily log) 2. Record strict I & O B. Assist patient with meals as needed C. Consult dietitian when appropriate D. Encourage frequent oral ingestion of high-calorie, high-protein foods and fluids E. If inadequate nutrition is noted, see SCP in Ch. 1: Nutrition, alteration in: less than body requirements F. Provide pediatric or adult menu, as desired	Patient will receive food/diet that will promote appetite and adequate intake
Body temperature, alteration in **Etiology** Infections of bone and/or organ infarcts Splenic infarction causes the spleen to lose its ability to filter bacteria Decreased splenic production	Persistent rise in body temperature to > 38.3° C (101° F) for 24-48 hours X-ray examination results of _____ Positive blood, urine, or sputum cultures	A. Monitor vital signs q.2-4h. paying attention to temperature B. Observe patient for excessive chills resulting from body's attempt to fight off fever C. Observe patient for profuse diaphoresis D. Assess joints for redness, warmth, and swelling E. Observe skin for any wounds with drainage F. Review patient's x-ray films and laboratory results with physician	A. Administer antipyretics as ordered B. Provide cool sponge baths C. Keep patient's body and linen clean and dry D. Administer antibiotics as ordered E. Push fluids as appropriate	Normal temperature will be maintained

Sickle Cell Pain Crisis: pediatric—cont'd

NURSING DIAGNOSIS/ PATIENT PROBLEM	DEFINING CHARACTERISTICS	NURSING ORDERS		EXPECTED OUTCOMES
		ASSESSMENT	INTERVENTIONS	

Coping, ineffective individual/family: potential
Etiology
Repeated hospitalizations; chronic status of disease
	Admitted weekly for crisis
	Poor attendance in school
	Falling grades
	No interest shown about problems in school
	Withdrawal
	Decrease in positive self-image
		A. Assess patient's ability to openly express feelings about disease
		B. Assess family involvement with patient care
			A. Provide a primary nurse relationship
			B. Set aside talk times when pain is being controlled
			C. Identify needs/provide information on coping mechanisms for patient and family
			  1. Outside activities
			  2. School extracurricular activities
			  3. Exercise programs (YMCA, health clubs)
			D. Inform patient/family of support systems available, e.g., National Association of Sickle Cell Anemia
			E. Use other resource persons
			  1. Pediatric nurse clinicians
			  2. Clinical specialists
			  3. Psychiatric liaison personnel
			  4. Social workers
				Parent/child will discuss methods of coping with a chronic, potentially life-threatening illness

Knowledge deficit
Etiology
Unfamiliarity with disease process, treatment, complications
	Inability to define sickle cell disease
	Inability to list signs and symptoms of crisis/infection
	Lack of understanding of self-care/preventive measures
		A. Assess child's level of understanding, patient developmental stage, and ability to learn
		B. Assess what the child already knows about the disease
			A. Explain to parents and child about sickle disease
			B. Instruct parent of signs of impending crisis
			  1. Verbal complaint of pain
			  2. Persistent low-grade temperature
			  3. Decreased appetite
			  4. Decreased fluid intake
			  5. Increased sleeping time
			  6. Swollen joints
			C. Instruct parents to inform physician of signs of infection, which may lead to crisis
			D. Instruct parents on importance of
			  1. Pushing fluids, water, and juice
			  2. Food high in carbohydrates and protein; three balanced meals per day
			  3. Keep child dressed warmly: hats, gloves, sweaters, rubber boots
			E. Inform parents of the importance of
			  1. Pain medications, dosage
			  2. Antiinflammatory agents
			F. Stress the importance of keeping clinic appointments and wearing Medic-Alert
			G. Inform patient/parents of support groups and importance of genetic counseling when planning families
				A. Parents/child will verbalize an understanding of
				  1. Sickle cell disease
				  2. Treatments/ procedures
				  3. Complications
				  4. Diet
				  5. Genetic counseling
				B. Parents/child will verbalize understanding of
				  1. Medications
				  2. Signs and symptoms of impending crisis
				  3. Home treatments
				  4. Medical emergency

THERAPEUTIC INTERVENTIONS

Chemotherapy

NURSING DIAGNOSIS/ PATIENT PROBLEM	DEFINING CHARACTERISTICS	NURSING ORDERS		EXPECTED OUTCOMES
		ASSESSMENT	INTERVENTIONS	
Anxiety/fear **Etiology** New procedure/treatment Change in health status Fear of death	Apprehension Withdrawal Excessive verbalization; questioning Facial tension Trembling	Assess for presence of anxiety (See Defining Characteristics)	See SCP in Ch. 1: Anxiety/fear	Anxiety will be relieved or minimized
Comfort, alteration in: nasuea and vomiting **Etiology** Side effects of chemotherapy	Report of patient/significant others Self-focusing Guarding	A. Assess history for side effects of chemotherapy and treatment measures that were effective B. Solicit patient's description, including 1. Onset 2. Severity 3. Duration 4. Precipitating factors	Arrange for measures to alleviate or minimize nausea, including A. Providing clean and odor-free environment B. Administering antiemetics (first dose should be given 2 hours before treatment, then q.4-6h., then as needed) C. Encouraging frequent mouth care with saline washes D. Limiting excessive activity and sudden rapid movements to minimize disturbances in equilibrium E. Adjusting diet to frequent small snacks such as crackers and fruit plate	Episodes of nausea and vomiting will be absent, minimized, or controlled
Injury: potential for **Etiology** Drug extravasation	Pain or burning at injection site Red or pink streaking extending from injection site along the individual vein Sluggish or absent blood return on aspiration	Observe infusion site closely throughout administration of drug	See hospital policy and procedure on chemotherapy drug extravasation management	Effects of drug extravasation will be minimized
Injury, potential for **Etiology** Chemotherapeutic drugs Antiemetic drugs	**Chemotherapeutic drugs** Restlessness Facial edema and flushing Wheezing Tachycardia Hypotension **Antiemetic drugs** Agitation Hypotension Irritability Spasm of neck muscles Dystonias	A. Check laboratory values before administration of drug B. Check for history of drug allergies C. Monitor vital signs q.4h. D. Be alert to signs and symptoms of drug hypersensitivity (see Defining Characteristics)	On indication of drug reaction, perform the following A. Stop infusion B. Notify physician C. Administer antidote as ordered D. Reassure patient	Injury from chemotherapeutic/antiemetic drugs will be minimized

Originated by **Concordia Solita, RN, BSN**
Resource persons: **Christa M. Schroeder, RN, MSN**
Jackie Suprenant, RN, BSN

Chemotherapy—cont'd

NURSING DIAGNOSIS/ PATIENT PROBLEM	DEFINING CHARACTERISTICS	NURSING ORDERS		EXPECTED OUTCOMES
		ASSESSMENT	INTERVENTIONS	
Fluid volume, deficit: potential **Etiology** Vomiting and diarrhea	Rapid respirations Decreased urine output Poor skin turgor Dry skin Irritability, restlessness Weakness	Assess hydration status (see Defining Characteristics)	See SCP in Ch. 1: Fluid volume deficit	Optimal hydration status will be maintained
Knowledge deficit **Etiology** New treatment (chemotherapy)	Multiple questions Lack of questions Apparent confusion over events	Assess patient's understanding of chemotherapy	A. Provide available patient teaching booklets B. Discuss pamphlets with patient/ significant others, and answer questions	Patient will verbalize an understanding of the major short- and long-term effects of chemotherapy and treatment schedule

Mastectomy: segmental and modified radical

NURSING DIAGNOSIS/ PATIENT PROBLEM	DEFINING CHARACTERISTICS	NURSING ORDERS		EXPECTED OUTCOMES
		ASSESSMENT	INTERVENTIONS	
Comfort, alteration in **Etiology** Contraction of tissue resulting from surgery and healing process Intraoperative arm position Possible injury to brachial plexus Lymphedema	Inability to move arm through full ROM Verbalized pain Increased circumference of affected arm	A. Note subjective reports of discomfort B. Assess neurovascular status of affected arm immediately after surgery and every ___ C. Measure arm circumference immediately after surgery and every shift	A. Avoid constriction of affected arm B. Keep arm elevated on two pillows while patient is in bed C. Protect affected arm from injury. Post notice at head of bed No BP reading No blood drawing No IVs D. Instruct and encourage patient in straight extension and abduction exercise (straight-elbow raises and wall climbing) on first postoperative day 1. 5-10 times/hour or as tolerated 2. Continue for 1 month postoperatively E. Obtain elastic sleeve for affected arm with severe lymphedema (per physician's order) F. Report signs of infection and/or phlebitis in affected arm	Discomfort to affected arm will be minimized

Originated by **Carol Burkhart, RN, BSN, CCRN**
 Virginia Cabongon, RN, BSN

Continued.

Mastectomy: segmental and modified radical—cont'd

NURSING DIAGNOSIS/ PATIENT PROBLEM	DEFINING CHARACTERISTICS	NURSING ORDERS		EXPECTED OUTCOMES
		ASSESSMENT	INTERVENTIONS	
Injury, potential for: seroma **Etiology** Altered lymph drainage Drain malfunction	Fluid accumulation under flap Flap tenderness Diminished or absent output from drain immediately after surgery	A. Immediately after surgery and every _____ , check drain for 1. Correct vacuum 2. Clots 3. Air leaks B. Assess for presence of fluid accumulation beneath flap	A. Milk/strip drain tubing every _____ B. Document amount of output from drain every _____ C. Notify physician if 1. Drain malfunctions 2. Fluid accumulates beneath flap	Potential for injury caused by presence of seroma will be minimized
Self-concept, disturbance in: body image/ role performance **Etiology** Excision of breast and adjunct tissue Asymetric breast Beginning scar tissue	Verbal identification of feelings about altered body part Focusing behavior on altered body part Verbalized concern regarding loss of femininity	Assess impact of change in patient's self-perception as a result of breast surgery	A. Encourage verbalization about perceived alteration in self (appearance, ability to carry out previous roles) B. Assist patient in gaining information regarding reconstruction (if desired) C. Contact Reach-To-Recovery volunteer; facilitate visit D. Assist patient in wearing temporary, nonweighted prosthetic insert at time of discharge E. Encourage family (especially husband) to provide positive input F. See SCP in Ch. 1: Body image: disturbance in	Patient will begin to acknowledge feelings about breast loss
Fear/anxiety **Etiology** Breast loss Diagnosis of cancer Uncertain prognosis	Questioning Crying Withdrawal Restlessness Inability to focus Insomnia	A. Assess level of anxiety B. Assess previous successful coping strategies	A. Encourage verbalization of feelings B. Reassure patient that anxiety is normal C. Assist patient in use of previously successful coping measures D. Involve other departments as indicated (psychiatry, social services) E. Support a realistic assessment of the situation; avoid false reassurance F. See SCP in Ch. 1: Anxiety/fear	Anxiety will be minimized to a manageable level

Mastectomy: segmental and modified radical—cont'd

NURSING DIAGNOSIS/ PATIENT PROBLEM	DEFINING CHARACTERISTICS	NURSING ORDERS		EXPECTED OUTCOMES
		ASSESSMENT	INTERVENTIONS	
Knowledge deficit **Etiology** Lack of previous similar experience	Verbalized knowledge deficit Demonstrated inability Questioning	A. Assess knowledge level regarding home care and health maintenance B. Determine ability to learn	Instructions for patient A. Wound/arm care 　1. Arm will be stiff and sore; stiffness will go away, but armpit numbness will not if nodes were dissected 　2. Continue exercises for at least 1 month 　3. Protect from injury: use electric razor when shaving; gloves when gardening, doing dishes; mitts for removing hot dishes from oven. No blood drawings, IVs/injections during subsequent hospitalizations/visits 　4. Deodorant is acceptable 　5. Avoid tight-fitting sleeves, watches 　6. Brassiere should be worn from time of discharge B. Follow-up care 　1. Importance of monthly breast examination 1 week following period 　2. Annual mammogram of remaining breast (increased risk of cancer in remaining breast) 　3. Reconstructive surgery (if desired) usually 3 months postoperatively 　4. Importance of being fitted for weighted prosthesis as soon as wound is healed C. Family needs 　1. Familial tendency toward breast cancer 　2. Women over 20 should examine breasts monthly 　3. Women over 35 should have annual mammogram D. Activity 　1. Return to all activities is possible 　2. Sexual activity as tolerated 　3. Swimming permitted after prosthesis is obtained 　4. Driving can be resumed as tolerated	Patient will verbalize importance of follow-up care and proper wound/arm care

CHAPTER ELEVEN

Eye, Ear, Nose, Throat

DISORDERS

Oral Thrush

NURSING DIAGNOSIS/ PATIENT PROBLEM	DEFINING CHARACTERISTICS	NURSING ORDERS		EXPECTED OUTCOMES
		ASSESSMENT	INTERVENTIONS	
Skin integrity, impairment of **Etiology** Lesions of oral cavity	White, flaky plaques covering tongue, mucous membranes, and gingiva Dryness of mouth and mucous membranes Presence of bleeding Pain Crying Irritability	A. Assess oral cavity q.4h. for 　1. Color 　2. Presence of lesions 　3. Changes in skin pigmentation 　4. Secretions 　5. Intactness of mucous membranes B. Evaluate effectiveness of nystatin and gentian violet treatment C. Refer to SCP in Ch. 1: Skin integrity, impairment of	A. Wash hands before and after patient contact B. Provide good oral hygiene after every feeding and q.4h. by 　1. Rinsing mouth with sterile water after each feeding 　2. Using half-strength 3% hydrogen peroxide to cleanse mouth 　3. Applying lemon-glycerin swabs C. Apply nystatin suspension or gentian violet 1% as ordered by physician	Oral lesions will be healed or improved
Nutrition, alteration in: less than body requirements **Etiology** Oral cavity discomfort	Sunken eyes and fontanel Poor skin turgor Dry lips and mucous membranes No tears Subnormal or abnormal temperature Irritability Listlessness Weight loss Poor appetite Poor sucking ability Poor nutritional history	A. Assess hydration status every shift 　1. Weight (AM only) 　2. Skin turgor 　3. Anterior fontanel 　4. Mucous membranes 　5. I & O B. Obtain nutritional history 　1. Eating habits 　2. Formula and feeding frequency 　3. Likes and dislikes C. Monitor caloric intake D. Refer to SCP in Ch. 1: Nutrition, alteration in: less than body requirements	A. Provide formula infant is currently taking B. Offer small, frequent feedings C. Encourage family participation, especially at mealtimes D. Consult with dietitian as needed	Infant will have adequate caloric intake to maintain present level of growth and development

Originated by **Andrea So, RN, BSN**
Resource person: **Ruth E. Novitt, RN, MSN**

Oral Thrush—cont'd

NURSING DIAGNOSIS/ PATIENT PROBLEM	DEFINING CHARACTERISTICS	NURSING ORDERS		EXPECTED OUTCOMES
		ASSESSMENT	INTERVENTIONS	
Comfort, alteration in: pain and discomfort **Etiology** Lesions in oral cavity	Crying Restlessness Irritability Moaning Decreased appetite Weight loss Difficult to soothe Tachycardia Poor sucking ability	A. Assess pain characteristics 1. Quality 2. Onset 3. Duration 4. Location B. Assess behavior characteristics 1. Irritability 2. Crankiness 3. Crying C. Refer to SCP in Ch. 1: Comfort, alteration in	A. Provide comfort measures 1. Mouth care by rinsing mouth after each feeding 2. Adequate rest periods during feedings 3. Stroking and holding infant B. Distract from pain with sensory stimulation 1. Visual: mobile with geometric shapes and colors 2. Auditory: radio, television, talking to infant C. Consult with physical/occupational therapist as needed D. Encourage family to visit and care for infant	Pain will be minimized or relieved as evidenced by a decrease and/or absence of pain characteristics
Parental knowledge deficit **Etiology** New condition	Hostility Anxiety Increased or decreased questioning Repetitive questioning Noncompliance	A. Assess parents' knowledge of illness B. Assess parent-infant relationship C. Evaluate family's ability to learn	A. Establish rapport with family B. Explain etiology of oral thrush C. Instruct family in infant's care 1. Good hand-washing technique 2. Formula preparation 3. Oral hygiene 4. Proper feeding 5. Proper administration of medications D. Refer to social worker/Visiting Nurses' Association, if needed	A. Parents will verbalize the etiology of oral thrush B. Parents will return demonstrate 1. Proper hand-washing technique 2. Formula preparation 3. Medication administration

Otitis Media: pediatric

NURSING DIAGNOSIS/ PATIENT PROBLEM	DEFINING CHARACTERISTICS	NURSING ORDERS		EXPECTED OUTCOMES
		ASSESSMENT	INTERVENTIONS	
Body temperature, alteration in **Etiology** Bacterial infection *Haemophilus influenzae* Beta-hemolytic streptococci Pneumococci	Skin warm and flushed Persistent rise in body temperature Irritability Drowsy Presence of drainage from middle ear(s) Tachycardia	A. Monitor vital signs q.4h., especially temperature. If > 38.5° C, monitor q.2h. B. Observe for chilling C. Assess previous history and physical, including 1. Age 2. Pattern of fever 3. Previous ear infections	A. Plot temperature curve, and observe for trends q.4h. B. Encourage oral fluids C. Use hypothermia blanket for elevated temperature as ordered D. Administer antipyretics as ordered E. Remove excessive clothing; use light blankets only if needed F. Maintain bedside humidifier G. Notify physician of temperature > 38.5° C	Child's body temperature will return to 37° C

Originated by **Andrea So, RN, BSN**
 Resource person: **Ruth E. Novitt, RN, MSN**

Continued.

Otitis Media: pediatric—cont'd

NURSING DIAGNOSIS/ PATIENT PROBLEM	DEFINING CHARACTERISTICS	NURSING ORDERS		EXPECTED OUTCOMES
		ASSESSMENT	INTERVENTIONS	

Airway clearance, ineffective
Etiology
Upper respiratory infection
	Coarse breath sounds
	Rales and/or rhonchi
	Upper airway congestion
	Congested cough (productive and nonproductive)
	Nasal drainage
		A. Assess respiratory status q.4h. and as needed for
		  1. Respiratory rate
		  2. Quality of respirations
		  3. Breath sounds
		  4. Retractions or nasal flaring
		  5. Cough (quality and frequency)
		  6. Rales and rhonchi
		B. Assess vital signs q.4h.
		C. Assess level of consciousness
		D. Refer to SCP in Ch. 1: Airway clearance, ineffective
			A. Maintain O_2 and humidity therapy as ordered by physician
			B. Position child for optimal breathing (upright, using infant seat, buggy, or pillows)
			C. Encourage deep breathing and position change q.2h.
			D. Monitor effectiveness of respiratory treatments
			  1. Chest percussion and drainage
			  2. Suctioning
			  3. Hand-held nebulizer
			E. Provide mouth care q.4h. and as needed
			  1. Rinse with water
			  2. Use lemon-glycerine swabs
				Child will have adequate oxygenation as evidenced by
				A. Respiratory rate within normal limits
				B. Clear breath sounds

Comfort, alteration in: pain **Etiology** Infected ears	Crying Irritability Restlessness Pulling of ear lobes Altered sleeping patterns Poor sucking ability Difficult to soothe	A. Assess child's level of comfort by observing both verbal and nonverbal behaviors (see Defining Characteristics) B. See SCP in Ch. 1: Comfort, alteration in: pain	A. Instill eardrops as ordered by physician B. Reposition child frequently to assist fluid drainage from ear C. Use warm moist compresses to affected ear(s) D. Administer analgesics as ordered by physician	Child will be comfortable and exhibit a decrease in pain behaviors

Knowledge deficit: parental
Etiology
Illness and hospitalization
	Hostility
	Suspiciousness
	Confusion
	Repetitive questions
	Lack of questions
	Disbelief
	Inconsistent visiting patterns
		A. Assess parents' knowledge of child's illness
		B. Assess parents' level of understanding
		C. Evaluate family's ability to learn
			A. Establish rapport with parents
			B. Provide information regarding cause of otitis media
			C. Instruct parents in the signs and symptoms of otitis media
			  1. Elevated temperature
			  2. Cold
			  3. Pulling of ear lobes
			  4. Ear drainage
			  5. Pain
			  6. Decreased appetite
			  7. Poor sucking ability
			D. Instruct parents in early home-management techniques
			E. Instruct parents in
			  1. Proper instillation of eardrops
			  2. Feeding and bubbling techniques
			  3. Prevention of upper respiratory infections
			F. Explain all diagnostic procedures
				A. Parents will list the signs and symptoms of otitis media
				B. Parents will describe the early interventions that could prevent ear damage

Visual Impairment

NURSING DIAGNOSIS/ PATIENT PROBLEM	DEFINING CHARACTERISTICS	NURSING ORDERS		EXPECTED OUTCOMES
		ASSESSMENT	INTERVENTIONS	

Sensory: perceptual alteration, visual
 Etiology
 Disease/trauma to the visual pathways/cranial nerves II, III, IV, and VI. Secondary to
 Stroke
 Intracranial aneurysms
 Brain tumor
 Trauma
 Myasthenia gravis
 Multiple sclerosis
 Glaucoma
 Cataract
	No eye-to-eye contact
	 Abnormal eye movements
	 Failure to locate distant objects
	 Squinting, frequent blinking
	 Bumps into things
	 Clumsy behavior
	 Closing one eye to see
	 Frequent rubbing of the eye
	 Deviation of the eye
	 Gray opacities of the eyes
	 Head tilt
		A. Assess the peripheral field of vision, corneal reflex, pupillary response, visual acuity, extraocular movements
		 B. Assess central vision with each eye individually and together
		 C. Determine the nature of visual symptoms, onset, and the degree of visual loss
		 D. Inquire about previous visual complaints, eye injury, or ocular pain
		 E. Assess the eye and lid for inflammation, edema, positional defects, and deviation
		 F. Inquire about any patient/family history of systemic or central nervous system disease
		 G. Evaluate the patient's ability to function within the limits of visual impairment
		 H. Assess factors/ aids that improve vision, such as glasses, contact lenses, bright lights
			A. Identify self to patient
			 B. Orient patient to the environment
			 C. Provide adequate lighting
			   1. Bright for patients with dimmed vision
			   2. Subdued for patients with photophobia
			 D. Place meal tray, tissues, water, and call light within patient's range of vision
			 E. Place sign over the bed indicating the type and degree of impairment and any contraindicated activities
			 F. If patient has a right-field cut, include in sign over the bed to approach the patient from the left
			 G. Provide an eye patch for the affected eye for a patient with diplopia
			 H. Instruct the patient with hemianopsia to visually scan his/her environment
			 I. Use visual aids such as magnifying glass, large-type printed books and magazines, when appropriate
			 J. If patient is blind
			   1. Place a sign in front of the chart
			   2. Keep him/her informed of date and time
			   3. Explain arrangement of food on tray and plate, using clockwise sequence
			   4. Place food on tray and plate in same place each meal
			   5. Encourage use of sense of touch to become familiar with new objects
			   6. Explain sounds
			   7. Encourage use of radios, tapes
			   8. Advise on the availability of "talking books" through the Library of Congress
				Optimal functioning within the limits of visual impairment will be achieved

Originated by **Maria Dacanay, RN**
 Resource persons: **Linda Arsenault, RN, MSN, CNRN**
          Connie Powell, RN, MSN

Continued.

Visual Impairment—cont'd

NURSING DIAGNOSIS/ PATIENT PROBLEM	DEFINING CHARACTERISTICS	NURSING ORDERS		EXPECTED OUTCOMES
		ASSESSMENT	INTERVENTIONS	
Injury: potential for **Etiology** Visual impairment	Stumbling into furniture Bruised legs Falls	A. Assess the need for assistive devices B. Inquire about previous fall history related to visual impairment C. Evaluate the patient's ability to mobilize within the environment D. Assess patient's fall-risk level	A. Place sticker in front of patient's chart and over the head of the bed indicating the type and degree of visual impairment B. Remove environmental barriers. If furniture or waste baskets are moved, notify patient of the changes C. Encourage patient's roommate and other patients to avoid leaving the doors partially open. Doors should be fully open or closed D. Maintain bed in low position with the side rails up, if appropriate. Keep bed in locked position E. Assist patient when ambulating, if appropriate F. Instruct patient to take hold of both arms of the chair before sitting G. Consult occupational therapy personnel for assistive devices and training in their use H. Supervise the patient when smoking	Risk of fall and injury will be minimized
Anxiety/fear **Etiology** Change in health status Visual impairment Change in role functioning Change in interaction patterns	Withdrawal Indifference Constant demands Uncooperative behavior Avoidance techniques Excessive napping Crying Sleepless nights	A. Recognize patient's level of anxiety (mild, severe) B. Assess patient's normal coping patterns (by interview with patient/ family/significant others/physician)	A. Display confident, calm manner and tolerant, understanding attitude B. Encourage ventilation of feelings/concerns/dependence; listen carefully. Give an unhurried, attentive appearance C. See SCP in Ch. 1: Anxiety/fear	Decreased level of anxiety will be evidenced by A. Calm, relaxed appearance B. Verbalization of fears and feelings C. Restful night
Self-concept, disturbance in **Etiology** Visual impairment	**Subjective** Patient/significant others report changes in self-esteem/personal identity **Objective** Withdrawn Irritable Tearful Anxious Denial of problem Insomnia Refusal to participate in teaching/learning experiences Self-maligning statements	Assess the following A. Patient's perception of self B. Patient's level of anxiety C. Verbalization by patient/significant others of change in self-concept D. Patient's affect, behavior, function E. Patient's previous methods of coping	A. Encourage patient to verbalize fears and concerns B. Include significant others in discussions when possible C. Support by positive reinforcement patient's effort to adapt to constructive changes D. Provide patient/significant others with opportunities to ask questions and verbalize feelings E. Use referral sources (other professionals or lay persons) when appropriate to facilitate patient's attempts at coping	Patient will verbalize positive expression of self-worth

Visual Impairment—cont'd

NURSING DIAGNOSIS/ PATIENT PROBLEM	DEFINING CHARACTERISTICS	NURSING ORDERS		EXPECTED OUTCOMES
		ASSESSMENT	INTERVENTIONS	
Knowledge deficit **Etiology** Change in health status	Questioning Misconceptions	A. Assess knowledge of patient/significant others concerning visual impairment B. Assess effects of visual impairment on ADL	A. Involve significant others in patient's care and instructions B. Help them understand the nature of the disease and its limitations C. Reinforce the physician's explanation of medical management and surgical procedures, if any D. Teach general eye care E. Demonstrate proper administration of eye drops or ointments F. Help family/significant others identify and make arrangements at home to provide for the patient's safety, if indicated G. Make appropriate referrals to home health agency for nursing and social service followup H. Reinforce the need to use community agencies, if indicated, such as American Foundation for the Blind Fifteen West 16th Street New York, NY 10011	Patient/significant others will demonstrate or verbalize knowledge of the disease and the care needed after discharge

THERAPEUTIC INTERVENTIONS

Cataract Extraction: with and without intraocular lens implant

NURSING DIAGNOSIS/ PATIENT PROBLEM	DEFINING CHARACTERISTICS	NURSING ORDERS		EXPECTED OUTCOMES
		ASSESSMENT	INTERVENTIONS	

Sensory-perceptual alteration: visual
 Etiology
 Opacity of the crystalline lens of the eye
 Congenital
 Senile/degenerative
 Metabolic (diabetes)
 Traumatic
 Toxic
	Gradual dimming, blurring of vision
	 Double vision
	 Progressive nearsightedness
	 Frequent need for new glasses
	 Glare noted in bright light
	 Inability to find lighting bright enough to read by
		A. Observe gross appearance of affected eye, particularly the pupil
		 B. Assess patient's level of daily functioning, need for assistance, etc.
			A. Orient patient to hospital environment
			   1. Walk patient around room and unit
			   2. Place objects (especially call light) within reach on unaffected side
			   3. Provide assistance with ADL as needed
			   4. Encourage patient to communicate concerns
			 B. Preoperative
			   1. Obtain surgical consent (includes special intraocular lens implant consent if applicable)
			   2. Instill mydriatic solution into ____ eye every ____ hours
			   3. Observe/document if pupil dilation occurs
			   4. Press inner canthus for about 30-60 sec to speed dilation, prevent systemic absorption, and prevent drops from running into nose
			   5. If more than one eye medication is to be given at one time, wait at least 3-5 min between dosages to allow for absorption of each successive medication
			   6. Darken room and caution patient to avoid bright lights
			 C. Provide verbal explanation of procedures/care
			   1. Inform patient that an eye patch and shield will cover eye postoperatively
			   2. Instruct patient not to touch, squeeze, or rub eye postoperatively
			   3. Instruct patient to avoid lying on the side of cataract extraction
			   4. Reassure patient that assistance will be given by nurses to meet physical needs after surgery
				A. Patient will be oriented to surroundings
				 B. Patient's anxiety will be diminished as evidenced by calm, relaxed appearance
				 C. Patient will verbalize concerns and fears
				 D. Patient will list precautions to be taken postoperatively

Originated by **Laura Vieceli-Brooks, RN, BSN**
Resource person: **Carol Burkhart, RN, BSN, CCRN**

Cataract Extraction: with and without intraocular lens implant—cont'd

NURSING DIAGNOSIS/ PATIENT PROBLEM	DEFINING CHARACTERISTICS	NURSING ORDERS		EXPECTED OUTCOMES
		ASSESSMENT	INTERVENTIONS	
Injury, potential for: to operative eye **Etiology** Increased intraocular pressure resulting from bleeding, edema, hematoma	Severe eye pain Eye hemorrhage Symptoms of damage to optic nerve (blindness)	A. Observe/document/report amount of drainage on eye patch and shield. Notify physician immediately if drainage is bright red and excessive B. Observe for and attempt to allay restlessness C. Report any complaints of eye pain (especially postoperative days 2 and 3) to physician since pain may indicate hemorrhage/infection D. If intraocular lens is implanted, observe/document/report presence of intraocular lens implant, signs and symptoms of eye inflammation, irritation, increased tearing, soreness, pain	A. Instruct patient to notify nurse if nausea or vomiting occurs. Administer antiemetic, as needed B. Reorient patient to physical surroundings C. Approach patient verbally, then touch. Announce yourself as you approach from unoperative side D. Place personal items (i.e., call light, urinal, bedpan) within reach on unaffected side E. Maintain quiet, relaxed atmosphere. Avoid jarring bed F. Elevate head of bed 30-45 degrees. Do not place patient flat in bed G. Position patient on nonoperative side or back, *never* on operative side H. Maintain bed rest with bathroom privileges; provide assistance I. Instruct patient to change position gradually J. Instruct patient in the following 1. Avoid rubbing, squeezing, scratching, or touching operative eye 2. Avoid nose blowing and coughing the first day after surgery 3. Avoid Valsalva's maneuver a. Administer stool softener as needed b. Avoid heavy lifting for 1 month 4. Avoid stooping and lowering head for 1 month. Use step-in slippers and shoes 5. Avoid turning head rapidly. No shaving, brushing teeth, combing hair, showering the first day after surgery. Provide mouthwash. Nurse will assist with morning care K. Medicate patient for discomfort, as needed	Physical injury because of increased intraocular pressure causing hemorrhage will be minimized as evidenced by A. Absence of symptoms of intraocular pressure B. Intact optic nerve (sight) C. Absence of nausea and vomiting or correction with antiemetics D. Eye patch and shield free of drainage E. With intraocular lens implant, lens is intact; no dislocation

Continued.

Cataract Extraction: with and without intraocular lens implant—cont'd

NURSING DIAGNOSIS/ PATIENT PROBLEM	DEFINING CHARACTERISTICS	NURSING ORDERS		EXPECTED OUTCOMES
		ASSESSMENT	INTERVENTIONS	
Knowledge deficit Etiology Unfamiliarity with postdischarge eye care	Asking many questions Misconceptions	Assess knowledge base of patient/significant others and readiness for learning	A. Teach specifics of eye care 1. Wear eye shield at night to prevent injury for approximately 1 month 2. Wear eye shield or glasses during the day. Wear old glasses for unoperated eye 3. With intraocular lens implant, wear old glasses for unoperated eye. Wear new temporary glasses, sunglasses, or eye shield for operated eye 4. Avoid heavy lifting, stooping, straining, bending for 4-6 weeks 5. Reading and light activity are permitted 6. Avoid falls and bumping or jarring head. Take care entering and leaving a car 7. Avoid squeezing, scratching, or rubbing the operative eye and lids 8. Instruct on proper eyedrop instillation 9. Call physician if patient experiences severe pain or sudden loss of vision 10. Avoid constipation B. Reassure patient that vision will gradually improve in a few weeks	Patient or significant others will have adequate knowledge to care for eye on discharge as evidenced by A. Accurate verbalizations and practice of precautions to be taken B. Written discharge instructions sent home with patient from nurse in eye room C. Return demonstration of eye drop instillation D. Carrying intraocular lens implant ID card

Tonsillectomy and Adenoidectomy: pediatric

NURSING DIAGNOSIS/ PATIENT PROBLEM	DEFINING CHARACTERISTICS	NURSING ORDERS		EXPECTED OUTCOMES
		ASSESSMENT	INTERVENTIONS	
Breathing pattern, ineffective **Etiology** History of tonsillitis Surgical removal of tonsils and adenoids	Dyspnea Tachypnea Nasal flaring Mouth breathing Enlarged tonsils Snoring	A. Assess respiratory rate and depth by listening to breath sounds every _____ hours B. Note retractions and/or nasal flaring C. Assess skin color, temperature, and capillary refill D. Note increased occurrence of mouth breathing E. Assess position patient assumes for normal/easy breathing F. Refer to SCP in Ch. 1: Breathing pattern, ineffective	A. Monitor changes in vital signs, especially in breathing patterns, and notify physician as necessary B. Elevate head of bed 30-40 degrees to ease breathing C. Monitor O_2 therapy as ordered per mask/tent	Improved respiratory status will be evidenced by A. Normal respiratory rate for age B. Absence of dyspnea C. Absence of cyanosis D. Decrease in incidence of mouth breathing

Comfort, alteration in: pain
Etiology
Tonsillitis
Surgical removal of tonsils and adenoids
	Patient/parent reports pain (sore throat, ear pain)
	Changes in behavior (moaning, crying, restlessness)
	Facial mask of pain
	Autonomic responses not seen in chronic stable pain (diaphoresis, changes in BP, pulse rate, increased or decreased respiratory rate)
	Difficulty swallowing
		A. Solicit patient's description of pain, if possible, documenting in patient's own words
		B. Assess pain characteristics
		  1. Quality (sharp, burning, etc.)
		  2. Severity (scale 1-3, 3 most severe)
		  3. Onset (gradual/sudden)
		  4. Duration (how long: intermittent/continuous)
		  5. Precipitating/relieving factors
			A. Anticipate need for analgesics and/or additional methods of pain relief
			B. Respond immediately to complaint of pain
			C. Give analgesics as ordered, evaluating effectiveness and observing for any signs/symptoms of adverse effects
			D. Use additional comfort measures when appropriate
			  1. Bedside humidifier for increased ease of respirations
			  2. Ice collar to throat
			  3. Encourage oral intake of cold fluids
			  4. Avoid intake of hot/spicy/acidic or hard (crumbly) foods
			  5. Discourage coughing/clearing of throat
			  6. Use of distractional devices
			  7. Use of psychosocial support system
			E. Refer to SCP in Ch. 1: Comfort, alteration in
				Pain will be relieved or decreased

Originated by **Susan Kansas, RN,C**
Resource person: **Michele Knoll-Puzas, RN,C BS**

Continued.

Tonsillectomy and Adenoidectomy: pediatric—cont'd

NURSING DIAGNOSIS/ PATIENT PROBLEM	DEFINING CHARACTERISTICS	NURSING ORDERS		EXPECTED OUTCOMES
		ASSESSMENT	INTERVENTIONS	

Fluid volume deficit: potential
Etiology
Decreased oral intake (resulting from post-operative discomfort)
	Decreased oral intake
	Decreased urine output
	Concentrated urine
	Thirst
	Dry mucous membranes
	Nausea/vomiting
		A. Assess hydration status
		  1. Skin turgor
		  2. Mucous membranes
		  3. I & O every _____ hours
		  4. Specific gravity every _____ hours
		B. Assess for nausea/emesis
		  1. Amount
		  2. Frequency
		  3. Blood tinged (small amount expected)
			A. Monitor strict I & O every _____ hours
			B. Administer parenteral fluids as ordered, monitoring IV flow rate until oral intake is adequate. Discontinue IV infusions when oral intake is adequate (at least _____ ml/hour)
			C. Provide clear, cold liquids as soon as child awakens; avoid acidic and hot liquids
			D. Notify physician if patient has not voided _____ hours after surgery
				Adequate fluid volume will be maintained as evidenced by
				A. Normal skin turgor
				B. Moist mucous membranes
				C. Normal urine specific gravity
				D. Absence of continued emesis

Anxiety/fear
Etiology
Hospitalization
Procedures
Separation from family
Loss of body parts
	Mild
	Withdrawal
	Restlessness
	Increased questioning
	Regressive behaviors
	
	Moderate/severe
	Insomnia
	Facial tension
	Overexcited
	Expressed concern
	Trembling
	Constant demands
		A. Recognize patient's level of anxiety (mild/severe). Note any signs/symptoms, especially nonverbal communication
		B. Assess patient's normal coping patterns by interview with patient/family/significant other/physician
			A. Display confident, calm manner and tolerant, understanding attitude
			B. Introduce self and personnel on unit
			C. Establish rapport with patient, especially through continuity of care
			D. Orient patient and family to environment
			E. Encourage patient to ask questions. Provide accurate information regarding medications, tests/procedures, self-care. Clarify misconceptions about loss of body parts
			F. Provide preoperative teaching
			  1. Arrange tour of holding area/recovery room
			  2. Explain postoperative expectations of IV infusions, sore throat, and slight (initial) nausea
			G. Allow family member/significant others to visit. Arrange for family member/significant other to remain overnight with child. Involve them in care as appropriate
			H. Reassure patient that it is allright to cry
			I. Use other supportive measures as indicated (medications, Child Life, Foster Grandparents). Assure patient that pain medications are readily available and will be provided promptly
			J. Provide diversional materials (television/books, favorite toys/games, stuffed animals/dolls)
			K. Monitor changes in level of anxiety. Assist in use of usual coping behaviors
				Decreased level of anxiety will be evidenced by
				A. Calm, relaxed appearance
				B. Verbalization of fears/feelings
				C. Restful night

Tonsillectomy and Adenoidectomy: pediatric—cont'd

NURSING DIAGNOSIS/ PATIENT PROBLEM	DEFINING CHARACTERISTICS	NURSING ORDERS		EXPECTED OUTCOMES
		ASSESSMENT	INTERVENTIONS	
Injury, potential for **Etiology** Postoperative hemorrhage (usually occurring within the first 8-12 hours after surgery)	Hematemesis of bright red blood Thrashing about in bed/restlessness Pallor Hypotension Increased pulse/respiratory rates Weakness Increased anxiety	A. Monitor amount, color, consistency of hematemesis. Expect a small amount of old blood B. Monitor vital signs every _____ hours for evidence of hemorrhage. Notify physician of 1. Heart rate < _____ or > _____ 2. Respiratory rate < _____ or > _____ 3. BP < _____ or > _____ C. Assess for increased restlessness and thrashing about in bed	A. Provide ice collar B. Discourage coughing, blowing nose, or clearing of throat C. Provide acetaminophen (Tylenol) for pain in place of aspirin products D. Remove straws from diet tray E. Check temperature (oral route is acceptable for the older child) F. Eliminate hot/acidic/hard (crumbly) foods or drinks from trays G. For slight bleeding 1. Apply cold compress or ice collar to throat 2. Pinch nostrils 3. Place on side to avoid aspiration H. For profuse, bright red bleeding, notify physician immediately	Patient's potential for bleeding will be minimized
Knowledge deficit related to follow-up care **Etiology** New procedures Unfamiliarity with follow-up care	Questioning Verbalizing misconceptions Not verbalizing feelings and/or questions	A. Assess physical/emotional readiness of patient/family to learn B. Assess patient/family understanding of diet, activity, analgesic, and signs/symptoms of hemorrhage	A. Teach patient/family diet to follow and foods to avoid 1. Begin with clear, cold liquids (popsicles, juices, carbonated beverages, gelatin) 2. After 24 hours, advance to milk and milk products (ice cream, egg nog, milk shakes) and soft foods (eggs, mashed potatoes, custards, soft white breads, as tolerated) 3. Avoid a. Hot foods such as soup, although foods may be warm b. Hard, dry foods such as toast, crackers, cookies c. Acidic or spicy foods such as citrus juices, fruits, or chili 4. Drink plenty of liquids B. Teach patient/family the progression of activity to follow 1. Bed rest or out of bed in a chair for a few hours each day initially 2. After 2 days, patient may be out of bed as much as tolerated, but no rough play, bending, lifting, or straining and no outdoor play, especially in cold weather 3. Patient may not return to school until permitted to do so by physician	A. Patient/significant other will communicate an understanding of recovery process, diet, activity, analgesics, and signs/symptoms of hemorrhage B. Patient will demonstrate adequate nutritional intake as indicated by 1. Tolerance of soft diet by the fourth day 2. Absence of signs/symptoms of dehydration 3. Absence of nausea/emesis C. Patient will resume normal quiet activities by the fourth day D. Surgical site(s) will heal without hemorrhage as indicated by absence of bright red blood E. Patient/family will verbalize signs/symptoms of hemorrhage and emergency treatment of hemorrhage

Continued.

Tonsillectomy and Adenoidectomy (Pediatric)—cont'd

NURSING DIAGNOSIS/ PATIENT PROBLEM	DEFINING CHARACTERISTICS	NURSING ORDERS		EXPECTED OUTCOMES
		ASSESSMENT	INTERVENTIONS	

			C. Teach patient/family signs/ symptoms of hemorrhage
			1. Watch for bright red blood coming from nose or mouth. Expect some old dark brown blood in saliva for 2-3 days
			2. Watch for pallor, thrashing about in bed, or increased restlessness during sleep
			3. For slight bleeding
			  a. Apply a cold compress or ice pack to throat
			  b. Elevate head
			  c. Place child on side
			  d. If bleeding persists more than 15 min, call physician
			4. For profuse bright red bleeding, notify physician immediately, or go to nearest emergency room
			D. Teach patient/family measures of easing discomfort
			1. Explain that some pain may occur in the throat, head, or ears, especially the ears. If occurring, it will usually be worse on the fifth or sixth day
			2. Use analgesics as prescribed
			3. Do *not* give aspirin or aspirin products
			4. Patient is not to use straws for drinking
			5. Use a room humidifier for 2-5 days to increase ease of breathing
			E. Patient may exhibit a low-grade temperature of 37°-38° C (99°-100.5° F) for 2-3 days. Explain correct method of taking oral temperature and interpreting results to patient/significant other
			F. Explain that a white membrane can be seen in the throat 10-14 days after the operation. This is normal and no cause for alarm; it will not interfere with the child's breathing
			G. Provide discharge instruction sheet summarizing diet, activity, and other teachings
			H. Instruct family to call physician for any problems/questions
				F. Patient will achieve optimal level of postoperative comfort as evidenced by
				1. Decreased need/use of analgesics
				2. Verbalization of decreased pain
				3. Increased appearance of relief and comfort
				G. Patient/family will demonstrate correct method of taking temperature and interpreting results

CHAPTER TWELVE

Psychosocial

DISORDERS

Child in Isolation

NURSING DIAGNOSIS/ PATIENT PROBLEM	DEFINING CHARACTERISTICS	NURSING ORDERS		EXPECTED OUTCOMES
		ASSESSMENT	INTERVENTIONS	
Fear: parent/child Etiology Isolation procedures Infectious disease process Unfamiliar procedures	Absence or excessive questioning Overly anxious or seeming indifference Inability to discuss new procedures Avoidance of learning isolation techniques Violation of isolation techniques Insomnia Hostility or tearfulness Child makes repetitive, unnecessary requests: water, toys, television, nurse	Assess child's Ability for play Pain Mood Behavior Previous experience with illness Family support Age Level of growth and development	A. With parent and child plan a daily schedule that alternates rest with play B. Encourage family calls/visits C. Provide age-appropriate activities: toys, books, games, television, coloring/drawing (must be disposable or cleanable) D. Consult child life therapist E. Consult schoolteacher F. Instruct parents of importance of maintaining contact with child, physically and emotionally	Premorbid level of growth and development will be maintained as evidenced by A. Use of coping diversional activities B. Appropriate behaviors for age
Knowledge deficit Etiology Unfamiliarity of procedure and need for infection control	Multiple questions Lack of questions Apprehension	Assess knowledge base and readiness for learning of child/parent	A. Provide explanations in simple accurate terms appropriate to child's and parent's level of understanding B. Provide adequate time for explanations and demonstrations C. Explain isolation and appropriate procedures 1. Rationale for isolation 2. Proper use of materials, i.e., gloves, masks, gowns, handwashing techniques D. Use a variety of instructional methods/aids 1. Demonstration 2. Discussion 3. Handouts/pamphlets on isolation procedures E. Explain "normal" disease course, treatment, and follow-up F. Arrange public health/social work follow-up as needed G. Instruct family concerning any special precautions/treatments necessary to prevent spread of disease in community 1. Refer to appropriate policy and procedure 2. Consult infection control clinician as necessary	Child/family will demonstrate understanding of appropriate infection control techniques

Originated by **Patricia Hasbrouck-Aschliman, RN, CCRN**
Resource persons: **Michele Knoll-Puzas, RN,C BS**
       Ann Filipski, RN, MSN, CS

Child in Isolation—cont'd

NURSING DIAGNOSIS/ PATIENT PROBLEM	DEFINING CHARACTERISTICS	NURSING ORDERS		EXPECTED OUTCOMES
		ASSESSMENT	INTERVENTIONS	

Diversional activity, deficit
Etiology
Removal from normal interpersonal and social contact
	Complaints of boredom, loneliness
	Lack of expression
	Regression in development
	Irritability
	Constant demands
		A. Assess current level of understanding
		  1. Need for isolation
		  2. Meaning of isolation
		  3. Current disease process
		  4. Developmental level
		B. Assess coping mechanisms being employed
		C. Assess current supports within the family
		D. Monitor changes in anxiety level
			A. Encourage questions/conversation/ventilation of feelings
			B. Address fears concerning communicability of disease
			C. Provide parents and child with information concerning progress, recovery, etc.
			D. Assure parents that optimal care is given to patients in isolation
			E. Adapt care to needs and routine of child/parents
			F. Allow family visitors, and involve them in patient's care
			G. Assist in identifying and using appropriate coping behaviors (see ''Knowledge deficit'')
				Anxiety will be decreased as evidenced by
				A. Calm, relaxed appearance
				B. Ability to verbalize fears/feelings
				C. Ability to verbalize reason for isolation
				D. Maintenance of isolation

Grief Over Long-Term Illness/Disability: psychosocial aspects

NURSING DIAGNOSIS/ PATIENT PROBLEM	DEFINING CHARACTERISTICS	NURSING ORDERS		EXPECTED OUTCOMES
		ASSESSMENT	INTERVENTIONS	
Grieving **Etiology** Altered body structure/function	Anger Depression Denial Crying Guilt Disgust Hostility Withdrawal Excessive fatigue Disturbed sleep patterns Weight gain or loss	Identify the following A. Behaviors that are suggestive of grieving (see Defining Characteristics) B. Patient's past responses to a loss C. The stage of grieving that the patient is experiencing (see Interventions) D. Potential pathologic grieving responses (see SCP in Ch. 1: Grieving, dysfunctional)	A. Establish a one-to-one relationship with patient B. Maintain a safe and private environment C. Encourage the verbalization of emotion through the use of open-ended questions D. Remain with patient throughout the expression of emotion (e.g., crying, anger) E. Assist patient in identifying feelings F. Avoid personalizing patient's behavior, i.e., avoid becoming angry with patient if he/she expresses anger that is vented toward you G. Respect patient's feelings H. Anticipate that patient may progress/regress in the grief process I. Encourage the use of coping mechanisms that have previously been useful J. Explain normal grief reactions to patient/significant others K. Recognize that each patient is unique and will progress through the process at his/her own pace	The patient will begin to A. Express grief B. Understand own stage of grief

Originated by **Margaret Williams, RN**
Resource persons: **Sue A. Conneighton, RN, MSN**
    Ann Filipski, RN, MSN, CS

Continued.

Grief Over Long-Term Illness/Disability: psychosocial aspects—cont'd

NURSING DIAGNOSIS/ PATIENT PROBLEM	DEFINING CHARACTERISTICS	NURSING ORDERS		EXPECTED OUTCOMES
		ASSESSMENT	INTERVENTIONS	

			Stages of grieving
			A. Shock and disbelief (patient's initial response to the loss): reality is overwhelming; denial, panic, and anxiety may be seen
			  1. Provide a safe environment for the expression of grief
			  2. Minimize environmental stresses/stimuli
			  3. Explain and remain with patient throughout procedures
			  4. Accept patient's need to deny the loss as part of the normal grief process
			B. Realization (occurs weeks to months following the loss): reality continues to be overwhelming; sadness, anger, guilt, and hostility may be seen
			  1. Anticipate an increase in affective expression and lability of behavior
			  2. Recognize patient's need to maintain hope for the future
			  3. Provide realistic information about health status without giving false reassurances or taking away patient's sense of hope
			C. Defensive retreat (occurs weeks to months following the loss): an attempt to maintain what has been lost; denial, wishful thinking, unwillingness to participate in self-care, and indifference may be seen
			  1. Recognize that regression may be an adaptive mechanism
			  2. Support and positively reinforce patient's efforts at remaining involved in self-care
			  3. Offer encouragement by pointing out patient's strengths and progress to date
			  4. Discuss with patient possible need for use of outside support systems (i.e., peer support, support groups, clergy)	

Grief Over Long-Term Illness/Disability: psychosocial aspects—cont'd

NURSING DIAGNOSIS/ PATIENT PROBLEM	DEFINING CHARACTERISTICS	NURSING ORDERS		EXPECTED OUTCOMES
		ASSESSMENT	INTERVENTIONS	
			D. Acknowledgement (occurs months to 1 year following the loss): patient slowly realizes the impact of the loss; depression, anxiety, and bitterness may be seen 1. Assist patient in listing importance of rehabilitation needs 2. Encourage patient/significant others to be actively involved with the rehabilitation team 3. Continue to reinforce patient's strengths and progress E. Adaptation (occurs during first year, or longer, following the loss): patient continues to reorganize resources, abilities, and self-image 1. Recognize patient's need to review (relive) the illness experience 2. Facilitate the reorganization process by reviewing patient's progress 3. Discuss with patient possible involvement with peers/ organizations (e.g., stroke club, arthritis foundation) that work with patient's medical condition	
Self-concept, disturbance in: body image, self-esteem, role performance, and personal identity **Etiology** Biophysical Cognitive/perceptual disturbance Psychosocial	Neglect of body part Refusal to discuss limitations/altered body function Staring at affected body part Unwillingness to look at or touch affected body part Disparaging remarks about personal appearance Refusal to accept or participate in rehabilitation efforts Withdrawal from social/personal role responsibilities Exaggerated attempts in directing own treatment Orientation to past rather than to present or future	Assess for the following: A. Any neurologic/ cognitive impairments leading to self-concept distortion B. Patient's verbalizations and perceptions about altered body structure or function C. Behavioral patterns suggesting an altered self-concept (see Defining Characteristics)	A. Provide an atmosphere that will allow the patient to discuss feelings, concerns, and perceptions about altered body structure/function 1. Provide privacy 2. Approach patient in an unhurried manner 3. Listen carefully to patient's attempts to verbalize feelings B. Explain to patient/significant others that physical condition may affect emotional status C. Provide information, and clarify any misconceptions that patient may have about health status D. Encourage patient to participate in grooming and hygiene activities E. Foster a sense of achievement by slowly providing patient with increasingly complex tasks	The patient will progress toward integration of altered self-concept

Continued.

Grief Over Long-Term Illness/Disability: psychosocial aspects—cont'd

NURSING DIAGNOSIS/ PATIENT PROBLEM	DEFINING CHARACTERISTICS	NURSING ORDERS		EXPECTED OUTCOMES
		ASSESSMENT	INTERVENTIONS	

			F. Provide an individualized approach to patient's care
			  1. Respect patient's need to be alone
			  2. Demonstrate sensitivity to patient's tolerance for information (avoid sensory overload)
			  3. Encourage patient to participate in the plan of care
			  4. Recognize patient's tolerance for hearing emotionally charged information
			  5. Plan routine activities to meet patient's needs
			G. Encourage family/significant others to actively participate in patient's care
			H. Use the resources of other health professionals: clergy, social workers, psychiatric liaison, vocational counselor	

Coping, ineffective individual: potential **Etiology** Situational crisis Maturational crisis Inadequate support system Inadequate coping methods	Verbalization of inability Change in usual communication patterns Inability to make decisions Altered behavior toward self or others Inability to meet basic needs Impaired concentration Inability to ask for help Emotional lability	Identify the following A. Behavioral cues suggestive of ineffective coping (see Defining Characteristics) B. Past coping mechanisms C. Patient's support systems	A. Listen carefully to patient's verbalization B. Observe patient's nonverbal communication C. Support patient's efforts to evaluate own behavior D. Encourage family/significant others to interact with patient E. Assist patient in problem-solving (e.g., identification of problem, alternatives) F. Encourage the use of coping mechanisms that have previously been helpful G. Support patient's constructive coping behaviors	The patient will begin to A. Verbalize emotions B. Identify constructive coping behaviors

Sexual dysfunction: potential
Etiology
Physiologic/psychosocial alteration of sexuality
	Verbalization of sexual dysfunction
	Expression of sexual dissatisfaction
	Decreased libido
	Impotence
	Change in sexual relationship with significant other
		Identify the following
		A. Previous level of sexual function and satisfaction
		B. Psychologic-physiologic factors that would compromise sexual function
		C. Cues suggesting sexual dysfunction
		D. Medication that might alter sexual function
			A. Encourage ventilation of feelings and concerns
			B. Provide an atmosphere that will allow patient to ask questions regarding sexual function
			C. Provide patient with accurate information regarding sexual dysfunction (e.g., cause, contributing factors, solutions)
			D. Encourage patient to decide (for self) what are acceptable sexual practices
			E. Avoid imposing your own sexual values and beliefs on the patient
			F. Use available resources
			  1. Sexual dsyfunction clinic
			  2. Written information
			  3. Community resources
			  4. See SCP in Ch. 1: Sexual dysfunction: alteration in sexual functioning
				Patient will begin to
				A. Explore emotions surrounding sexual dysfunction
				B. Integrate information about sexual dysfunction

Grief Over Long-Term Illness/Disability: psychosocial aspects—cont'd

NURSING DIAGNOSIS/ PATIENT PROBLEM	DEFINING CHARACTERISTICS	NURSING ORDERS		EXPECTED OUTCOMES
		ASSESSMENT	INTERVENTIONS	

Coping, ineffective family: potential
Etiology
Temporary family disorganization and role changes
Family crises
Prolonged disability that exhausts supportive capacity
	Limited involvement or noninvolvement with patient
	Expressed hopelessness
	Refusal to participate in patient's rehabilitation
	Distortion of reality (regarding patient health)
	Prolonged denial of patient's health status
	Verbalization of inability to cope
	Emotional lability of family members
		Identify
		A. Behavioral cues suggestive of ineffective coping (see Defining Characteristics)
		B. Past coping mechanisms
			A. Create a supportive environment for the family
			  1. Orient family to the hospital (e.g., visiting hours, cafeteria, how to contact the nursing unit and physician)
			  2. Allow family some private time to spend with patient
			B. Acknowledge the family's feelings
			C. Provide realistic information about patient's health status without giving false reassurances
			D. Encourage the use of coping mechanisms that have previously been helpful
			E. Acknowledge the family's strengths
			F. Encourage the family members to discuss their feelings about patient's hospitalization. Remember that the family may experience the same stages of grieving either at the same or different time than patient
			G. Teach the family about patient's physical health status
			H. Involve the family in patient's care when possible
			I. Consider referring the family to other sources (when their problems extend beyond nursing expertise): family therapist, psychiatric liaison, social worker, self-help groups, clergy
				The family will begin to
				A. Verbalize emotions
				B. Identify constructive coping behaviors

CHAPTER THIRTEEN

Emergency/Trauma

Drug Overdose: adolescent

NURSING DIAGNOSIS/ PATIENT PROBLEM	DEFINING CHARACTERISTICS	NURSING ORDERS		EXPECTED OUTCOMES
		ASSESSMENT	INTERVENTIONS	
Tissue perfusion, alteration in: cardiopulmonary (potential) **Etiology** Drug ingestion	Change in level of consciousness Hyperventilation or hypoventilation Tachycardia and hypertension Bradycardia and hypotension	A. Assess vital signs on admission; reassess 1. Temperature every _____ 2. Heart rate every _____ 3. Cardiac rhythm every _____ 4. Respiratory rate and pattern every _____ 5. BP every _____ B. Assess for open airway every _____	A. Place patient on cardiorespiratory monitor B. Keep Ambu bag at bedside C. Place patient in semi-Fowler's position D. Administer O_2 as necessary at _____ L/min as ordered E. Maintain quiet environment F. Notify physician of changes in vital signs G. Place crash cart at bedside if condition warrants	Patient's cardiopulmonary status will remain within normal limits as evidenced by temperature, pulse, respiration, and BP within normal limits for age
Consciousness: altered levels of **Etiology** Drug ingestion	Marked constriction or dilation of pupils Lethargy, confusion, disorientation Coma (likely with ingestion of salicylate sedatives, narcotics, narcotic-like drugs, anticholinergic and cholinergic agents)	Assess neurologic status q.2h., including A. Level of consciousness B. Pupil size and reactivity C. Visual acuity D. Muscle strength E. Behavioral changes, irritability F. Headache G. Response to stimuli H. Orientation I. Tinnitus	A. Avoid excessive stimulation by 1. Dimming lights 2. Limiting visitors 3. Maintaining quiet environment B. Provide seizure precautions 1. Keep side rails up at all times; pad if necessary 2. Keep bed in lowest position 3. Keep head of bed slightly elevated C. Record responses to questions D. Reorient to environment as needed	Maximal neurologic function will be established
Injury, potential for: self **Etiology** Further absorption of ingested drugs	Progressive decline in neurologic status (see preceding Nursing Diagnosis for neurologic assessment)	A. Obtain symptoms of ingestion B. Assess time of onset, estimated time of ingestion C. Obtain patient's age and weight D. Assess prior attempts at treatment E. Assess type and amount of drug ingested 1. Send blood and urine for toxicology screening immediately	A. Induce emesis as ordered per physician 1. Do not attempt if patient is convulsing or if neurologic status is significantly depressed 2. Do not induce if ingested substance is caustic 3. Provide ipecac, as ordered for emesis induction 4. Provide abundant clear liquids if ipecac is given B. Provide gastric lavage as ordered (effective in patients with significantly depressed level of consciousness; method of choice if ingested substance is caustic)	Risk of further injury will be minimized

Originated by **Janet McCants, RN, BSN**
Resource persons: **Michele Knoll-Puzas, RN,C BS**
      Ann Filipski, RN, MSN, CS

Drug Overdose: adolescent—cont'd

NURSING DIAGNOSIS/ PATIENT PROBLEM	DEFINING CHARACTERISTICS	NURSING ORDERS		EXPECTED OUTCOMES
		ASSESSMENT	INTERVENTIONS	

		2. Ask for note, if any, left by patient
		3. Ask for empty bottles left nearby; question if any drugs are missing from home
		4. Ask if patient is taking any prescription drugs and, if so, what type
			1. Attempt nasogastric insertion after checking gag reflex; if sluggish, patient should be intubated first (notify physician)
			2. Provide appropriate size nasogastric tube; check for placement before beginning lavage
			C. Administer absorption-inhibiting medications, as ordered and as appropriate for type of ingestion, at safe dosage for patient's age and weight
			  1. Administer activated charcoal within 1 hour of aspirin ingestion
			  2. Administer acetylcysteine (Mucomyst) q.4h. for 24 hours if patient has ingested acetaminophen
			D. Promote catharsis as ordered
			  1. Provide medications as ordered; drug of choice is magnesium sulfate solution
			  2. Tell patient to expect abdominal cramping, diarrhea-like symptoms
			  3. Provide privacy, bedpan, cleaning materials
			  4. Assist as needed
			E. Promote diuresis as ordered
			  1. Push oral fluids if patient is alert
			  2. Maintain IV fluids if level of consciousness is depressed (usually 1½ times maintenance fluid required for weight)
			  3. Assist with bedpan/urinal
			  4. Catheterize if necessary
			  5. Maintain I & O during renal excretion of toxins
			  6. Repeat urine/blood toxicology levels as ordered	

Continued.

Drug Overdose: adolescent—cont'd

NURSING DIAGNOSIS/ PATIENT PROBLEM	DEFINING CHARACTERISTICS	NURSING ORDERS		EXPECTED OUTCOMES
		ASSESSMENT	INTERVENTIONS	
Fluid volume deficit Etiology Side effects of ingested toxins or treatment modalities	Increased pulse Hypotension Decreased urine output Increased urine specific gravity Elevated serum Na Dry mucous membranes Weakness Decreased fluid intake	A. Monitor for nausea and vomiting B. Check laboratory values 1. CBC 2. Electrolytes 3. Toxicology levels C. Assess vital signs q.2h., minimally D. Assess level of hydration q.2h. 1. Urine specific gravity 2. Urine pH 3. Skin turgor 4. Mucous membranes 5. I & O	A. Maintain fluid intake, oral if possible, or IV fluids as ordered B. Measure and record type of emesis C. Keep patient NPO, and advance gradually as tolerated D. See SCP in Ch. 1: Fluid volume deficit	Fluid and electrolytes will return to normal limits for age and weight
Coping, ineffective family: compromised Etiology Temporary family separation/disorganization Situational crisis	Parent or guardian Verbalizes inadequate understanding of situation Displays inappropriate or overly protective behaviors Appears withdrawn Appears preoccupied with personal guilt, fears, and grief	A. Assess the family's immediate understanding of patient's situation/ physical status B. Assess available coping mechanisms and supports	A. Provide family with support personnel, clergy, ombudsman, volunteer, psychiatric nurse liaison, physician B. Keep family informed of patient's status and of care being provided C. Allow visitors when possible D. Provide privacy during discussion of further treatment, hospitalization, follow-up with physician, psychiatric nursing E. Support family's use of adaptive coping mechanisms	Family members will display appropriate coping behaviors as evidenced by A. Verbalization of understanding of current crisis situation B. Ability to ask appropriate questions C. Ability to provide support for adolescent child

Hypovolemic Shock: acute care

NURSING DIAGNOSIS/ PATIENT PROBLEM	DEFINING CHARACTERISTICS	NURSING ORDERS		EXPECTED OUTCOMES
		ASSESSMENT	INTERVENTIONS	
Fluid volume deficit **Etiology** 15%-25% estimated blood volume loss	Thirst Dry mouth Dizziness, light-head- edness Cool, clammy skin Tachycardia <120 BPM Anxiety Decrease in CVP <5 mm/Hg Flat neck veins Capillary refill >2 seconds Tachypnea >20 Increased diastolic pressure Decreased pulse pres- sure <40 mm Hg Postural hypoten- sion >10 mm Hg Slow speech	A. Evaluate and doc- ument the extent of patient's inju- ries related to air- way, breathing, and circulation (including source and extent of hem- orrhage) B. Perform secondary assessment, using head to toe exami- nation C. Assess early warn- ing signs of vol- ume loss 1. Skin pale 2. Coolness of lower extremi- ties 3. Tachycardia under 120 BPM 4. Subtle changes in BP 5. Slow capillary refill D. Assess all possible causes of tachy- cardia, and alle- viate, if possible 1. Anxiety 2. Fear 3. Hypovolemia 4. Pain E. Assess CVP to distinguish be- tween hypovole- mic and cardio- genic shock F. Assess I & O from IV infusions, Fo- ley catheter, naso- gastric (NG) tube, chest tube, vomi- tus as appropriate	A. Maintain airway B. Attempt to control source of bleeding. If *external,* apply di- rect pressure, pressure dressing; if *internal,* control source as or- dered such as NG tube: flush with saline until clear C. Monitor continued blood loss closely D. Initiate O_2 on all patients per physician's order. Suction as needed E. Initiate IV therapy with lactated Ringer's solution or normal sa- line as ordered 1. Replacement therapy should be 3 ml per 1 ml lost (po- tential 2-4 L) 2. Patient exhibiting these signs and symptoms of hy- povolemia should have ei- ther two large-bore IV cath- eters or one large-bore pe- ripheral IV catheter in addition to central line or cutdown F. Obtain initial spun Hct, and reevaluate q.1-4h. Hct will drop with fluid replacement G. Obtain admission blood sam- ples, and type and cross-match for at least 4 units of packed RBCs as ordered H. Obtain urine sample and send to laboratory for urinalysis. Check urine for blood I. Monitor for arrhythmias J. Monitor vital signs and CVP every 15 min K. Offer reassurance, and explain procedures to patient	Shock will be reversed within 10-15 min, within limits of con- dition

Originated by **Christine Jutzi, RN, BS**
Resource person: **Helen Snow-Jackson, RN, BSN, TNS, CEN**

Continued.

Hypovolemic Shock: acute care—cont'd

NURSING DIAGNOSIS/ PATIENT PROBLEM	DEFINING CHARACTERISTICS	NURSING ORDERS		EXPECTED OUTCOMES
		ASSESSMENT	INTERVENTIONS	
Potential for alteration in tissue perfusion because of decompensated (late) hypovolemic shock **Etiology** >30% blood volume lost (>1500 ml) Profound hemorrhage affecting major organs	Rapid (>120 BPM), weak, or very slow pulse Decreased urine output Anuria Decrease in systolic blood pressure to <100 mg Hg Decrease in pulse pressure to <20 mm Hg Inability to sit up CVP of 0 Change in patient sensorium (belligerent, restless, uncooperative) Poor capillary refill Tachypnic >30 Shallow, rapid respirations or Cheyne-Stokes respirations Electrolyte imbalances Decrease in Hct Deterioration in ABGs Arrhythmias Cardiac arrest	A. Continue ongoing assessment as described in Nursing Orders for Fluid volume deficit B. Anticipate potential causes of shock state from ongoing assessment C. If only visible injury is head injury, look for other cause of hypovolemia, e.g., internal injuries (isolated head trauma does not usually lead to shock) D. Assess urine output (minimally adequate urine output is 0.5 ml/kg/hour) E. Assess baseline ABGs for increasing acidosis and hypoxia. Assess patency of airway	A. Continue as in Nursing Interventions for Fluid volume deficit B. Prepare for possible intubation C. Maintain lactated Ringer's IV infusions wide open until patient's BP is 90 mg Hg (systolic) (massive fluid resuscitation needed of at least 4 L of lactated Ringer's solution) D. For severe hypovolemia with massive injuries: prepare for 2 or 3 cutdowns and peripheral lines E. Apply MAST suit as ordered when systolic BP falls <90 mm Hg. Deflate when systolic BP is >100 mm Hg or the patient is in the OR F. Position patient with lower extremities elevated about 20-30 degrees G. Transfuse the patient with whole blood or packed RBCs, using a blood pump H. Check urine output every _____ with Foley catheter I. Prepare for possible interventions, e.g., chest tube insertion, pericardiocentesis, abdominal tap J. Prepare patient for OR if indicated K. Initiate CPR, treatment of arrythmias, administration of drugs according to Advanced Cardiac Life Support (ACLS) standards. (Focus should be correction of underlying problem causing arrest)	Complications of hypovolemic shock will be minimized
Anxiety/fear **Etiology** Acute injury	Restlessness Crying Agitation Increased pulse Increased BP Increased respirations Irrational thought process Patient admits anxiety Patient/significant others question patient's condition	Assess level of anxiety of patient/significant others according to Defining Characteristics	A. Reduce anxiety of patient/significant others by explaining all procedures/treatment. Keep explanations basic B. Maintain confident, assured manner C. Reduce unneccessary external stimuli, e.g., clear unnecessary personnel from room, decrease volume of cardiac monitor D. Reassure patient/significant others as appropriate E. Provide a quiet, private place for significant others to wait F. Refer to other support systems as appropriate, e.g., clergy, social worker, other family/friends	Ability of patient/significant others to cope will be maximized

Hypovolemic Shock: acute care—cont'd

NURSING DIAGNOSIS/ PATIENT PROBLEM	DEFINING CHARACTERISTICS	NURSING ORDERS		EXPECTED OUTCOMES
		ASSESSMENT	INTERVENTIONS	
Comfort, alteration in: pain (potential) **Etiology** Acute injury	Anxiety Crying Uncooperative behavior Thrashing about Increase in respirations Tachycardia Verbalization of pain or discomfort	A. Maintain an ongoing assessment of patient's complaints and description of pain (helpful in determining internal injuries) B. Assess and document all obvious injuries	A. Attempt to reduce anxiety as described in preceding problem to decrease patient's perception of pain B. Use positioning and immobilization as appropriate: _____ C. Use analgesic and narcotics to decrease pain and anxiety. NOTE: Give only after cleared by physician for patients with internal injuries, those scheduled for impending surgery, and those who are hypotensive D. Reassure and explain all procedures to patient	Patient will verbalize less pain or discomfort

Lead Poisoning: pediatric

NURSING DIAGNOSIS/ PATIENT PROBLEM	DEFINING CHARACTERISTICS	NURSING ORDERS		EXPECTED OUTCOMES
		ASSESSMENT	INTERVENTIONS	
Hematologic status, alteration in **Etiology** Ingestion of substances containing lead	Decreased Hct Decreased Hb Increased lead level >15-40 mg/100 ml History of pica	A. Check vital signs, with BP q.4h. B. Monitor daily laboratory values, i.e., CBC, lead level C. Observe skin for pallor/anemia	A. Administer chelating agents such as dimercaprol (BAL in Oil) or edetate calcium disodium (Ca EDTA) B. Monitor for side effects/complications of these agents (see p. 342: Urinary elimination, alteration in pattern of: potential)	Blood lead level will be decreased
Consciousness, altered levels of: potential **Etiology** Chronic lead ingestion	Falling, clumsiness, loss of coordination Irritability Seizures Drowsiness, coma Peripheral nerve palsy	A. Assess level of consciousness q.4h. or more frequently if any deterioration, increased toxicity, or encephalopathy is noted B. Assess vital signs, especially, respiratory status q.2h.-q.4h. C. Compare present neurologic assessment to previous level from history	A. Document neurologic assessment B. Use seizure precautions and safety measures, i.e., side rails up and padded C. If *actual* alteration in level of consciousness is noted 1. Obtain emergency equipment; place Ambu bag at bedside 2. Report to physician 3. Institute SCP in Ch. 3: Consciousness, alteration in level of 4. Consult neurologic clinical specialist	A. Maximal neurologic functioning will be maintained B. Injury will be prevented

Originated by **Karen Kushibab, RN, BSN**
Resource person: **Michele Knoll-Puzas, RN,C BS**

Continued.

Lead Poisoning: pediatric—cont'd

NURSING DIAGNOSIS/ PATIENT PROBLEM	DEFINING CHARACTERISTICS	NURSING ORDERS		EXPECTED OUTCOMES
		ASSESSMENT	INTERVENTIONS	
Comfort, alteration in Etiology Multiple injections	Irritability Crying Decreased play activities Swelling, inflammation, and redness at the injection site	Observe injection areas for swelling, redness, inflammation, abscess formation	A. Palpate muscle area before preparing site to locate/avoid fibrous tissue from previous injections B. Rotate all injection sites; use large muscle groups (e.g., gluteus, vastas lateralis) C. Obtain order for use of local anesthetic with injections (draw up last in syringe and do not mix) D. Administer BAL and Ca EDTA by deep IM injection as ordered (last may be given IV if ordered to avoid traumatic injections) E. Apply warm soaks to injection sites as needed F. Tailor child's activity to include rest periods G. Inform parents of type of treatment and possible physical and psychologic response from child H. Involve parents in comforting child after injection I. Consult with child life worker to start play therapy with needle	A. Discomfort and complications from injections will be minimized B. Parents will verbalize understanding of treatment and the necessity for injections even though child may be asymptomatic C. Child will be able to express anger over injections
Urinary elimination, alteration in pattern of: potential Etiology Toxic levels of BAL and/or Ca EDTA	Decreased urine output Proteinurea Hematuria	A. Monitor vital signs q.4h. (especially for increased heart rate and change in BP) B. Monitor I & O q.8h. C. Check specific gravity and dipstick for protein/ blood every void	A. Know potential renal side effects of all drugs used before administration B. Monitor laboratory results (urinalysis, electrolytes, BUN, creatinine) C. Do not administer Ca EDTA to dehydrated patients D. Force fluids at least _____ every shift E. Maintain patent IV if child does not have adequate oral intake F. Report any significant change in intake/output ratio or a urine output <30 ml/hour G. Explain to parents the rationale for increased fluid intake (fluids will maintain excretion of the lead via the urine)	A. Complications related to toxic drug levels will be prevented B. Fluid balance and hydration will be adequate C. Parents will understand rationale for nursing measures regarding fluid balance/hydration

Lead Poisoning: pediatric—cont'd

NURSING DIAGNOSIS/ PATIENT PROBLEM	DEFINING CHARACTERISTICS	NURSING ORDERS		EXPECTED OUTCOMES
		ASSESSMENT	INTERVENTIONS	
Knowledge deficit **Etiology** Unfamiliarity with diagnosis, source of exposure Continued exposure with repeated hospitalization	**Subjective** Parents indicate lack of understanding of diagnosis and its cause through their questions or comments **Objective** Repeated episodes of ingestion	A. Assess parental knowledge of lead poisoning and source of ingestion B. Assess child for pica behavior and observe mother/ child interaction C. Screen all siblings for increased lead levels	A. Explain the etiology of lead poisoning to the parents (i.e., pica behavior) B. Explain the environmental factors that contribute to lead poisoning C. Review and emphasize the hazards of lead, signs of lead intoxication, and long-term complications D. Inform parents of the importance of proper medication administration at home E. Initiate referrals with social worker, public health nurse, Board of Health, and other agencies that can assist in overall management F. Emphasize to parents the need for continuous follow-up to monitor lead levels G. Give parents telephone number for local emergency room and regional number for poison control	Parents will verbalize an understanding of A. Lead poisoning/ pica behavior B. Environmental hazard C. Long-term complications D. Medications E. Resource people for follow-up

Near Drowning: pediatric

NURSING DIAGNOSIS/ PATIENT PROBLEM	DEFINING CHARACTERISTICS	NURSING ORDERS		EXPECTED OUTCOMES
		ASSESSMENT	INTERVENTIONS	

Gas exchange, impaired
Etiology
Surfactant elimination
Bronchospasm
Aspiration
Pulmonary edema
	Cyanosis
	Retractions
	Tachypnea
	Stridor
		A. Assess breath sounds every _____ hours
		B. Assess for signs of respiratory distress
		  1. Retractions
		  2. Stridor
		  3. Nasal flaring
		  4. Use of accessory muscles
		C. Assess for signs of hypoxemia
		  1. Alteration in level of consciousness
		  2. Tachycardia
		  3. Deteriorating ABGs
		  4. Tachypnea
		  5. Cyanosis
		  6. Increasing respiratory distress
		D. Assess serial chest x-ray examination reports
			A. Place child in high Fowler's position
			B. Notify physician of any changes in respiratory status
			C. Administer humidified O_2 at rate of _____ L/min
			D. Draw serial ABGs as ordered
			E. Monitor for signs of pneumothorax
			F. Monitor for evidence of increasing pulmonary edema
			G. Suction only as necessary
				Child will maintain adequate oxygenation as evidenced by
				A. ABGs within normal limits
				B. Adequate breath sounds

Cerebral perfusion, alteration in
Etiology
Impaired gas exchange
Increased intracranial pressure
	Deficit in cranial nerve responses
	Altered level of consciousness
	Inappropriate behavior
	Altered pupillary response
		A. Assess neurologic signs q.1h. until stable, then every _____
		B. Monitor for increasing intracranial pressure
		  1. Intracranial pressure monitor readings
		  2. Narrowed pulse pressure and decreased heart and respiratory rates
		  3. Alteration of pupil response
		  4. Alteration in level of consciousness from admission
		C. Assess for seizure activity
		D. Assess environment for degree of stimulation
			A. Elevate head of bed 30 degrees, and maintain midline head and body alignment
			B. Notify physician of any signs of increasing intracranial pressure
			C. Administer seizure medications as ordered
			D. Maintain seizure precautions
			E. Minimize frequency of suctioning
			F. Minimize exposure to noxious stimuli
			G. Sedate child before proceeding with noxious stimuli as ordered (i.e., blood drawing, x-ray examinations, invasive procedures)
			H. Administer medication as ordered per physician to maintain patient in barbiturate coma
			I. Maintain child's temperature at _____ °C
				Alteration in cerebral perfusion will be minimized as evidenced by
				A. Normal BP and heart rate for age
				B. Normal intracranial pressure monitor readings

Originated by **Patricia Hasbrouck-Aschliman, RN, CCRN**
Resource persons: **Janice L. Miller, RN,C MSN**
    Ruth E. Novitt, RN, MSN

Near Drowning: pediatric—cont'd

NURSING DIAGNOSIS/ PATIENT PROBLEM	DEFINING CHARACTERISTICS	NURSING ORDERS		EXPECTED OUTCOMES
		ASSESSMENT	INTERVENTIONS	
Fluid volume, alteration in: excess **Etiology** Aspiration of fresh water Fluid shift from interstitial to intravascular space	Abnormal vital signs Poor peripheral vascular tone leading to edema Arrhythmias	A. Assess serial electrolytes B. Assess pH results for acidosis/alkalosis C. Assess Hct D. Assess urine output q.1h. E. Assess specific gravity every _____ hours F. Assess urine electrolytes, BUN, and creatinine G. Assess weight on admission, then every day once neurologic signs are stable	A. Maintain accurate I & O readings B. Record all laboratory results C. Notify physician of laboratory results and any cardiac arrhythmias D. Administer IV fluids as ordered	Alteration in fluid/electrolyte balance will be minimized as evidenced by A. Normal laboratory values B. Adequate urine output and specific gravity
Injury, potential for: infection **Etiology** Ingestion of contaminated water Multiple invasive procedures Bed rest	Increased temperature Red, swollen sites at areas of invasive procedures Pain or drainage at sites of invasive procedures Rales, rhonchi in lungs Positive cultures	A. Monitor temperature q.2h.-q.4h., then _____ B. Monitor results of cultures and WBC counts C. Assess for increased respiratory distress	A. Monitor vital signs every _____ hours B. Obtain serial CBCs C. Obtain cultures as ordered D. Obtain chest x-ray examinations E. Record color, odor, and amount of sputum and urine F. Maintain sterile technique with all invasive procedures	Risk of infection will be minimized
Skin integrity, impairment of: potential **Etiology** Imposed hypothermia Immobility	Reddened areas of skin Rashes Edema Blisters	A. Assess rectal temperature every _____ hour(s) B. Assess child every _____ hours for pressure areas, redness, blisters, edema, rashes	A. Maintain child's temperature at _____ B. Reposition child q.2h. C. Protect bony prominences with padding D. Apply lotion to pressure areas E. See SCP in Ch. 1: Skin integrity, impairment of: potential	Child's skin will remain intact
Anxiety/fear: family's **Etiology** Near drowning Child's critical status Admission to ICU	Continuous questions Excessive talking Constant demands Inability to come into unit Pacing Withdrawal Inability to leave child's bedside	A. Assess degree of stress B. Assess support systems available C. Assess level of understanding about child's illness and hospitalization D. Assess understanding of prognosis E. Assess degree of involvement in child's care	A. Establish a good rapport B. Encourage expression of feelings about illness and hospitalization C. Reassure and support parents D. Allow for questions, and answer as honestly as possible E. Include family in patient's care F. Include minister and social worker in meetings with family G. Assist family in anticipating mourning H. See SCP in Ch. 1: Anxiety/fear	Family's anxiety/fear will be decreased as evidenced by A. Ability to talk about accident B. Ability to verbalize feelings

CHAPTER FOURTEEN

General Surgery

Child (through age 6) and Surgery

NURSING DIAGNOSIS/ PATIENT PROBLEM	DEFINING CHARACTERISTICS	NURSING ORDERS		EXPECTED OUTCOMES
		ASSESSMENT	INTERVENTIONS	
Anxiety of patient/ parents: potential **Etiology** Diagnosis and/or impending surgery	**Child** Apprehensive Tearful Holds on to/cries out for parents Withdrawn **Parent(s)** Trembling Tearful Multiple questions Lack of questions Verbalizes fear Verbalizes need for more information	A. Assess growth and development of infant/toddler to determine level of understanding and knowledge B. Assess parents' knowledge and understanding of impending surgery	A. Greet infant/toddler and parent(s) in holding area; introduce self and other surgical team members B. Explain purpose, procedures of holding area, waiting room, and recovery room C. Offer emotional support to patient and parent(s) D. Allow parent to remain with child until child is transferred to OR suite	Anxiety will be decreased as evidenced by improved interaction of patient and parents with surgical team
Injury, potential for **Etiology** Improper identification of child	Incorrect/incomplete identification band Discrepancy between identification band and consent Consent differs from OR schedule Child fails to answer to name called	Assess child's identity via parent and chart	A. Verify surgical consent with surgeon's orders, OR schedule, written history, and physical examination B. Verify procedure with parent(s), if available C. Identify child by comparing hospital admission number to child's identification band	Risk of injury because of misidentification will be eliminated
Injury, potential for **Etiology** Risk of falling Improper body alignment Use of equipment	Child thrashing about on cart Reddened, blistered, or bruised skin	A. Assess safety of child's environment B. Assess body alignment C. Assess skin for presence of potential pressure points	A. Remain with child during transport, induction, and extubation B. Request assistance for difficult child C. Maintain correct body alignment D. Pad pressure points E. Secure grounding pad to fleshy part F. Maintain temperature of K-pad between 35.0 and 36.7° C G. Ensure that there is no pooling of fluids beneath child	Risk of falling will be minimized and skin will remain intact
Body temperature, potential alteration in: hypothermia **Etiology** Cool OR suite Length of surgical incision Size of child Exposure of child Cool solutions used	Body temperatures decreased from baseline	Assess child's body temperature throughout procedure	A. Increase OR suite temperature to 22°-26° C (72°-80° F) B. Place K-pad on table, and turn on before child's arrival C. Use overhead warmer for newborns before incision and after completion of surgery D. Provide warm preparation and irrigating solutions E. Prevent pooling of liquids beneath child F. Cover child with warmed blankets when indicated G. Place infant in Isolette, if indicated. Maintain temperature of Isolette at 31.1° C (88° F)	Body temperature will be maintained within normal limits during and after surgery

Originated by **Jacqueline Monaco, RN**
Resource person: **Katie Wyatt, RN**

Child (through age 6) and Surgery—cont'd

NURSING DIAGNOSIS/ PATIENT PROBLEM	DEFINING CHARACTERISTICS	NURSING ORDERS		EXPECTED OUTCOMES
		ASSESSMENT	INTERVENTIONS	
Fluid volume (excess/ deficit) potential **Etiology** Fluid therapy during procedure Loss of body fluids during procedure	**Deficit** Increased heart rate Decreased BP Decreased urine output Increased temperature Decreased turgor **Excess** Increased BP Increased heart rate Increased urine output Distended neck veins Rales Edema	A. Assess I & O throughout procedure B. Monitor vital signs throughout procedure C. Assess laboratory values before beginning of surgery	A. Confer with anesthesiologist regarding abnormal laboratory values B. Check amount of available blood C. Calculate and document amount of blood loss on sponges and laps D. Monitor irrigation amounts	Optimal fluid volume will be maintained
Potential for ineffective airway clearance/ altered breathing pattern/impaired gas exchange **Etiology** Misplaced or dislodged endotracheal tube Laryngeal spasm Aspiration	Increased or decreased respiratory rate Absent or decreased breath sounds after intubation or extubation Wheezing Altered ABGs	A. Assess rate, depth, and quality of respirations before surgical procedure B. Check baseline ABGs if available C. Auscultate breath sounds before procedure	A. Provide holding area nurse with O₂ tank and Ambu bag for intubated child B. Assist anesthesiologist with changing endotracheal connectors C. Verify NPO status preoperatively D. Assist anesthesiologist with induction and extubation E. Monitor respiratory pattern during procedure F. Position child on side during transport to recovery room	Child's airway and oxygenation will be maintained throughout procedure
Injury, potential for: wound infection **Etiology** Altered skin integrity (surgical incision) Invasive technique	Red, painful wound Positive cultures Purulent drainage Increased WBC Unhealed wound	A. Assess maintenance of aseptic technique throughout procedure B. Assess appearance of wound 72 hours postoperatively	A. Correct breaks in aseptic technique B. Check all indicators in pack and trays to ensure sterility C. Observe preparation and draping of child D. Keep OR suite traffic and conversation to minimum	There will be no evidence of wound infection 72 hours postoperatively
Injury, potential for: intraoperative injury **Etiology** Retained foreign body in wound	Pain not related to incision site X-ray film positive for foreign body Incorrect sponge, needle, or instrument count	Count sponges, needles, blades, and instruments used for procedure, according to policy	Document counts at end of procedure	Risk for intraoperative injury will be minimized

Low Anterior Resection: perioperative care

NURSING DIAGNOSIS/ PATIENT PROBLEM	DEFINING CHARACTERISTICS	NURSING ORDERS		EXPECTED OUTCOMES
		ASSESSMENT	INTERVENTIONS	
Anxiety **Etiology** Diagnosis and impending surgery	Appears nervous Trembling Wringing hands Multiple questions Lack of questions	Assess patient's knowledge and understanding of impending surgery	A. Interview patient preoperatively B. Provide information about intraoperative care C. Encourage patient to express self D. Maintain a quiet OR environment E. Support patient before and after intubation	Patient will be relaxed and comfortable before induction, as noted by body position and verbalization
Anxiety: potential **Etiology** Delay in beginning procedure because of inadequate room setup	Verbalization of fear Appears nervous Increased questioning	A. Assess OR suite preparation B. Note changes in patient's anxiety level	A. Reassure patient that the delay is resulting only from equipment unreadiness B. See preceding Interventions column	Patient will verbalize understanding of necessary delay
Injury: potential for **Etiology** Urinary catheterization Lithotomy position	**Urinary catheterization** Cloudy, foul-smelling urine Positive urine cultures Frequency and/or burning on urination **Lithotomy position** Numbness, tingling Pain, swelling of lower extremities	A. Monitor technique used during catheterization B. Assess patient's body alignment	A. Maintain asepsis during catheterization B. Position catheter to avoid disconnection, tension, or backflow of urine C. Apply padded knee-foot crutches before positioning patient D. Pad bony prominences E. Adjust arm boards to avoid hyperextension of arms F. Secure arm to side of patient with drawsheet G. Raise and lower patient's legs simultaneously and slowly during sign checks H. Maintain leg position by use of Ace bandage or Kerlix bandage I. Remind surgical team not to lean on arms or legs during procedure	Patient will exhibit no signs of postoperative urinary tract infection or neurovascular/muscular alteration
Body temperature, alteration in: potential hypothermia/ hyperthermia **Etiology** *Hypothermia* Use of anesthetic agent(s) Cool OR environment Length of incision	**Hypothermia** Decreased baseline temperature Postoperative shivering Decreased BP Abnormal ABGs and electrolytes	Monitor patient's temperature throughout surgical procedure	**Hypothermia** A. Place hyperthermia blanket on OR bed, and turn on before patient's arrival B. Place blankets to be used during and immediately after the procedure in the warmer C. Use warm irrigation solutions D. Consult with anesthesiologist regarding use of humidified air delivered via ventilator and warmed IV solution via blood warmers	Patient will exhibit minimal change in baseline body temperature during procedure

Originated by **Jacqueline Monaco, RN**
Resource person: **Katie Wyatt, RN**

Low Anterior Resection: perioperative care—cont'd

NURSING DIAGNOSIS/ PATIENT PROBLEM	DEFINING CHARACTERISTICS	NURSING ORDERS		EXPECTED OUTCOMES
		ASSESSMENT	INTERVENTIONS	
Hyperthermia Use of anesthetic agent(s) Family history positive for hyperthermic reaction to anesthetic agent(s)	**Hyperthermia** Increased baseline temperature Elevated heart rate Hyperventilation Muscle vesiculation Electrolyte imbalance Arrhythmias		**Hyperthermia** A. Assist anesthesiologist to discontinue anesthesia and administer emergency drugs B. Turn Blanketrol unit to cool C. Remove IVs from blood warmers D. Hang cold IV fluids from refrigerator E. Place ice packs around patient F. Prepare iced gastric lavage G. Send ABGs and electrolytes to laboratory for evaluation H. Assist surgical team to complete procedure as quickly as possible	
Fluid volume deficit: potential **Etiology** Blood loss	Decreased BP Increased pulse Decreased CVP Decreased urine output Decreased Hct	A. Assess vital signs throughout procedure B. Monitor and record accurate I & O during procedure	A. Check availability of blood; have half sent to OR B. Maintain accurate sponge and lap count C. Administer fluids and/or blood products as ordered D. Send appropriate specimens for laboratory evaluation	Blood loss will be minimized
Wound infection, abdominal (potential) **Etiology** Leakage of bowel contents Length of procedure Use of staple guns through rectum	Wound drainage Incisional redness, swelling, pain Fever Positive wound culture Elevated white blood count	A. Assess aseptic technique throughout procedure B. Observe for breaks in technique	A. Correct breaks in technique when observed B. Administer antibiotics as ordered	Abdominal wound will be free of signs of infection 72 hours postoperatively
Injury, potential for **Etiology** Malfunctioning of nondisposable staple gun Misfiring of staple gun Incomplete line of available staples	Gun misfires Anastomosis insecure	A. Assess readiness of equipment B. Assess knowledge of surgical team in use of staple guns C. Assemble and check metal gun D. Check disposable gun against manufacturer's package enclosure E. Observe that tissue donots are whole	A. Obtain all sizes of disposable guns B. Obtain metal staple gun and disposable staples C. Review use of staple gun with surgical team D. Set up and maintain back table separate from main tables E. Assemble sterile procto set F. Assist team with operation of gun G. Remove tissue donots from anvil and cartridge H. Have suture material ready I. Irrigate abdominal table with warm solution to check for leaks in staple line	End to end anastomosis will be completed without intraoperative complications

Routine Perioperative Plan

NURSING DIAGNOSIS/ PATIENT PROBLEM	DEFINING CHARACTERISTICS	NURSING ORDERS		EXPECTED OUTCOMES
		ASSESSMENT	INTERVENTIONS	

Anxiety/fear **Etiology** Impending surgery Perceived threat of pain, disfigurement, death No previous operative experience *or* memories of negative experience	Appears forlorn or upset Weeping Avoids staff Irritability Aggression	A. Observe expressions of feelings: inadequacy, frustration, fear, hostility B. Assess patient's level of comprehension C. Assess degree of insight concerning the surgical procedure D. Identify erroneous perceptions and exaggerated fears	A. Visit patient preoperatively to initiate a nurse/patient interaction (If a preoperative visit was not made on the unit, use the holding area to initiate interactions)
			  1. Demonstrate calmness
			  2. Express warmth and friendliness
			  3. Provide an atmosphere of acceptance
			  4. Touch patient judiciously
			B. Encourage patient to verbalize feelings and concerns
			  1. Listen attentively
			  2. Offer feedback to expressed feelings
			C. Solicit patient's questions
			  1. Refer any questions that you are unable to answer to the surgeon
			  2. Inform the surgeon that patient has questions
			  3. Avoid leaving questions unanswered
			D. If family members are present, encourage their participation
			E. Confer with unit nurse to share findings and exchange relevant data
			F. Explain sensory experiences related to surgery: what the client will see, hear, and feel
			G. Explain what to expect (and why) in the environment: holding area, attire, sounds, temperature, bright lights, roles of personnel
			H. Provide printed material to reinforce instructions
				Patient will verbalize a reduction of fear/anxiety

Anxiety: potential **Etiology** Prolonged OR experience because of Incomplete chart Questionable identification Incomplete/inappropriate consent Inadequate room setup	Looks anxious Asks reasons for delay Verbalizes misconceptions as to reason for delay Questions biopsy results Misinterprets delay as, "It must be something bad"	Review orders and nursing notes to ensure that all preoperative orders have been completed and all supplies and equipment are assembled	A. Confer with anesthesiologist concerning course of action if laboratory values are not acceptable B. Take appropriate action to ensure correct identification C. Verify surgical site with orders and OR schedule D. Obtain all equipment and supplies needed before admission to OR E. Remain with patient, and give emotional support throughout intubation period	A. Patient will verbalize an understanding of cause for delay; anxiety is minimized B. Anxiety will be minimized as the result of a timely diagnosis based on properly handled tissue specimen

Originated by **Katie Wyatt, RN**
Resource person: **Louise Rzeszewski, RN, BSN**

Routine Perioperative Plan—cont'd

NURSING DIAGNOSIS/ PATIENT PROBLEM	DEFINING CHARACTERISTICS	NURSING ORDERS		EXPECTED OUTCOMES
		ASSESSMENT	INTERVENTIONS	
Medical/surgical treatment delays resulting from mishandled, lost, or improperly labeled specimen		Determine need for appropriate labels, containers, solutions before beginning of procedure	F. Gather appropriate specimen containers and preservatives G. Ask the surgeon how the specimen should be labeled H. Check label with scrub person I. Route specimen to appropriate laboratory J. Send all tissue/objects removed from patient's body to surgical pathology department	
Injury, potential for **Etiology** Prolonged surgical position Improper body alignment Improper use of positioning apparatus	Pain unrelated to incision site postoperatively Foot drop, wrist drop	A. Assess ROM before positioning patient B. Assess skin integrity before positioning patient	A. Document ROM and skin integrity B. Maintain anatomically correct body alignment C. Pad all bony prominences that may contact other body or table parts D. Use padded positioning assistive devices as needed: pillows, sandbags, footboard, side arm supports, donuts, tape, and special table attachments E. Ensure that area beneath patient remains dry and free of solutions F. Ensure that operative team does not lean on patient during procedure G. Remain alert to and correct any positional changes during procedure	Potential for injury will be minimized
Injury, potential for: postoperative infection **Etiology** Surgical incision Use of electrical equipment Multiple portals of entry for pathogens	Redness, swelling, pain at incision site Purulent drainage Increase WBC Denuded/discolored area corresponding to size, shape, and site of ground pad or electrodes	A. Identify patients at risk (e.g., from obesity, aging, poor nutritional status) B. Assess condition of all electrical equipment to be used C. Assess incision sites and areas of possible electrical contact before OR discharge and postoperatively 24 to 48 hours D. Monitor housekeeping procedures	A. Become acquainted with and adhere to the principles and practices of aseptic technique B. Ensure proper surgical preparation C. Control traffic in suite D. Use only electrical equipment that has been certified safe E. Inspect all electrical apparatus for intactness and proper operation before each use F. Remove and report any malfunctioning or defective electrical apparatus immediately G. Monitor electrical equipment throughout procedure for: smoking, fraying cords, kinks, disconnections, or breakage	Potential for postoperative infection will be minimized
Injury, potential for **Etiology** Retained needles, sponges, instruments	Postoperative pain, above levels commonly occurring for that procedure Postoperative infection X-ray examination reveals presence of foreign object in patient Discovery of foreign object on subsequent surgery	A. Assess which counts are appropriate for procedure according to policy B. Assess complaints of pain and signs of infection on postoperative visit	A. Count instruments, needles, and sponges with scrub personnel according to procedure B. Never take instruments, needles, or sponges from OR for any reason during a procedure C. Use only x-ray detectable sponges in the wound D. Account for, in their entirety, any broken instrument or needle and any severed sponge E. Initiate x-ray procedure for any incorrect count	Potential for injury resulting from retained needles, sponges, or instruments is eliminated

Same-Day Surgery, Pediatric: preoperative preparation

NURSING DIAGNOSIS/ PATIENT PROBLEM	DEFINING CHARACTERISTICS	NURSING ORDERS		EXPECTED OUTCOMES
		ASSESSMENT	INTERVENTIONS	
Knowledge deficit of parent/child **Etiology** Unfamiliarity with surgical correction	Asking repetitive questions Anxious Silent Hostile Not seeking information concerning procedure or cause of problem Denial of need Noncompliance with earlier therapy Refusal to sign consent	A. Assess level of parents' and child's knowledge 1. Parents' and child's past experience with surgical procedure or illness 2. Child's ideas or feelings concerning problem (age appropriate) B. Assess family system 1. Communication patterns between parents, child, or significant others 2. Past experience with stressful situations and coping mechanisms 3. Resources available to family 4. Interaction between parent and child, both verbal and nonverbal	A. Develop team approach with surgeon, resident, and clinic staff to provide consistent and appropriate teaching for parents and child B. Use appropriate teaching material to describe related concerns, e.g., present condition (or problem), surgical correction C. Encourage parents/child to ask questions D. Discuss the requirements of both the parents and the child preoperatively 1. Child should be kept NPO after midnight 2. Child should be bathed night before surgery 3. Parents should arrive at surgery 2 hours before surgical time 4. Parent/legal guardian should sign surgical consent form E. Describe events that will occur postoperatively (while in recovery room and on discharge) 1. Parents will not be able to see child until child is awake and stable in recovery room 2. Child will most likely have an IV 3. Child will have a dressing on the area of the operation 4. Dressing may have small areas of blood, which is normal 5. The surgeon and the anesthesiologist will evaluate the child before discharge, for evidence that the child has a. Urinated b. Taken oral fluids c. Had no apparent bleeding from surgical site d. Awakened and is responsive to staff	Parents/child will verbalize an understanding of present problem, purpose of surgery, surgical procedures, preoperative/postoperative care and discharge instructions

Originated by **Judith Kenney, RN, MSN**
Resource person: **Ruth E. Novitt, RN, MSN**

Same-Day Surgery, Pediatric: preoperative preparation—cont'd

NURSING DIAGNOSIS/ PATIENT PROBLEM	DEFINING CHARACTERISTICS	NURSING ORDERS		EXPECTED OUTCOMES
		ASSESSMENT	INTERVENTIONS	
			F. Reinforce physician's discharge instructions 　1. Follow-up in surgery clinic within 4 to 7 days 　2. Child may be bathed after 24 hours 　3. Wound closure strips should not be removed from incision 　4. Area may be covered with bandage 　5. Physical activity should be limited as instructed until follow-up in clinic 　6. Diet should be advanced from liquids to soft diet to normal diet	
Injury, potential for: infection at surgical site **Etiology** Surgical interruption of skin and tissue integrity	Incisional site red, tender, swollen Drainage from site Elevation in body temperature Complaints of increased pain or fullness at surgical site	A. Assess parent's knowledge of the signs of infection and routine care for incisions B. Assess parent's previous experiences with caring for infection C. Assess patient's knowledge and skill for taking both oral and rectal temperatures	A. Discuss with parents and illustrate proper techniques for dressing changes done daily B. Discuss importance of reducing child's exposure to those with colds or infections and of trying to avoid crowds C. Review with parents the proper method for taking the child's temperature D. Discuss with parents any unusual events following surgery that may indicate infection 　1. Sudden decrease in appetite 　2. Decrease in activity 　3. Elevation in body temperature 　4. Complaints of pain at operative site or near surrounding area 　5. Drainage from site 　6. Incisional site red, tender, swollen	A. Parents will notify physician or clinic staff if 　1. Surgical site appears red, tender, swollen, or has drainage 　2. Child complains of pain or of not feeling well B. Parents will be able to take child's temperature correctly and to know appropriate parameters
Comfort, alteration in: potential **Etiology** Surgical pain	Parents/child report pain or discomfort Restlessness Increase in irritability Facial expressions of discomfort Relief/distraction behavior e.g., crying, moaning, rocking	A. Assess parents' and child's past experience with pain or discomfort B. Assess parents' and child's past experience with methods used to help alleviate or control pain	A. Discuss with parents and child the different characteristics of pain 　1. Quality (sharp, burning, shooting) 　2. Location 　3. Time of onset 　4. Duration 　5. What seems to help B. Discuss with parents the type of pain frequently experienced and the need for analgesics C. Instruct parents on proper administration of analgesics	Child's pain experience will be minimized

Trauma Patient: perioperative care

NURSING DIAGNOSIS/ PATIENT PROBLEM	DEFINING CHARACTERISTICS	NURSING ORDERS		EXPECTED OUTCOMES
		ASSESSMENT	INTERVENTIONS	
Anxiety Etiology Emergency surgery	Nervous appearance Increased BP Increased heart rate Multiple questions Lack of questions	A. Assess patient's understanding of impending surgery B. Assess anxiety level	A. Introduce self and other team members B. Explain procedures C. Allow verbalization D. Offer emotional support E. Minimize activity in OR	Patient will appear less anxious as evidenced by body posture and verbalization before induction
Injury, potential for Etiology Hurried arrival to OR or undiagnosed patient Emergent nature of impending procedure	Bruises, abrasions Swollen areas Deformed extremities Abnormal laboratory results	Obtain history using AMPLE method (*A*llergies, *M*edications, *P*ast Illness, *L*ast meal, *E*vents prior to injury)	When moving and/or positioning patient, maintain alignment to prevent additional injury	Potential for inadvertent injury will be minimized

Fluid volume deficit: potential
Etiology
Blood loss
	Increased heart rate
	Increased respiratory rate
	Decreased BP
	Decreased urine output
	Decreased CVP
	Cool, clammy, pale skin
	Confusion, disorientation
		A. Assess vital signs every _____
		B. Monitor I & O every _____
		C. Assess amount of obvious blood loss
		D. Note changes in behavior
			A. Document ongoing blood loss by maintaining accurate sponge count
			B. Administer IV therapy as indicated
			  1. Assist in starting additional IVs
			  2. Monitor flow rate of existing peripheral and central IVs
			  3. Keep additional lactated Ringer's and normal saline solutions on hand
			  4. Determine fluid replacement needs based on weight and blood loss
			C. Administer blood component therapy
			  1. Use universal donor blood for critical patients
			  2. Obtain blood from blood bank as soon as available
				Perioperative fluid volume deficit will be prevented/corrected

Body temperature, alteration in: potential
Etiology
Anesthetic agents
Family history positive for hyperthermic episodes
Fluid/blood therapy
Length of incision
Exposure
Shivering
	Increased or decreased body temperature
	Cyanosis
	Cool or warm skin
	Increased heart rate
	Hyperventilation
		Monitor patient's temperature throughout procedure via esophageal or rectal probe	A. Hypothermia
			  1. Place hyperthermia blanket on OR bed and turn on before beginning of procedure
			  2. Consult with anesthesia about humidifers and blood warmers
			  3. Cover patient with warmed blankets
			  4. Warm all irrigation solutions
			B. Hyperthermia
			  1. Assist anesthesiologist in discontinuing anesthetic agents and administering emergency drugs
			  2. Remove or discontinue all warming agents/devices
			  3. Institute cooling measures
				Body temperature will be maintained near baseline throughout surgical procedure

Originated by **Jacqueline Monaco, RN**
Resource person: **Katie Wyatt, RN**

Trauma Patient: perioperative care—cont'd

NURSING DIAGNOSIS/ PATIENT PROBLEM	DEFINING CHARACTERISTICS	NURSING ORDERS		EXPECTED OUTCOMES
		ASSESSMENT	INTERVENTIONS	
Fluid volume, alteration in: excess (potential) **Etiology** Overaggressive fluid therapy	Increased CVP Distended neck veins Increased pulmonary wedge pressure Swollen eyelids Peripheral edema	A. Assess vital signs every _____ B. Monitor I & O	A. Document evidence of fluid volume excess B. Administer diuretic therapy as ordered; monitor results	Fluid volume excess will be avoided both intraoperatively and postoperatively

Potential ineffective airway clearance/impaired gas exchange
 Etiology
 Misplaced and/or dislodged endotracheal tube
 Pneumothorax or hemothorax
 Aspiration before or during intubation attempts
 Chest injuries
	Restlessness, agitation
	 Absent or decreased breath sounds
	 Rales
	 Cyanosis
	 Abnormal ABGs
		A. Assess rate, rhythm, quality of respiration
		 B. Auscultate breath sounds before and following intubation
		 C. Note obvious chest injuries
		 D. Note behavior changes
			A. Prevent/anticipate aspiration
			   1. Verify with patient, nurse from ward or emergency room, and/or physicians the NPO status of patient
			   2. Insert NG tube to empty stomach contents
			   3. Note patient's blood alcohol level
			 B. Assist with intubation
			   1. Encourage awake patient's cooperation
			   2. Assist anesthesiologist with changing endotracheal connections
			   3. Obtain oxygen tank and Ambu bag for any intubated patient
			   4. Obtain sterile tracheostomy tray if indicated
			   5. Send blood gas sample every _____
			 C. Set up chest tube tray if indicated
			 D. Initiate, assist with, and document resuscitative measures as indicated
				Effective airway will be maintained; gas exchange will be maximized

Injury, potential for
 Etiology
 Incompatible blood products
 Massive transfusion
	Increased temperature
	 Chills
	 Hives or rash
	 Hemodynamic instability
	 Hematuria
		A. Monitor vital signs every _____
		 B. Monitor temperature via esophageal probe
		 C. Note chills, rash
		 D. Monitor I & O every _____
		 E. Note color of urine
			A. Administer blood, blood components, according to policy
			   1. Obtain blood as soon as available
			   2. Check identification number of blood and patient identification with _____
			   3. Record all blood components on appropriate record
			 B. Send blood sample to monitor platelet count every _____
			 C. Administer drugs as ordered
				Potential for injury resulting from transfusion therapy will be minimized

Continued.

Trauma Patient: perioperative care—cont'd

NURSING DIAGNOSIS/ PATIENT PROBLEM	DEFINING CHARACTERISTICS	NURSING ORDERS		EXPECTED OUTCOMES
		ASSESSMENT	INTERVENTIONS	
Anxiety: potential **Etiology** Insufficient OR suite preparation Insufficient OR staff because of emergent nature of case Inadequate instrumentation	Patient questions delay in beginning Patient interprets hurried preparation for lack of concern	A. Assess patient's anxiety level B. Assess readiness of OR suite in view of patient's condition/needs	A. See SCP in this chapter: Routine perioperative care B. Explain procedures/room preparation to patient as condition allows	Anxiety will be minimized
Injury, potential for: wound infection **Etiology** Penetrating trauma (stabs, gunshot wound) Unprepared surgical area	Drainage from wound 24-72 hours postoperatively Red wound edges Fever Increased WBC	A. Assess type and location of wound/ injury B. Monitor aseptic technique throughout procedure	A. Provide preparation for skin B. Clean debris from wound C. Administer antibiotics as ordered	Potential for wound infection will be minimized

CHAPTER FIFTEEN

Obstetric/Gynecologic

DISORDERS/CONDITIONS

Abruptio Placentae

NURSING DIAGNOSIS/ PATIENT PROBLEM	DEFINING CHARACTERISTICS	NURSING ORDERS		EXPECTED OUTCOMES
		ASSESSMENT	INTERVENTIONS	
Knowledge deficit **Etiology** New condition	Apparent confusion over events Multiple questions or lack of questions Patient expresses need for more information	A. Assess the patient's knowledge base regarding abruptio placentae B. Assess to what degree the patient's anxiety, level of discomfort, or level of consciousness may compromise or influence the patient's ability to understand explanations	Provide information regarding A. How placenta is effected B. Possible effects on labor C. Possible maternal consequences D. Possible fetal consequences	The patient will verbalize an understanding of abruptio placentae

Anxiety
 Etiology
 Unfamiliarity with nursing procedures
	Extreme restlessness
	 Regressed, childlike behavior
	 Resistance
	 Anger
		Assess the patient's knowledge regarding nursing procedures	A. Include significant others in explanations of all actions taken
			   1. Rationale behind the procedures performed
			   2. Manner in which procedures are to be performed
			   3. Options available
			   4. Expected outcome to be realized from the procedure
			 B. Reinforce the physician's explanations
			 C. Simplify explanations and repeat them when necessary
			 D. Proceed with care measures in a calm and assured fashion
			 E. Institute a teaching plan for the type of delivery anticipated
				The patient will verbalize an understanding of
				 A. Rationale behind the procedures
				 B. Manner in which the procedure is to be performed

Comfort, alteration in
 Etiology
 Manifestations of abruptio placentae
	Extreme tenderness of fundus of the uterus
	 General or localized pain uncharacteristic of uterine contractility
	 Lack of relaxation periods between contractions
		A. Assess the patient's understanding of how the pain associated with abruptio placentae may differ from that associated with the usual contractile pattern
		 B. Solicit the patient's perception of discomfort
		   1. Length of contractions
		   2. Frequency of contractions
		   3. Quality of pain
		   4. Location of pain
			A. Explain how discomfort in abruptio placentae may differ from normal uterine contractions
			 B. Minimize or eliminate when possible the factors that may be contributing to the patient's discomfort
			 C. Provide positive reinforcement and personal contact
			 D. Use nonpharmacologic comfort measures when appropriate
			   1. Position changes
			   2. Relaxation techniques
			   3. Breathing modifications
			   4. Distraction techniques
				A. The patient will verbalize an understanding of why she is experiencing this particular type of discomfort
				 B. The patient will verbalize that the discomfort is experienced less or is more manageable

Originated by **Deidra Gradishar, RNC BA**
Resource person: **Jane Parker, RNC BAN**

Abruptio Placentae—cont'd

NURSING DIAGNOSIS/ PATIENT PROBLEM	DEFINING CHARACTERISTICS	NURSING ORDERS		EXPECTED OUTCOMES
		ASSESSMENT	INTERVENTIONS	
		5. Intensity of pain 6. Presence/absence of periods of uterine relaxation C. Assess other factors which may be contributing to discomfort, i.e., fear, loneliness D. Evaluate the mechanisms that the patient currently uses to manage discomfort E. Observe patient for changes in her coping mechanisms		

Injury, potential for: to the fetus
Etiology
Hemorrhage
	Hyperactive fetus
	Fetal bradycardia
	Presence of late decelerations
	Loss of fetal heart tones
	Increasing baseline fetal heart rate (FHR) with decreasing variability
		Continuously monitor fetal heart tones electronically by either internal or external devices every 15 min. Document
		A. Baseline FHR
		B. Baseline FHR variability
		C. Presence and type of periodic patterns noted
		D. Recovery time for decelerations
			A. If tracing denotes the presence of fetal distress, institute SCP in this chapter: Fetal distress
			B. Notify physician of any change in baseline FHR parameters
			C. Prepare for the delivery of a neonate that may be compromised
			  1. Notify physician
			  2. Check emergency pediatric equipment
			  3. Check transporter
				Injury to fetus will be minimized

Fluid volume deficit: potential
Etiology
Hemorrhage
	Board-like rigidity of uterus
	Increase in fundal height or abdominal girth
	Vaginal bleeding in excess of normal bloody show
	Shock
	Oliguria progressing to anuria
	Dry mucous membranes
		A. Assess and document color and amount of vaginal bleeding
		B. On admission, measure and record abdominal girth. Mark fundal height and document. Assess and record these parameters q. $\frac{1}{2}$h.
		C. Monitor and record BP, pulse, and respirations q. $\frac{1}{2}$h. and more frequently when indicated
		D. Assess Hb, Hct, PT, PTT, and fibrinogen as ordered by the physician
		E. Monitor and document CVP q. $\frac{1}{2}$h. when applicable
			A. Inform physician of changes in vital signs or if
			  1. The uterus fails to relax between contractions
			  2. The patient reports greater abdominal pain
			  3. The patient's level of consciousness or behavior state changes
			  4. Vaginal bleeding increases
			  5. Urinary output decreases
			B. Maintain complete bed rest
			C. Administer parenteral fluids, volume expanders, blood, and blood components, as ordered by the physician
			D. Institute an intensive care flow sheet if applicable
			E. On order of physician, prepare the patient for an emergency cesarean section
				The injurious effects of fluid volume deficit resulting from hemorrhage will be minimized, as evidenced by
				A. Normal laboratory studies
				B. Urine output at least 30 ml/hour
				C. Balanced I & O
				D. Normal skin turgor
				E. Moist mucous membranes
				F. Normal urine specific gravity
				G. Stable vital signs

Abruptio Placentae—cont'd

NURSING DIAGNOSIS/ PATIENT PROBLEM	DEFINING CHARACTERISTICS	NURSING ORDERS		EXPECTED OUTCOMES
		ASSESSMENT	INTERVENTIONS	

		F. Assess and document the patient's level of consciousness q.1h.
		G. Observe condition of skin and mucous membranes, and record observations q.1h.
		H. Ask patient to verbalize change in her perception of abdominal pain
		I. Continuously monitor contractions electronically with either internal or external devices. Observe and document the following q.$\frac{1}{2}$h. or more frequently when indicated
		  1. Frequency and duration of contractions
		  2. Presence/absence of resting tone between contractions
		  3. Strength of contractions if an internal pressure transducer is used		

Bartholinitis: acute

NURSING DIAGNOSIS/ PATIENT PROBLEM	DEFINING CHARACTERISTICS	NURSING ORDERS		EXPECTED OUTCOMES
		ASSESSMENT	INTERVENTIONS	
Comfort, alteration in **Etiology** Infectious process	Reports acute, throbbing pain between labia, especially when walking or sitting Reports burning pain on urination and defecation Unilateral or bilateral swelling over site of infected gland Palpable, tender inguinal nodes Redness and stretching of overlying skin Edema of labia and surrounding tissues Purulent drainage (spontaneous or expressed) from duct Nonverbal physiologic expressions or pain, i.e., crying, grimacing, moaning, tenseness, extreme restlessness or absolute stillness with body in protective position	A. Assess pain experience as reported or manifested by patient 1. Location: identify point of origin 2. Intensity: on a scale of 0-5 with 5 as most severe (mild, discomforting, intense, excruciating) 3. Temporal pattern: time of onset and associated events; trigger zones 4. Description of quality of pain B. Assess the effects of pain C. Assess effectiveness of measures used to relieve pain; include undesired effects	A. Accept and understand pain as patient feels it B. Anticipate need for and provide analgesia C. Compare behavioral responses before and after intervention D. Encourage bed rest to prevent further irritation E. Apply moist heat compresses or provide sitz baths for symptom relief F. Help patient focus her attention on a well-defined set of stimuli G. Observe effects of antibiotic therapy H. Prepare for possible incision and drainage	A. Patient will verbalize relief following comfort measures B. Patient will be able to resume ADL
Self-concept, disturbance in **Etiology** Shame/embarrassment	Describes feelings of shame or embarrassment Uses negative self-labeling Avoids eye contact, turns face away, twists fingers or hands, shuffles feet, has an embarrassed laugh, hand tremors, exaggerated "chin up" posture masking feelings of shame, change in voice and speech pattern	A. Identify situations that could evoke shame or embarrassment B. Identify shame/ embarrassment behaviors (verbal and nonverbal)	A. Maintain and respect individuality of patient. Call her by name B. Maintain privacy; avoid inadvertent exposure during procedures and treatments that focus on the pelvic region C. Encourage patient to acknowledge feelings to another person, i.e., significant other D. Discuss shame/embarrassment situations and behavior	Patient will acknowledge shame/embarrassment and begin to establish dignity and self-respect

Originated by **Fe Corazon R. Mendoza, RN, BSN**
Resource person: **Jackie Suprenant, RN, BSN**

Continued.

Bartholinitis: acute—cont'd

NURSING DIAGNOSIS/ PATIENT PROBLEM	DEFINING CHARACTERISTICS	NURSING ORDERS		EXPECTED OUTCOMES
		ASSESSMENT	INTERVENTIONS	
Knowledge deficit **Etiology** Unfamiliarity with diagnosis	Verbalizes lack of understanding of diagnosis and treatment plan Asks many questions or no questions Noncompliance with prescribed treatment Distrustful and angry	A. Assess patient's perception and knowledge of symptoms, disease process, and specific treatment plans B. Identify learning needs	A. Take time to explain procedures, policies, and hospital routines B. Describe infectious process, treatment involved, and probable outcome C. Provide reliable information about gonorrhea if this organism is involved D. Ask questions and encourage verbalization of concerns E. Provide instruction in daily health and hygiene practices F. Teach patient how to distinguish between normal and abnormal vaginal discharges and how to recognize signs of infection in partner, especially if sexually active G. Stress importance of seeking medical attention as soon as signs of infection develop	A. Patient will be able to describe disease process and explain reasons for treatment B. Patient will be able to describe how infection occurs, spreads, and ways to prevent reinfection C. Patient will be able to describe how daily health practices influence control of infection
Sexual dysfunction **Etiology** Diagnosis Hospitalization and physical condition preclude sexual activity and may interfere with role as sexual partner	Expresses concerns about ability to maintain sexuality Verbalizes concerns about social or sexual habits Verbalizes fear that venereal disease may exist Reports of dyspareunia	Assess patient's perception of her sexuality	A. Initiate discussion and explore issues of potential concern to patient, i.e., extent to which sexual abstinence is possible and alternative methods (e.g., use of condom until symptoms of infection disappear) B. Use careful, tactful questions C. Provide accepting atmosphere and understanding for patient's personal feelings D. Communicate through verbal and nonverbal cues your knowledge and comfort in discussing sexuality E. Assure confidentiality	A. Patient will explore with her partner any adaptations in sexual behavior brought about by her illness and hospitalization B. Patient will begin to relate knowledge of venereal disease prevention to personal relationships

Breast Engorgement in Breast-Feeding Mother

NURSING DIAGNOSIS/ PATIENT PROBLEM	DEFINING CHARACTERISTICS	NURSING ORDERS		EXPECTED OUTCOMES
		ASSESSMENT	INTERVENTIONS	
Comfort, alteration in **Etiology** Breast engorgement	Breasts distended and hard Mother reports breast discomfort	A. Assess breasts daily for signs/symptoms of engorgement B. Identify factors contributing to engorgement	A. Teach mother the following preventive measures, as appropriate 1. Give the baby early, frequent feedings from birth 2. Do not skip or delay feedings 3. Do not restrict sucking time. Allow at least 5 minutes on each side, right from the first feeding 4. Avoid sugar water supplements B. If engorgement develops, teach mother the following treatment measures, as appropriate 1. Encourage short, frequent feedings (every $1\frac{1}{2}$ to 3 hours) that continue through the day and night. Baby should nurse on both breasts at each feeding 2. Apply moist heat for fifteen minutes before each feeding. Follow this with breast massage all around the breast, moving from the outer margin towards the nipple 3. If necessary, soften the areola before each nursing by expressing a little milk 4. Use the electric breast pump following feeding if the baby nursed lazily, slept, or took from one side only 5. Avoid nipple shields 6. Take pain medication (per physician's order) if needed C. Explain cause of engorgement and that condition is temporary D. Provide emotional support. Reassure mother that she can continue breast-feeding	A. Mother will demonstrate proper preventive measures B. If engorgement develops, mother will use appropriate treatment measures

Originated by **Jackie Suprenant, RN, BSN**

Fetal Distress

NURSING DIAGNOSIS/ PATIENT PROBLEM	DEFINING CHARACTERISTICS	NURSING ORDERS		EXPECTED OUTCOMES
		ASSESSMENT	INTERVENTIONS	
Knowledge deficit **Etiology** Unfamiliarity with condition of fetal distress	Apparent confusion over events Multiple questions Lack of questions Expressed need for more information	A. Assess patient's understanding of fetal distress B. Assess to what degree anxiety or the level of discomfort may compromise or influence the patient's ability to understand explanations	A. Provide information regarding 1. Known or possible causes of fetal distress 2. Misconceptions B. Include significant other when possible	The patient will verbalize an understanding of fetal distress
Injury, potential for: to the fetus **Etiology** Uteroplacental insufficiency Cord compression or occlusion Maternal hypotension as a result of major regional anesthesia	Fetal bradycardia Fetal tachycardia Passage of meconium-stained amniotic fluid in the absence of breech presentation Baseline variability <5 BPM Late decelerations Variable decelerations that last more than 1 minute or fall to < 60 BPM. Any variable deceleration with a late component	A. Assess and record continuous electronic fetal monitoring either by internal or external devices every 15 min 1. Baseline fetal heart rate 2. Baseline variability 3. Presence and type of periodic patterns noted, i.e., variables, lates, sinusoidal B. Observe contraction pattern for evidence of hyperstimulation, which may lead to fetal compromise 1. Nonachievement of baseline tone 2. High amplitude 3. Increased frequency 4. Increased duration	A. Notify physician of any changes in baseline fetal heart parameters B. Maintain patient in the left or right lateral position C. Administer O_2 per rebreather mask at _____ L/min D. Increase nonoxytocin IV infusion E. Discontinue oxytocin infusion if in use and notify physician F. Prepare for delivery of potentially compromised fetus G. Evaluate patient for possible prolasped cord 1. Check introitus for cord 2. If cord is present, palpate for pulsation 3. Place patient in knee chest position or elevate presenting part 4. Call for help H. Reassure patient with calm manner I. Begin to prepare patient for the type of delivery anticipated	Injury to fetus will be minimized

Originated by **Paulette N. Kelleher, RN,C BSN**
Resource person: **Jane Parker, RNC BAN**

Fetal Distress—cont'd

NURSING DIAGNOSIS/ PATIENT PROBLEM	DEFINING CHARACTERISTICS	NURSING ORDERS		EXPECTED OUTCOMES
		ASSESSMENT	INTERVENTIONS	
Knowledge deficit **Etiology** Unfamiliarity with nursing procedures	Noncompliance Repetitive questioning Inattentive Angry Demanding	A. Assess patient's knowledge regarding nursing procedures B. Assess patient's knowledge of hospital environment	A. Explain all actions taken (include significant other if possible) 1. Rationale behind the procedure performed 2. Manner in which procedures are to be performed 3. Available options 4. Expected outcome to be realized from the procedure B. Simplify explanations and repeat them when necessary	The patient will verbalize a basic understanding of A. The manner in which the procedure is to be performed B. Rationale behind the procedure C. Expected outcomes
Anxiety/fear **Etiology** Uncertain outcome for infant	Trembling Tearfulness Restlessness Depression Expressed fear Expressed sense of impending doom	A. Assess patient's perception of current status of infant B. Observe for nonverbal signs of fear/anxiety	A. Provide patient with realistic, factual information regarding the status of her infant B. Provide information regarding neonatal intensive care unit. Reassure patient that emergency equipment and appropriate personnel are available C. Encourage patient to verbalize concerns **Post delivery** A. Allow parents to see infant before transport to nursery B. Allow mother to stroke infant, if possible C. Give realistic information on possible outcome for neonate	Patient will be provided with the opportunity to verbalize fears and concerns regarding infant

Fourth Stage of Labor

NURSING DIAGNOSIS/ PATIENT PROBLEM	DEFINING CHARACTERISTICS	NURSING ORDERS		EXPECTED OUTCOMES
		ASSESSMENT	INTERVENTIONS	
Knowledge deficit **Etiology** Unfamiliarity with purpose of constant care environment and procedures	Apparent confusion over events Multiple questions Lack of questions Expressed need for more information	Assess patient's understanding of the physical facilities, policies, procedures and purpose of the Constant Care Unit (CCU)	Orient patient to CCU, explaining policies, procedures, and purpose	Patient will verbalize an understanding of the physical facilities, policies, and procedures related to the fourth stage of labor

Comfort, alteration in
 Etiology
 Involution of uterus
 Episiotomy
	Verbalizing discomfort
	 Moaning
	 Restlessness
		A. Assess patient's perception of discomfort
		   1. Location
		   2. Intensity
		   3. Quality
		 B. Determine other factors that may contribute to discomfort
		   1. Hunger
		   2. Fatigue
		   3. Distended bladder
		 C. Assess condition of perineum every 15 min for 1 hour, then every $\frac{1}{2}$ hour for
		   1. Swelling
		   2. Presence of hematoma
		   3. Episiotomy
		 D. Palpate bladder for distention every 15 min for 1 hour, then every $\frac{1}{2}$ hour
			A. Apply ice pack to perineum (as ordered)
			 B. Explain reason for afterbirth pains when appropriate
			 C. Encourage patient to void. Catheterize patient if necessary, per physician's order
			 D. Administer pain medication as ordered, noting effect
			 E. Notify physician of presence of hematoma
			 F. Minimize other factors that may be contributing to discomfort
				Patient will verbalize that the discomfort experienced is lessened or more manageable

Originated by **Imelda Fahy, RN**
Resource person: **Jane Parker, RNC BAN**

Fourth Stage of Labor—cont'd

NURSING DIAGNOSIS/ PATIENT PROBLEM	DEFINING CHARACTERISTICS	NURSING ORDERS		EXPECTED OUTCOMES
		ASSESSMENT	INTERVENTIONS	
Fluid volume deficit: potential **Etiology** Hemorrhage (>500 ml)	Hypotension Tachycardia Dyspnea Pallor Syncope	A. Assess uterine status every _____ 1. Tone 2. Fundal height 3. Position B. Assess amount and color of vaginal bleeding and the presence of clots C. Palpate and percuss urinary bladder for distention D. Assess condition of perineum 1. Swelling 2. Ecchymosis 3. Episiotomy E. Assess possibility of bleeding from cervical, vaginal, or perineal tears (firm uterus but continued oozing of bright red blood) F. Monitor and record BP, pulse, and respiration every _____ G. Observe strict peripad count H. Assess results of Hb and Hct when ordered I. Review delivery notes for documentation of sponge count	A. Report deviations from baseline parameters to physician B. See SCP in this chapter: Hemorrhage following vaginal delivery	A. Injury to patient will be minimized B. Optimal fluid volume will be maintained
Self-concept, disturbance in **Etiology** Birthing experience	Withdrawal Expressed disappointment Self-deprecating statements Overt expressions of guilt or blame	A. Assess mother's feelings regarding her role in the birth process B. Assess to what degree the husband or significant other influenced her feelings	A. Encourage mother to verbalize feelings B. Include significant other in discussions as appropriate C. Encourage the presence of the significant other as appropriate D. Explain to mother the normalcy of her feelings/behavior	Mother will be provided the opportunity to verbalize concerns

Genital Herpes: postpartum care

NURSING DIAGNOSIS/ PATIENT PROBLEM	DEFINING CHARACTERISTICS	NURSING ORDERS		EXPECTED OUTCOMES
		ASSESSMENT	INTERVENTIONS	

Tissue integrity, alteration in
Etiology
Herpes infection
	First stage (average duration: 6 days for primary lesion, 2 days for secondary lesion)
	Tender inguinal nodes
	Formation of extremely tender and painful vesicles
	Fever, malaise, dysuria
	
	Second stage (average duration: 6 days)
	Broken vesicles; formation of a wet ulcer (shallow crater with yellow border)
	Severe pain
	
	Third or final stage (average duration: 8 days)
	Formation of dry crusts
	Reepithelialization
		A. Assess condition of herpes lesion and determine whether it is primary or secondary
		B. In patients with herpes history without evidence of infection, be alert to presence of prodromal symptoms, including
		  1. Itching
		  2. Tingling
		  3. Pain
		  4. Increased sensitivity at infection site (secondary or recurrent genital herpes infection usually begins with a prodromal period lasting 1-2 days)
		C. Assess for signs of systemic illness: fever, headache, malaise, chills, enlarged inguinal nodes, or general adenopathy
			A. Instruct mother on the following infection control guidelines
			  1. Follow good handwashing technique after voiding and before handling infant
			  2. Wear fresh cover gown when handling infant
			  3. Restrict tub baths unless in private room
			  4. Keep lesion dry to decrease the period of viral shedding
			  5. Use good personal hygiene measures, including daily shower and perineal care after each void
			  6. Avoid hand contact with the lesion
			B. Administer acyclovir as ordered (this is not a cure but may increase healing and decrease viral shedding time)
			C. Wear gloves or use no-touch technique when handling soiled dressing or pads
				Mother will correctly demonstrate infection control guidelines

Comfort, alteration in **Etiology** Herpes lesion	Facial mask of pain Restlessness, irritability Alteration in sleep pattern Patient soliciting techniques to relieve pain	Assess pain characteristics A. Quality: sharp, burning B. Severity (scale 1-10, 10 most severe) C. Onset: gradual or sudden D. Duration: intermittent or continuous E. Precipitating factors or relieving factors	A. Administer topical anesthetics (lidocaine jelly) or mild analgesics as ordered. Evaluate effectiveness B. Encourage sitz baths morning and evening for 15 to 20 min C. Instruct patient to dry the infected area with a blow dryer on low heat setting. Corn starch is also effective for this purpose D. Advise patient to wear loose or well-ventilated clothing	Pain will be minimized or relieved

Originated by **Monalisa S. Bron, RN, BSN**
Resource person: **Jackie Suprenant, RN, BSN**

Genital Herpes: postpartum care—cont'd

NURSING DIAGNOSIS/ PATIENT PROBLEM	DEFINING CHARACTERISTICS	NURSING ORDERS		EXPECTED OUTCOMES
		ASSESSMENT	INTERVENTIONS	
Urinary elimination, alteration in patterns: retention **Etiology** Dysuria, edema, and voiding hesitancy	Absence of urinary output for more than 8 hours Suprapubic fullness/ tenderness Decrease in volume and force of the urinary stream Sensation of incomplete bladder emptying	A. Palpate for bladder distention or elevated deviated fundus B. Assess for tendency to hold urine because of discomfort associated with voiding C. Assess for signs/ symptoms of urinary tract infection	A. Encourage voiding while sitting in sitz bath to decrease dysuria B. Advise the use of peri-bottle to stimulate urination with less pain C. Encourage frequent voiding to ensure complete emptying of bladder and decrease the incidence of urinary tract infection D. Push fluids (2000-3000 ml/day)	Patient will demonstrate ability to void freely and with minimal discomfort
Knowledge deficit **Etiology** New condition	Lack of questions Apparent confusion over events Expressed need for more information	Assess patient's knowledge base regarding genital herpes	A. Provide information on herpes, based on assessment data. Dispel any myths patient may have B. Provide postdischarge health teaching to patient and her partner: sexual abstinence when symptoms are present and the use of a condom when there are no symptoms	Patient will verbalize understanding of the nature of herpes and the appropriate precautionary measures
Self-concept, disturbance in **Etiology** Herpes	Refusal to make eye contact Overt expression of guilt and blame Self-maligning statements	A. Assess patient's perception of self B. Identify patient's level of anxiety C. Assess patient's normal coping pattern	A. Display confident, calm manner and tolerant, understanding attitude B. Encourage ventilation of feelings and concern. Include significant other whenever possible. Listen carefully. Give an unhurried, attentive appearance C. Concentrate on patient's strengths to help alleviate anxiety and poor self-image associated with the disease D. Consult with psychiatric liaison or social worker as needed E. Encourage getting in touch with support groups such as HELP, after discharge	A. Patient will recognize self-maligning statements B. Patient will begin to verbalize positive expressions of self-worth

Hyperemesis Gravidarum

NURSING DIAGNOSIS/ PATIENT PROBLEM	DEFINING CHARACTERISTICS	NURSING ORDERS		EXPECTED OUTCOMES
		ASSESSMENT	INTERVENTIONS	

Fluid volume deficit: potential
Etiology
Hyperemesis
	Oliguria
	Concentrated urine
	Presence of acetone in urine
	Hypotension
	Syncope
	Dry mucous membranes
	General malaise
		A. Obtain subjective data base
		  1. Onset of emesis
		  2. Frequency of emesis
		  3. Duration of emesis
		  4. Amount of emesis
		  5. Approximate food and fluid intake
		  6. Precipitating factors (i.e., smoking, aroma of certain foods)
		  7. Past history of "morning sickness"
		  8. Past use of nonmedical modalities
		    a. Carbonated beverage (7-Up)
		    b. Crackers
		    c. Toast
		    d. Position changes
		B. Assess emesis for
		  1. Color
		  2. Consistency
		  3. Presence of blood
		C. Observe episodes of vomiting, and document findings. Note
			A. Administer antiemetic as ordered by physician
			B. Document any changes after antiemetic is given
			C. Administer fluids via IV every ____ as ordered by physician
			D. See SCP in Ch. 1: Fluid volume deficit (as needed)
				Fluid volume deficit will be minimized as evidenced by Normal laboratory results
				Urine output of ≥30 ml/hour
				Sp. gr. of 1.010-1.030
				Moist mucous membranes

Originated by **Yvette Roberts, RN,C BSN MHA**
Resource person: **Jane Parker, RNC, BAN**

Hyperemesis Gravidarum—cont'd

NURSING DIAGNOSIS/ PATIENT PROBLEM	DEFINING CHARACTERISTICS	NURSING ORDERS		EXPECTED OUTCOMES
		ASSESSMENT	INTERVENTIONS	
		1. Time of day 2. Amount of emesis 3. Color of emesis 4. Precipitating factors D. Check skin for evidence of ecchymosis or petechiae E. Check condition of skin for signs of dehydration F. Monitor and record the amount of urine every ___ G. Document specific gravity every ___ H. Observe and document the presence of acetone in urine I. Monitor electrolyte results J. Monitor and record BP, pulse, respirations, temperature every ___ K. Monitor laboratory results for changes in Hct L. Observe and document patient's tolerance of oral fluids		
Knowledge deficit **Etiology** Unfamiliarity with condition	Apparent confusion over events Multiple questions or lack of questions Patient expresses a need for more information	A. Assess the patient's knowledge base regarding hyperemesis B. Assess to what degree the patient's anxiety and level of discomfort may compromise or influence her ability to understand explanations	Provide information regarding A. Physiology of hyperemesis B. Possible effects of hyperemesis on pregnancy and fetus	Patient will verbalize an understanding of hyperemesis

Continued.

Hyperemesis Gravidarum—cont'd

NURSING DIAGNOSIS/ PATIENT PROBLEM	DEFINING CHARACTERISTICS	NURSING ORDERS		EXPECTED OUTCOMES
		ASSESSMENT	INTERVENTIONS	
Knowledge deficit **Etiology** Unfamiliar personnel, procedures New environment	Inability to concentrate Inability to retain information given Inability to communicate	A. Assess patient's level of concentration B. Assess patient's knowledge regarding nursing procedures C. Assess patient's knowledge of unfamiliar surroundings	A. Encourage patient to verbalize concerns B. Provide an environment that is conducive to communication C. Orient to environment and personnel D. Explain rationale for all tests and procedures, including the manner in which they will be done E. Include significant other when possible	Patient will verbalize an understanding of A. Rationale behind procedures B. Manner in which procedures are done

Comfort, alteration in
Etiology
Episodes of emesis
	Complaints of
	  Sore throat
	  Sour taste in mouth
	  Soreness in abdominal muscles
	  Generalized weakness
	  Ptyalism
		A. Elicit patient's perception of discomfort related to emesis
		B. Determine contributing factors that may alter patient's comfort
			A. Use nonpharmacologic measures when appropriate
			  1. Positioning
			  2. Muscular relaxation techniques
			  3. Breathing techniques
			  4. Distraction techniques
			  5. Application of cold towel to forehead, neck
			  6. Mouth care
			  7. Supportive contact
			B. Eliminate or minimize other factors that may be contributing to discomfort
				Patient will verbalize that discomfort is decreased or is more manageable

Self-concept, disturbance in **Etiology** Interruption in normal pregnancy course	Minimal eye contact Self-deprecating statements Overt expressions of guilt or blame Anger	A. Assess patient's perception of self B. Assess degree to which patient assumes responsibility for condition C. Assess and evaluate the availability of support systems	A. Assist patient to express her feelings B. Assist patient to verbalize feelings of guilt and blame C. Maintain an open nonjudgmental approach to communication D. Respect and support patient's choice to be introspective at various times E. Include significant other in discussions F. Provide positive feedback to the patient for seeking early intervention G. Provide suggestions and methodologies for resumption of ADL	A. Patient acknowledges self-maligning statements and behavior B. Patient begins to verbalize positive expressions of continued self-worth

Hypertension: pregnancy-induced

NURSING DIAGNOSIS/ PATIENT PROBLEM	DEFINING CHARACTERISTICS	NURSING ORDERS		EXPECTED OUTCOMES
		ASSESSMENT	INTERVENTIONS	
Knowledge deficit **Etiology** Unfamiliarity with condition	Noncompliance Apparent confusion over events Multiple questions Lack of questions Expressed need for more information	A. Assess patient's understanding of pregnancy-induced hypertension B. Assess degree to which signs and symptoms interfere with patient's ability to understand	A. Provide information regarding pregnancy-induced hypertension 1. Causes 2. Signs and symptoms 3. Possible treatment B. Include significant other in information session C. Reinforce physician's information and explanations	The patient will verbalize an understanding of A. Causes B. Treatment C. Procedure
Cardiovascular instability **Etiology** Pregnancy-induced hypertension	Rapid weight gain: 2 pounds/week—suspicious; 3 pounds/week—alarming Edema, especially face (periorbital), hands, fingers, pitting edema in legs Proteinuria: > +1 Oliguria: <30 ml/ hour Epigastric pain Hypertension: a rise of 30 mm Hg or more systolic, 15 mm Hg diastolic from normal BP (refer to prenatal record) *or* >140/90	Assess patient's physical status, document baseline findings, and report significant changes every ____ min Pulse rate Respiratory rate BP: manual or arterial line CVP, pulmonary artery pressure, pulmonary capillary wedge pressure (every ____) Skin color, temperature, moisture Fluid balance (I & O) Pain (epigastric, contractions) Edema Laboratory values (electrolytes, BUN, creatinine, uric acid, SGOT, magnesium sulfate level, Ca level, PT, PTT, fibrinogen, CBC with platelets)	A. Administer appropriate medication as ordered by physician B. Report and record any side effects and/or toxicity C. Maintain fluid intake at ____ ml/hour D. Maintain urinary output >____ ml/hour E. Position patient in left lateral position F. If there is a decreased cardiac output, see SCP in Ch. 1: Cardiac output, alteration in: decreased	The patient will maintain cardiovascular stability as evidenced by Pulse _____ Respiration _____ BP: Systolic _____ Diastolic _____ CVP _____ Pulmonary artery pressure _____ Pulmonary capillary wedge pressure _____ Urine output >____ ml/hour

Originated by **Paulette N. Kelleher, RN,C BSN**
Resource person: **Jane Parker, RNC BAN**

Continued.

Hypertension: pregnancy-induced—cont'd

NURSING DIAGNOSIS/ PATIENT PROBLEM	DEFINING CHARACTERISTICS	NURSING ORDERS		EXPECTED OUTCOMES
		ASSESSMENT	INTERVENTIONS	

Injury, potential for: seizures
 Etiology
 CNS irritability
	CNS irritability
	 Deep tendon reflexes: +3 to +4
	 Clonus may be present
	 Nervousness
	 Headache: frontal-occipital
	 Vertigo
	 Changes in level of consciousness
	 Visual disturbances
	 Epigastric pain
		Assess patient's neurologic status. Report and record changes from baseline information every ____ minutes/hour
		 A. Level of consciousness
		 B. Deep tendon reflexes
		 C. Clonus (beats)
		 D. Vital signs
			A. Place patient in quiet, nonstimulating environment and subdued lighting
			 B. Maintain bed rest
			 C. Observe seizure precautions
			   1. Ensure an adequate airway; keep airway at bedside
			   2. Protect patient from injury
			     a. Padded side rails
			     b. Side rails on bed pulled up
			     c. Bed in low position
			   3. Have emergency equipment available
			     a. Suction
			     b. Crash cart
			     c. Cardiac monitor/defibrillator
			     d. Emergency drug box
			 F. Administer medications as ordered by physician, and observe for untoward effects
			   1. Magnesium sulfate: respiratory depression, depressed deep tendon reflexes
			   2. Calcium gluconate: nausea and vomiting, cardiac arrest, tissue necrosis
			   3. Valium: respiratory depression, hypotension, possible cardiac arrest
			 G. Have call light within reach
				Potential for seizure activity will be minimized as evidenced by
				 A. Deep tendon reflexes: 1+ to 2+
				 B. Lack of clonus
				 C. Full consciousness: awake, alert, and oriented

Injury, potential for: to fetus **Etiology** Decreased placental perfusion	Fetal bradycardia Presence of late decelerations Decreased baseline variability: <5 beats/min Loss of fetal heart tones Meconium-stained amniotic fluid	Continuously monitor fetal heart rate by electronic means; assess and record every ____ A. Baseline fetal heart rate B. Baseline variability C. Presence and type of periodic patterns noted	A. Notify physician of any changes in baseline fetal heart parameters B. Maintain patient in the left lateral position C. Administer O_2 via rebreather mask at ____ L/min D. Prepare for delivery of potentially compromised fetus E. Institute care plan for type of delivery anticipated	Injury to fetus will be minimized

Knowledge deficit
 Etiology
 Unfamiliarity with nursing procedures
	Noncompliance
	 Somatic complaints
	 Demanding
	 Repetitious questions
	 Inattentive
		A. Assess the patient's knowledge regarding nursing procedures
		 B. Assess patient's knowledge of hospital environment
			A. Explain the following (include significant other when possible)
			   1. Rationale behind the procedure performed
			   2. Manner in which procedures are to be performed
			   3. Available options
			   4. Expected outcomes to be realized from the procedures
			 B. Reinforce the physician's explanations
			 C. Explain at patient's present level of understanding
			 D. Proceed with nursing care in a calm and assured manner
			 E. Involve patient in her own care when appropriate
				The patient will verbalize basic understanding of
				 A. The manner in which the procedure is to be performed
				 B. Rationale behind the procedures
				 C. Expected outcomes

Insulin-Dependent Diabetes: intrapartum care

NURSING DIAGNOSIS/ PATIENT PROBLEM	DEFINING CHARACTERISTICS	NURSING ORDERS		EXPECTED OUTCOMES
		ASSESSMENT	INTERVENTIONS	
Knowledge deficit **Etiology** Changes in diabetic regimen during labor	Multiple questions Lack of questions Apparent confusion over events Expressed need for more information	A. Assess patient's knowledge about diabetic management during labor B. Assess to what degree anxiety or discomfort may influence patient's ability to understand explanations C. Assess educational background and maturational stage	Provide explanation about diabetic care during labor A. Nothing by mouth B. Changes in insulin requirements (because of stress of labor and NPO) C. Changes in method of insulin administration D. More frequent blood glucose determinations	Patient will verbalize an understanding of changes in diabetic regimen
Injury, potential for: to mother **Etiology** Hypoglycemia/hyperglycemia	**Hypoglycemia** Blood glucose level < _____ Cold clammy skin Perspiration Weakness Tremors Irritability **Hyperglycemia** Blood glucose level > _____ Plasma glycosuria and ketonuria Acidosis	A. Assess patient's knowledge of signs of hypoglycemia, and ascertain which generally occur during an episode B. Assess urine sugar/acetone every _____ C. Assess blood glucose level per physician's order every _____ via 1. Chemstrip 2. Laboratory determination of blood glucose 3. Glucose meter (patient/RN) D. Assess for symptoms of hypoglycemia E. Monitor I & O every _____ F. Monitor temperature, pulse, respirations, BP every _____ G. Observe for increasing physical/ emotional stress of labor	A. Administer insulin per physician's order B. Administer IV fluids at _____ ml/hour per physician's order C. Notify physician of changes in baseline parameters D. Compare Chemstrip fingersticks with laboratory blood glucose determinations E. Maintain flow sheet of Chemstrips for comparison F. Instruct patient to notify staff of early symptoms of hypoglycemia	Injury to the mother will be minimized

Originated by **Sarah Cohen, RN**
Resource person: **Jane Parker, RNC BAN**
      Christina L. Valenta, RN, BS

Continued.

Insulin-Dependent Diabetes: intrapartum care—cont'd

NURSING DIAGNOSIS/ PATIENT PROBLEM	DEFINING CHARACTERISTICS	NURSING ORDERS		EXPECTED OUTCOMES
		ASSESSMENT	INTERVENTIONS	
Injury, potential for: to the fetus **Etiology** Macrosomia Uteroplacental insufficiency	**Macrosomia** Early decelerations in beginning first stage of labor Failure of descent of fetal head **Uteroplacental insufficiency** Late decelerations Decreased baseline variability (<5) Meconium-stained amniotic fluid	A. Continuously monitor fetal heart rate by electronic means; assess and record every _____ 1. Baseline fetal heart rate 2. Baseline variability 3. Presence of periodic patterns B. Review antepartum records for 1. Gestational date/size confirmation 2. Studies of fetal well-being	A. Notify physician of any changes in fetal heart rate parameters B. For late decelerations 1. Turn mother to lateral recumbent position 2. Administer O_2 per rebreather mask at _____ L/min C. See SCP in this chapter: Fetal distress D. Prepare for delivery of a potentially compromised infant	Injury to the fetus will be minimized.
Anxiety/fear **Etiology** Uncertain outcome for infant/self	Restlessness Crying Trembling Expressed fear	A. Assess patient's perception of current status of herself and fetus B. Observe for non-verbal signs of fear/anxiety C. Assess to what degree coping with the stress of a chronic illness may be influencing fear/anxiety D. Assess support systems currently available to patient	A. Provide patient with realistic, factual information regarding current status of herself and infant (include significant other when possible) B. Institute a teaching plan to prepare patient for 1. Serial induction 2. Vaginal delivery 3. Cesarean section as appropriate C. Keep patient informed regarding 1. Labor status 2. Fetal status 3. Diabetic status D. Provide information regarding neonate ICU as appropriate E. If necessary, provide information regarding special needs for infant to be under observation 1. Prematurity 2. Hypoglycemia 3. Hyperbilirubinemia F. Encourage patient to verbalize concerns G. Promote maternal/infant bonding when possible (see SCP in this chapter: Maternal/infant bonding)	Patient will be provided with the opportunity to verbalize fears, anxiety, concerns about: A. Herself B. Unborn baby C. Neonate

Insulin-Dependent Diabetes: intrapartum care—cont'd

NURSING DIAGNOSIS/ PATIENT PROBLEM	DEFINING CHARACTERISTICS	NURSING ORDERS		EXPECTED OUTCOMES
		ASSESSMENT	INTERVENTIONS	
Injury, potential for: to mother **Etiology** Microvascular/macro-vascular complications of diabetes in pregnancy	**Pregnancy-induced hypertension** Hypertension (rise of 30 mm Hg systolic; 15 mm Hg diastolic) Complaint of headache, visual disturbances, epigastric pain Hyperreflexia **Acute renal failure** Hypertension Oliguria progressing to anuria Hematuria Edema	A. Assess BP and pulse every _____ B. Measure I & O every _____ C. Observe for subjective symptoms of preeclampsia every _____ D. Assess deep tendon reflexes every _____ E. Monitor urine for protein every void or every _____ F. Observe patient for edema G. See previous SCP: Pregnancy-induced hypertension	A. Report changes in baseline parameters to physician immediately B. Maintain intake at _____ ml/hour and output at _____ ml/hour C. See previous SCP: Pregnancy-induced hypertension	Potential for injury will be minimized

Infertility as Emotional Crisis

NURSING DIAGNOSIS/ PATIENT PROBLEM	DEFINING CHARACTERISTICS	NURSING ORDERS		EXPECTED OUTCOMES
		ASSESSMENT	INTERVENTIONS	

Coping, ineffective
Etiology
Childlessness
	Verbalization of inability to cope or inability to ask for help
	Inability to meet normal role expectations
	Inability to meet basic needs
	Inability to problem-solve
	Alteration in societal participation
		A. Note expressed feelings of hopelessness, helplessness, and powerlessness
		B. Observe for inappropriate expression of anger/hostility and/or loss of control
		C. Note weeping, irritability, and expressed feelings of incompetence
		D. Assess noncompliant or other problematic behavior
		E. Assess ability to plan and make decisions
		F. Note statements of work, social, or family withdrawal or incompetent performance
			A. Provide emotional support
			  1. Create environment conducive to expression of feelings
			  2. Provide frequent patient contact in an unhurried manner
			  3. Avoid excessive focus on physical tasks
			  4. Emphasize the person's value as an individual
			  5. Offer feedback of the patient's feelings
			  6. Provide interest, concern, and understanding
			B. Encourage the use of past adaptive coping mechanisms
			C. Provide attention to the concerns of each individual (husband/wife)
			D. Attempt to clarify feelings/behavior
			E. Provide supportive silence to permit the person to continue a response when description is difficult
				A. The couple will use adaptable defense mechanisms to cope with stress
				B. The couple will demonstrate less hostility and more cooperation as evidenced by
				  1. Good communication with the staff
				  2. A calm, reassured, unthreatened approach to diagnostic testing and treatments
				  3. Proper use of referrals

Originated by **Anita C. Houtsma, RN**
Resource person: **Helen Snow-Jackson, RN, BSN, TNS, CEN**

Continued.

Infertility as Emotional Crisis—cont'd

NURSING DIAGNOSIS/ PATIENT PROBLEM	DEFINING CHARACTERISTICS	NURSING ORDERS		EXPECTED OUTCOMES
		ASSESSMENT	INTERVENTIONS	
		G. Observe for evidence of decreased self-esteem 1. Poor hygiene 2. Poor job performance 3. Poor sexual performance 4. Feelings of guilt and unworthiness H. Assess ability to comprehend or follow-through I. Observe for expressed overdependency J. Assess the level of social and family acceptance, and note descriptions of "family pressures" to have children K. Observe for isolation or statements of need to withdraw from family/ friends/environments that are child-centered L. Note descriptions that reflect secrecy about the infertility problem or the inability to talk about the problem	F. Confront when necessary to focus attention on feelings or behavior G. Refer to infertility support group, if available, or to social service personnel for individual therapy as needed H. Facilitate communication between partners by including each individual in all aspects of care	
Self-concept/body image, disturbance in: actual/potential **Etiology** Belief that pregnancy is critical to one's own personal/social fulfillment as a woman Psychosocial pressures to conceive Biophysical imperativeness to conceive while pregnancy is physically possible Cultural or religious mandates that make pregnancy imperative	Responses to actual or perceived change in structure and/or function A. Verbalization of injury to sense of self 1. Feelings of bodily damage/ invasiveness 2. Feelings of incompetence (hampered work/family performance) 3. Feelings of loss of identity; not feeling totally "female" or "male"	A. Assess level of social, intellectual, intrapersonal, physical, and emotional function B. Observe for changes in affect, behavior, cognition, perception and/or level of function 1. Note quality and quantity of verbalizations regarding the self (see Defining Characteristics)	A. See Interventions (ineffective coping) B. Discuss with the couple "normal" emotional reactions to the state of childlessness C. Provide accurate information D. Provide information/assistance to begin adoptive proceedings as possible alternative to the infertility workup E. Promote warm, communicating relationship through effective verbal and nonverbal (touching) exchanges F. Refer for sexual counseling as needed	A. The couple will be able to function at an adequate level at work, with the family, and in society B. The individual will display a minimum of change in affect, behavior, cognition, perception, and/or level of function C. The couple will resolve conflicts of values while continuing infertility therapy and testing

Infertility as Emotional Crisis—cont'd

NURSING DIAGNOSIS/ PATIENT PROBLEM	DEFINING CHARACTERISTICS	NURSING ORDERS		EXPECTED OUTCOMES
		ASSESSMENT	INTERVENTIONS	
	4. Distorted perceptions: ''the whole world is pregnant except for me'' 5. Obsession/ preoccupation with infertility and body function 6. Grieving the loss of a potential life B. Conflicts involving values 1. Verbalization of threatened religious, cultural, or legal beliefs concerning the infertility procedures/treatments 2. Nonverbal response to actual/perceived change in structure and/ or function a. Poor eye contact b. Preoccupied c. Discontent d. Noncompliant e. Selfdestructive f. Nonparticipation in therapy g. Not taking responsibility for selfcare h. Signs of initiation of grief: weeping, sobbing, physical symptoms such as loss of appetite, exhaustion, choking or tightness in throat	2. Observe for help-seeking behaviors such as crying, attention-seeking, touching persons/objects, seeking someone to talk to 3. Observe for overt behaviors as stated under nonverbal responses (see Defining Characteristics) C. Assess level/presence of grieving the loss of children; loss of genetic continuity; loss of fertility; loss of the pregnancy experience D. Note religious/cultural background and potential conflicts with values or treatments E. Observe for statements that project the psychologic inability to be a good parent (''I cannot conceive because God knows I will be a poor parent'') F. Observe for statements of a change in sexual behaviors 1. Intercourse with prostitutes 2. Extramarital affairs 3. Impotence 4. Frigidity 5. Inability to achieve erection or orgasm 6. Vaginismus 7. Premature ejaculation 8. Ejaculatory incompetence 9. Statements of denial or verbalization of loss	G. Stress the importance of spouse support. Expressing acceptance of one another can help the body image and self-image of each partner H. Reinforce appropriate emotional responses; redirect inappropriate negative response I. Advise that negative responses from others be regarded with minimal significance J. Reinforce reality without giving false reassurance K. Provide safety from self-destructive behaviors L. Provide alternative methods for obtaining semen (seminal pouch) to patients with threatened religious/cultural values M. Assist the couple through grief: to recognize, work through, and overcome the intense/painful feelings of loss	D. The couple will display a minimum of sexual problems and maintain an open, communicating awareness with self and partner E. The couple may successfully attain a state of resolution

Continued.

Infertility as Emotional Crisis—cont'd

NURSING DIAGNOSIS/ PATIENT PROBLEM	DEFINING CHARACTERISTICS	NURSING ORDERS		EXPECTED OUTCOMES
		ASSESSMENT	INTERVENTIONS	

	3. Denial of role; refusal to verify actual change in reproductive capacity
	4. Negative feelings about body: increased verbalization of self-destruction and self-derogatory statements
	5. Verbalization regarding the change in personal identity and role performance
	  a. Expressed inability to perform on the job
	  b. Inappropriately blaming personal inadequacies for the infertility
	  c. Descriptions of sexual inadequacies/dysfunctions			

Knowledge deficit
Etiology:
 	
Lack of exposure to information
Poor recall
Misinterpretation of information
Cognitive limitation
Lack of interest in learning
Lack of familiarity with information
	Verbalization of problem
	Inaccurate follow-through of instruction
	Inappropriate or exaggerated behaviors, e.g., hysterical, hostile, anxious, apathetic
	Repetitive questions
		A. Assess need for teaching/counseling and the patient's level of understanding of the disease process, treatments, emotional reactions
		B. Assess level of anxiety
		C. Assess level of education
			A. Assist couple to maintain reproductive function by eliminating anxiety through teaching/awareness of the reproductive process, anatomy, and physiology
			B. Explain diagnostic tests/procedures
			C. Relate diagnostic testing to the normal physiology of the body
			D. Teach techniques for taking basal body temperatures, how to read a thermometer, and correct recording measures. Encourage the couple's involvement in their care
			E. Teach techniques/give knowledge needed for home care
			  1. Medications, side effects, mode of action, and method of administration
			  2. Rest and good nutrition
			  3. Menstrual calendar
			F. Observe for a favorable response to teaching
				The couple will demonstrate
				A. Workable knowledge of normal reproductive anatomy/physiology
				B. Knowledge of their diagnosis and relation to the treatment plan
				C. Better cooperation with taking/recording the basal body temperatures, keeping appointments, and undergoing diagnostic testing
				D. Less anxiety from fear of the unknown

Intrapartum Patient, Care of

NURSING DIAGNOSIS/ PATIENT PROBLEM	DEFINING CHARACTERISTICS	NURSING ORDERS		EXPECTED OUTCOMES
		ASSESSMENT	INTERVENTIONS	
Knowledge deficit **Etiology** Unfamiliarity of the labor process	Multiple questions Expressed need for more information Fearfulness Noncompliance	A. Assess patient's knowledge of the labor process B. Assess educational knowledge base affecting comprehension of teaching C. Assess the effect of anxiety and discomfort from labor on the patient's ability to comprehend teachings	A. Provide basic explanations on the physiologic and psychologic changes throughout all stages of labor B. Use visual aids as necessary C. Use terminology comprehensible to the patient D. Reinforce or repeat previous teachings as necessary; allow for feedback E. Use short, direct terminology during progressive phases of labor F. Keep patient and significant other informed of labor progress	The patient and significant other will verbalize an understanding of the labor process
Knowledge deficit **Etiology** Unfamiliarity with hospital and nursing procedures	Multiple questions Noncompliance Anxiety Anger	A. Assess knowledge of patient and significant other concerning hospital and nursing procedures B. Determine effect of labor on patient's ability to comprehend teachings	A. Provide explanation to patient and significant other before performing procedures 1. Give rationale for the procedure 2. State manner of performing the procedure 3. Inform patient of expected outcome B. Reinforce previous teachings when necessary C. Allow for feedback and clarification of explanations	Patient/significant other will verbalize an understanding of hospital and nursing procedures
Comfort, alteration in **Etiology** Contractions	Verbalizing discomfort Moaning Crying Restless	A. Determine patient's level of discomfort related to labor B. Determine physical factors contributing to discomfort C. Identify other variables adding to discomfort	A. Allow ambulation and position changes B. Encourage use of relaxation and comfort measures 1. Perform massage according to patient's desire 2. Teach effleurage 3. Encourage muscle relaxation C. Teach breathing modifications when appropriate 1. Slow, deep chest 2. Accelerated/decelerated 3. Modified panting 4. Patient's own relaxation breathing technique D. Provide pharmacologic interventions per physician's order; then observe and document 15 and 30 min after administration 1. Fetal heart rate pattern 2. Contraction pattern 3. BP and pulse 4. Patient's perception of pain	Patient will verbalize that the discomfort is lessened or more manageable

Originated by **Bernadette Keller, RNC**
Resource person: **Deidra Gradishar, RNC, BA**

Continued.

Intrapartum Patient, Care of—cont'd

NURSING DIAGNOSIS/ PATIENT PROBLEM	DEFINING CHARACTERISTICS	NURSING ORDERS		EXPECTED OUTCOMES
		ASSESSMENT	INTERVENTIONS	

			E. Assist significant other in providing support to the patient
			F. Minimize external factors contributing to discomfort
			  1. Decrease excessive noises
			  2. Provide soft lighting
			  3. Promote privacy
			  4. Minimize temperature extremes
			G. Maintain hydration and elimination
			  1. Hydration
			    a. Provide ice chips and clear liquids if ordered
			    b. Administer parenteral fluids as ordered
			  2. Elimination
			    a. Encourage voiding every 1-3 hours, as necessary
			    b. Observe for bladder distention
			H. Provide frequent hygienic measures
			  1. Oral hygiene q.2h. as needed. Apply petroleum jelly to lips if needed
			  2. Body hygiene
			    a. Assist patient to bathe q.8h.
			    b. Provide frequent perineal care q.2-3h.
			    c. Maintain dry, wrinkle-free linen	

Injury, potential for: to the fetus
Etiology
Physiologic stress of labor
	Fetal bradycardia
	Meconium-stained amniotic fluid
	Presence of periodic patterns indicating fetal distress: late decelerations, variable decelerations
	Baseline variability <5 BPM
		A. Assess and document fetal heart rate every 30 min
		  1. Baseline rate
		  2. Baseline variability
		  3. Presence and type of periodic pattern
		B. Assess and document contractions every 30 min
		  1. Intensity
		  2. Frequency
		  3. Duration
			A. Inform physician of any change in
			  1. Baseline fetal heart rate parameters
			  2. Uterine hyperactivity
			B. If fetal heart rate pattern is indicative of fetal distress, institute SCP in this chapter: Fetal distress
			C. Document interventions and response to treatment
				Potential for injury to the fetus will be minimized

Intrapartum Patient, Care of—cont'd

NURSING DIAGNOSIS/ PATIENT PROBLEM	DEFINING CHARACTERISTICS	NURSING ORDERS		EXPECTED OUTCOMES
		ASSESSMENT	INTERVENTIONS	

Injury, potential for: to the mother
Etiology
Infection
Hemorrhage
Hypertension
	Infection
	Elevated temperature
	Tachycardia
	Fetal tachycardia
	Diaphoresis
	Chills
	Vaginal discharge
	
	Hemorrhage
	Vaginal bleeding
	Tachycardia
	Hyperpnea
	Diaphoresis
	Restlessness
	Hypotension
	Decreased urinary output
	
	Hypertension
	Elevated BP
	Epigastric pain
	Edema
	Proteinuria (+ 1)
	Epigastric pain
		A. Infection. Assess and document temperature q.4h. or, on rupture of membranes, q.2h.
		B. Hemorrhage
		  1. Observe for excessive vaginal bleeding
		  2. Monitor BP, pulse, respiration, and fetal heart rate every 15-30 min in the presence of excessive vaginal bleeding
		  3. Institute pad count if indicated
		  4. Record I & O
		C. Hypertension
		  1. Assess and document BP, pulse, respiration, temperature q.4h. routinely
		  2. Assess and document BP every 30 min if BP is >140/90 or if a 30 mm systolic or 15 mm diastolic deviation from baseline is noted
		  3. Check for proteinuria
		  4. Check for hyperreflexive deep tendon reflexes
		  5. Determine if any visual disturbances or epigastric pain is present
			A. Infection
			  1. Maintain asepsis in performing procedures
			  2. Notify physician of
			    a. Temperature >37.5° C
			    b. Fetal tachycardia, fetal heart rate >160 BPM
			    c. Maternal tachycardia
			    d. Malodorous vaginal discharge
			B. Hemorrhage
			  1. Institute administration of IV fluids or increase in drip rate
			  2. Place bed in Trendelenburg's position
			  3. Administer O_2 at 10 L/min
			  4. Prepare for emergency delivery of a potentially compromised fetus
			C. Hypertension. Institute SCP in this chapter: Hypertension: pregnancy-induced (if indicated)
				Potential for injury to the patient will be minimized

Intrauterine Fetal Demise (IUFD)

NURSING DIAGNOSIS/ PATIENT PROBLEM	DEFINING CHARACTERISTICS	NURSING ORDERS		EXPECTED OUTCOMES
		ASSESSMENT	INTERVENTIONS	

Knowledge deficit
Etiology
Unfamiliarity with causes of intrauterine fetal demise
Unfamiliarity with nursing procedures
	Apparent confusion over events
	Multiple questions
	Lack of questions
	Expressed need for more information
	Resistance
	Anger
	Inability to retain information given
	Inability to communicate
	Inability to concentrate and/or understand explanations
	Putting call light on frequently
		A. Assess patient's knowledge base regarding IUFD
		B. Assess to what degree fear or the level of discomfort may compromise or influence the patient's ability to understand the explanations
		C. Assess the patient's knowledge regarding nursing procedures
			A. Provide information regarding
			  1. Known causes of IUFD
			  2. Myths
			B. Explain all actions taken; include significant other if and when possible
			  1. Rationale behind the procedure performed
			  2. Manner in which procedures are to be performed
			  3. Available options
			  4. Expected outcome to be realized from the procedure
			C. Reinforce the physician's explanations
			D. Simplify explanations, and repeat them when necessary
			E. Proceed with care measures in a calm and assured manner
			F. Institute a teaching plan for the type of delivery planned
				The patient will verbalize an understanding of
				A. Some known causes of IUFD
				B. Myths
				The patient will verbalize an understanding of
				A. Rationale behind nursing procedures
				B. Manner in which the procedures are to be performed

Comfort, alteration in
Etiology
Uterine contractions
	Verbalized pain
	Thrashing in bed
	Facial grimacing
	Hyperventilation/hypoventilation
	Muscle tension
		A. Elicit patient's perception of discomfort related to uterine contractions
		  1. Length of contractions
		  2. Frequency of contractions
		  3. Quality of pain
		  4. Location of pain
		  5. Intensity of pain
		B. Assess patient's understanding of contractile pattern and its role in discomfort
		C. Assess other factors that may be contributing to discomfort, e.g., grieving, fear, loneliness
		D. Evaluate the mechanisms the patient currently uses to manage discomfort
		E. Observe patient for changes in her coping mechanisms
		F. Assess duration of induction/augmentation
			A. Explain role of uterine contractions in terminating pregnancy
			B. Explain cyclic nature of uterine contraction pattern
			C. Use nonpharmacologic comfort measures when appropriate
			  1. Position changes
			  2. Relaxation techniques
			  3. Breathing techniques
			  4. Distraction techniques
			  5. Presence of support person
			D. Minimize or eliminate, when possible, other factors that may be contributing to discomfort
			  1. Encourage frequent voiding
			  2. Explain all procedures before and as they occur
			  3. Keep patient informed of labor process
			E. Provide positive reinforcement and personal contact
			F. Administer analgesic medications as ordered
			  1. Evaluate effectiveness
			  2. Evaluate duration of effectiveness
			  3. Observe for untoward reactions
			G. Explain the possibility of a prolonged induction/augmentation because of an unripe cervix
				A. The patient will verbalize an understanding of the discomfort associated with the labor process
				B. The patient will be able to verbalize and display a decreased or lessened discomfort state

Originated by **Linda Escobar, RN, BSN**
Resource person: **Jane Parker, RNC BAN**

Intrauterine Fetal Demise (IUFD)—cont'd

NURSING DIAGNOSIS/ PATIENT PROBLEM	DEFINING CHARACTERISTICS	NURSING ORDERS		EXPECTED OUTCOMES
		ASSESSMENT	INTERVENTIONS	
Self-concept, disturbance in **Etiology** Perception of role in IUFD	Self-maligning statements Overt expression of guilt and blame Refusal to make eye contact	A. Assess patient's perception of herself B. Assess degree to which patient assumes responsibility for fetal loss	A. Assist patient to express feelings about herself B. Assist patient to verbalize feelings of guilt and blame C. Maintain open, nonjudgmental approach to communication D. Respect and support patient's choice to be introspective at various times	A. Patient will acknowledge self-maligning statements and behavior B. Patient will begin to verbalize positive expressions of continued self-worth

Grieving
Etiology
Perception and anticipation of a loss
Loss of fetus
	Anger
	Bargaining
	Crying
	Denial
	Disbelief
	Shock
	Screaming
		A. Assess maternal response to IUFD
		B. Assess maternal support system
		  1. Husband or significant other
		  2. Family
		  3. Friends
		C. Assess maternal developmental stage
		D. Assess influence, if any, of culture and/or religion on grieving process
		E. Assess maternal state in grieving process
			A. Assist patient to identify and verbalize her feelings about
			  1. Feeling cheated
			  2. Fairness
			  3. Anger
			  4. Helplessness, powerlessness
			  5. Strangeness of own feelings
			  6. Seeing other infants and mothers. Confirm or reinforce the normalcy of these feelings
			B. Provide physical care, and meet dependency needs in a thoughtful and unhurried manner
			C. Do not attempt to minimize event
			D. Be accepting of any behavior that is not self-destructive
			E. Encourage presence of husband or significant other
			F. Encourage mother and significant other to view fetus to
			  1. Minimize continuing denial
			  2. Minimize forming unreal mental images of fetus now or at a later time
			  3. Promote separation of infant from self
			  4. Promote reality versus fantasy
			G. Prepare mother and significant other for appearance of fetus
			H. Provide adequate time and privacy for mother and significant other to view fetus, if they desire
			I. Accept mother's decision not to view fetus
			J. Arrange for baptismal rites or last rites if mother so desires
			K. Proceed with postmortem care in a respectful and dignified manner
			L. Refer to social worker for follow-up: Obtain infant footprint sheets and file in the labor rooms for social worker access
			M. See SCP in Ch. 1: Grieving, dysfunctional
				The patient will begin to verbally express an awareness of the loss and its impact

Continued.

Intrauterine Fetal Demise (IUFD)—cont'd

NURSING DIAGNOSIS/ PATIENT PROBLEM	DEFINING CHARACTERISTICS	NURSING ORDERS		EXPECTED OUTCOMES
		ASSESSMENT	INTERVENTIONS	
Injury, potential for: to mother **Etiology** Prolonged retention of products of conception	**Sepsis** Elevated temperature Elevated WBCs Abnormal clotting index, PT, PTT, fibrinogen Persistent bleeding from venipuncture or parenteral sites Inappropriate bleeding from mucous membranes	A. Monitor and record temperature every _____ B. Review result of WBCs as ordered by the physician C. Assess for malodorous vaginal discharge every _____ D. Observe for signs and symptoms of chills, flushing, tachycardia every _____ E. Assess and document amount of vaginal bleeding every _____ F. Assess and document prolonged bleeding from venipuncture and parenteral sites G. Assess and document inappropriate bleeding from orifices H. Review results of clotting studies as ordered by physician	Inform physician of changes in baseline parameters A. Temperature above: ____ B. Vital signs C. Bleeding D. Abnormal WBC: ____ E. Abnormal clotting studies PT: ____ PTT: ____ Fibrinogen: ____	Injury to the mother will be minimized

Iron Deficiency Anemia: postpartum care

NURSING DIAGNOSIS/ PATIENT PROBLEM	DEFINING CHARACTERISTICS	NURSING ORDERS		EXPECTED OUTCOMES
		ASSESSMENT	INTERVENTIONS	
Nutrition, alteration in: less than body requirements **Etiology** Iron deficiency anemia	Pallor, especially lips and palm of hands Poor appetite Bleeding gums Dyspepsia Increased sensitivity to cold Hb <12, Hct <37 Verbalizes poor understanding of food values	A. Observe for signs and symptoms of iron-deficiency anemia (see Defining Characteristics) B. Monitor for decreasing Hb/Hct values C. Assess level of understanding of nutritional requirements	A. Assist with menu selection, encouraging high-iron foods such as liver, meat, egg yolk, whole wheat, legumes, seafoods, dark green vegetables, and dried fruits B. Involve family member in patient education; provide information on 1. Maintenance of dietary intake 2. Signs and symptoms of iron deficiency anemia C. Provide sample menu(s) to attain therapeutic and individual goals	A. The patient will demonstrate ability to select iron-rich foods from menu B. The patient will verbalize understanding of the role of nutrition in the prevention of iron-deficiency anemia

Originated by **Monalisa S. Bron, RN, BSN**
Resource person: **Jackie Suprenant, RN, BSN**

Iron Deficiency Anemia: postpartum care—cont'd

NURSING DIAGNOSIS/ PATIENT PROBLEM	DEFINING CHARACTERISTICS	NURSING ORDERS		EXPECTED OUTCOMES
		ASSESSMENT	INTERVENTIONS	
		D. Assess patient's physical and emotional readiness to learn	D. Encourage good oral hygiene, using mild mouth wash or warm saline gargle several times a day E. Keep mealtime free from distracting hospital procedures F. Administer iron-rich medication with orange juice or tomato juice (vitamin C enhances absorption) after meals to prevent GI tract disturbance G. Explain that stool color will become dark green and that mild constipation or loose stools may occur as side effects of iron medication H. Consult dietitian as indicated	
Activity intolerance **Etiology** Diminished physical stamina	Reluctance to attempt movement Irritability Verbal report of fatigue, weakness, dizziness Abnormal heart rate or BP response to activity	A. Assess patient's respiratory/cardiac status before activity B. Observe and document response to activity. Report 1. Pulse >120 BPM 2. Palpitations 3. Weakness, dizziness 4. Dyspnea 5. Changes in skin color	A. Provide assistance with ambulation as needed to prevent accidental falls B. Encourage adequate naps or rest periods, especially before activity C. Encourage patient to seek assistance with household responsibilities after discharge. Inform significant other of need for rest D. Provide support and positive feedback for every effort at self-care E. Provide assistance and emotional support with infant care	The patient will evidence increased activity tolerance
Injury, potential for: puerperal infection **Etiology** Decreased body resistance	Fever: temperature ≥38.5° C Pulse >100 BPM Foul-smelling lochia Uterine tenderness Poor wound healing	A. Monitor vital signs as scheduled and as necessary B. Assess lochia. With infection, appearance varies depending on causative organism. May appear normal, profuse, bloody, and foul-smelling; may be scant and serosanguineous to brownish C. Examine fundus for uterine tenderness D. Observe wounds (episiotomy or abdominal incision) for signs of infection, including inadequate approximation, redness, edema, purulent drainage, and excessive pain E. Monitor for severe afterpains	A. Observe aseptic technique when handling incisional dressings B. Instruct patient on measures to prevent/minimize infection C. Report signs/symptoms of infection to physician	Normal progression of involution without evidence of infection will occur

Newborn, Assessment and Stabilization of

NURSING DIAGNOSIS/ PATIENT PROBLEM	DEFINING CHARACTERISTICS	NURSING ORDERS		EXPECTED OUTCOMES
		ASSESSMENT	INTERVENTIONS	

Potential for maladaptation to extrauterine life
Etiology
Alteration in respiratory system
	Cyanosis other than acrocyanosis
	Retractions
	Nasal flaring
	Grunting
	Tachypnea
	Bradypnea
	Absence of cry
	Choking
	Excessive secretions
		A. Assess respiratory status immediately after admission to the nursery
		B. Assess factors affecting respiratory status, i.e., prematurity, maternal premedication, presence of fetal distress during labor and/or delivery
		C. Evaluate need for ventilatory assistance
		D. Perform Chemstrip test to assess if respiratory distress is a result of hypoglycemia
			A. Maintain patent airway
			  1. Suction nose and oropharynx per bulb syringe or DeLee trap as needed
			  2. Position infant on side or abdomen to drain any secretions
			B. Institute measures to relieve respiratory distress
			  1. Stimulate crying by gently tapping feet
			  2. Administer free O_2 per tube at 10 ml/min 1-2 inches from nose
			  3. Notify pediatrician to evaluate infant
			  4. If infant remains unresponsive, begin bag and mask ventilation with O_2 at a rate of 50 times/min
			  5. Maintain stable body temperature
				Respiratory rate of 40-60/min after birth will be established and maintained

Etiology Alteration in cardiovascular system	Heart rate <100/min Cyanosis Hyporeflexia Edema Irregular rhythm Abnormal heart sounds Signs of shock: diaphoresis, cold, clammy skin	A. Assess infant for signs of cardiovascular dysfunction (see Defining Characteristics) B. Evaluate vital signs on admission to the nursery C. Note decrease or absence of reflexes D. Note infant's color	Notify pediatrician to evaluate infant when signs/symptoms of cardiovascular dysfunction are present	Establishment and maintenance of proper cardiovascular function after birth will be evidenced by A. Heart rate: 120-160/min B. Color: pink
Etiology Hypothermia	Axillary temperature <36° C Cyanosis Decreased or shallow respirations Retractions Bradycardia Decreased reflexes Nasal flaring	A. Assess newborn for signs of hypothermia (see Defining Characteristics) B. If hypothermia is present, perform Chemstrip test to assess for hypoglycemia	A. Place infant in radiant warmer on admission, and monitor temperature. When temperature is stable—36.4° C or above, admission bath may be given B. Place cap on infant's head C. Check temperature 30 min after bath; if above 36.5° C, infant may be warmly wrapped and placed in open crib D. Monitor temperature twice a day until third day, then daily, unless ordered otherwise	Loss of body heat will be minimized

Originated by **Josephine C. Anderson, RN**
Resource person: **Jackie Suprenant, RN, BSN**

Newborn, Assessment and Stabilization of—cont'd

NURSING DIAGNOSIS/ PATIENT PROBLEM	DEFINING CHARACTERISTICS	NURSING ORDERS		EXPECTED OUTCOMES
		ASSESSMENT	INTERVENTIONS	
Etiology Alteration in neurologic system	Unusual size or shape of head Paralysis of face and extremities Poor reflexes Lethargy Shrill cry Poor temperature control	A. Assess infant for normal/abnormal neurologic development B. Assess effect of maternal medication or history of drugs or alcohol abuse C. Observe infant's response to stimulation D. Evaluate muscle tone E. Note presence or absence of sucking, grasping, and Moro's reflex	A. Measure head circumference B. Gently palpate head for sunken fontanels and for overriding or closed sutures C. Stimulate cry by gently tapping feet D. Notify pediatrician of abnormally large or small head measurement	Maintenance of neurologic function will be evidenced by A. Appropriate muscle tone B. Reflex response within normal limits

Etiology
Alteration in skin integrity
	Rash
	Lacerations
	Forcep marks
	Condition of cord
	Birthmarks
	Plethora
	Pallor
	Blisters
	Pustules
	Petechiae
	Scalp electrode site
		Assess infant for signs of any deviation from normal skin integrity (see Defining Characteristics)	A. Apply alcohol to cord after admission bath and after each diaper change
			B. Provide special skin care
			  1. Lacerations. Apply povidone-iodine (Betadine) every shift
			  2. Rash on buttocks. Apply ointment as needed/as ordered
			C. Notify physician if blisters, pustules, petechiae, pallor, or plethora present
				A. Skin integrity will be promoted
				B. Cord will be dry by third day of life

Etiology Alteration in GI system	Cleft lip or palate Vomiting Imperforate anus Abnormal or absence of stools Abdominal distention Tracheoesophageal fistula	A. Assess infant for normal GI functions and signs of abnormalities B. Observe for initial passage of meconium stool C. Measure abdominal girth if abdomen appears distended; then check every shift as ordered	A. Use lamb's nipple or cleft palate nurser for infant with cleft lip or palate, and observe for problems with secretions B. If vomiting occurs, document color, consistency, amount, and note if projectile C. Document consistency, size, color, odor, and frequency of stools	Maintenance of infant's GI function will be evidenced by A. Passage of meconium within 24 hours B. Abdomen soft without distention
Etiology Alteration in genitourinary function	Abnormal genitalia Abnormal urinary function Anuria Abnormal number of vessels in cord	A. Assess infant for normal/abnormal urinary function B. Observe for voiding within first 24 hours C. Assess penis for hypospadias or epispadias D. Observe for abnormal or absent external genitalia E. Check cord for proper number of vessels	Document color, concentration, and frequency of urine output	Maintenance of urinary function of infant will be evidenced by passage of urine within 24 hours

Continued.

Newborn, Assessment and Stabilization of—cont'd

NURSING DIAGNOSIS/ PATIENT PROBLEM	DEFINING CHARACTERISTICS	NURSING ORDERS		EXPECTED OUTCOMES
		ASSESSMENT	INTERVENTIONS	
Potential for maladaptation to extrauterine life—cont'd **Etiology** Alteration in musculoskeletal system	Fractured clavicle Polydactyly Absent or malformed extremities Hip dysplasia Meningocele Omphalocele	A. Assess infant for normal/abnormal musculoskeletal function (see Defining Characteristics) B. Note presence of all extremities and digits C. Check alignment of trunk and extremities	A. Move all extremities through normal ROM B. Document any deviation in normal physical status	Maintenance of musculoskeletal development of infant will be evidenced by A. Free movement of all extremities B. Proper number of digits
Etiology Alteration in nutrition	Poor sucking Color change Choking Regurgitation Lethargy Weight loss >10% of birth weight Incomplete closure of lip or palate	Assess infant for signs of poor feeding (see Defining Characteristics)	A. Unless ordered otherwise, institute and maintain feedings per appropriate policy and procedure B. Weigh infant every day	A. Loss of body weight will be <10% of birth weight B. Infant will be sucking well and retaining feedings
Hyperbilirubinemia: potential **Etiology** Physiology Pathology Prematurity ABO incompatability Rh incompatability	Skin: yellow Sclera: yellow Poor feeder Lethargic	A. Assess infant for signs of hyperbilirubinemia (see Defining Characteristics) B. Assess predisposing factors: perinatal asphyxia, respiratory distress syndrome, intrapartum diabetes mellitus, prematurity, physiologic jaundice, bruising, polycythemia, hematoma, and bruising C. Observe for passage of meconium stool	A. Provide adequate feedings as infant requires B. Check laboratory results; notify pediatrician of elevated bilirubin levels C. If ordered, prepare infant for phototherapy D. Inform parents of infant's condition and provide educational material	Hyperbilirubinemia will be minimized
Knowledge deficit: potential **Etiology** Unfamiliarity with newborn care	Multiple questions Lack of questions Confusion Verbalizes anxiety Expresses need for more information	Assess mother's ability to care for infant	A. Instruct parents on the following 1. Hand-washing technique 2. Crib supplies 3. Feedings 4. Diapering 5. Cord care 6. Bathing 7. Dressing 8. Safety measures B. Measure parents' understanding of instructions by allowing a return demonstration whenever possible	Parents will demonstrate ability to care for infant

Pelvic Inflammatory Disease: adolescent

NURSING DIAGNOSIS/ PATIENT PROBLEM	DEFINING CHARACTERISTICS	NURSING ORDERS		EXPECTED OUTCOMES
		ASSESSMENT	INTERVENTIONS	

Comfort, alteration in
 Etiology
 Pelvic cavity inflammation
	Low abdominal pain
	 Abdominal distention
	 Back pain
		A. Assess patient for low abdominal and back pain
		   1. Type: sharp/dull
		   2. Quality: severe/mild
		   3. Duration _____
		 B. Assess patient's abdomen for
		   1. Abdominal girth every ___ hours
		   2. Bowel sounds every_____ hours
			A. Administer analgesics for pain as ordered
			 B. Assess for side effects of medications used
			 C. Provide external comfort measures
			   1. Heating pad on low temperature
			   2. Positioning with extra pillows
			   3. Turning every _____ hours
			   4. Activity tolerance
			     a. Bed rest _____
			     b. Bed rest with bathroom privileges ____
			     c. Ambulation _____
				Relief or minimization of pain will be evidenced by
				 A. Verbalization of relief
				 B. Appearance of improved comfort

Fluid volume deficit: potential
 Etiology
 Vomiting
	Abnormal electrolytes
	 Decreased urine output (< 30 ml/hour)
	 Poor skin tugor
	 Dry mucous membranes
	 Increased urine specific gravity (> 1.020)
		A. Monitor patient for vomiting
		 B. Check output of emesis
		   1. Amount _____
		   2. Color _____
		   3. Consistency
		 C. Hematest emesis
		 D. Monitor I & O
		 E. Monitor IV fluids
		 F. Check urine every ____ hours
		   1. Specific gravity _____
		   2. Dipstick _____
		 G. Monitor laboratory values for abnormal
		   1. Electrolytes _____
		   2. CBC _____
			A. Administer antiemetics
			 B. Keep patient NPO, or give clear liquids until nausea and vomiting decrease
			 C. Give small amounts of ice chips, sips of water, or carbonated beverages (not colas) until nausea and vomiting subside
			 D. See SCP in Ch. 1: Fluid volume deficit
				Fluid volume and electrolyte balance will be maintained as evidenced by
				 A. Normal electrolytes
				 B. Urine output at least 30 ml/hour
				 C. Normal skin turgor
				 D. Moist mucous membranes
				 E. Normal specific gravity and urine dipstick

Originated by **Caramen Billheimer, RN, BSN**
Resource persons: **Mary Muse, RN,C BSN**
    Michele Knoll-Puzas, RN,C BS
    Jackie Suprenant, RN, BSN

Continued.

Pelvic Inflammatory Disease: adolescent—cont'd

NURSING DIAGNOSIS/ PATIENT PROBLEM	DEFINING CHARACTERISTICS	NURSING ORDERS		EXPECTED OUTCOMES
		ASSESSMENT	INTERVENTIONS	

Injury, potential for: actual infection and potential spreading of infection
 Etiology
 Gonococcal infection of
   Fallopian tubes (salpingitis)
   Ovaries (oophoritis)
   Uterus (endometritis)
	Vaginal discharge
	 Increased body temperature
	 Positive cultures
		A. Check vital signs every _____ hours (pay attention to spiking temperatures)
		 B. Assess gynecologic examination and cultures
		 C. Assess for malodorous vaginal discharge in copious amounts
			A. Institute enteric precautions
			 B. Discard soiled perineal pads in isolated containers
			 C. Maintain strict hand-washing technique for all persons in contact with patient
			 D. Administer antibiotics as ordered
			 E. Administer perineal care after each pad is changed and after bedpan use
			 F. Cleanse all equipment used with disinfectant i.e., bedpan, tub, and toilet seat
			 G. Use utensil or gloves when handling soiled materials
			 H. Make sure patient does not use tampons
			 I. Position patient in sitting position every _____ hours
				Spread of infection will be minimized

Anxiety/fear: potential
 Etiology
 Parental reactions
 Hospitalizations
 Treatment
	Expressing anger
	 Nonverbalization with withdrawal
	 Crying when discussing medical treatment or hospitalization
	 Agitation
	 Embarrassment
		Assess for
		 A. Patient's normal coping patterns by interview with patient, family, significant others
		 B. Changes in behavior patterns of the patient (see Defining Characteristics)
		 C. Parental knowledge of patient's sexual activity
		 D. History of urinary or reproductive tract infections
		 E. Past hospitalizations
		 F. Treatment for gonorrhea or syphillis
		 G. Use of contraceptives
			A. After diagnosis is confirmed, talk with parents (particularly if patient is a minor) concerning their feelings and concerns
			 B. Elicit patient and family feelings about the effects of pelvic inflammatory disease
			   1. Recurrences of infection
			   2. Normal sexual functioning
			   3. Surgical intervention
			   4. Normal childbearing
			 C. Allow parents and adolescent to talk out their feelings and concerns to one another
			 D. Be supportive and nonjudgmental of patient's behavior
			 E. Explain all tests and procedures to patient before they are done
			   1. Blood and urine test
			   2. Pregnancy test
			   3. Gynecologic examination
			   4. X-ray studies
			   5. IV fluids
			   6. Medications
			   7. Provide physical and emotional support as needed during examinations
				Decreased anxiety will be evidenced by
				 A. Calm, relaxed appearance
				 B. Verbalization of fears or feelings
				 C. Restful sleep

Pelvic Inflammatory Disease: adolescent—cont'd

NURSING DIAGNOSIS/ PATIENT PROBLEM	DEFINING CHARACTERISTICS	NURSING ORDERS		EXPECTED OUTCOMES
		ASSESSMENT	INTERVENTIONS	

Knowledge deficit
 Etiology
 Unfamiliarity with cause of disease, medical management, prevention
	Questioning
	 Silence during questioning about illness
	 Frequent complaints
		A. Assess level of knowledge
		 B. Assess level of comprehension
		 C. Assess developmental level of patient and parents
			A. Explain to patient and parents how pelvic inflammatory disease is acquired and prevented
			 B. Explain to patient that sexual contact(s) may need to be notified so they can receive treatment
			 C. Instruct patient and parents on the importance of proper administration of medication
			   1. Type of medication
			   2. Dosage
			   3. Side effects
			 D. Instruct patient and parents to notify physician if
			   1. Symptoms reappear
			   2. Menstruation does not occur
			   3. Occurrence of bleeding other than menstruation
			   4. Severe abdominal cramps
			 E. Inform patient of the importance of refraining from sexual intercourse until follow-up visit with physician is completed
			 F. Discuss the use of contraceptives if patient plans to continue sexual activities
			 G. Inform patient and parents of resource personnel available to assist them
			   1. Family planning
			   2. Adolescent groups
			   3. Social worker
				A. Patient and parents will verbalize an understanding of
				   1. Pelvic inflammatory disease
				   2. Causes
				   3. Complications
				   4. Treatment
				   5. Prevention
				 B. Parents and patient will verbalize an understanding of
				   1. Medication
				   2. Dosage
				   3. Side effects
				   4. When to notify physician
				 C. Patient and parents will verbalize an understanding of
				   1. Resource people within the hospital or in the city
				   2. The importance of having other resources for assistance

Placenta Previa: acute

NURSING DIAGNOSIS/ PATIENT PROBLEM	DEFINING CHARACTERISTICS	NURSING ORDERS		EXPECTED OUTCOMES
		ASSESSMENT	INTERVENTIONS	
Knowledge deficit **Etiology** New condition Unfamiliarity with nursing/hospital procedures/environment *Population at risk:* individuals with Multiparity Advancing age Previous cesarean section or uterine surgery Previous defective vascularization of the decidua as result of infection or atrophic changes Large placenta resulting from fetal erythroblastosis or multiple fetuses	Confusion over events Multiple questions Expressed need for more information Inability to concentrate Inability to retain information given Restlessness	A. Assess patient's knowledge base regarding placenta previa B. Assess patient's knowledge regarding nursing procedures C. Assess patient's knowledge of unfamiliar surroundings D. Assess patient's capacity for understanding events E. Assess patient's level of concentration	A. Encourage patient to verbalize concerns B. Provide an environment that encourages communication C. Orient to environment and personnel D. Explain rationale for all tests, and explain the manner in which they will be done E. Include significant other when possible F. Give rationale for being closely monitored G. Institute teaching plan for anticipated method of delivery H. Provide information regarding 1. Physiology of placenta previa 2. Possible effects it could have on pregnancy and eventual delivery of child (emergent/premature) 3. Possible effects on type of delivery (cesarean section) 4. Possible effect on fetus	The patient will verbalize an understanding of A. Rationale behind procedures B. The manner in which procedure is to be performed C. The nature of placenta previa
Injury, potential for: to mother **Etiology** Hemorrhage	Uterus non-tender Painless bleeding Bleeding occurring before expected date of confinement (most often between 24-48 weeks gestation) Oliguria or anuria Cyanosis of mucous membranes of lips and of the nail beds of the hands	A. Obtain subjective data base 1. Patient's estimate of the amount of blood loss 2. When bleeding began 3. Whether or not pain accompanied the bleeding 4. Color of the blood 5. What patient had done for the bleeding B. Assess for vaginal bleeding 1. Quality 2. Color	A. Institute perineal pad count B. Monitor pulse, respirations, and BP every 15 min until stable, than every _____ C. Review results of Hb and Hct as ordered D. Record I & O every _____ E. Monitor uterine contractions/irritability by electronic device	Potential for injury will be minimized

Originated by **Joanne Coleman, RN**
Resource person: **Jane Parker, RNC, BAN**

Placenta Previa: acute—cont'd

NURSING DIAGNOSIS/ PATIENT PROBLEM	DEFINING CHARACTERISTICS	NURSING ORDERS		EXPECTED OUTCOMES
		ASSESSMENT	INTERVENTIONS	

Injury, potential for: to fetus
 Etiology
 Uteroplacental insufficiency
	Fetal tachycardia
	 Decreased baseline variability
	 Absence of fetal heart tones
		Monitor fetal heart tones electronically, and assess every
		 _____
		 A. Baseline rate
		 B. Baseline variability
		 C. Presence of periodic patterns
			A. Notify physician of any change in fetal heart tones from baseline
			 B. In the event of fetal distress
			   1. Have mother assume left lateral position
			   2. Increase IV flow rate
			   3. Administer O_2 by rebreather mask at _____ L/min
			 C. If delivery is planned, prepare for a possibly compromised infant
				Injury to fetus will be minimized

Anxiety/fear **Etiology** Uncertain outcome for infant/self	Trembling Restlessness Expressed sense of impending doom	A. Obtain patient's perception of current status of infant and self B. Observe for nonverbal signs of fear/anxiety	A. Provide patient with realistic factual information regarding her status and that of her infant (include significant other when possible) B. Provide information regarding neonatal ICU (arrange tour, if possible) C. Encourage patient to verbalize concerns	Patient will be provided with opportunity to verbalize fears/ concerns regarding herself and infant

Postpartum Adolescent

NURSING DIAGNOSIS/ PATIENT PROBLEM	DEFINING CHARACTERISTICS	NURSING ORDERS		EXPECTED OUTCOMES
		ASSESSMENT	INTERVENTIONS	
Coping, ineffective individual: potential **Etiology** Situational maturational crisis of adolescent parenting	Verbalization of inability to cope Inability to meet role expectations Inability to meet basic needs of self and infant Low self-esteem	A. Assess patient's need/resources for financial/emotional support B. Identify educational plans/goals C. Assess concerns related to role changes associated with motherhood D. Assess awareness of access to "helping" community agencies regarding employment, day care, and welfare	A. Spend extra time with patient to facilitate a trust relationship B. Explore with patient her strengths, and provide information regarding resources available within the community, e.g., financial services, young parent centers, Catholic charities, Department of Health and Human Services C. Encourage patient to continue in school or to receive vocational training whenever possible. Discuss with patient, and make necessary referrals D. Teach a realistic approach from the standpoint of priorities and available budget E. Provide anticipatory guidance or discussion to promote self-confidence and build self-esteem	Patient will verbalize community and family resources available to assist her
Knowledge deficit **Etiology** Unfamiliarity with normal infant growth and development Lack of previous experience	Asks many questions or no questions Expresses need for more information Verbalizes unrealistic expectations of infant development	A. Assess learning needs of patient B. Assess level of understanding C. Ascertain the accuracy of patient's understanding of normal infant growth and development	A. Initiate discussions with patient regarding infant growth and development B. Encourage patient to verbalize concerns related to newborn behavior and characteristics C. Provide concrete explanation of basic infant growth and development D. Introduce patient to other teenage patients on unit for support and to exchange points of view E. Advise patient of infant's need for touch and interaction in the promotion of growth and development	The patient will verbalize an understanding of basic normal infant growth and development
Etiology Unfamiliarity with contraception and family planning	Asks many questions or no questions Expresses need for more information Verbalizes unrealistic expectations of infant development	A. Assess the patient's knowledge, attitudes, and concerns about her sexuality and family planning methods B. Assess methods used in the past C. Assess degree of sexual activity D. Assess the patient's thoughts regarding the following: family size, burden of more children, hazards of additional pregnancy during adolescent years	A. Help patient in selecting a method suited to her needs B. Include sexual partner or mother in discussion whenever possible C. Encourage patient to share information of method used with her partner or mate D. Explain that repeat pregnancy in the teen years is a hazard to herself and the unborn child E. Reinforce teaching from family planning clinic	Patient will verbalize an understanding of the following A. Selected family planning methods B. Need to avoid future pregnancy during teenage years

Originated by **Manee Omsin, RN, BSN**
Resource person: **Jackie Suprenant, RN, BSN**

Postpartum Adolescent—cont'd

NURSING DIAGNOSIS/ PATIENT PROBLEM	DEFINING CHARACTERISTICS	NURSING ORDERS		EXPECTED OUTCOMES
		ASSESSMENT	INTERVENTIONS	
Nutrition, alteration in: less than body requirements **Etiology** Pregnancy and adolescent growth requirements Poor dietary habits Misinformation about nutrition	Iron deficiency anemia: Hb <12, Hct <37 ≥10%-20% under appropriate body weight	A. Assess patient's nutritional status Skin Mucous membranes Tongue Eyes Hair Weight/height Weight gain pattern B. Obtain nutritional history as appropriate C. Assess patient's nutritional knowledge	A. Provide patient with necessary information based on nutritional assessment 1. Four basic food groups 2. Eating patterns that will promote weight gain (if appropriate) 3. Importance of maintaining adequate caloric intake B. Assist patient with selection of appropriate foods from each food group on menu C. Educate the patient to take daily vitamin with iron pill if prescribed D. Provide positive feedback when appropriate E. Refer to SCP in Ch. 15: Iron deficiency anemia: postpartum care, as necessary	Patient will verbalize and demonstrate proper nutritional patterns
Self-concept, disturbance in: body image **Etiology** Physical and psychosocial changes related to delivery	Verbalizes displeasure with body Overt expression of guilt and blame Fear of rejection or reaction by others Preoccupation with body changes	A. Assess the patient's perception of self B. Assess patient's normal coping pattern	A. Approach patient unhurriedly, and demonstrate accepting attitude B. Encourage patient to verbalize her feelings and listen attentively. Offer feedback to the patient's expressed feelings C. Explain reason for episiotomy or Cesarean section, and encourage patient to look at episiotomy or C-section incision D. Encourage exercise. Develop a postpartum exercise program suited to individual needs. Include such exercises as Kegal, abdominal curl-up, and walking E. Instruct patient to seek physician approval before resuming physical education activities in school	Patient will begin to verbalize positive feelings about self

Postpartum Hemorrhage Following Vaginal Delivery

NURSING DIAGNOSIS/ PATIENT PROBLEM	DEFINING CHARACTERISTICS	NURSING ORDERS		EXPECTED OUTCOMES
		ASSESSMENT	INTERVENTIONS	

Fluid volume deficit
Etiology
Rapid loss of blood (>500 ml)
 	
Patients at risk
Those with overdistended uterus because of large baby, multiple pregnancies or polyhydramnios, multiparity, prolonged or precipitous labor, fibromyoma, augmented labor, forceps delivery, general anesthesia, placenta previa, abruptio placentae
	Hypotension
	Rapid pulse
	Dyspnea
	Pallor
	Syncope
		A. Assess uterine status every _____
		  1. Tone
		  2. Fundal height
		  3. Position
		B. Assess amount and color of vaginal bleeding and the presence of clots
		C. Palpate and percuss urinary bladder for distention
		D. Assess condition of perineum
		  1. Swelling
		  2. Ecchymosis
		  3. Approximation of episiotomy
		E. Assess possibility of bleeding from cervical, vaginal, or perineal tears (firm uterus but continued oozing of bright red blood)
		F. Monitor and record BP, pulse, and respiration every
		
		_____
		G. Observe strict perineal pad count
		H. Assess results of Hb and Hct when ordered
		I. Review delivery notes for documentation of sponge count
			A. Massage uterine fundus until firm
			B. Increase flow rate of IV fluids
			C. Notify physician of deviations from baseline parameters
			D. Administer oxytocic agents per physician's order
			E. Encourage patient to void; catheterize if necessary (as ordered)
			F. Prepare for second IV line; transfuse per physician's order
			G. Prepare for examination, dilation and curettage, repair of laceration or episiotomy, or possible abdominal surgery, as indicated
				Optimal fluid volume will be maintained

Comfort, alteration in
Etiology
Uterine massage and contraction of uterus
	Verbalizing pain
	Uncooperative during examinations
	Elevated BP and/or tachycardia
		A. Elicit patient's description of pain related to uterine massage
		  1. Quality
		  2. Severity
		  3. Frequency: during examinations and/or constant
		B. Assess means by which patient presently deals with discomfort
			A. Explain purpose of assessments
			  1. Palpation of fundus for height, position, and tone
			  2. Uterine massage if necessary
			B. Allow patient to palpate fundus and learn what good uterine tone feels like. Encourage patient to check fundus periodically and to massage if needed
			C. Minimize other factors that may be contributing to discomfort
				Patient will verbalize that discomfort is decreased or is more manageable

Originated by **Theresa Vanderhei, RN**
Resource person: **Jane Parker, RNC, BAN**

Postpartum Hemorrhage Following Vaginal Delivery—cont'd

NURSING DIAGNOSIS/ PATIENT PROBLEM	DEFINING CHARACTERISTICS	NURSING ORDERS		EXPECTED OUTCOMES
		ASSESSMENT	INTERVENTIONS	
		C. Assess other reasons for discomfort 1. Distended bladder 2. Episiotomy pain 3. "Afterbirth" pain	1. Encourage frequent voiding 2. Apply ice pack to perineum as needed 3. Promote comfort by change in position 4. Encourage patient to rest between examinations D. Provide emotional support, especially if analgesic is contraindicated at this time E. Administer analgesia as ordered by physician. Observe for any untoward reactions	
Knowledge deficit **Etiology** Unfamiliarity with postpartum hemorrhage, its causes, and treatment	Frequent questioning, or lack of questions Confusion Fear	A. Assess patient's knowledge of postpartum hemorrhage, its causes and treatment B. Assess physical and emotional parameters that may affect patient's ability to understand	A. Explain briefly possible causes of postpartum hemorrhage B. Allow patient to ask questions about treatment and procedures C. Explain oxytocic agents and their role in promoting uterine involution D. Explain all necessary procedures thoroughly before initiation 1. Catheterization and the effects of distended bladder on the uterus 2. Other possible procedures (as appropriate) a. Manual exploration b. Repair of episiotomy or lacerations c. Dilation and curettage d. Hysterectomy in severe cases E. Explain importance of continued observation to detect any further bleeding episodes	Patient will verbalize understanding of postpartum hemorrhage, its treatment, and follow-up care

Premature Labor

NURSING DIAGNOSIS/ PATIENT PROBLEM	DEFINING CHARACTERISTICS	NURSING ORDERS		EXPECTED OUTCOMES
		ASSESSMENT	INTERVENTIONS	
Knowledge deficit **Etiology** Unfamiliarity with premature labor	Multiple questions Patient expresses a need for more information Confusion about early hospitalization	A. Assess the patient's knowledge base regarding premature labor B. Assess the patient's maturational stage and educational background	A. Provide information and rationale for 1. Causes of premature labor 2. Treatment of premature labor a. Drug of choice b. Other treatment modalities B. Discuss development at the gestational stage of the fetus C. Explain the need for hospitalization	Patient will verbalize an understanding of A. Causes of premature labor B. Rationale regarding the treatment of premature labor

Originated by **Yvette Roberts, RN,C, BSN, MHA**
Resource person: **Jane Parker, RNC BAN**

Continued.

Premature Labor—cont'd

NURSING DIAGNOSIS/ PATIENT PROBLEM	DEFINING CHARACTERISTICS	NURSING ORDERS		EXPECTED OUTCOMES
		ASSESSMENT	INTERVENTIONS	
Knowledge deficit— cont'd **Etiology** Unfamiliarity with hospital environment and nursing procedures	Restlessness Apprehension Agitation Selective inattention	Assess the patient's knowledge regarding hospital environment and nursing procedures	A. Encourage the patient to verbalize concerns B. Provide an environment that is conducive to communication C. Explain to patient and significant other 1. Rationale behind the procedures performed 2. Manner in which procedures are to be performed D. Reinforce the physician's explanations E. Give rationale for close observation by various personnel	The patient will verbalize an understanding of A. Rationale behind the procedure B. The manner in which the procedure is to be performed
Comfort, alteration in **Etiology** Uterine contractions	Facial grimacing Thrashing in bed Lack of relaxation during contractions	A. Assess the patient's perception of discomfort of uterine contractions B. Assess and document every 30 minutes 1. Length of contractions 2. Frequency of contractions 3. Location of pain 4. Intensity of pain C. Assess patient's past and present patterns of coping with discomfort D. Assess and document other stressors that may be contributing to discomfort	A. Use nonpharmacologic measures when appropriate 1. Positioning 2. Muscular relaxation techniques 3. Breathing techniques 4. Distraction techniques B. Eliminate or minimize, when possible, other factors that may be contributing to discomfort 1. Encourage patient to void frequently 2. Explain all procedures before executing them 3. Answer all questions if possible 4. Keep patient and significant other informed of labor and fetal status C. Explain to patient why analgesic agents may not be appropriate 1. Effect on fetal heart rate 2. Possibility of masking contractions 3. Combined side effects of the tocolytic agents to inhibit labor and analgesia D. Provide positive reinforcement and personal contact E. Plan nursing care to provide rest periods to facilitate comfort, sleep, and relaxation	Patient will verbalize that the discomfort experienced is minimized or more manageable
Self-concept, disturbance in **Etiology** Interruption of perception of the birth process	Minimal eye contact Self deprecating statements Overt expressions of guilt/blame Anger	A. Assess and document how the patient feels about herself and her role in the birthing process B. Assess to what degree the patient feels responsible for premature labor C. Assess and evaluate the availability of support systems	A. Encourage patient to verbalize her fears and concerns B. Include significant other in discussion C. Provide factual information regarding patient's lack of responsibility for the initiation and continuation of uterine contractions D. Provide positive feedback to the patient for seeking early intervention	Patient will begin to verbalize positive expressions of continued self-worth

Premature Labor—cont'd

NURSING DIAGNOSIS/ PATIENT PROBLEM	DEFINING CHARACTERISTICS	NURSING ORDERS		EXPECTED OUTCOMES
		ASSESSMENT	INTERVENTIONS	
Injury, potential for: to the fetus **Etiology** Preterm contractions accomplishing cervical dilation/effacement	Gestation of < 36 weeks Uterine contractions leading to dilation and effacement of cervix	A. Assess for burning sensation and frequency or urgency on urination B. Assess for presence of low back pain, flank pain, or "pressure in the vagina" C. Obtain a clean-catch urine specimen D. Assess the time of onset of contractions E. Elicit from patient her perception of occurrence and intensity of uterine contractions F. Continuously monitor and document 1. Frequency of contractions 2. Intensity of contractions G. Continuously monitor fetal heart rate, and document every 30 min 1. Baseline fetal heart rate 2. Baseline fetal heart rate variability H. For patients receiving tocolytic agents (e.g., ritodrine) 1. Monitor K+ and glucose 2. Maintain strict I & O 3. Observe for severe tachycardia (pulse > 130 BPM) 4. Observe for hypotension (BP < 80/60) 5. Refer to drug protocol	A. Administer IV fluids and antibiotics as ordered B. Apply continuous electronic fetal monitor C. Encourage patient to maintain left lateral recumbent position D. Administer tocolytic agents as ordered E. Discuss the potential side effects of the drug and their relationship to the treatment of premature labor F. Report and document side effects of the drug G. In the event that uterine contractions are not halted, prepare for delivery of the premature infant	Injury to the fetus will be minimized

Prolapsed Cord (Viable Infant)

NURSING DIAGNOSIS/ PATIENT PROBLEM	DEFINING CHARACTERISTICS	NURSING ORDERS		EXPECTED OUTCOMES
		ASSESSMENT	INTERVENTIONS	
Injury, potential for: to fetus **Etiology** Cord compression Uteroplacental insufficiency	Protrusion of cord from vagina Palpation of cord on vaginal examinations Sudden morbid and precipitous decrease in fetal heart rate with prolonged bradycardia Absence of fetal heart tones	Assess and record the following every _____ minutes A. Baseline fetal heart rate B. Baseline variability C. Presence and type of periodic patterns noted	A. Notify physician of any evidence of prolonged bradycardia or alterations in fetal heart rate B. Evaluate patient for possible prolapsed cord 1. Check introitus for cord 2. If cord is present, palpate for pulsations 3. Place patient in knee-chest position or elevate presenting part 4. Call for help C. Prepare for the immediate delivery of a potentially compromised fetus 1. Refer to SCP in this chapter for emergency cesarean section 2. Transfer the patient to the OR if a vaginal delivery is anticipated	Potential for injury to fetus will be minimized
Fear/anxiety **Etiology** Potential loss of fetus Increased activity and rapid sequence of events	Multiple questions Lack of questions Lack of cooperation Crying	A. Assess patient's awareness and understanding B. Assess the importance of the significant other in obtaining the patient's cooperation C. Observe for non-verbal signs of fear/anxiety D. Refer to SCP in Ch. 1: Anxiety/ fear	A. Explain all actions taken, and include the significant other when possible. Provide patient with the rationale for all procedures performed B. Repeat explanations when necessary C. Reassure the patient that she is in no way responsible for the occurrence of the cord prolapse D. Encourage patient to verbalize concerns **After delivery** A. Allow parents to see infant before it is transported to the nursery, whenever possible B. Allow mother to have tactile contact with infant if possible C. Provide realistic information on the probable outcome for the neonate D. See patient on the postpartum unit to review labor/delivery events	Anxiety will be minimized as a result of patient's ability to comprehend the events that are occurring

Originated by: **Cheryl A. King, RN, BSN**
Resource person: **Deidra Gradishar, RNC BA**

Prolapsed Cord (Viable Infant)—cont'd

NURSING DIAGNOSIS/ PATIENT PROBLEM	DEFINING CHARACTERISTICS	NURSING ORDERS		EXPECTED OUTCOMES
		ASSESSMENT	INTERVENTIONS	
Knowledge deficit Etiology New condition/procedures regarding fetal distress	Apparent confusion over events Multiple questions Lack of questions Expressed need for more information	A. Assess patient's understanding of fetal distress B. Assess anxiety and discomfort as possible deterrents to understanding explanations C. Refer to SCP in this chapter: Fetal distress	Provide information (include significant other) regarding A. Known/possible causes of fetal distress B. Misconceptions	Patient will verbalize an understanding of fetal distress

Sore Nipples in the Breast-Feeding Mother

NURSING DIAGNOSIS/ PATIENT PROBLEM	DEFINING CHARACTERISTICS	NURSING ORDERS		EXPECTED OUTCOMES
		ASSESSMENT	INTERVENTIONS	
Comfort, alteration in Etiology Sore nipples	Nipples red Nipples cracked Mother complains of nipple discomfort throughout breast-feeding session	A. Assess nipples daily B. Identify factors contributing to sore nipples	A. Teach mother the following preventive measures, as appropriate 1. Follow prenatal conditioning exercises, i.e., nipple rolling, Hoffman technique, milk cups 2. Use no soap, alcohol, or petroleum-based products on nipple 3. Air-dry nipples 10-15 min after nursing at least four times a day 4. Apply a scant amount of Massé cream or A and D ointment after air-drying. Vitamin E oil 400 IU may also be used 5. Feed the baby on demand (usually q.2-3h.) 6. Do not allow breasts to become overly full, as this flattens out nipples, making them more difficult to grasp 7. Use proper nursing position (see LaLeche League Reprint No. 11: "Managing Nipple Problems")	A. Mother will demonstrate proper preventive measures B. If sore nipples develop, mother will use appropriate treatment measures

Continued.

Sore Nipples in the Breast-Feeding Mother—cont'd

NURSING DIAGNOSIS/ PATIENT PROBLEM	DEFINING CHARACTERISTICS	NURSING ORDERS		EXPECTED OUTCOMES
		ASSESSMENT	INTERVENTIONS	
			8. Allow unlimited sucking time after ensuring correct position 9. Break suction correctly 10. Change nursing position periodically to distribute the sucking pressure to different parts of the nipple 11. Avoid nipple shields B. If sore nipples develop, teach mother the following treatment measures, as appropriate 　1. Nurse on the least sore side first 　2. Adjust position at the breast so that the baby's jaws exert pressure on the least tender spots 　3. If necessary, soften the areola before each nursing by expressing a little milk 　4. Use relaxation-breathing techniques to encourage letdown 　5. Do not pull away when putting baby to breast. Some women unconsciously move back as the infant begins to draw the nipple into his/her mouth 　6. Apply expressed breast milk to nipples, and allow them to dry, or use a hair dryer on low/warm setting. This will promote healing and is especially good for cracked nipples 　7. Apply crushed ice in cold washcloth to the nipples immediately before nursing. This eases nipple pain and also helps to bring out nipples C. Provide emotional support. Reassure the mother that she can continue breast-feeding	

Originated by **Jackie Suprenant, RN, BSN**

ASSESSMENTS/THERAPEUTIC INTERVENTIONS

Cesarean Birth, Acute/Emergency: preoperative

NURSING DIAGNOSIS/ PATIENT PROBLEM	DEFINING CHARACTERISTICS	NURSING ORDERS		EXPECTED OUTCOMES
		ASSESSMENT	INTERVENTIONS	

Knowledge deficit
 Etiology
 Unfamiliarity with procedure
	Expresses need for more information
	 Multiple questions or lack of questions
	 Confusion
		A. Assess patient's knowledge regarding cesarean section
		 B. Identify priorities for patient teaching based on patient need, preference, and available time/ resources
			A. Discuss with mother/significant other the reason for cesarean section
			 B. Explain "normal" preoperative procedures and modifications for current situation
			   1. Obtaining consent form and baseline vital signs
			   2. Drawing blood for CBC, electrolytes, type, and screen
			   3. Obtaining urine for urinalysis
			   4. Insertion of Foley catheter
			   5. Choosing type of anesthesia (general, spinal, or epidural)
			   6. Maintaining NPO status
			   7. Performing abdominal preparation
			   8. Administering IV fluids
			   9. Removing dentures, contact lenses, jewelry, fingernail polish
			 C. Inform patient that husband/ significant other *may* be present in the OR as appropriate
				Patient will verbalize understanding of/ and rationale for cesarean section procedure

Anxiety/fear **Etiology** Uncertain outcome for infant	Ambivalence Inability to communicate Disappointment Expressed fear Restlessness Tearfulness Trembling	Assess mother's understanding of present status and expected outcome of infant	A. Encourage patient to verbalize concerns B. Provide patient with realistic information regarding status of infant C. Inform patient that pediatric resident will be present during cesarean section and that emergency equipment will be available D. Encourage husband/significant other to be present in OR (as indicated)	Patient will be provided the opportunity to verbalize fears and concerns regarding infant
Self-concept, disturbance in **Etiology** Interruption in anticipated birth plan	Verbalizing sense of failure at not delivering "normally" Feelings of being cheated/disappointed Feelings of intrusion from surgical procedure	A. Identify verbal/ nonverbal behaviors that may suggest patient feels responsible for cesarean section B. Assess patient's perception of herself and usual coping abilities	A. Encourage and allow patient to ventilate fears and feelings of guilt and blame B. Provide support through reassurance and open nonjudgmental approach C. Include husband or significant other in discussions D. Provide positive feedback to patient and significant other	Patient will begin to verbalize expressions of continued self-worth

Originated by **Elicita A. Chaves, RN**
Resource person: **Jane Parker, RNC BAN**

Cesarean Birth: postpartum care

NURSING DIAGNOSIS/ PATIENT PROBLEM	DEFINING CHARACTERISTICS	NURSING ORDERS		EXPECTED OUTCOMES
		ASSESSMENT	INTERVENTIONS	
Impairment of uterine involution: potential **Etiology** Bladder distention Uterine atony Retained placental fragments/infection	Boggy, displaced uterus Persistent discharge of lochia rubra or return of lochia rubra Hemorrhage Foul-smelling lochia Uterine tenderness	A. Assess fundus, lochia, and bladder B. Evaluate vital signs for evidence of infection or hemorrhage	A. Massage fundus if not firm B. Notify physician of deviations from baseline parameters	Involution progressing normally as evidenced by A. Firm fundus B. Lochia change from rubra to serosa by third to fourth postpartum day
Injury, potential for: infection **Etiology** Altered skin integrity: incisions	Redness Tenderness Reports of pain Seropurulent discharge Elevated temperature Swelling	A. Observe incision for signs of infection (see Defining Characteristics) B. Monitor vital signs for evidence of infection	Change dressing as needed or per physician's order	Incision will be healing well as evidenced by absence of signs/symptoms of infection
Urinary elimination, altered patterns: potential **Etiology** Edema Hyperemia of bladder Increased capacity and decreased sensation of bladder filling	Bladder distention Uterus elevated and deviated from midline Inability to void (reports by patient)	A. Palpate bladder for distention B. Assess for signs/symptoms of urinary infection: urgency, frequency, burning on urination, fever C. Measure urinary output as indicated	A. Encourage voiding q.4-6h. during the day B. Employ techniques to facilitate voiding as needed C. Explain perineal care procedure	Patient will void spontaneously and without discomfort
Bowel elimination, alteration in: constipation (potential) **Etiology** Decreased hormonal levels Decreased muscle tone in the intestine Decreased intraabdominal pressure	Straining at stool Hard, formed stool	A. Assess for presence of bowel sounds daily until bowel function is established B. Ask patient if she is passing flatus or belching C. Monitor intake and tolerance of each dietary change	A. Encourage patient to 1. Ambulate as tolerated 2. Increase intake of fluids when permitted (2000-3000 ml daily) 3. Include fruit and roughage in diet B. Give stool softener/laxative as ordered, and monitor effectiveness	Patient will have bowel movement within 3-5 days after surgery
Airway clearance, ineffective: potential **Etiology** Surgery Immobility Pain	Increased respiratory rate Nonproductive cough Audible rhonci Congestion	Assess respiratory status (see Defining Characteristics)	A. Encourage patient to cough, turn, and deep breathe q.2h. during first postoperative day, then as needed B. Demonstrate splinting as a method to support incision during this activity C. Encourage use of incentive spirometer D. Encourage ambulation	Respiratory congestion/infection will not occur

Originated by **Paulette E. Brevard, RN, BSN**
Resource person: **Jackie Suprenant, RN, BSN**

Cesarean Birth: postpartum care—cont'd

NURSING DIAGNOSIS/ PATIENT PROBLEM	DEFINING CHARACTERISTICS	NURSING ORDERS		EXPECTED OUTCOMES
		ASSESSMENT	INTERVENTIONS	
Comfort, alteration in **Etiology** Incisional or afterbirth pains	Reports of pain at incisional site/abdomen Facial mask of pain Decreased mobility Relief/distraction behavior	A. Assess location, intensity, and duration of pain B. Assess effects of pain on ADL, including ability to provide infant care C. Assess predisposing factors that lead to pain	A. Anticipate need for analgesics and/or additional methods of pain relief B. Administer pain medication as ordered and evaluate its effectiveness C. Provide other comfort measures that may be helpful, such as repositioning, or changing environment	Patient will verbalize minimization of pain following pain-relief measures
Etiology Breast engorgement	Breasts distended and hard Patient reports breast discomfort	Palpate the breasts daily, checking for engorgement, heat, and tenderness	A. Instruct mother to wear supportive bra 24 hours a day B. If engorgement develops in bottle-feeding mother, apply breast binder and ice packs as needed and administer pain medication if necessary. In lactating mother, see SCP in this chapter: Breast engorgement in breast-feeding mother C. Explain cause of engorgement and that it will disappear within 48-72 hours	The patient, on discharge, will experience minimal or no breast engorgement as evidenced by A. Minimal or no reports of breast discomfort B. No signs/symptoms of engorgement on examination
Circulation, alteration in: peripheral/tissue (deep vein thrombosis, pulmonary embolism) (potential) **Etiology** Increased coagulation factors Decreased mobility	**Deep vein thrombosis** Localized tenderness Calf pain Redness Swelling Elevated temperature Positive Homans' sign **Pulmonary embolism** Chest pain Dyspnea Tachycardia Change in BP	Assess for signs and symptoms of pulmonary embolism and deep vein thrombosis (see Defining Characteristics)	A. Assist with early ambulation B. Provide appropriate patient teaching 1. No leg crossing for 1 week 2. Elevate feet as needed	A. The patient will ambulate within 12 hours of delivery or as ordered by the physician B. The patient will exhibit no signs and symptoms of pulmonary embolism or deep vein thrombosis during hospitalization
Knowledge deficit **Etiology** Unfamiliarity with self-care and infant care	Multiple questions Confusion	Assess learning needs of mother regarding self-care and infant care	A. Provide teaching based on mother's learning needs B. Encourage mother and significant other to participate in infant care. Provide assistance as needed	Patient will demonstrate appropriate self-care and infant care
Development of mother-infant attachment **Etiology** Parenting role	Holds infant close to body Establishes eye contact with infant Talks to infant in soothing or playful manner	Observe maternal/infant interactions	A. Provide opportunity for maternal/infant interactions. Involve father or significant other whenever possible B. Provide support and encouragement as the parents begin to interact and care for the infant	Patient will demonstrate appropriate attachment behavior with infant

Continued.

Cesarean Birth: postpartum care—cont'd

NURSING DIAGNOSIS/ PATIENT PROBLEM	DEFINING CHARACTERISTICS	NURSING ORDERS		EXPECTED OUTCOMES
		ASSESSMENT	INTERVENTIONS	
Emotional adjustment **Etiology** Childbirth experience Parenting role	The patient will process and verbalize feelings regarding Childbirth Ability to parent Changes in interpersonal relationships	A. Assess emotional status B. Assess mother's feelings regarding a cesarean delivery rather than a vaginal delivery	A. Allow free discussion of real and perceived problems B. Provide opportunity for labor review. Help mother internalize the reality of her labor and delivery experience C. Provide reassurance in patient's ability as a mother D. Accept emotional ups and downs of postpartum period, and explain that such changes are common at this time E. Encourage mother to rest periodically throughout the day	Patient will begin to demonstrate effective emotional adjustment

Dilation and Curettage (D & C) and Cone Biopsy

NURSING DIAGNOSIS/ PATIENT PROBLEM	DEFINING CHARACTERISTICS	NURSING ORDERS		EXPECTED OUTCOMES
		ASSESSMENT	INTERVENTIONS	
Knowledge deficit **Etiology** New surgical procedure	Verbalizes lack of knowledge about nature of D & C and cone biopsy Asks numerous questions or none at all Puts call light on frequently	Assess patient's knowledge about nature of D & C and cone biopsy, including postoperative expectations	A. Provide careful explanations regarding procedures involved, amount of vaginal drainage expected, and restriction on activity B. Instruct patient to notify staff if excessive, bright-red vaginal drainage occurs C. Instruct patient to refrain from sexual activity, vaginal douching, and tampons until advised by physician	Patient will verbalize an understanding of D & C and cone biopsy procedure
Fluid volume deficit: potential **Etiology** Excessive vaginal bleeding	Reports faintness, dizziness, apprehension, and thirst Saturates perineal pads easily (a blood loss of at least 60 ml is required to saturate a perineal pad) Weak, rapid pulse, and rapid respirations that become progressively shallow; early slight rise in BP Decrease in urinary output	A. Assess vaginal bleeding, noting amount of volume lost (spotting, mild, moderate, or profuse) and number of perineal pads used B. Observe for changes that may indicate active bleeding (see Defining Characteristics)	A. Notify physician of excessive vaginal bleeding, marked changes in vital signs, and abnormal Hb and Hct values B. See SCP in Ch. 1: Fluid volume deficit	Fluid volume deficit will be minimized

Originated by **Fe Corazon R. Mendoza, RN, BSN**
Resource person: **Jackie Suprenant, RN, BSN**

Dilation and Curettage (D & C) and Cone Biopsy—cont'd

NURSING DIAGNOSIS/ PATIENT PROBLEM	DEFINING CHARACTERISTICS	NURSING ORDERS		EXPECTED OUTCOMES
		ASSESSMENT	INTERVENTIONS	
Anxiety: potential Etiology New diagnosis	Restlessness Increased awareness Increased questioning Withdrawal	A. Assess patient's level of anxiety (mild, moderate, severe, panic) B. Identify factors causing or contributing to anxiety	A. Provide a therapeutic climate and encourage patient to express her feelings and ask questions B. Recognize the uniqueness of the surgical experience to the patient. Listen to what the patient says C. Provide reasonable explanations that are reality based. Correct misconceptions and misinformation D. Provide only the information that patient wants, needs, and can interpret E. See SCP in Ch. 1: Anxiety/fear	Anxiety level will be minimized

Laparoscopy, Hysteroscopy, and Endometrial Biopsy: postoperative care

NURSING DIAGNOSIS/ PATIENT PROBLEM	DEFINING CHARACTERISTICS	NURSING ORDERS		EXPECTED OUTCOMES
		ASSESSMENT	INTERVENTIONS	
Knowledge deficit Etiology Surgical procedure and follow-up home care	Verbalizes lack of knowledge Expresses a need for more information Asks repetitive questions	A. Assess need for teaching in terms of patient's understanding of procedure B. Assess level of education C. Encourage patient and family members to ask questions and express concerns	A. Provide preoperative teaching, using teaching manual and surgical program on closed-circuit television B. Discuss preoperative procedures and postoperative expectations in terms suited to intellectual/cognitive level of patient C. Respond appropriately to questions and concerns D. Provide going-home instructions when patient demonstrates readiness to learn E. Include information on 1. Nutritional needs 2. Activity level 3. Incision care 4. Vaginal discharge 5. Resumption of intercourse 6. Avoidance of tampons and douching 7. Follow-up appointment with physician	Patient will verbalize a basic understanding of A. Surgical experience B. Going-home instructions
Fluid volume deficit: potential Etiology NPO Poor appetite Nausea and vomiting	Decreased urine output Decreased venous filling Decreased skin turgor	A. Assess hydration status, skin turgor, mucous membranes, I & O as indicated B. Assess tolerance to oral fluids when instituted	See SCP in Ch. 1: Fluid volume deficit	Adequate fluid volume balance will be evidenced by A. Urine output >30 ml/hour B. Normal skin turgor C. Moist mucous membranes

Originated by **Lydia Serra, RN**
Resource person: **Jackie Suprenant, RN, BSN**

Continued.

Laparoscopy, Hysteroscopy, and Endometrial Biopsy: postoperative care—cont'd

NURSING DIAGNOSIS/ PATIENT PROBLEM	DEFINING CHARACTERISTICS	NURSING ORDERS		EXPECTED OUTCOMES
		ASSESSMENT	INTERVENTIONS	
Comfort, alteration in **Etiology** Surgical procedure and intubation	Reports pain in incisional site and/or shoulders Evidences decreased mobility Reports sore throat	A. Assess location, duration, quality, and intensity of pain B. Assess effect of pain reliever(s)	A. Apply heating pad for shoulder discomfort B. Offer throat lozenges and warm NS solution gargle for sore throat C. See SCP in Ch. 1: Comfort, alteration in: pain	Patient will verbalize minimization of pain following relief measures
Injury, potential for: **wound infection** **Etiology** Altered skin integrity	Redness Tenderness Swelling Pain Elevated temperature	Evaluate vital signs and incision site for indications of infection (see Defining Characteristics)	A. Change dressing as needed as ordered by physician B. Notify physician when evidence of infection is present	Incision will be clean and dry with no sign of infection
Anxiety/fear **Etiology** Uncertainty of surgical diagnostic results	Chain smoking Crying Constant talking on telephone Nonconversant with staff or roommate Isolates self by drawing drapes around bed Agitation Restlessness	A. Assess patient and significant others for signs and symptoms of anxiety (see Defining Characteristics) B. Note degree of anxiety (mild, moderate, severe)	See SCP in Ch 1: Anxiety/fear	Anxiety/fear will be minimized or prevented
Coping, ineffective: **potential** **Etiology** Difficult adaptation to infertility	Verbalization of inability to cope Inability to meet basic needs Noncompliance with treatment plan	A. Note expressed feeling of hopelessness, helplessness, and powerlessness B. Observe for inappropriate expression of anger/hostility/loss of control C. Note weeping, irritability, and expressed feelings of incompetence D. Observe for expressed overdependency E. Assess noncompliance with treatment plan or other problematic behavior	See SCP in this chapter: Infertility as emotional crisis	Patient will demonstrate a calm, unthreatened approach to diagnostic testing

Maternal/Infant Bonding

NURSING DIAGNOSIS/ PATIENT PROBLEM	DEFINING CHARACTERISTICS	NURSING ORDERS		EXPECTED OUTCOMES
		ASSESSMENT	INTERVENTIONS	
Development of parent-infant attachment **Etiology** Delivery of newborn	Initial face-to-face (visual) contact between parents and infant Initial tactile contact (postpartum) between parents and infant Initial auditory contact (postpartum) between parents and infant	A. Assess patient's knowledge base regarding bonding with infant B. Assess patient's readiness/desire to bond with infant C. Assess factors that may interfere with bonding process 1. Physical 2. Psychosocial	A. Place mirror or position patient (and significant other) for viewing delivery of infant when requested/possible B. Allow patient to hold infant immediately after delivery when possible; assist when necessary C. Allow patient to see and, if possible, to hold stabilized infant as soon as possible D. Encourage/aid patient to visually examine infant (head to toe) E. Encourage/aid patient to touch infant F. Encourage patient to talk to infant G. Aid father/significant other with Leboyer bath if desired H. Allow breast-feeding when requested. Aid patient when necessary I. Allow patient and infant to remain together in constant care unit when requested (per physician's order) or allow patient/significant other and infant time alone (in viewing room) J. Hold infant at eye level for patient unable to hold, e.g., because of anesthesia, surgery K. Encourage father/significant other to hold infant in delivery room, especially at times when patient is unable, e.g., during cesarean section, repair of episiotomy L. Bring infant from nursery (if possible) to patient who must remain in labor rooms because of complications of pregnancy/delivery, e.g., postpartum pregnancy-induced hypertension M. Bring picture of compromised infant from special care nursery to patient who must remain in labor room N. Inform patient and significant other that, as condition permits, they can go to special care nursery to see infant at any time. Accompany when necessary O. Encourage reluctant patient/significant other to bond with infant P. Reinforce/commend positive bonding behavior Q. Document bonding behaviors in newborn nursery nursing notes	Opportunity to establish communication/bonding between mother/significant other and infant will be offered and evidenced by visual, tactile, and auditory contact

Originated by **Kathy V. Stewart, RN**
Resource person: **Jane Parker, RNC BAN**

Neonate, Evaluation of: in delivery room

NURSING DIAGNOSIS/ PATIENT PROBLEM	DEFINING CHARACTERISTICS	NURSING ORDERS		EXPECTED OUTCOMES
		ASSESSMENT	INTERVENTIONS	

Respiratory dysfunction: potential
 Etiology
 Transition to extra-uterine life
	Cyanosis (other than acrocyanosis)
	 Retractions
	 Nasal flaring
	 Grunting
	 Tachypnea ($\geq$60/min)
	 Bradypnea ($\leq$ 40/min)
	 Absence of cry
	 Absent respirations
		A. Assess for visible anomalies affecting normal respiratory function
		 B. Assess factors affecting respiratory status: e.g., prematurity, meconium-stained amniotic fluid, type of delivery, maternal premedication, presence of fetal distress during labor
		 C. Evaluate need for ventilatory assistance
			A. Assemble resuscitation equipment before delivery
			 B. Maintain patency of airway
			   1. Suction nose and oropharynx with bulb syringe or DeLee trap
			   2. Position infant in modified Trendelenburg's position
			 C. Stimulate crying by gently tapping feet or rubbing sternum
			 D. Institute measures to relieve respiratory distress
			   1. Administer free O_2 per tube at 10 L/min with tube at an angle and 1-2 inches from nose for cyanosis, nasal flaring, or mild retractions
			   2. Begin ventilatory assistance with Ambu bag (40 to 60/min) for slow or absent respiratory effort
			 E. Notify pediatrician to evaluate infant
			 F. Maintain stable body temperature (see following Nursing Diagnosis)
				Respirations of 40-60/min will be established and maintained after birth

Hypothermia: potential
 Etiology
 Altered environment
	Temperature <37° C
	 Cyanosis
	 Decreased or shallow respirations
	 Retractions
	 Bradycardia
	 Decreased reflexes
	 Nasal flaring
		Assess newborn for signs of hypothermia (see Defining Characteristics)	A. Dry infant with warm blankets (especially the head) immediately after delivery
			 B. Place infant in heated radiant warmer
			   1. Preset temperature at 37° C (98.6° F)
			   2. Expose infant's unwrapped body to radiant heat
			   3. Tape temperature probe to abdomen
			   4. Place cap on infant's head
			 C. Provide for temperature maintenance during bonding
			   1. Dry infant during or before bonding
			   2. Allow maternal/infant skin-to-skin contact
			   3. Cover both with warm, dry blankets
			 D. Maintain temperature during transport
			   1. Use prewarmed Isolette
			   2. Keep portholes closed
				Loss of body heat associated with change in environment will be minimized

Originated by **Bernadette Keller, RNC**
Resource person: **Jane Parker, RNC BAN**

Neonate, Evaluation of: in delivery room—cont'd

NURSING DIAGNOSIS/ PATIENT PROBLEM	DEFINING CHARACTERISTICS	NURSING ORDERS		EXPECTED OUTCOMES
		ASSESSMENT	INTERVENTIONS	
Injury, potential for: **to infant** **Etiology** Difficulty in adapting to extrauterine live Presence of birth trauma or anomalies	**Respiratory** Slow, irregular respiratory pattern Blocked airway Excess secretions **Cardiovascular** Slow heart rate Cyanosis Hyporeflexia Number of vessels in cord Edema **Neurologic system** Unusual size and shape of head Paralysis of face or extremities Poor reflex response **Musculoskeletal** Polydactyly Absent or malformed extremities Hip dysplasia Meningocele or omphalocele **Skin integrity** Rash Lacerations Forcep marks **Genitourinary system** Abnormal genitalia Urinary function (abnormal) **Gastrointestinal system** Cleft palate Abnormal stools	A. Assign and document Apgar score at 1 and 5 min. If score is below 7, repeat scoring again at 10 min B. Evaluate physical status immediately after birth and document abnormalities 1. Respiratory system 2. Cardiovascular function 3. Neurologic system 4. Musculoskeletal system 5. Skin integrity 6. Genitourinary system 7. Gastrointestinal system	A. Establish and maintain adequate respiration (see first Nursing Diagnosis) and circulation 1. Apgar score of 7-10: no special interventions required 2. Apgar of 4-6: ensure patent airway; provide ventilatory support 3. Apgar of 0-3: institute resuscitative measures immediately (see hospital policy concerning CPR) B. Apply sterile dressing moistened with saline to exposed external organs as indicated C. Inform parents of visible anomalies before bonding. Provide emotional support D. Notify pediatrician for further evaluation of any suspected irregularities E. Document in nursing notes any deviations in physical status F. Transfer infant to special care nursery as soon as possible (if indicated)	Potential for injury to the infant will be minimized

Oxytocin Induction/Augmentation of Labor

NURSING DIAGNOSIS/ PATIENT PROBLEM	DEFINING CHARACTERISTICS	NURSING ORDERS		EXPECTED OUTCOMES
		ASSESSMENT	INTERVENTIONS	
Knowledge deficit **Etiology** Unfamiliarity with induction/augmentation of labor procedure	Apparent confusion over events Multiple questions or lack of questions Expressed need for more information Expressed fear over chemical stimulation of labor	Assess patient's knowledge regarding oxytocin induction of labor	A. Provide environment conducive to learning B. Reinforce physicians' explanations C. Explain at patient's present level of understanding D. Provide information regarding 1. Indications for procedure 2. Methodology of administration 3. Expected effects of oxytocin induction/augmentation of labor 4. How induction/augmentation differs from normal spontaneous contractions	Patient will verbalize understanding of A. Indications B. Methodology C. Expected effects of oxytocin induction/augmentation of labor
Injury, potential for **Etiology** Hyperstimulation Abruption Uterine rupture	**Hypertonicity** Failure to establish uterine resting tone between contractions Contraction frequency every 2 min Contraction duration of 90 seconds **Abruption** Rising uterus Severe restlessness Fundal pain Vaginal pain Shock **Uterine rupture** Vaginal bleeding Cessation of pain Shock	A. Monitor contractions electronically. Observe and document the following, per protocol 1. Length of contractions 2. Frequency of contractions 3. Intensity of contractions 4. Periods of uterine relaxation B. Assess and document color and amount of vaginal bleeding C. Monitor and record BP, pulse, and respirations every _____ if patient is in shock D. Measure fundal height and abdominal girth every _____ E. Assess and document patient's level of consciousness	A. On written order of physician, administer the oxytocin by Harvard pump at prescribed rate. Refer to policy and procedure manual B. Discontinue infusion, and notify physician immediately if 1. The uterus fails to relax between contractions 2. Patient reports changes in her perception of abdominal pain 3. There is a change or increase in fundal height or abdominal girth C. Inform physician of changes in 1. Vital signs 2. Level of consciousness 3. Behavior D. Maintain complete bed rest E. Administer parenteral fluids as ordered by the physician F. If symptoms of shock occur, institute the appropriate SCP for the treatment, e.g., SCP in Ch. 13: Hypovolemic shock; or SCP in this chapter: Abruptio placentae G. On order of the physician prepare the patient for an emergency cesarean section (see SCP in this chapter: Cesarean birth, acute/emergency: preoperative)	Injury to the mother will be minimized

Originated by **Mary Chris McCarthy, RN, BSN**
Resource persons: **Jane Parker, RNC BAN**
    Deidra Gradishar, RNC BA

Oxytocin Induction/Augmentation of Labor—cont'd

NURSING DIAGNOSIS/ PATIENT PROBLEM	DEFINING CHARACTERISTICS	NURSING ORDERS		EXPECTED OUTCOMES
		ASSESSMENT	INTERVENTIONS	
		F. Ask patient to verbalize changes in her perception of contractions; she may 1. Experience sharp and shooting continuous pain 2. Cry out "Something tore inside me" 3. Experience sudden relief from pain 4. Have cessation of uterine contractions		
Injury, potential for: to the fetus **Etiology** Uteroplacental insufficiency	Significant changes in baseline fetal heart: fetal tachycardia; fetal bradycardia Late decelerations Variable decelerations that last more than 1 min and/or fall below 60 BPM Baseline variability <5 BPM	A. Assess fetal heart rate by electronic monitoring for 15 min before initiation of oxytocin infusion B. Assess and document, with each increase/decrease of infusion pump (or more frequently if indicated) 1. Baseline fetal heart rate 2. Baseline fetal heart rate variability 3. Periodic patterns: absence or presence 4. Contraction frequency; resting tone	A. Discontinue oxytocin immediately, and notify physician in the event of untoward changes in fetal heart rate parameters B. If tracing denotes the presence of fetal distress, institute SCP in this chapter: Fetal distress C. Prepare for the delivery of a compromised neonate 1. Notify pediatrician 2. Check pediatric boards (emergency equipment for infant resuscitation) 3. Check transporter	Injury to the fetus will be minimized
Comfort, alteration in **Etiology** Uterine contractions	Patient verbalizes severe pain Thrashing in bed Facial grimacing Hyperventilation/hypoventilation	A. Elicit patient's perception of discomfort related to uterine contractions B. Assess other factors that may be contributing to discomfort C. Assess mechanisms patient uses to manage discomfort D. Assess patient's understanding of contractile pattern in labor	A. Explain cyclic nature of uterine contraction pattern B. Use nonpharmacologic comfort measures when appropriate C. Eliminate or minimize, when possible, other factors that may be contributing to discomfort 1. Encourage frequent voiding 2. Keep patient informed of labor and fetal status D. Administer analgesic medication as ordered E. Provide positive reinforcement and personal contact F. Encourage presence of support person	Patient will verbalize an understanding of why she is experiencing the discomfort associated with labor process

Tubal Pregnancy: preoperative care

NURSING DIAGNOSIS/ PATIENT PROBLEM	DEFINING CHARACTERISTICS	NURSING ORDERS		EXPECTED OUTCOMES
		ASSESSMENT	INTERVENTIONS	
Comfort, alteration in Etiology Tubal pregnancy	**Prodromal** Low abdominal pain and tenderness that may be unilateral or general **Ruptured** Severe lower abdominal pain; may be sudden and stabbing Rectal pressure Referred supraclavicular pain Rebound tenderness, guarding Pain with movement of cervix during vaginal examination	A. Elicit patient's description of discomfort or pain 1. Location 2. Quality 3. Severity 4. Correlation with examinations B. Assess the mechanisms the patient presently uses to deal with discomfort or pain C. Assess other factors that may be contributing to discomfort, e.g., fear and anxiety	A. Minimize or eliminate possible factors that may be contributing to discomfort B. Use nonpharmacologic comfort measures such as 1. Position change 2. Relaxation techniques 3. Distraction techniques C. Provide emotional support, especially if analgesia is contraindicated at this time D. Administer analgesia as ordered by physician. Observe for any untoward reactions	Patient will be able to A. Describe pain B. Verbalize changes in pain sensations
Fluid volume deficit: potential Etiology Ruptured fallopian tube	Tachycardia Hypotension Dyspnea Cyanosis of mucous membranes and nail beds Vaginal bleeding Palpation of fluid-filled rigid mass **Signs and symptoms of shock** Decreasing arterial pressures Increasing pulse rate Cold, clammy skin Alterations of neurologic status Decreasing urine volume Sharp intense sensation of pain	A. Monitor pulse, BP and respiration every 15 min until stable, then every _____ B. Review results of Hb and Hct, and notify physician of deviations C. Assess level of consciousness D. Assess quality and color of vaginal bleeding every _____ E. Initiate peri-pad use F. Assess I & O every _____ G. Assess mucous membranes, nail beds, and skin turgor every _____	A. Maintain complete bed rest B. Notify physician of deviations from baseline parameters C. If symptoms of shock occur, prepare for second intravenous line for administration of volume expanders/blood and blood components as ordered by physician D. Prepare patient for possibility of surgical intervention 1. Obtain consent form 2. Draw blood for CBC, electrolytes, type and screen/type and cross-match, VDRL* test as ordered by physician 3. Obtain urine for urinalysis/dipstick as ordered by physician 4. Maintain NPO status 5. Prepare and shave abdomen as ordered by physician 6. Obtain chest x-ray examination and ECG as ordered by physician 7. Complete preoperative checklist	A. Potential for severe fluid loss will be minimized B. Adequate tissue perfusion will be maintained as evidenced by 1. Normal skin turgor and color 2. Stable vital signs 3. Adequate urinary output

Originated by **Denise Pang, RN, BSN**
Resource person: **Deidra Gradishar, RNC BA**
*Venereal Disease Research Laboratories.

Tubal Pregnancy: preoperative care—cont'd

NURSING DIAGNOSIS/ PATIENT PROBLEM	DEFINING CHARACTERISTICS	NURSING ORDERS		EXPECTED OUTCOMES
		ASSESSMENT	INTERVENTIONS	
Grieving **Etiology** Loss of pregnancy Loss of reproductive potential	Verbal expression of distress over loss Anger Sadness, crying Regression Alterations in thought process Guilt or rumination Inappropriate affect	Observe for verbal or nonverbal expression of grief	See SCP in Ch. 1: Grieving, dysfunctional: failure to grieve	Patient will begin to verbally express feelings of grief and loss of pregnancy
Knowledge deficit **Etiology** Unfamiliarity of tubal pregnancy, its causes, treatment, and outcome	Overt confusion over events Inability to comprehend or retain information Multiple questions or lack of questions Patient expresses need for more information	A. Assess patient's knowledge base regarding ectopic pregnancy B. Assess patient's level of understanding and educational background C. Assess to what degree anxiety or level of discomfort may influence patient's capacity to understand explanations and events D. Identify priorities for patient teaching based on patient's needs and availability of time and resources	A. Provide information regarding 1. Possible causes of tubal pregnancy 2. Reasons for hospitalization and possibility of surgery B. When applicable, explain procedures that will aid in diagnosis such as 1. Vaginal/speculum examination 2. Culdocentesis 3. Pregnancy test 4. Ultrasonography 5. Laparoscopy C. Explain the treatment and nursing interventions of tubal pregnancy 1. Frequent nursing surveillance 2. Preoperative procedures to prepare for surgical intervention 3. Postoperative procedures D. Reinforce the physician's explanations E. Simplify explanations and repeat when necessary F. Include the significant other when possible	Patient will verbalize a basic understanding of tubal pregnancy and nursing interventions related to tubal pregnancy

Vaginal Delivery, Normal Spontaneous: postpartum care

NURSING DIAGNOSIS/ PATIENT PROBLEM	DEFINING CHARACTERISTICS	NURSING ORDERS		EXPECTED OUTCOMES
		ASSESSMENT	INTERVENTIONS	
Uterine involution, impairment of: potential **Etiology** Bladder distention Uterine atony Retained placental fragments and/or infection	Boggy, displaced uterus Persistent discharge of lochia rubra or return of lochia rubra Hemorrhage Four-smelling lochia Uterine tenderness	A. Assess fundus, lochia, and bladder (see hospital policy and procedure manual regarding care of the postpartum patient) B. Monitor vital signs for evidence of infection or hemorrhage	A. Massage fundus if not firm. Mother may be taught self-massage B. If bladder is distended, encourage patient to void (see also Nursing Diagnosis on urinary elimination later in this SCP) C. In case of postpartum hemorrhage, see SCP earlier in this chapter: Postpartum hemorrhage following vaginal delivery	A. Fundus will be firm and without pain B. Fundal height will progressively descend
Injury, potential for: infection **Etiology** Episiotomy/laceration(s)	Fever Seropurulent discharge Redness	Examine episiotomy/ lacerations for redness, edema, discharge, ecchymosis, and approximation	A. Instruct patient on perineal care (see hospital policy and procedure manual on perineal self-care) B. Instruct patient on use of sitz bath	Episiotomy/lacerations will heal without evidence of infection
Comfort, alteration in: potential **Etiology** Episiotomy and/or afterbirth pains	Patient reports pain Guarding behavior Facial mask of pain	A. Solicit patient's description of pain B. Assess pain characteristics (quality, severity, location, onset, duration, precipitating factors) C. Assess effects of pain on ADL, including ability to provide infant care	A. Anticipate need for analgesics/ additional methods of pain relief B. Administer pain medication as ordered and evaluate its effectiveness C. For episiotomy discomfort, instruct mother to squeeze buttocks together when sitting down D. For afterbirth pains during breast-feeding, encourage mother to use relaxation breathing techniques learned in childbirth class	Patient's pain will be relieved or minimized
Bowel elimination, alteration in: constipation (potential) **Etiology** Decreased hormonal levels Decreased muscle tone in intestine Decreased intraabdominal pressure	Patient reports abdominal pain, back pain, and/or headache Straining at stool Hard-formed stool	A. Assess bowel function daily B. Assess for presence of hemorrhoids, and treat as ordered	A. Give stool softener or laxative as ordered B. Encourage patient to 1. Ambulate as tolerated 2. Increase intake of fluids (2000-3000 ml daily) 3. Include fruit and roughage in diet	The patient will demonstrate measures that will prevent constipation
Urinary elimination, alteration in patterns: potential **Etiology** Edema Hyperemia of bladder Increased capacity of bladder Decreased sensation of bladder filling	Bladder distention Uterus elevated and deviated from midline Patient reports inability to void	A. Evaluate bladder for distention B. Assess for signs/ symptoms of urinary infection (urgency, frequency, burning, fever) C. Measure urinary output as indicated	A. Encourage patient to void q.4-6h. throughout the day B. Employ techniques to facilitate voiding as needed	Patient will void spontaneously and without discomfort

Originated by **Jackie Suprenant, RN, BSN**

Vaginal Delivery, Normal Spontaneous: postpartum care—cont'd

NURSING DIAGNOSIS/ PATIENT PROBLEM	DEFINING CHARACTERISTICS	NURSING ORDERS		EXPECTED OUTCOMES
		ASSESSMENT	INTERVENTIONS	
Comfort, alteration in: breast discomfort (potential) **Etiology** Engorgement	Breasts distended and hard Patient reports discomfort	Palpate the breasts daily, checking for distention, heat, and tenderness	A. Instruct mother to wear supportive brassiere 24 hours/day B. If engorgement develops in bottle-feeding mother, apply breast binder and ice packs as needed, and administer pain medication if necessary. In the lactating mother, see SCP in this chapter: Breast engorgement in breast-feeding mother	Patient will demonstrate proper breast care
Circulation, interruption in: peripheral/ pulmonary (potential) deep vein thrombosis/ pulmonary embolism **Etiology** Increased coagulation factors	**Deep vein thrombosis** Localized tenderness Calf pain Redness Swelling Elevated temperature Positive Homans' sign **Pulmonary embolism** Chest pain Dyspnea Tachycardia Change in BP	Assess for signs and symptoms of pulmonary embolism and deep vein thrombosis (see Defining Characteristics)	A. Assist with early ambulation B. Provide appropriate patient teaching 1. No leg crossing for 1 week 2. Elevate feet as necessary	A. Patient will ambulate within 12 hours of delivery or as ordered by the doctor B. Patient will exhibit no signs and symptoms of pulmonary embolism or deep vein thrombosis during hospital stay
Knowledge deficit **Etiology** Unfamiliarity with infant and self-care	Multiple questions Confusion	Assess learning needs of mother regarding self and infant care	A. Provide teaching based on mother's learning needs B. Inform mother of educational programs on hospital television channel C. Encourage mother and significant other to participate in infant care. Provide assistance as needed	Patient will demonstrate self-care and infant care appropriately
Attachment, development of: mother-infant **Etiology** Parenting role	Holds infant close to body Establishes eye contact with infant Talks to infant in soothing or playful manner	Observe maternal/infant interactions	A. Provide opportunity for maternal/infant interactions. Involve father or significant other whenever possible B. Provide support and encouragement as the parents begin to interact and care for the infant	Patient will demonstrate appropriate behavior with infant
Adjustment, emotional **Etiology** Childbirth experience Parenting role	Patient processes and verbalizes feelings regarding childbirth experience and ability to parent Patient experiences fatigue and resultant changes in interpersonal relationships	Assess emotional status	A. Allow for discussion of real and perceived problems B. Help mother internalize the reality of her labor and delivery experience C. Provide reassurance in patient's ability as a mother D. Help patient accept emotional ups and downs of postpartum period, and explain that such changes are common at this time E. Encourage periodic rest throughout the day	Patient will begin to demonstrate effective emotional adjustment

Continued.

Vulvectomy

NURSING DIAGNOSIS/ PATIENT PROBLEM	DEFINING CHARACTERISTICS	NURSING ORDERS		EXPECTED OUTCOMES
		ASSESSMENT	INTERVENTIONS	

Knowledge deficit
Etiology
Unfamiliarity with surgery and diagnosis
	Expresses lack of understanding of diagnosis and surgical intervention plan
	Asks many questions or no questions
	Expresses negative feelings
		A. Identify patient's learning needs and ability to comprehend
		B. Assess readiness to learn. Establish priorities for patient teaching based on patient need and preference
			A. Provide information at the appropriate time regarding
			  1. Diagnosis and reason for surgery
			  2. Preoperative preparation
			  3. Intraoperative procedure
			  4. Postoperative therapy
			B. Involve family members as much as possible in teaching
			C. Provide all explanations and information within a supportive environment
				Patient will be able to verbalize an understanding of
				A. Nature and extent of disease
				B. Surgical treatment plan and any other additional therapy

Anxiety/fear: potential Etiology Diagnosis Surgical experience Fear of unknown	Restlessness Alteration in vital signs (BP, pulse) Expressed concern Constant demands Poor eye contact Insomnia Facial tension Increasing silence or excessive talking	A. Assess patient and significant others for signs and symptoms of anxiety (see Defining Characteristics) B. Note level of anxiety/fear (e.g., mild, moderate, severe)	A. Display confident, calm, tolerant, and understanding attitude B. Establish rapport with patient and significant others C. Use other supportive staff (clergy, social worker) as needed D. See SCP in Ch. 1: Anxiety/fear	Patient will display decreased level of anxiety by A. Relaxed appearance B. Verbalization of fears/feelings C. Restful night

Self-concept, disturbance in: body image
Etiology
Surgical procedure
	Expresses fear of loss of strength and ability to work
	Verbalizes feelings of helplessness, hopelessness in relation to body
	Describes feelings of guilt, shame, grief related to physical disfigurement, and loss of body part associated with sexuality
	Verbalize negative feelings about body (dirty, unsightly)
	Poor eye contact
	Weeping
	Noncompliant
		A. Assess cohesiveness of significant others. Note the amount of support they are able to provide
		B. Identify physiologic and psychologic fears
		C. Assess patient knowledge of sexuality
		D. Assess level of social, intellectual, intrapersonal, physical, and emotional function
		E. Observe for changes in affect, behavior, cognitive perception, and/or level of function
		  1. Note quality and quantity of verbalization regarding self (see Defining Characteristics)
		  2. Observe for help-seeking behaviors such as crying, attention seeking, touching, and/or seeking someone to talk to
			A. Encourage patient to express feelings about disfiguring and defeminizing type of surgery
			B. Provide teaching of significant others as needed
			C. Support significant others, and help them develop strengths needed to cope with patient's problems
			D. Promote warm communicating relationship through effective verbal and nonverbal (touching) exchanges. Stress the importance of support by spouse/ significant other
			E. Reinforce appropriate emotional response, and redirect inappropriate negative response
			F. Encourage self-care activities, and provide positive reinforcement accordingly
			G. Refer to social services as needed
				Patient will demonstrate an active adaptive process to accept altered body image as evidenced by
				A. Verbalizing feelings of body loss to staff and significant others
				B. Participating in self-care activities

Originated by **Rosita Sortijas, RN, BSN**
Resource person: **Jackie Suprenant, RN, BSN**

Vulvectomy—cont'd

NURSING DIAGNOSIS/ PATIENT PROBLEM	DEFINING CHARACTERISTICS	NURSING ORDERS		EXPECTED OUTCOMES
		ASSESSMENT	INTERVENTIONS	
Comfort, alteration in Etiology Postoperative pain	Reports of pain Tension, crying, moaning Irritability Facial mask of pain Refusal to cough Limited movement	A. Assess pain characteristics (quality, severity, location, duration, precipitating factor) B. Solicit patient description of pain	A. Anticipate need for analgesics, and evaluate their effectiveness B. See SCP in Ch. 1: Comfort, alteration in: pain	Patient will evidence relief or minimization of pain by comfortable appearance and verbalization of comfort
Fluid volume deficit: potential Etiology NPO Hemovac Nasogastric drainage	Decreased urinary output Concentrated urine Decreased skin turgor, hypotension Decreased pulse pressure Dry mucous membranes Increased serum sodium Increased drainage from Hemovac and nasogastric tube	Assess hydration status: skin turgor, mucous membranes, drainage from Hemovac and nasogastric tube, vital signs, I & O as needed (see Defining Characteristics)	See SCP in Ch. 1: Fluid volume deficit	Patient will demonstrate adequate fluid and electrolyte balance as evidenced by A. Normal electrolytes B. Moist mucous membranes C. Normal skin turgor

Gas exchange, impaired: potential
 Etiology
 Anesthesia
 Limited mobility
	Diminished breath sounds
	 Increased respiratory rate
	 Audible rales
		Assess patient's respiratory status as indicated (see Defining Characteristics)	A. Instruct patient in the following
			   1. Use of pillow or hand splints when coughing
			   2. Use of spirometer
			   3. Importance of early ambulation
			 B. Encourage patient to turn, couth, and deep breathe q.1-2h. while awake in the early postoperative period and as necessary
			 C. Assist with early ambulation and position changes
				A. Patient will participate in measures designed to enhance pulmonary function
				 B. Pulmonary complications will be prevented or minimized

Injury, potential for wound and bladder infection Etiology Surgical procedures	**Systemic** Increased WBC Increased RBC Elevated temperature Increased respiratory rate **Wound** Swelling and tenderness in the surgical area and its immediate surroundings Postoperative drainage from incision with unusual odor and color **Bladder** Urinary urgency and frequency (after Foley catheter is discontinued) Urinalysis reveals hematuria, pyuria, bacteriuria	A. Assess patient's vital signs every _____ , and report any abnormalities B. Assess patient for signs/symptoms of infection (see Defining Characteristics)	A. Use good hand-washing technique B. Irrigate vulvar wound with prescribed antiseptic solution as ordered by physician C. Keep wound clean, dry, and free from rectal contamination D. Maintain patency of Foley catheter, and perform Foley catheter care every _____ E. Position patient to prevent tension from suture lines and further trauma to vulvar tissue F. For bladder infection, see SCP in Ch. 6: Urinary tract infection	Wound and bladder complications will be prevented/minimized

Continued.

Vulvectomy—cont'd

NURSING DIAGNOSIS/ PATIENT PROBLEM	DEFINING CHARACTERISTICS	NURSING ORDERS		EXPECTED OUTCOMES
		ASSESSMENT	INTERVENTIONS	

Self-care deficit
Etiology
Postoperative recovery
	Verbalized change in life-style
	Inability to perform total self-care and ADL
		A. Identify patient's ability to perform self-care and ADL
		B. Assess willingness and ability of significant others to provide home health care and assistance with ADL
			A. Involve patient and significant others as much as possible in discharge planning, individualizing a program that will meet their needs accordingly
			B. Discuss with patient/significant others
			  1. Activity level
			  2. Dressing changes/cleansing of wounds
			  3. Provision and management of general housekeeping tasks (e.g., cooking, cleaning)
			C. Encourage significant others to emphasize patient's remaining strengths and achievements
				Arrangements will be made with patient and significant others for provision of continuity of care at home

CHAPTER SIXTEEN

High-Risk Neonatal

DISORDERS/CONDITIONS

Anemia in Growing Premature Infant

NURSING DIAGNOSIS/ PATIENT PROBLEM	DEFINING CHARACTERISTICS	NURSING ORDERS		EXPECTED OUTCOMES
		ASSESSMENT	INTERVENTIONS	
Decreased oxygen-carrying capacity **Etiology** Insufficient number of RBCs secondary to Frequent blood sampling Relative underproduction of RBCs compared to rapid somatic growth of the premature infant	Hct below _____ Suboptimal reticulocyte count Tachypnea Tachycardia Episodes of apnea and bradycardia Pallor Decreased perfusion Prolonged O$_2$ dependence in the absence of bronchopulmonary dysplasia or other pulmonary pathology Respiratory compromise as evidenced by grunting, flaring, retracting Lethargy Temperature instability Failure to gain weight despite adequate cal/kg/day	A. Assess Hct by heelstick every _____ B. If Hct is ____, check CBC and reticulocyte count as ordered C. Assess heart rate for tachycardia (rate above ____) D. Assess respiratory status every ____ for 1. Grunting 2. Nasal flaring 3. Retractions 4. Tachypnea (above ____) E. Record amount of blood drawn for laboratory sampling on I & O record, and note daily total on 24-hour fluid balance sheet F. Calculate amount of blood drawn since last transfusion G. Notify physician if blood drawn is ≥10% of normal circulating blood volume H. Assess infant's color for pallor I. Observe for decrease in infant's activity level; with oral feeding, note decreased ability to suck, increase in feeding time, cyanosis, or pallor with feeding	A. Decrease energy expenditure 1. Minimize handling of infant 2. Maintain neutral thermal environment 3. Initiate nasogastric feedings (until after transfusion) if infant is compromised during oral feeding B. Provide supportive O$_2$ therapy as ordered C. Consider supplementation with vitamin/iron drops D. Assist with packed RBC transfusion as ordered	The infant's oxygen-carrying capacity will be optimized as evidenced by A. Hct increased to ____ % B. Improved skin color (pink)

Originated by **Mary Lawson-Carney, RN**
Resource person: **Diane Gallagher, RN, BSN**

Anemia in Growing Premature Infant—cont'd

NURSING DIAGNOSIS/ PATIENT PROBLEM	DEFINING CHARACTERISTICS	NURSING ORDERS		EXPECTED OUTCOMES
		ASSESSMENT	INTERVENTIONS	
		J. Evaluate weight gain pattern over past week, using Dancis curve K. Check blood gases (arterial or capillary) if infant appears to be in respiratory distress		

Parents' anxiety/fear of blood transfusion
Etiology
Religious beliefs (Jehovah's Witness)
Fear of possibility of transfusion-transmitted disease (AIDS, cytomegalovirus, hepatitis)
Previous association with transfusion signifying death/poor prognosis
	Refusal to consent to transfusion
	Multiple questions
	Verbalization of anxiety/fear about transfusion-transmitted disease
		A. Evaluate parents' understanding of infant's need for transfusion
		B. Determine parents' previous experience with blood transfusions
		C. Identify reason for fear and/or refusal to sign consent
		D. Assess family support systems
			A. Demonstrate a nonjudgmental supportive attitude toward parents
			B. If parents' refusal results from religious beliefs, consult with attending physician, social worker, and legal affairs personnel to
			  1. Assist with arrangements for temporary guardianship
			  2. Inform parents of the reasons for the actions being taken on their child's behalf
			C. If fear stems from transfusion-transmitted disease
			  1. Inform parents that they may, within blood bank guidelines, select a blood donor known to them to reduce the risk of transfusion-transmitted disease (guidelines include: 17-65 years of age; in good health; not taking any medication except those approved by blood bank; no history of hepatitis, jaundice, malaria, syphilis. Contact blood bank for further restrictions)
			  2. Determine parents' willingness/ability to find an acceptable donor of the appropriate group and Rh type
			D. Report to parents the results of transfusion (improved color, increased Hct) as applicable after transfusion
				Parental anxiety will be reduced as evidenced by
				A. Verbalization of specific concerns regarding transfusion
				B. Acceptance of bonding with infant after transfusion
				C. Verbalization of reduced anxiety by parents

Bacterial Meningitis, Acute: neonate

NURSING DIAGNOSIS/ PATIENT PROBLEM	DEFINING CHARACTERISTICS	NURSING ORDERS		EXPECTED OUTCOMES
		ASSESSMENT	INTERVENTIONS	
Consciousness, altered levels of **Etiology** Inflammation of meninges	Temperature instability Nuchal rigidity Irritability Bulging fontanel High-pitched cry Seizure activity	See SCP later in this chapter: Seizures: neonate. Monitor daily weights and head circumference, and plot both on graph; palpate anterior fontanel	A. See SCP: Seizures: neonate B. Practice careful hand washing to prevent spread of infection C. Assist with complete diagnostic workup as ordered 1. Blood glucose 2. CBC with platelets 3. Serum electrolytes 4. Blood cultures 5. Urine: culture and sensitivity; counterimmunoelectrophoresis D. Record results on appropriate chart forms (laboratory sheets, bedside Kardex) E. Maintain parenteral fluids at ____ ml/kg/24 hours F. Administer prescribed antibiotics immediately after cultures are obtained G. Maintain antibiotics ____ mg/kg/24 hours for ____ days per infectious disease consultation H. Consider neonate as potential candidate for percutaneous central venous catheter	Alteration in level of consciousness will be minimized
Fluid volume, excess: potential **Etiology** Inappropriate secretion of antidiuretic hormone	Oliguria Increased specific gravity of urine Hyponatremia Hypoosmolality Weight gain Edema Low Hct, low total serum solute Increased blood volume Low BP Pulmonary edema Cardiac failure	A. Assess hydration status (see Defining Characteristics) B. Assess respiratory status. Monitor for pulmonary edema/cardiac failure C. Assess neurologic status 1. Palpate for bulging fontanel and split sutures 2. Assess level of consciousness 3. Assess PERRLA* 4. Monitor for seizures D. Assess daily weights; notify physician of sudden increase in weight E. Assess skin turgor; document pitting edema	A. Maintain fluids at ____ ml/kg/24 hours B. Position neonate every ____ hours, and place on sheepskin to prevent pressure ulcers C. Administer blood products or volume expanders as ordered	Potential for fluid volume excess will be minimized

Originated by **Ellen T. McSwiney, RN, BSN**
Resource person: **Diane Gallagher, RN, BSN**
*Pupils equal, round, reactive to light, accommodative.

Bacterial Meningitis, Acute: neonate—cont'd

NURSING DIAGNOSIS/ PATIENT PROBLEM	DEFINING CHARACTERISTICS	NURSING ORDERS		EXPECTED OUTCOMES
		ASSESSMENT	INTERVENTIONS	

		F. Assess and document I & O; assess specific gravity
		G. Assess the following laboratory parameters
		  1. Serum electrolytes
		  2. Urine electrolytes
		  3. Hct and total serum solute
		  4. Serum and urine osmolality		

Breathing pattern, ineffective **Etiology** Infection	Periodic breathing Apnea Tachycardia Cyanosis	A. Refer to SCP in Ch. 1: "Breathing pattern, ineffective" B. Assess serial blood gases (arterial or capillary)	A. Observe neonate closely for apnea. Document on apnea and bradycardia flow sheet B. Place neonate on cardiorespiratory graph monitor C. Provide appropriate resuscitation D. Suction as necessary E. Maintain ventilation as ordered	Respiratory status will be improved

Nutrition, alteration in: less than body requirements
Etiology
Feeding intolerance
	Lack of interest in feeding, tires easily
	Poor suck
	Abdominal distention
	Vomiting
		A. Determine appropriate feeding route based on
		  1. Gestational age
		  2. Sensitivity of gag reflex
		  3. Ability to coordinate suck and swallow
		  4. Level of activity and alertness
		B. Assess neonate's ability to tolerate feeding
		  1. Observe for vomiting
		  2. Observe for amount of residual feedings in stomach before meals if nasogastric feedings are used
		  3. Measure abdominal circumference every _____
		C. Assess pattern of weight gain based on daily weights compared to Dancis curve
			A. During acute phase of illness, monitor administration of IV fluids
			  1. Monitor intake
			  2. Provide _____ ml/kg/24 hours
			  3. Maintain _____ cal/kg/24 hours
			B. Initiate oral feedings when neonate's condition improves. Begin offering small quantities of formula, observing for
			  1. Vomiting
			  2. Abdominal distention
			  3. Inability to suck or poor irregular suck
			C. Provide nasogastric feedings as needed
			D. Advance to regular feeding schedule as tolerated
				Caloric requirements of neonate will be attained, as evidenced by
				A. Weight gain of _____ g/day
				B. Normal Chemstrip and normal blood sugar

Continued.

Bacterial Meningitis, Acute: neonate—cont'd

NURSING DIAGNOSIS/ PATIENT PROBLEM	DEFINING CHARACTERISTICS	NURSING ORDERS		EXPECTED OUTCOMES
		ASSESSMENT	INTERVENTIONS	
Parenting, alteration in **Etiology** Separation/hospitalization of neonate	Verbal/nonverbal expression of fear and anxiety about intensive care environment Self-blame for neonate's condition Report of guilt feelings for having a "less than perfect" neonate	Assess for presence of Defining Characteristics	See SCP later in this chapter: Parenting	Alteration in parenting will be minimized

Breast-Feeding the Infant Requiring Special Care

NURSING DIAGNOSIS/ PATIENT PROBLEM	DEFINING CHARACTERISTICS	NURSING ORDERS		EXPECTED OUTCOMES
		ASSESSMENT	INTERVENTIONS	

Potential inability to initiate or maintain milk production
Etiology
Anxiety and stress over infant's condition
Physical separation from infant
Incomplete or irregular emptying of breasts
Inadequate fluid/caloric intake
Lack of knowledge of the breast-feeding process
Lack of motivation
	Delayed or absent letdown
	Low milk supply
	Engorged breasts
	Lack of rest
		A. Ascertain that adequate fluid and calories are being consumed
		B. Evaluate sleep and rest patterns
		C. Measure quantity of milk, if any, being produced
		D. Assess knowledge of process of lactation and benefits of breast milk for special care infants
		E. Note condition of breasts and nipples
			A. Provide teaching based on assessment data*
			B. Explain proper care of breasts (see SCPs in Ch. 15 on engorgement, sore nipples, and postpartum care)
			C. Instruct in techniques for hand expression and use of breast pumps*
			D. Instruct in aseptic collection and storage of milk
			E. Outline an optimal pumping schedule. Pump every ＿＿ hours while awake and once at night if possible. Pump each breast each time
			   5 min 1st day
			   8 min 2nd day
			   10 min 3rd day
			   10-15 min 4th day
			F. Demonstrate breast massage*
			G. Explain caloric and fluid requirements of nursing mother
			H. Explain role of stress/emotions in milk production
			I. Reassure mother with explanations of infant's care and condition
			J. Encourage mother to handle infant and participate in care as much as possible to promote bonding
			K. Emphasize the contribution breast milk makes to infant's recovery
				Mother's milk supply will be maximized to the best of her ability

Originated by **Laura L. Rybicki, RN, BSN**
Resource person: **Diane Gallagher, RN, BSN**
*Refer to booklet: "Breastfeeding Your Special Care Baby." Copies may be obtained from Administrative Assistant, Special Care Nursery, Michael Reese Hospital and Medical Center, Lake Shore Drive at 31st St., Chicago, IL 60616.

Breast-Feeding the Infant Requiring Special Care—cont'd

NURSING DIAGNOSIS/ PATIENT PROBLEM	DEFINING CHARACTERISTICS	NURSING ORDERS		EXPECTED OUTCOMES
		ASSESSMENT	INTERVENTIONS	

			L. Explain need for adequate rest
			M. Suggest activities to enhance milk flow
			  1. Comfortable position
			  2. Nap before pumping
			  3. Breast massage
			  4. Back rub with or during pumping
			  5. Looking at picture of baby while pumping
			  6. Applying heat to breasts to promote let-down (heating pad, bath, shower)
			  7. Soft music
			  8. Glass of wine/beer (maximum 1 glass/day)
			N. Reassure mother that milk supply increases and let-down occurs more quickly when infant begins nursing	

Alteration in infant's ability to breast-feed
Etiology
Prematurity
Low birth weight
Medications
CNS damage
Congenital heart disease
Respiratory problems
Congenital anomalies
Initial oral feedings taken from bottle
	Poor suck and swallow
	Duskiness or bradycardia with feeding
	Failure to coordinate breathing and sucking
		Evaluate infant's short-term ability to nurse
		A. Respiratory rate
		B. Color during feeding
		C. Ability to maintain temperature
		D. Gestational age
		E. Weight
		F. Tolerance of feeding by bottle
		G. Anatomic abnormalities
			A. Provide nonnutritive sucking opportunities for infant, using Nuk pacifier
			B. Use Nuk nipples on bottles to facilitate transition to breast
			C. Schedule first nursing attempts between feedings to avoid frustration in a hungry infant
			D. Provide frequent, short opportunities to nurse
			E. Recognize cumulative effects of breast-feeding that indicate intolerance
			  1. Temperature instability
			  2. Decreased weight gain, secondary to excessive caloric needs
			  3. Refusal to suck at subsequent feedings
			F. Reassure mother that a "get acquainted" period is necessary before nursing will progress
			G. Encourage mother to spend as much time as possible on unit, so she is available when infant is hungry
			H. Instruct mother on ways to encourage sucking
			  1. Attempt nursing during alert periods
			  2. Pump/express small amount of milk after putting infant to breast
			    a. To ensure that let-down has occurred
			    b. To bring out nipple
			    c. To soften full, hard breast so that premature infant can grasp nipple
			  3. Position infant to easily reach nipples
				Infant will nurse to the best of his/her ability

Continued.

Breast-Feeding the Infant Requiring Special Care—cont'd

NURSING DIAGNOSIS/ PATIENT PROBLEM	DEFINING CHARACTERISTICS	NURSING ORDERS		EXPECTED OUTCOMES
		ASSESSMENT	INTERVENTIONS	
			4. Rub nipple over infant's lip and cheek 5. Put drop of milk or glucose water on lips to stimulate infant's interest 6. Use nipple shield at *start* of feeding to ease transition to breast 7. Stimulate sucking by stroking feet 8. Change position to wake sleepy infant 9. Unwrap infant to increase wakefulness if condition permits 10. Hold infant as upright as possible to facilitate swallowing 11. Stop feeding frequently to allow for rest and breathing 12. Burp frequently to avoid abdominal distention and subsequent pressure on diaphragm 13. Administer O_2 during feeding, as indicated 14. Schedule medications that affect alertness so they are least likely to cause drowsiness at feeding time 15. Explain how the special implications of the infant's disease/condition will influence nursing	

Fluid/caloric balance, alteration in: potential
 Etiology
 Prematurity
 Hyperbilirubinemia
 Diuretic therapy
	Inadequate weight gain
	 Low output with high specific gravity
		A. Assess fluid balance
		   1. Maintain output at _____ ml/kg/day
		   2. Maintain sp. gr. between 1.003-1.009
		   3. Evaluate skin turgor
		 B. Assess adequacy of weight gain
		   1. Weigh *once* daily
		   2. Compare weight gain to Dancis curve
			A. Observe quality and duration of sucking
			 B. Note length of time infant is satisfied between feedings
			 C. Check creamatocrit to assess caloric content
			 D. Suggest diet improvements to maintain adequate caloric content of milk
			 E. Notify physician of insufficient weight gain
			 F. Feed by nasogastric tube until infant can nurse without excessive caloric usage, and supplement nursing with nasogastric feeding as necessary
			 G. Minimize infant's caloric expenditure by maintaining temperature within normal limits
			 H. Instruct mother to pump after infant nurses as a method of assessing amount infant took from breast
			 I. Instruct mother on interventions *A, B, D, F, G*
				A. Infant will maintain adequate fluid balance
				 B. Infant will demonstrate steady, adequate weight gain

Cleft Lip and Palate

NURSING DIAGNOSIS/ PATIENT PROBLEM	DEFINING CHARACTERISTICS	NURSING ORDERS		EXPECTED OUTCOMES
		ASSESSMENT	INTERVENTIONS	
Coping, ineffective family: compromised **Etiology** Temporary preoccupation by parent(s) trying to manage the emotional conflict of having an infant with a visible defect Temporary disorganization of the family	Parents express a concern about others' response to infant's defect Parents describe preoccupation with personal reactions, e.g., shock, disbelief, inability/reluctance to look at and interact with infant, guilt feelings, and feelings of loss of the perfect child	A. Assess the following 1. Understanding/ knowledge by parents/family of the nature of cleft lip and palate 2. Degree of the family's anxiety and level of discomfort 3. Interpersonal relationship among family members 4. The family reaction to the infant B. Identify the existing support systems within the family	A. Support the open visiting policy B. Encourage parents to 1. Verbalize their feelings 2. Participate in the support group of parents with infants in the special care nursery 3. Participate in caretaking activities, e.g., diapering, feeding, bathing, and holding infant C. Explore potential use of other support systems, e.g., parent-to-parent referral or use of other family members	The family's coping ability will be maximized
Knowledge deficit of parents/family **Etiology** Lack of previous exposure to this problem	Inappropriate or exaggerated behaviors, e.g., verbalization of fear that the "baby might die," lowered self-esteem, and hesitancy in bonding with infant Request for information	Assess understanding/ knowledge of parents/family of the nature of the cleft lip and palate	A. Let parents see and hold infant as soon as possible after the birth. With infant present, discuss the problems, as well as the infant's normal attributes B. In conjunction with the appropriate physician, provide information regarding 1. Occurrence of cleft lip and palate 2. Etiology and nature of the defect 3. Needs of the infant 4. Available support group systems C. Encourage questions D. Give the parents the booklet, "Your Cleft Lip and Palate Child" (Mead Johnson & Co.)	Parents will verbalize an understanding of the nature and sequela of the defect
Nutrition, alteration in: less than body requirements **Etiology** Difficulty ingesting food	Inability to form an adequate nutritive seal for sucking Failure to gain weight according to the growth curve Documented inadequate caloric intake	A. Assess fluid and caloric intake daily B. Assess weight pattern according to the Dancis curve C. Observe the following during the feeding 1. Respiration 2. Color 3. Nutritive sucking ability	A. Provide _____ cal/kg/day and _____ ml/kg/day B. Facilitate breast-feeding (see previous SCP: Breast-feeding the infant requiring special care) 1. Encourage the mother to massage the breast before nursing to bring milk to the surface. This will make the breast full and hard, which will help the infant hold the nipple in his/her mouth	The infant will achieve optimal weight gain as indicated per Dancis growth curve

Originated by **Apolonia Tinio, RN, BSN**
Resource person: **Karen Kavanaugh, RN, MSN**

Continued.

Cleft Lip and Palate—cont'd

NURSING DIAGNOSIS/ PATIENT PROBLEM	DEFINING CHARACTERISTICS	NURSING ORDERS		EXPECTED OUTCOMES
		ASSESSMENT	INTERVENTIONS	
			2. Hold the infant in a semisitting or upright position to make swallowing easier and to reduce the amount of milk that may come out of the nose because of the defect	
			3. If the infant has difficulty holding the nipple in his/her mouth, have the mother apply pressure to the areola with her fingers. It may be necessary for the mother to guide the nipple to the side of the mouth and hold it there during the entire feeding. The baby will then be able to "milk" the nipple with his/her gums	
			4. Burp the infant frequently, since babies with clefts swallow more air during feeding	
			5. Contact the La Leche League* for the name of support person for the mother	
			6. Give the mother a handout on breast-feeding a baby with a cleft of the soft palate	
			7. If the infant is unable to breast-feed because of the defect, consider using a LactAid until the defect is surgically repaired	
			C. Bottle feeding adjustments	
			1. Hold infant in an upright or semisitting position	
			2. Place the nipple against the inside cheek toward the back of the tongue. If a regular nipple is inadequate, use a nipple designed for premature infants, and enlarge the hole. A cleft palate nurser may even be necessary. If the infant is still having problems, use a soft plastic bottle to squeeze the formula into baby's mouth	
			3. Feed small amounts slowly	
			4. Burp frequently, as often as after each 10-15 ml of milk	
			5. If infant is not able to take all feedings orally, consider a combination of oral and nasogastric feedings	

*La Leche League International Inc., 9616 Minneapolis Ave., Franklin Park, IL 60131.

Cleft Lip and Palate—cont'd

NURSING DIAGNOSIS/ PATIENT PROBLEM	DEFINING CHARACTERISTICS	NURSING ORDERS		EXPECTED OUTCOMES
		ASSESSMENT	INTERVENTIONS	
Injury, potential for: infection **Etiology** Accumulated formula in the oral cavity	Tender, reddened areas on the lip and palate	A. Assess the general hygiene, nutrition, and feeding techniques used B. Assess oral cavity (see Defining Characteristics)	A. Cleanse the cleft areas by giving 5-10 ml of water after each feeding B. If a crust has already formed, use a cotton tipped applicator or swab to apply a peroxide solution (1:1 water and peroxide) to loosen the crust C. If the cleft area becomes dry, keep it moist with mineral oil, glycerine, or petrolatum D. If the cleft or lip areas become infected or irritated, contact the physician for further treatment orders	Signs of infection will be identified early so that complications can be minimized
Airway clearance, ineffective: potential **Etiology** Aspiration of breast milk/formula or mucus because of the anatomic defect	Abnormal breath sounds Tachypnea/dyspnea Nasal flaring Retractions Cyanosis	Assess the following A. Respiratory rate B. Presence of nasal flaring or retractions C. Skin color and capillary refill D. Breath sounds	A. Check vital signs every _____ hour B. Suction oropharynx and nasopharynx as needed C. Maintain adequate airway by positioning the infant on his/her abdomen during periods of sleep D. Burp frequently during feeding with the infant in an upright position E. Pace activities (feeding, bathing, handling) to avoid distress F. Provide high humidity or O_2 therapy as ordered by physician	A patent airway will be maintained

Home maintenance management, impaired: potential **Etiology** Defect of infant Inadequate community resources	Parents express difficulty in preparing their home for infant Parents request a delay in the discharge Parents decrease their calls/visits as the discharge date approaches	A. Assess the general home condition and the availability of any necessary equipment
		B. Assess other family member's reactions to, acceptance of, and willingness to participate in infant's care
			A. Encourage parents to verbalize their degree of preparation
			  1. Psychologically
			  2. Physically
			  3. Financially
			B. Along with the social worker and visiting nurse, assist the parents in preparing the home for the infant
			C. Have parents assume total caretaking responsibilities for an extended period before discharge
			D. Provide the telephone number of the physician or clinic for follow-up care
			E. Advise parents of potential problems that necessitate professional evaluation before the scheduled follow-up visit
				A. Parents will demonstrate home care activities
				B. Infant will be discharged to parents who are prepared to be primary caretakers

Congestive Heart Failure

NURSING DIAGNOSIS/ PATIENT PROBLEM	DEFINING CHARACTERISTICS	NURSING ORDERS		EXPECTED OUTCOMES
		ASSESSMENT	INTERVENTIONS	
Breathing pattern, ineffective **Etiology** Pulmonary-venous congestion	Tachypnea >60/min Rales Retractions Cyanosis	A. Count respirations for 1 full min B. Auscultate breath sounds in all lung fields, noting aeration/presence of rales C. Note any nasal flaring or retractions, including location and severity D. Note general skin and mucous membrane color	A. Maintain infant in semi-Fowler's position or in infant seat B. Place small linen roll under infant's shoulders C. Suction as needed (endotracheal, oropharyngeal, nasopharyngeal) D. Provide O_2 as needed to maintain PaO_2 at prescribed level E. Monitor blood gases (arterial and capillary) to evaluate metabolic/respiratory status F. Maintain axillary temperature at 36.4°-36.8° C G. Organize care to minimize handling and provide for long rest periods H. Observe infant for early signs and symptoms of superimposed infection 　1. Temperature instability/hypothermia 　2. Peripheral vasoconstriction 　3. Need for increased amount of O_2 and/or increased ventilator pressure	A. The infant will breathe with less difficulty as evidenced by decrease in 　1. Respiratory rate 　2. Severity of retractions B. Blood gases will show 　pH: _____ 　$PaCO_2$: _____ 　PaO_2: _____
Cardiac output, decreased **Etiology** Decreased contractility	Presence of or change in quality/radiation of murmur Presence of ventricular gallop Tachycardic rhythm Bounding peripheral pulses Hepatomegaly >2 cm below right costal margin Oliguria (<0.5-1 ml/kg/hr) Peripheral vasoconstriction A. Skin and nail-beds pale and mottled B. Cool extremities C. Prolonged capillary refill time (>3 seconds)	A. Count heart rate for 1 full min every _____ B. Assess heart sounds every _____ C. Palpate liver edge at right costal margin D. Note strength of peripheral pulses every _____ E. Assess capillary refill every _____ F. Assess temperature and color of extremities every _____ G. Assess for periorbital or dependent edema every _____	A. Monitor weight once or twice daily B. Document strict I & O C. Obtain specific gravity and Labstix each shift D. Restrict fluids as ordered to meet infant's needs E. Mark liver edge daily; verify with nurse or physician F. For infants receiving furosemide (Lasix) 　1. Monitor electrolytes 　2. Assess and document 　　a. Time of administration 　　b. Quantity of urine output after furosemide G. For infants receiving digoxin 　1. Before administering digoxin 　　a. Note recent digoxin level 　　b. Note recent potassium 　　c. Observe infant for hypokalemia 　　d. Document heart rate; notify physician if heart rate is <100 or 30 beats below baseline 　　e. Recheck dosage	A. Infant will have improved cardiac output as evidenced by 　1. Normal heart rate (120-160) 　2. Adequate urine output (0.5 ml/kg/hour) 　3. Good perfusion B. The infant will have normal electrolytes as evidenced by 　1. Potassium: 3.5-5.0 　2. Sodium: 135-145 C. Digoxin level will be noted 　1. Therapeutic (1-2) 　2. Overlap (2-3) 　3. Toxic (>3.3)

Originated by **Terri L. Russell, RN**
Resource person: **Martina Evans, RN, BS**

Congestive Heart Failure—cont'd

NURSING DIAGNOSIS/ PATIENT PROBLEM	DEFINING CHARACTERISTICS	NURSING ORDERS		EXPECTED OUTCOMES
		ASSESSMENT	**INTERVENTIONS**	

			2. Observe infant for toxic effects of digoxin
			   a. Bradycardia
			   b. Arrhythmias
			   c. Anorexia
			   d. Vomiting
			   e. Diarrhea
			3. If digoxin toxicity is suspected
			   a. Notify physician
			   b. Hold medication	

Nutrition, alteration in
Etiology
Dyspnea
	Increased tachypnea with feedings
	Increase in severity of retractions with feedings
	Cyanosis
		Assess respiratory status and activity during feedings	A. Provide infant with 100-150 cal/kg/day
			B. Organize care to provide longer rest periods between feedings
			C. Keep infant in upright position during feedings
			D. Feed infant q.3h. as needed
			E. Use nipple for premature infants, and enlarge the hole
			F. Allow for frequent stops/rest periods during feeding
			G. If infant is distressed, finish feedings by gavage
			H. Initiate scheduled gavage feedings as needed
			I. Plot weight daily on Dancis curve
			J. Calculate cal/kg/day
			K. Consider MCT Oil, Polycose, or 24-hour calorie formula for infants with slow or absent weight gain
				A. The infant will have adequate caloric intake as evidenced by steady weight gain
				B. The infant will tolerate feedings as evidenced by no or minimal change in
				  1. Respiratory rate and effort
				  2. Color

Knowledge deficit **Etiology** New condition (congestive heart failure) Special situation affecting infant care	Many questions Lack of questions Afraid to care for infant	A. Assess parent's level of knowledge related to illness B. Assess parent's comprehension level	A. Explain to parents the symptoms of heart failure the infant is exhibiting B. Explain how the physical characteristics affect the special needs of the baby (e.g., feeding, rest, medication) C. Assist parents with infant feeding and care D. Begin documenting information in planning tool soon after admission E. Involve social services in infant's care early in hospitalization	A. Parents will verbalize understanding of infant's condition as it relates to heart failure B. Parents will be able to care for infant

Glucose and Calcium Metabolism: alterations in

NURSING DIAGNOSIS/ PATIENT PROBLEM	DEFINING CHARACTERISTICS	NURSING ORDERS		EXPECTED OUTCOMES
		ASSESSMENT	INTERVENTIONS	
Glucose metabolism, alterations in: hypo-glycemia **Etiology** Intrauterine malnutrition resulting from prematurity, post-maturity, or small-for-gestational age Increased use of blood glucose resulting from respiratory distress, hypothermia, or infant of diabetic mother Iatrogenic causes Inadequate glucose intake	Dextrostix <40 Jitteriness Lethargy Refusal to suck Hypotonia Apnea or cyanosis High-pitched cry Abnormal eye movements Temperature instability	A. Assess possible cause of hypoglycemia B. Monitor Chemstrip bG every 15-30 min until stable	A. Obtain blood sample to check glucose level with Chemstrip bG ≤20-40 B. Initiate early feeding if infant is at risk for hypoglycemia C. Administer IV dextrose fluids when Chemstrip bG ≤20-40 (as ordered) D. Minimize energy needs 1. Maintain neutral thermal environment 2. Minimize handling 3. Coordinate care and procedures to limit energy expenditure E. Continue to monitor Chemstrip bG every _____ F. Support infant with O$_2$ therapy as needed	A. Chemstrip bG will be between 40-120 mg% B. Neurologic sequelae will be minimized
Glucose metabolism, alteration in: hyper-glycemia **Etiology** Extreme prematurity Sepsis Respiratory distress Stress Iatrogenic cause	Jitteriness Glycosuria greater than trace Chemstrip bG ≥120	A. Assess possible cause of hyperglycemia B. Monitor Chemstrip bG every 30 min to 1 hour, or more often until stable C. Monitor urine Labstix every void. If urine glucose is ≥1$^+$, check Chemstrip bG D. Note the amount of glucose present in the IV fluid	A. Maintain IV fluids with ____ ml/kg/day of D5W B. Record Chemstrip bG and urine Labstix q.1-2h.	Chemstrip bG will be between 40-120 mg%
Calcium metabolism, alterations: hypocalcemia **Etiology or predisposing factors** Maternal causes Diabetes and toxemia Dietary deficiency of calcium Hyperparathyroidism Intrapartum causes Perinatal asphyxia Prematurity	Irritability Jitteriness Seizures Cyanosis Feeding intolerance Calcium level <7 mg%	A. Assess infant for predisposing factors (see Etiology) B. Observe infant for jitteriness or irritability C. Monitor blood calcium level as indicated by *A* and *B*	A. Notify resident if blood calcium level is <8.0 B. Establish placement of umbilical vein catheter or umbilical artery catheter if used for calcium infusion C. Administer 10% calcium gluconate solution as ordered 1. Calculate dose to determine appropriateness: 200 mg/kg dose immediately, then 500 mg/kg/day maintenance 2. Infuse calcium slowly over 20 min 3. Do not infuse calcium with IV solutions containing sodium bicarbonate D. Check calcium level every 24 hours	Blood calcium level will be stable at 8-10 mg%

Originated by **Evangeline Pintang, RN, BSN**
Resource person: **Diane Gallagher, RN, BSN**

Glucose and Calcium Metabolism: alterations in—cont'd

NURSING DIAGNOSIS/ PATIENT PROBLEM	DEFINING CHARACTERISTICS	NURSING ORDERS		EXPECTED OUTCOMES
		ASSESSMENT	INTERVENTIONS	

Postnatal causes
  Hypoxia
  Shock
  Sepsis
  Metabolic acidosis
    treated with so-
    dium bicarbonate
  Respiratory distress
  Administration of
    citrated blood
			E. Check magnesium and phos-
			phorus levels if calcium level is
			not improved after 24-hour cal-
			cium therapy	

Injury, potential for: **to the infant** **Etiology** Calcium administra- tion	Calcium burn Bradycardia or other cardiac arrhythmias	A. Determine the pa- tency of the IV in- fusion B. Assess peripheral IV site for redness or blanching dur- ing infusion C. Monitor heart rate during calcium in- fusion. Observe for bradycardia D. Observe IV line for presence of precipitant	A. Discontinue peripheral IV line if redness or blanching occurs during calcium infusion B. Stop infusion when heart rate <100, and notify physician C. Stop infusion if precipitant is present	Complications from calcium administra- tion will be prevented
Parental knowledge **deficit** **Etiology** Newness of patient's condition	Anxiety Frequent questioning Repetitive questioning Lack of questions Inconsistent visiting patterns	A. Assess parent's level of under- standing and knowledge of pa- tient's condition B. Assess parent's knowledge of pro- cedures and equip- ment	A. Explain equipment and nursery routine B. Provide parents with the unit booklet C. Explain infant's condition spe- cifically, i.e., change in neuro- logic status and plan of care D. Refer parents to physician for further questions as needed	Parents will be able to verbalize knowledge and understanding of infant's condition

Hyperbilirubinemia

NURSING DIAGNOSIS/ PATIENT PROBLEM	DEFINING CHARACTERISTICS	NURSING ORDERS		EXPECTED OUTCOMES
		ASSESSMENT	INTERVENTIONS	

Injury, potential for: secondary to onset of jaundice within 24 hours of life
Etiology
Intravascular hemolysis
Infection
	Hct $\leq$ 40%
	Serum bilirubin level of 5-10 mg%
	Marked left shift in differential count of WBCs
	Reticulocyte count elevated
	Total serum solute $\leq$ 4.0
	Metabolic acidosis
	Apnea
	Cardiac failure
	Hepatomegaly
	Hypovolemia
	Massive generalized edema
		A. Note age of infant at onset of increased serum bilirubin level
		B. Review maternal/fetal history and clinical data to determine etiology
		C. Send initial blood work
		  1. Type and Coombs' test, using cord blood
		  2. CBC with reticulocyte count and differential
		  3. Cultures as ordered
		  4. ABG as needed
		  5. Fractionated serum bilirubin
		D. Assess presence of hematoma and bruising
		E. Monitor vital signs with BP closely q.2h. to determine early signs of
		  1. Cardiac failure
		  2. Hypovolemia
		  3. Respiratory failure
			A. Maintain accurate I & O
			B. Record specific gravity every void
			C. Monitor hemolytic process
			  1. Obtain serum bilirubin every _____ hours
			  2. Fractionate bilirubin every _____ hours if bilirubin rise is > 0.5 mg//hour and close to exchange level
			  3. Check Hct every _____ hours
			  4. Check Chemstrip every _____ hours
			  5. Check total serum solute every _____ hours
			D. Assist with partial exchange transfusion as ordered
			E. Record the bilirubin level at which the infant will receive an exchange transfusion as determined by the physician
			F. Assist in exchange transfusion as needed
			G. Initiate phototherapy as ordered
			H. Provide good skin care
			I. Observe for signs/symptoms of encephalopathy (kernicterus)
			  1. *Early signs*
			    a. Poor feeding
			    b. Vomiting
			    c. Lethargy
			    d. High-pitched voice
			    e. Hypotonia
			    f. Decreased Moro's reflex
			  2. *Later signs*
			    a. Opisthotonus posturing
			    b. Apnea
			    c. Irritability
			    d. Seizures
			J. Note skin color/sclera
				Potential for kernicterus will be minimized

Injury, potential for: secondary to onset of jaundice on the second to seventh day of life **Etiology** Perinatal asphyxia Respiratory distress syndrome Infant of diabetic mother Prematurity Physiologic jaundice	Jaundice noted on the second day Indirect serum bilirubin: $\geq$ 12 mg% Rate of bilirubin increase: 5 mg%/day (for bilirubin considered high, refer to protocol manual) Peak bilirubin level of *full-term infant:* 6 mg% by 48-72 hours	See preceding Assessment *A, B, D, E*	A. Follow preceding Interventions *A-C* and *E-I* B. Provide early feedings as tolerated C. Withhold intralipids while infant is under phototherapy as ordered D. Record stooling pattern. Perform rectal stimulation if no stool for 2-3 days	Potential for kernicterus will be minimized

Originated by **Rosetonia Sapaula, RN, BSN**
Resource person: **Karen Kavanaugh, RN, MSN**

Hyperbilirubinemia—cont'd

NURSING DIAGNOSIS/ PATIENT PROBLEM	DEFINING CHARACTERISTICS	NURSING ORDERS		EXPECTED OUTCOMES
		ASSESSMENT	INTERVENTIONS	
Hemolysis resulting from birth trauma (bruising) Polycythemia Increased enterohepatic circulation Delayed stooling pattern	*Premature infant:* 10-15 mg% peaking by 4-6 days Lethargy Poor feeding pattern Dark stools Dark, amber, concentrated urine			
Injury, potential for: secondary to jaundice related to use of breast milk	Jaundice occurring on the fourth to seventh day Indirect bilirubin of 15-25 mg% Serum bilirubin declines 2.4 mg% after milk is discontinued	A. Correlate the presence of jaundice and the use of breast milk B. Obtain fractionated serum bilirubin as ordered	A. Follow first Interventions under Hyperbilirubinemia: *A, B; G-I* B. Interrupt feeding breast milk for 2-5 days C. Repeat serum bilirubin on the fifth day D. Resume offering breast milk on the fifth or ninth day if serum bilirubin level decreases to ____ mg%	Risks of kernicterus will be minimized
Injury, potential for: secondary to late onset or failure to resolve jaundice **Etiology** Organic causes: red cell deficiency and biliary obstruction Liver damage secondary to total parenteral nutrition Metabolic and endocrine disturbances	Absence of glucose 6-phosphate dehydrogenase Elevated liver enzyme tests Bilirubin levels > 15 mg%	A. Assess infant's clinical course B. Assess and review all laboratory data available	A. Follow first Interventions under ''Hyperbilirubinemia'': *A-B* and *G-I* B. Obtain fractionated serum bilirubin every ____ hours. Send specimen to adult biochemistry C. Discontinue total parenteral nutrition and intralipids until further orders	Risks of kernicterus will be minimized
Fluid volume deficit: potential **Etiology** Use of radiant warmers Use of phototherapy Loose stools	Urine output < 1-1.5 ml/kg/hour Urine sp gr: >1.010-1.012 5% weight loss per 24-hour period Dry skin and mucous membranes Thick secretions Serum Na > 145 Polycythemia Rise of bilirubin despite other treatment	Assess hydration status based on A. Daily weights B. Skin turgor C. Fontanels D. Electrolytes every ____ hours E. Specific gravity every ____ with Labstix F. Urine output every ____ G. Recorded I & O every ____ hours	A. Maintain adequate fluid intake to provide ____ ml/kg/day 1. Infants receiving phototherapy need 1½ maintenance fluid 2. Infants with low birth weight may require higher fluid requirement (a maximum of ____ ml/kg/day) B. Observe closely for signs of fluid overload	Optimal hydration will be attained

Continued.

Hyperbilirubinemia—cont'd

NURSING DIAGNOSIS/ PATIENT PROBLEM	DEFINING CHARACTERISTICS	NURSING ORDERS		EXPECTED OUTCOMES
		ASSESSMENT	INTERVENTIONS	
Nutrition, alteration in: less than body requirements (potential) **Etiology** Nothing by mouth Total parenteral nutrition Poor oral feeding Increased peristaltic activity	Weight loss Sunken orbits Hypoglycemia Restlessness Irritability Emesis Diarrhea Documented inadequate caloric intake	A. Assess patterns of weight loss/weight gain based on daily weights. Compare to Dancis curve B. Assess caloric intake compatible for weight gain C. Assess feeding tolerance by 1. Recording abdominal girth q.3h. 2. Testing stools by Hematest and reducing substance every _____ hours 3. Recording type of stools, frequency, and amount	A. Provide approximately _____ cal/kg/day with formula or breast milk feedings B. Evalute infant's ability to be fed orally 1. Feed via nasogastric tube if infant is unable to complete oral feeding 2. Use continous nasogastric feeding for premature infants below 1000 g	Caloric requirement of infant will be attained
Knowledge deficit: of parents **Etiology** Unfamiliarity with hyperbilirubinemia	Withdrawn and unable to verbalize understanding of infant's condition Anxious and extremely worried when Breast-feeding withheld Infant placed back on nothing by mouth Subsequent exchange transfusion needed	A. Assess level of knowledge and educational background B. Assess parents' 1. Strengths and weaknesses 2. Resources for information 3. Acceptance of infant's present condition 4. Comprehension of information given	A. Provide parents with information regarding infant's 1. Diagnosis and treatment 2. Current condition by means of a. Handout on neonatal jaundice b. Explanation of specific etiology and management plan B. Encourage parents to ask questions C. Encourage parents to attend parents' class or support group	Parent's ability to comprehend infant's illness will be optimal
Parenting, alteration in **Etiology** Separation of parent and infant because of Critically ill infant Critically ill mother Transfer of infant from another hospital	Infrequent visits and telephone calls Delayed display of interactive and fondling behavior Display of discomfort in handling infant Display of hostile and demanding behavior in terms of infant care and information Questions that focus on equipment instead of infant	A. Evaluate mother's emotional state. Signs of tension include 1. Rapid breathing 2. Muscle tension; arms stiff; tires easily 3. Perspiration 4. Rapid or stilted conversation B. Observe and evaluate parent-infant interactions C. Evaluate and document in appropriate chart forms 1. Frequency of calls 2. Family members who visit	A. Explain visitation and telephone call policies to parents B. Encourage early visits C. Give handout on special care to the parents D. Provide parents with infant's picture E. When parents visit 1. Turn off bili-lite 2. Take off infant's eyepads 3. Encourage touching and handling 4. Allow parents to a. Hold and/or feed infant b. Change infant's diapers and apply lotion c. Bathe infant as condition permits 5. Encourage parents to discuss their support systems F. Request social worker referral as needed	Optimal parent-infant bonding will be achieved

Meconium Aspiration

NURSING DIAGNOSIS/ PATIENT PROBLEM	DEFINING CHARACTERISTICS	NURSING ORDERS		EXPECTED OUTCOMES
		ASSESSMENT	INTERVENTIONS	
Breathing pattern, ineffective **Etiology** Meconium aspiration	Tachypnea Grunting Nasal flaring Retractions Mild to profound cyanosis Rales Chest hyperexpanded and barrel-shaped	A. Assess vital signs and BP B. Assess for presence of grunting. Document if audible with or without stethoscope C. Assess for presence of nasal flaring D. Assess depth and location of retractions 1. Mild, moderate, or severe 2. Substernal or subcostal E. Assess for cyanosis (room air, O$_2$) F. Assess breath sounds and air entry 1. Equality 2. Rales (fine, coarse) G. Assess blood gas (arterial or capillary)	A. Document presence of grunting, nasal flaring, retractions, or cyanosis B. Maintain patent airway 1. Chest physical therapy/postural drainage 2. Suction C. Monitor arterial or capillary blood gases q.4h. and as needed D. Monitor transcutaneous Po$_2$ during suctioning or during periods of agitation E. Minimize handling to avoid agitation with subsequent hypoxia F. Maintain O$_2$ therapy, continuous positive airway pressure, or ventilatory settings as ordered by physician G. Prevent pulmonary vasoconstriction 1. Provide neutral thermal environment 2. Monitor ABGs; in addition a. Maintain alkalotic pH ____ b. Keep infant well oxygenated c. Maintain arterial Pco$_2$ ____ d. Maintain HCO$_3$ ____ 3. For persistent hypoxia administer pancuronium (Pavulon) per physician's order NOTE: Infants receiving Pavulon must be maintained on mechanical ventilation as ordered per physician. Observe for sudden deterioration, suction oropharynx as needed, administer methylcellulose eye drops q.2h. and as needed, and reposition infant q.1-2h.	Minimal respiratory compromise will be evidenced by A. ABG or CBG within limits B. Respiratory rate ____ C. Absence of retractions D. Absence of grunting E. Absence of nasal flaring F. Absence of rales G. Pink color H. Equal breath sounds
Injury, potential for: complications **Etiology** Meconium aspiration	**Metabolic complications** Metabolic acidosis Hypocalcemia Hypoglycemia/hyperglycemia Electrolyte imbalance **Neurologic complications** Postasphyxia cerebral edema Syndrome of inappropriate antidiuretic hormone Seizures	Assess the following A. Serum calcium B. Chemstrip bG or serum glucose C. Peripheral perfusion, total serum solute, and presence of edema D. Hct E. Urine output F. Urine specific gravity and Labstix G. Abdominal circumference	A. Auscultate breath sounds q.2h. and as necessary B. Document location of points of maximum impulse C. Monitor ABGs. Maintain Po$_2$ ____ Pco$_2$: ____ pH: ____ HCO$_3$: ____ D. Administer Na HCO$_3$ per order E. Monitor serum Ca and electrolytes every ____. Maintain Na: ____ K: ____ Cl: ____. Administer calcium gluconate per order; do not infuse calcium gluconate and bicarbonate together	Complications will be minimized

Originated by **Debby Rickard, RN, BSN**
Resource person: **Martina Evans, RN, BS**

Continued.

Meconium Aspiration—cont'd

NURSING DIAGNOSIS/ PATIENT PROBLEM	DEFINING CHARACTERISTICS	NURSING ORDERS		EXPECTED OUTCOMES
		ASSESSMENT	INTERVENTIONS	
	Circulatory complications Profound hypoxia Hypovolemia Fluid shifts Anemia Disseminated intravascular coagulation Hematuria Oliguria Anuria Necrotizing enterocolitis **Respiratory complications** Respiratory acidosis Hypercapnia Persistent pulmonary hypertension Pneumothorax Pneumopericardium	H. Stools and/or gastric drainage for bleeding I. Weight every _____ J. Other laboratory tests as needed	F. Document type and duration of seizure activity G. Document accurate I & O with specific gravity and Labstix every void H. Monitor pulse and capillary refill I. Note presence and location of edema	

Fluid volume deficit: potential
 Etiology
 Increased H$_2$O loss via respiratory tract in tachypneic infant
 Use of radiant warmer
	Poor tissue turgor
	 Decreased urine output
	 Increased specific gravity
	 Weight loss
	 Sunken fontanels
	 Tacky mouth secretions
		Assess hydration status
		 A. Skin turgor
		 B. Mucous membranes
		 C. Quality of mouth secretions
		 D. I & O
		 E. Specific gravity
		 F. Fontanels
			A. Maintain IV rate to provide appropriate fluid and electrolyte requirements
			  1. _____ ml/kg/24 hours first day of life
			  2. _____ ml/kg/24 hours second day of life
			  3. _____ ml/kg/24 hours thereafter
			  4. Restrict fluids to _____ ml/kg/24 hours in cases of inappropriate antidiuretic hormone or cerebral edema
			 B. Assess I & O q.1-2h.
			  1. Document urine output < 1 ml/kg/hour
			  2. Maintain specific gravity: _____
			  3. Monitor urine Labstix for presence of protein, blood, and glucose
			 C. Monitor serum electrolytes q.12-24h.
			 D. Monitor Chemstrip bG or serum glucose
			 E. Monitor daily weight. Document excessive weight gain or loss
				Appropriate fluid volume will be maintained as evidenced by
				 A. Normal skin turgor
				 B. Nontacky mouth secretions
				 C. Moist mucous membranes
				 D. Soft fontanel
				 E. Urine output > 1 ml/kg/hour
				 F. Normal specific gravity
				 G. Normal electrolytes
				 H. Normal vital signs

Meconium Aspiration—cont'd

NURSING DIAGNOSIS/ PATIENT PROBLEM	DEFINING CHARACTERISTICS	NURSING ORDERS		EXPECTED OUTCOMES
		ASSESSMENT	INTERVENTIONS	
Knowledge deficit: meconium aspiration **Etiology** New condition	Asking same questions of different members of health team Apparent confusion over events Lack of questions Expressed need for more information	A. Assess parents' experience with well and ill children B. Assess parents' knowledge of infant's illness and condition C. Assess parents' knowledge of procedures and equipment	A. Orient parents to 1. Unit 2. Staff 3. Procedures and equipment B. Provide parents with unit booklet C. Provide parents with information regarding 1. Meconium aspiration as it relates to their child's illness 2. Rationale behind procedures 3. How procedures are performed 4. Expected outcomes regarding infant's condition D. Provide explanations appropriate for parents' level of understanding E. Encourage parents to ask questions F. Reinforce information given by other members of health care team	Knowledge deficit will be minimized or reduced as evidenced by parents' verbalized understanding of A. Infant's illness and condition B. Rationale behind procedures C. How procedures are performed D. Expected outcomes regarding infant's condition
Parenting, alteration in: potential **Etiology** Interruption of normal adaptation of new family unit	Withdrawal Grief Indifference Sadness Limited involvement with infant Delay in choosing a name for infant	A. Assess parental developmental age B. Assess degree of parental self-esteem C. Assess maternal support system 1. Husband or significant other 2. Other family members 3. Friends/peers 4. Religious beliefs D. Assess infant's growth and development E. Assess parents' degree of involvement with infant F. Assess parents' need for referrals to other services 1. Social services 2. Dysfunctional child center	A. Encourage parents to express feelings B. Facilitate open lines of communication between parents and health care team C. Demonstrate nonjudgmental supportive attitude D. Encourage parents to visit and telephone. Document on flow sheet E. Encourage attendance and participation in parents' support group F. Make referrals as needed G. Encourage parents to interact with infant as physical condition permits H. Emphasize positive aspects of infant I. Encourage parents to choose name	Potential alteration in parenting will be minimized as evidenced by A. Initiation of parent-infant bonding 1. Looks at infant 2. Touches infant 3. Asks to hold infant 4. Talks to infant 5. Participates in care 6. Brings toy for bed 7. Selects name B. Attendance and participation in parents' support group

Pulmonary Hypertension: persistent

NURSING DIAGNOSIS/ PATIENT PROBLEM	DEFINING CHARACTERISTICS	NURSING ORDERS		EXPECTED OUTCOMES
		ASSESSMENT	INTERVENTIONS	
Inadequate pulmonary blood flow **Etiology** High pulmonary vascular resistance	Tachypnea Cyanosis Possible murmur Hepatomegaly Hypoxia despite maximal ventilatory support	A. Review perinatal history B. Assess cardiac status 1. Rate 2. Variability 3. Absence or presence of murmur 4. Points of maximum impulse 5. Perfusion 6. BP every _____ C. Assess respiratory status 1. Spontaneous respiration 2. Respiratory effort 3. Breath sounds 4. Chest expansion 5. Grunting, flaring, retracting D. Assess need for chest physiotherapy; adapt procedure based on infant's tolerance level and need E. Assess tolerance of activity: degree of duskiness or cyanosis with increased handling or activity F. Assess blood gases every _____ 1. Correlate with transcutaneous Po_2 monitor 2. Notify physician if respiratory or metabolic acidosis develops	A. Minimize handling B. Maintain clear airway 1. Reposition infant q.2h. 2. Suction every _____ 3. Perform gentle chest physiotherapy as necessary C. Document urine output. Notify physician of urine specific gravity _____ or urine output _____ D. Collect laboratory data as needed 1. Hct every _____ 2. Chemstrip bG every _____ 3. Electrolytes every _____ E. Maintain IV fluids at _____ ml/ kg/day	Optimal cardiopulmonary status will be maintained

Originated by **Vanida Komutanon, RN**
Resource person: **Martina Evans, RN, BS**

Pulmonary Hypertension: persistent—cont'd

NURSING DIAGNOSIS/ PATIENT PROBLEM	DEFINING CHARACTERISTICS	NURSING ORDERS		EXPECTED OUTCOMES
		ASSESSMENT	INTERVENTIONS	
Injury, potential for **Etiology** Side effects of tolazoline hydrochloride (Priscoline) therapy	**Side effects** GI bleeding Decrease in cardiac output Skin rash or flushed skin Renal failure, hematuria Thrombocytopenia Pulmonary hemorrhage Hypotension and shock Diarrhea Tachycardia	A. Assess for side effects and/or complications of Priscoline B. Correlate BP with Priscoline infusion rate	A. Calculate appropriate dose: ____ mg/kg/hour B. Add medication to 50 ml D5W C. Infuse medication into upper extremities or scalp veins to avoid generalized vasodilation	Complications will be minimized
Knowledge deficit: parental **Etiology** Unfamiliarity with persistent pulmonary hypertension	Frequent questioning Lack of questions Repetitive questions	Assess parents' understanding of infant's condition	A. Explain infant's condition and plan of care to parents B. Refer parents to physician for questions as necessary C. Explain equipment and nursery routine	Parents will be able to verbalize understanding of infant's condition
Anxiety: parental **Etiology** New condition Change in health status	Afraid to touch infant Infrequent calling Expression of guilt feelings Critical about care given to infant Silence	A. Assess coping mechanism of family B. Assess family-infant interactions	A. Encourage parents to 1. Touch infant 2. Talk to infant 3. Call and visit whenever they can 4. Participate in care (e.g., breast-feeding, blood donor program) 5. Bring toys B. Encourage parents to verbalize concerns C. Refer to special care nursery parents' support group	A. Parents will touch infant and visit more frequently B. Parents will demonstrate appropriate infant stimulation techniques

Seizures: neonate

NURSING DIAGNOSIS/ PATIENT PROBLEM	DEFINING CHARACTERISTICS	NURSING ORDERS		EXPECTED OUTCOMES
		ASSESSMENT	INTERVENTIONS	
Consciousness, altered levels of **Etiology** Seizures **Risk factors for development of neonatal seizures** Perinatal asphyxia Intracranial hemorrhage Metabolic disturbance Intracranial infection Drug withdrawal/drug overdosage problems Developmental defects Other less frequent causes such as pyridoxine deficiency, amino acid imbalance, and kernicterus	Apnea or transient alteration in respiration Sudden eye opening or eye blinking Vasomotor movements like chewing and sucking Tonic-clonic movement Limpness Facial twitching Abnormal cry Drooling ''Bicycle''-like movements Agitation Change in alertness	A. Verify seizure activity, using Defining Characteristics, noting location, activity involved, duration, and effect on patient B. Differentiate whether movements are indicative of jitteriness or seizures C. Assess alteration in level of responsiveness 1. Change in level of alertness as determined by evaluation of spontaneous activity and response to external stimulation 2. Pupillary reaction 3. Hypotonia/hypertonia 4. Muscle flaccidity 5. Asymmetry 6. Absence of developmental reflexes 7. Tight and tense anterior fontanel 8. Abnormal respiratory pattern and periods of apnea and bradycardia 9. No oculovestibular reaction or doll's eyes sign	A. Monitor vital signs and neurologic status every ____, and report significant changes to the physician B. Minimize stimulation; keep handling and noise to a minimum C. Observe if seizure is related to such activities as feeding or agitation D. Monitor Chemstrip bG every ____ . Notify physician if <40 mg E. Monitor serum calcium every ____ . Notify physician if <8 F. Administer appropriate medication as ordered G. Monitor Hct. Notify physician if there is significant drop from previously recorded Hct H. Maintain patent airway 1. Position infant on side or abdomen, with neck slightly hyperextended 2. Suction secretions 3. Assist with ventilation as needed I. Assist in completing diagnostic workup as ordered 1. Blood culture 2. Lumbar puncture 3. CBC 4. Electroencephalogram 5. Skull films 6. Transillumination 7. Torch titers 8. Ultrasound	Potential for injury will be minimized

Originated by **Ruby Rotor-Cajindos, RN, BSN**
Resource persons: **Karen Kavanaugh, RN, MSN**
Martina Evans, RN, BS
Diane Gallagher, RN, BSN

Seizures: neonate—cont'd

NURSING DIAGNOSIS/ PATIENT PROBLEM	DEFINING CHARACTERISTICS	NURSING ORDERS		EXPECTED OUTCOMES
		ASSESSMENT	INTERVENTIONS	
		D. Determine etiology by reviewing maternal and neonatal history, performing physical examination of baby, and drawing blood for metabolic workup. Consider contributing factors to any changes, e.g., medications		
Injury, potential for: to the infant **Etiology** Side effects of phenobarbital	Drowsiness Diarrhea and other GI symptoms Aggravated psychomotor seizure	Assess for side effects and/or complications of phenobarbital	A. Administer phenobarbital loading dose: 5-10 mg/kg/dose, slow IV per physician's order 1. If seizures continue, repeat dose 2. If seizures persist, give 10 mg/kg 3. If tonic-clonic movements are accompanied by respiratory depression, repeat phenobarbital 5 mg/kg for the third time for a maximum of 15 mg/kg B. If seizure subsides, maintain phenobarbital 5 mg/kg/24 hours IV or IM in two divided doses q.12h. C. Monitor serum phenobarbital level after ___ hours, and notify physician if serum level is below or above the therapeutic level (15-40 mg/ml)	Side effects will be minimized
Etiology Side effects of phenytoin (Dilantin)	Drowsiness Nausea and vomiting Hypotension Hypotonia Gastritis Liver damage Cardiovascular collapse	Assess for side effects and/or complications of Dilantin therapy	A. Administer loading dose of 15 mg/kg in normal saline (over 2-3 min) per physician's orders, and give maintenance dose of 5-8 mg/kg/12 hours as ordered B. Monitor Dilantin level after ___ hours, and notify physician if nontherapeutic or toxic	Side effects will be minimized
Mobility, impaired physical: potential **Etiology** Sedation Decreased muscle tone and strength Impaired coordination High phenobarbital or Dilantin level	Inability to nipple feed (poor suck and swallow reflex, inability to keep tongue down) Limited ROM Decreased muscle control	A. Assess respiratory rate, rhythm, amplitude every ___ hours B. Auscultate breath sounds every ___ hours C. Assess skin integrity D. Assess nutritional needs as they relate to immobility. Determine need for nipple or nasogastric feeding	A. Turn and position q.2h. B. Maintain limbs in functional alignment with pillows, sandbags (consult with physical therapy department) C. Use antipressure devices (sheepskin, special mattress) D. Clean, dry, and moisturize skin every ___ hours E. Perform chest physiotherapy and suctioning every ___ hours F. Establish degree of wakefulness (may need readjustment in medication, i.e., phenobarbital/Dilantin)	Optimal mobility will be maintained and potential complications prevented

Continued.

Seizures: neonate—cont'd

NURSING DIAGNOSIS/ PATIENT PROBLEM	DEFINING CHARACTERISTICS	NURSING ORDERS		EXPECTED OUTCOMES
		ASSESSMENT	INTERVENTIONS	
			G. Observe respiratory and neurologic status during feeding, and make adjustments as needed 1. Feed in upright position 2. Put extra hole in nipple 3. Use nipple designed for premature infants H. Insert nasogastric tube as needed, and gavage feed until able to feed by mouth I. Observe for abdominal distention and vomiting J. Monitor weight every _____ K. Monitor I & O L. Instruct parents on how to feed infant by nipple or nasogastric route M. Encourage parent participation in feeding, giving medication as needed, performing ROM exercises (consult with physical/occupational therapy personnel) N. Reinforce teaching before discharge, and arrange for discharge follow-up	
Parent-infant bonding, alteration in: potential **Etiology** Separation Fear of the unknown	Change in visiting and calling patterns Unrealistic expectations of baby and self Lack of physical contact with baby (touching and holding) Verbalization of feelings of detachment because of fear of death, permanent brain damage, or mental retardation Lack of or inappropriate response to infant Verbalization of resentment towards baby Verbalization of lack of knowledge about disease entity	A. Assess parental developmental stage B. Assess parents' degree of involvement with infant	A. Encourage visiting and calling as much as possible, and give an accurate description of baby's appearance and condition B. Encourage touching and holding when possible, especially during feedings C. Recognize any support system, and encourage parents to verbalize feelings of anxiety and guilt D. Explain to parents and significant others the disease process 1. Signs and symptoms 2. Possible complications 3. Treatment and procedures E. Encourage participation in the care of baby by letting them perform simple tasks they can succeed in doing F. Assist parents to make decisions for long-term care, as needed	A. Parents will demonstrate bonding behaviors to infant B. Parents will demonstrate infant caretaking activities C. Parents will verbalize a description of the disease process

Skin Integrity, Impairment of: potential

NURSING DIAGNOSIS/ PATIENT PROBLEM	DEFINING CHARACTERISTICS	NURSING ORDERS		EXPECTED OUTCOMES
		ASSESSMENT	INTERVENTIONS	
Potential impairment Disruption of skin surface Destruction of skin layers	**Etiology** A. Internal (somatic) factors 1. Extremely premature infant 2. Altered tissue perfusion 3. Altered nutritional status 4. Altered immunologic state (microbial colonization) 5. Generalized edema 6. Gelatinous-transparent skin 7. Hypothermia/ hyperthermia 8. Alteration in skin turgor B. External (environmental) factors 1. Mechanical factors a. Shearing forces from adhesives b. Pressure c. Use of restraints d. Use of extremely warm compresses e. Use of monitoring devices 2. Chemical factors: infusion and transfusion infiltrations 3. Physical immobility secondary to use of a. Anesthesia b. Paralyzing drugs such as pancuronium (Pavulon) c. Barbiturates	A. Review maternal and fetal history 1. Gestational age 2. Trauma in delivery, bruising or hematoma 3. Use of invasive monitoring device B. Assess skin 1. Color 2. Temperature 3. Texture 4. Turgor 5. Moisture 6. Presence/absence of skin breakdown 7. Edema 8. Perfusion C. Assess nutritional status 1. Daily weight and growth pattern (see Dancis curve) 2. Total fluid intake per 24 hours 3. Total caloric intake per 24 hours 4. Use of total parenteral nutrition and fresh frozen plasma 5. Accurate I & O 6. Clinical status and medical management D. Establish medical and surgical risk factors to document etiology (see Defining Characteristics) E. Assess current skin care rendered F. Evaluate laboratory data 1. Total serum solute 2. Chemstrip every _____ 3. Hct every _____	A. Document signs of tissue ischemia, redness, and changes in skin color. Notify physician of observations B. Clean skin according to institution's bath policy and procedure C. Place infant in appropriate neutral thermoregulation (see NCP in this chapter on thermoregulation) D. Administer adequate nutritional and hydration requirements as ordered E. Record accurate I & O, specific gravity, and Labstix q.4-6h. F. *Limit use of adhesives* 1. Use needle electrodes on infants with a birth weight <1 kg (change electrodes every 3 days; label site with date, time, and initials) 2. Use Karaya-base electrodes (e.g., Syn-cor) on infants >1 kg who have sensitive skin 3. Remove adhesives and electrodes with water-soaked cotton balls *Do not peel off!* 4. When a transcutaneous P_{O_2} and P_{CO_2} monitor is used, place disposable discs on thoracoabdominal area, and rotate sites q.2-4h. as needed 5. As an alterative to Band-Aids, apply pressure with sterile gauze (2 × 2) to stop bleeding from heel-sticks, needle punctures, and IV sites. If *bleeding persists,* wrap area with gauze and apply tape over it 6. Tape nasogastric tubes 1-2 mm away from septum, avoiding displacement of nostril	Optimal skin integrity will be maintained

Originated by **Rosetonia Sapaula, RN, BSN**
Resource persons: **Diane Gallagher, RN, BSN**
        Karen Kavanaugh, RN, MSN

Continued.

Skin Integrity, Impairment of: potential—cont'd

NURSING DIAGNOSIS/ PATIENT PROBLEM	DEFINING CHARACTERISTICS	NURSING ORDERS		EXPECTED OUTCOMES
		ASSESSMENT	INTERVENTIONS	

	4. Irritations caused by excretions
	  a. Stoma drainage
	  b. Gastric drainage
	  c. Urine
	  d. Loose, watery stools
	5. Humidity and excessive heat from
	  a. Oxygen hood
	  b. Body hood
	  c. Isolette
			7. Use water-type skin barriers (e.g., Stomahesive, Duoderm)
			  a. On skin area where tape is frequently used (cheeks, upper lips, temples). Apply tape over skin barrier, and change only as necessary (no more frequently than every 4 days)
			  b. Use on skin exposed to irritating secretions/ excretions
			8. Use permeable skin barriers or Kling dressing to immobilize dressings or IV infusions
			9. Cover operative site with Tegaderm if areas are at risk for friction (e.g., elbows, knees)
			10. Check IV patency before administering drugs and blood/blood products
			11. Monitor IV sites every hour and document
			12. Rinse off povidone-iodine (Betadine) with water on completion of procedure
			13. Record temperature q.2h. of oxygen hoods, body hoods, ventilator
			14. Apply warm compress to sites of IV infiltrations if markedly edematous or swollen
			15. Change infant's position q.2h.
			  a. Gently massage around pressure areas
			  b. Perform passive ROM exercises (especially when immobile)
			16. Provide prophylactic use of sheepskin
			17. Use liquid film barriers on skin or protective skin barriers when securing endotracheal tubes
			18. Use only wide, soft restraints to immobilize an infant	

Substance Abuse Withdrawal: infant

NURSING DIAGNOSIS/ PATIENT PROBLEM	DEFINING CHARACTERISTICS	NURSING ORDERS		EXPECTED OUTCOMES
		ASSESSMENT	INTERVENTIONS	
Breathing patterns, ineffective **Etiology** Inhibitory effects of maternal drug ingestion	Respiratory rate >60 per minute Respiratory alkalosis Increased secretions Rales Retractions Cyanosis	A. Review maternal drug history B. Count respirations for 1 full min C. Auscultate all lung lobes and compare breath sounds D. Observe location and severity of retractions E. Observe color of trunk, face, extremities, nail beds, and mucous membranes F. Monitor ABG results G. Observe amount and nature of secretions	A. Perform chest physiotherapy, and suction as needed B. Reposition infant frequently, keeping neck slightly hyperextended C. Place bed in semi-Fowler's position, or use infant seat	Improved respiratory status will be evidenced by A. Pink color B. Decrease in severity of retractions C. Resolution of alkalosis (pH value of _____ to _____)
Fluid volume deficit: potential **Etiology** Effects of drug withdrawal: vomiting, diarrhea, and profuse sweating	Excessive weight loss Poor skin turgor Decreased urine output Increased urine specific gravity Decrease or concentration of mouth secretions Lethargy Electrolyte imbalance Diarrhea Sweating Vomiting Sunken fontanels Poor perfusion Hypotension Increased heart rate	A. Observe skin turgor B. Assess I & O status C. Assess fontanels: Are fontanels sunken? Do sutures overlap? D. Assess the tenacity and amount of secretions E. Observe activity level F. Monitor electrolyte values G. Monitor vital signs	A. Weigh every _____ hours B. Adjust IV or feedings to provide _____ ml/kg/day on first day of life, _____ ml/kg/day on second day of life, and _____ ml/kg/day thereafter. *Plus,* add 10%-20% based on severity of dehydration C. Observe strict I & O D. Check urine specific gravity every _____ hours E. Monitor serum electrolytes every _____ to _____ hours F. Continue to monitor vital signs, including BP	Optimal fluid balance will be evidenced by A. Minimal weight loss (<_____ g) B. Loosening of secretions C. Normal skin turgor D. Normal fontanels E. Increase in alertness or activity F. Normal electrolytes G. Urine output > _____ ml/kg/ hour H. Urine sp. gr. between _____ and _____ I. Improvement in perfusion and BP (_____ to _____)

Originated by **Christine Todd, RN**
Resource person: **Martina Evans, RN, BS**

Continued.

Substance Abuse Withdrawal: infant—cont'd

NURSING DIAGNOSIS/ PATIENT PROBLEM	DEFINING CHARACTERISTICS	NURSING ORDERS		EXPECTED OUTCOMES
		ASSESSMENT	INTERVENTIONS	
Nutrition, alteration in: less than body requirements (potential) **Etiology** Inability to feed, secondary to Irritability Lethargy Vomiting Uncoordinated suck/swallow Respiratory distress Increased secretions Hypersensitive gag reflex Abdominal cramps	Weight loss of _____ Inability to feed	A. Assess ability to handle secretions secondary to inability to swallow B. Determine appropriate feeding route based on 1. Gestational age 2. Sensitivity of gag reflex 3. Ability to coordinate suck and swallow 4. Respiratory rate 5. Level of activity/alertness C. Assess infant's ability to tolerate feedings 1. Observe for vomiting 2. Observe amount of residual gastric content before meals if nasogastric feedings are used 3. Measure abdominal circumference every _____	A. Encourage oral formula feedings when appropriate, using Assessment data and following criteria 1. Gestational age $\geq$ 32 weeks 2. Respiratory rate of _____ to _____ 3. Infant's tolerance of 5-10 ml B. Offer pacifier with nasogastric feedings C. Check abdominal circumference every _____ to _____ hours D. Check residual gastric content before nasogastric feedings. Hold feedings and notify physician if residual is $\geq$ _____ ml	Minimized or reduced nutritional deficit will be evidenced by A. Caloric intake of at least _____ cal/kg/day B. Steady weight gain C. Coordinated, nutritive suck D. Tolerance of formula feedings without vomiting
Comfort, alteration in **Etiology** Withdrawal of the drug	Irritability or hyperactivity Disorganized, vigorous sucking Tremors or hypertonicity Hyperphagia Exaggerated reflexes Fever Sneezing Hiccups Yawning Short, restless sleep Drooling Sensitive gag reflex Abdominal cramps Stuffy nose Flushing	A. Assess level of activity B. Assess reactions to stimuli	A. Use calming techniques 1. Swaddle infant 2. Place in prone position 3. Hold and cuddle as often as possible B. Satisfy sucking desire, using pacifier or infant's hands C. Reduce environmental stimuli 1. Dim lights near bed if possible 2. Limit activity and noise near bedside whenever possible 3. Organize care to limit amount of invasive procedures	Infant will be more comfortable as evidenced by A. Longer periods of sleep B. Reduction in hyperactive symptoms

Substance Abuse Withdrawal: infant—cont'd

NURSING DIAGNOSIS/ PATIENT PROBLEM	DEFINING CHARACTERISTICS	NURSING ORDERS		EXPECTED OUTCOMES
		ASSESSMENT	INTERVENTIONS	

Parental knowledge deficit
Etiology
Lack of understanding of infant's condition
	Inappropriate or repetitive questions
	Hostility or suspicion toward staff
	Anxiety
	Disbelief
		A. Observe attitude of parents as expressed by comments and behavior
		B. Assess the level of parents' knowledge as expressed by the appropriateness of their questions
		C. Observe parental reactions to changes in infant's condition or treatment
			A. Encourage parents to discuss their feelings and concerns regarding infant and his/her condition
			B. Offer information and ask for feedback regarding
			  1. Baby's condition
			  2. Unit policies
			  3. Role/responsibilities of unit personnel
			C. Contact social service personnel, if indicated
				Knowledge deficit will be minimized or reduced as evidenced by
				A. Parents continuing to ask appropriate questions
				B. Parents verbalizing
				  1. Rationale for treatment
				  2. Purpose of unit policies regarding infant's care
				  3. Roles/responsibilities of various unit personnel
				C. Appropriate reactions to changes in infant's condition

Parenting, alteration in: potential
Etiology
Interruption of normal adaptation of new family unit
	Inconsistency or disinterest in visiting or calling
	Disinterest or uneasiness in handling infant
	Nonverbal/verbal expression of concern about infant's condition
	Guilt, hostility, or suspicion
		A. Observe frequency of visits or calls
		B. Observe interaction of parents with infant
		C. Assess developmental stage of parents
		D. Assess support system of parents
		  1. Other family members
		  2. Friends
		  3. Religious beliefs
		E. Assess emotional response of parents regarding infant's reason for hospitalization
			A. Initiate calls to parents if necessary, and encourage them to visit
			B. Encourage parents to hold infant and do as much of care as possible
			C. Encourage parents to express their feelings regarding their drug addiction
			D. Stress the positive aspects of infant's condition
			E. Make referrals as indicated
			  1. Social services
			  2. Parent support group
			  3. Drug rehabilitation program
				Initiation of parental infant bonding will be evidenced by
				A. Frequent visits or calls
				B. Interest in handling and caring for infant

Terminally Ill Infant: care of family of

NURSING DIAGNOSIS/ PATIENT PROBLEM	DEFINING CHARACTERISTICS	NURSING ORDERS		EXPECTED OUTCOMES
		ASSESSMENT	INTERVENTIONS	
Grieving, anticipatory: of the family **Etiology** Infant's moribund condition	Repetitious and inappropriate questions Inability to comprehend explanations Afraid to touch infant Infrequent calls and visits Silence Critical about care given to infant Denial of potential loss Alteration in sleeping pattern Altered communication among family members Expressions of affect: crying, sadness, silence	A. Assess infant's condition B. Assess parents' 1. Involvement with the infant 2. Response to infant's condition 3. Existing support system 4. History of other losses, including perinatal losses 5. Needs for referral to other services, e.g., social service	A. Communicate with parents on a daily basis. Alter the frequency of these contacts depending on infant's condition B. If the mother remains hospitalized, contact the nurse caring for the mother to facilitate communication with the family C. Give the parents a picture of the baby D. Encourage parents 1. To name the infant 2. To visit with siblings and other family members 3. To hold the infant 4. To photograph the infant with or without the family members E. Allow parents to spend extended periods of uninterrupted time with the infant	Family will be provided with opportunity to discuss the loss in a supportive environment
Grieving, dysfunctional: family (potential) **Etiology** Infant's death	Hostility toward health professionals and themselves Anger at God Guilt Expression of unresolved issues Difficulty in expressing loss Idealization Expressions of affect: crying, rage, depression, fear Denial of loss Alteration in eating habits and sleep pattern Interference with life functioning Reliving of past losses	A. Assess parents' 1. Response to infant's death 2. Way of coping with the loss 3. Existing support systems B. Assess if parents are at high risk for dysfunctional grieving 1. Lack of resolution of previous grieving response 2. Poor support systems 3. History of multiple losses	A. With the physician, inform at least two individuals of the infant's death. When only one parent is present, have one of the professional staff stay with the parent. Call a clergyman if so desired B. Explain what happened. Keep explanation simple C. Verbalize your concern and offer yourself by using such statements as 1. "I don't know how you feel, but I'm sure it must be so painful" 2. "I'm sorry. I know this is a bad time for you" 3. "Is there anything I could do for you?" 4. "Can I call anyone for you?" D. Avoid phrases that will downplay grief, such as 1. "You can have other children" 2. "The baby would have been abnormal anyway" 3. "Angel in heaven" 4. "It was for the best" 5. "You are lucky you are alive" 6. "It wasn't a real baby anyway" 7. "God wanted it that way" E. Explain infant's appearance F. Prepare the infant's body by cleaning and wrapping in a blanket G. Allow the parents to see the dead infant	The potential for family's dysfunctional grieving will be minimized

Originated by **Digna Limjoco, RN**
Resource person: **Karen Kavanaugh, RN, MSN**

Terminally Ill Infant: care of family of—cont'd

NURSING DIAGNOSIS/ PATIENT PROBLEM	DEFINING CHARACTERISTICS	NURSING ORDERS		EXPECTED OUTCOMES
		ASSESSMENT	INTERVENTIONS	

			H. Provide opportunities for parents to
			1. Hold and touch the infant
			2. Take pictures
			3. Spend time alone with the infant (stay with the family if so requested)
			I. Give momentos to the parents
			1. Crib card with birth date, time of birth, weight and length of the infant
			2. Identification bands
			3. Footprint sheet
			4. Toys and other personal items
			5. Lock of hair
			J. If parents refuse the above items, let them know that they will be kept on file and they can call anytime in the future if they want these items. Then place them in box with name, date of birth, and any other important information
			K. Describe burial options. Ask parents if they want a private or a hospital burial
			1. *Private.* Encourage parents to seek assistance from family/friends in planning the type of service. If additional information is needed, refer to ''When an Infant Dies'' by Compassionate Friends, Inc. (National Headquarters, P.O. Box 3696, Oak Brook, IL 60522)
			2. *Hospital.* Inform parents of the following
			  a. There is no memorial service
			  b. The body is buried in a common burial site by the county morgue
			  c. The city contracts with cemeteries, and the cemetery location changes every 2 years
			  d. The parents must go to the Bureau of Vital Statistics to obtain a death certificate, which will have the cemetery location but not the plot number
			  e. The bodies are in unmarked graves	

Continued.

Terminally Ill Infant: care of family of—cont'd

NURSING DIAGNOSIS/ PATIENT PROBLEM	DEFINING CHARACTERISTICS	NURSING ORDERS		EXPECTED OUTCOMES
		ASSESSMENT	INTERVENTIONS	

			L. Assist the physician/clinician with autopsy counseling
			M. Encourage therapeutic ventilation of feelings
			N. Anticipate disturbed behavior
			O. Facilitate religious or cultural customs. Be sympathetic and adaptable
			P. Demonstrate caring and concern, especially immediately after the loss. Use touch to show support
			Q. Send a personalized sympathy card
			R. Determine the need for follow-up support
			  1. Call the parents the day after the baby's death
			  2. Encourage parents to openly discuss and express feelings about the loss. Offer booklets and books to facilitate this
			  3. Support parents in seeking psychologic support from clergy or mental health professional during bereavement, as needed
			  4. Make a referral to support groups as needed, e.g., Compassionate Friends, The Caring Connection
			  5. Provide anticipatory guidance and support. Let the parents know that they will experience the resurgence of grief on anniversaries, holidays, and other significant dates
			  6. Encourage attendance at the autopsy conference in 4-6 weeks. It will help the parents better understand the problems of the baby and will assist them in family planning	

Terminally Ill Infant: care of family of—cont'd

NURSING DIAGNOSIS/ PATIENT PROBLEM	DEFINING CHARACTERISTICS	NURSING ORDERS		EXPECTED OUTCOMES
		ASSESSMENT	INTERVENTIONS	

Grieving, dysfunctional (of the siblings): potential
 Etiology
 Infant's death
	Less than 4 years old
	 Sense a change in behavior
	 May have nightmares
	 Fear of separation
	
	 4-6 years old
	 May think they will die
	 Become more dependent
	 Magical thinking that leads to guilt
	 Unable to comprehend the finality of death
	
	 7-11 years old
	 Acting out behavior
	 School problems
	 More sensitive to relationships
	
	 11 and older
	 Aware of others' feelings
	 Sensitive
	 Understands that death is final
		A. Assess the chronologic and psychologic ages of the child
		 B. Assess the parents' knowledge of how to inform the child or children of the death
			A. Reinforce the importance of sibling visitation before the infant's death
			 B. Let the parents offer explanations in the words the child can understand. Keep explanations simple
			 C. If it is hard for the parents to tell the children about death, have them use appropriate booklets such as
			   1. Coloring book: *The Frog Family's Baby Dies*
			   2. *Where's Jess?*
			   3. *Tell Me, Papa*
			 D. Tell the parents to avoid phrases that could trigger feeling of fear, such as
			   1. "The baby went to sleep." (This could lead to sleep disturbance)
			   2. "God took the baby to heaven because He loved or needed the baby more than we did." (This may cause resentment against God or a conflict in the child)
			 E. Reassure the child that the infant had a problem that the sibling will not acquire
			 F. Explain to the child that no family member could have caused or prevented the death by their actions, thoughts, and wishes
			 G. Help siblings understand what death means by
			   1. Relating death to stories, books, miniatures, drawings, etc.
			   2. Reminding them of a dead animal or fading flowers
			   3. Reminding them of what living means (e.g., breathing and walking) and that absence of these signs means death
			 H. Advise the parents to let the child or children go to the funeral. If they don't want to, don't insist
			   1. Explain the ritual
			   2. Letting an adult close to the child accompany him/her to answer questions and to reassure the child if he/she becomes fearful
			 I. Encourage parents to express emotions with the children
				Potential for siblings' dysfunctional grieving will be minimized

THERAPEUTIC INTERVENTIONS

Neonate, Care of: after cardiac surgery

NURSING DIAGNOSIS/ PATIENT PROBLEM	DEFINING CHARACTERISTICS	NURSING ORDERS		EXPECTED OUTCOMES
		ASSESSMENT	INTERVENTIONS	

Gas exchange, impaired
Etiology
Pneumothorax
Hemothorax
Atelectasis
	Hypercapnea
	Hypoxia
	Ineffective spontaneous respirations
	Increased need for ventilatory support
	Decreased or absent breath sounds on affected side
	Positive transillumination of chest
	Asymmetrical chest movement
	Decrease in BP
		A. Assess respiratory status q.1-2h.: rate, grunting, flaring, retracting, breath sounds, chest movement
		B. Transilluminate chest as necessary
		C. Assess color—central and peripheral
		D. Assess oxygenation
		  1. Transcutaneous (tc) Po_2 and $tcPco_2$ monitor
		  2. ABGs q.1-2h. and as necessary
		E. Monitor chest x-ray examination immediately after surgery, and follow up as necessary
			A. Avoid chest physiotherapy unless radiographic evidence of atelectasis. If indicated use toothbrush only for percussion and vibration
			B. Suction endotracheal tube q.2h. and as necessary
			C. Change position q.1-2h.
			D. Keep temperature of inspired air at _____
			E. Maintain ventilatory support
			F. Strip thoracic drain
			  1. Every 15-20 min when draining fresh blood
			  2. Every 1h. when draining serosanguinous drainage
			G. Notify physician if thoracic drainage ≥____ (suggested ≥5 ml/kg/hour for 1 hour or ≥3 ml/kg/hour for 3 hours)
			H. Maintain water seal at ____ mm Hg (recommended: 10-15 mm Hg)
				Effects of impaired gas exchange will be minimized

Breathing pattern, ineffective
Etiology
Neuromuscular impairment
Decreased lung expansion
	Inadequate/ineffective spontaneous respiration
	Abnormal ABGs
	Cyanosis
		A. Assess respiratory status q.1-2h.: rate, grunting, flaring, retracting, breath sounds, chest movement
		B. Transilluminate chest as necessary
		C. Assess color—central and peripheral
		D. Assess oxygenation
		  1. $tcPo_2$ and $tcPco_2$ monitor
		  2. ABGs q.1-2h. and as necessary
			Wean infant from ventilator quickly when awake and having spontaneous and effective respirations
			A. Decrease intermittent mandatory ventilation by ____ every _____
			B. Decrease FIo_2 by ____ every _____
			C. Decrease peak inspiratory pressure by ____ every _____
				Optimal respiratory effort will be achieved

Origianted by **Laura L. Rybicki, RN, BSN**
Resource persons: **Diane Gallagher, RN, BSN**
      Terry Griffin, RN
      Karen Kavanaugh, RN, MSN

Neonate, Care of: after cardiac surgery—cont'd

NURSING DIAGNOSIS/ PATIENT PROBLEM	DEFINING CHARACTERISTICS	NURSING ORDERS		EXPECTED OUTCOMES
		ASSESSMENT	INTERVENTIONS	

Fluid volume deficit
 Etiology
 Blood loss
 Inadequate fluid replacement
	Decreased urine output
	 Rising or stable Hct in spite of blood loss
	 Low BP
	 Poor perfusion
	 Metabolic acidosis
	 Increased drainage from thoracic drain
	 Inadequate pulses
	 Pallor
	 Prolonged bleeding time
	 Bloody nasogastric drainage
	 Edema
	 Depressed fontanel
	 Low platelet count
		A. Assess vital signs, including BP and CVP, q.1-2h.
		 B. Obtain report of blood loss from OR and type and amount of fluid replacement
		 C. Assess color and perfusion
		   1. Temperature of extremities
		   2. Capillary refill
		   3. Peripheral pulses
		 D. Monitor I & O q.1h.
		   1. Urine specific gravity and Labstix
		   2. Type and amount of thoracic drainage
		   3. Blood loss (laboratory needs; loss from other sites)
		 E. Monitor laboratory data
		   1. Hct on admission and q.2-4h. until stable
		   2. CBC on admission and as necessary
		   3. BUN and creatinine on admission and as necessary
		 F. Assess for presence of edema
		 G. Assess condition of fontanel
			A. Administer parenteral fluids to provide _____ ml/kg/day (usually ⅔ maintenance)
			 B. Maintain urine output at 1-2 ml/kg/hour
			 C. Maintain sp. gr. between 1003-1010. (Expect increased sp. gr. for 24 hours after cardiac catheterization.) Report sp. gr. >1010 or output <1 ml/kg/hour to physician
			 D. Observe for alternate sites of bleeding (e.g., nasogastric, chest tube, puncture sites)
			 E. Administer volume expanders and/or blood products as ordered
			 F. Report thoracic drainage ≥5 ml/kg/hour for one time or 3 ml/kg/hour for three times
				Optimal cardiac output will be evidenced by
				 A. Adequate tissue perfusion
				 B. Blood gas
				   pH: _____
				   Po_2: _____
				   Pco_2: _____
				 C. Vital signs
				   Heart rate: _____
				   BP: _____
				   CVP: _____

Continued.

Neonate, Care of: after cardiac surgery—cont'd

NURSING DIAGNOSIS/ PATIENT PROBLEM	DEFINING CHARACTERISTICS	NURSING ORDERS		EXPECTED OUTCOMES
		ASSESSMENT	INTERVENTIONS	
Cardiac output, alteration in: decreased (potential) **Etiology** Ineffective contractility secondary to tamponade	Increased respiratory rate Tachycardia Decreased BP Narrowing pulse pressure Distant heart sounds Abrupt decrease in thoracic drainage Widening mediastinal shadow Decreased QRS voltage Decreased peripheral perfusion	A. Assess respiratory rate, apical pulse, BP, CVP q.1h. B. Assess peripheral perfusion and pulses C. Assess for cessation or significant decrease in thoracic drainage D. Follow chart x-ray reports E. Observe ECG configuration F. Follow Hct G. Assess clinical status (see Defining Characteristics)	Notify physician of abrupt decrease in chest tube drainage and/or presence of symptoms listed under Defining Characteristics	Alterations in cardiac output will be minimized
Alteration in cardiac electrical conduction, rate, or rhythm **Etiology** Low calcium levels Central venous line Digoxin toxicity Acidosis High or low potassium levels Myocardial dysfunction	Irregular pulse ECG changes Tachycardia >160 Bradycardia <100	A. Assess calcium and electrolytes on admission as needed B. Assess chest x-ray film on admission and as necessary for central venous line placement C. Monitor ECG configuration D. Monitor digoxin level if toxicity suspected	A. Document arrhythmias with rhythm strip B. Give calcium gluconate as ordered C. Supplement electrolytes as ordered	Optimal cardiac rhythm will be maintained
Cardiac output, alteration in: decreased (potential) **Etiology** Shunt too large	Change in quality or radiation of murmur Tachycardia Bounding peripheral pulses Ventricular gallop Hepatomegaly >2 cm below right costal margin Oliguria Peripheral vasoconstriction Tachypnea >60 Rales Retractions Cyanosis	See SCP earlier in this chapter: Congestive heart failure	See SCP earlier in this chapter: Congestive heart failure	Optimal cardiac output will be maintained

Neonate, Care of: after cardiac surgery—cont'd

NURSING DIAGNOSIS/ PATIENT PROBLEM	DEFINING CHARACTERISTICS	NURSING ORDERS		EXPECTED OUTCOMES
		ASSESSMENT	INTERVENTIONS	
Cardiac output, alteration in: decreased (potential) Etiology Shunt inadequate— secondary to size and/or occlusion	Clinical deterioration with decreased pO_2, pH, and platelet count	A. Assess ABGs on admission and q.1-2h. as necessary B. Assess vital signs, including BP and CVP, on admission, and q.1h. and as necessary C. Assess color, perfusion, and capillary refill	A. Maintain Hct between 45 and 60 B. Administer prostaglandin E at 0.05-0.1 µg/kg/min if it is determined that shunt is nonfunctional C. Titrate prostaglandin E at lowest dose that maintains oxygenation	Optimal cardiac output will be maintained
Consciousness, altered levels of: potential Etiology Impaired cerebral blood flow	Seizure activity Flaccidity and/or lethargy not attributable to drug therapy Extreme irritability Fluctuations in BP, heart rate, perfusion Change in pupil size and/or reactivity to light Hemiparesis	A. See SCP earlier in this chapter: Seizures: (neonate) B. Document type/ amount of anesthetic agents and medications given C. Observe for unexplained changes in BP, heart rate, oxygenation, perfusion D. Check pupils for size and reactivity to light	A. Keep Hct >45 and <60 B. Do not allow any air to enter arterial circulation C. Do not allow air to enter venous circulation (particularly important if infant has right-to-left shunt)	Neurologic impairment will be minimal
Injury, potential for: infection Etiology Surgical procedure Decreased resistance secondary to compromised infant	Temperature instability Increased or decreased WBC Inflammation of and/ or drainage from incision Foul-smelling or green/yellow drainage from endotracheal tube or thoracic drain	A. Assess vital signs, including temperature, q.1-2h. B. Assess all skin incisions for signs of inflammation or drainage C. Note color, type, and amount of thoracic drainage D. Monitor CBC and assess culture results	A. Culture suspicious drainage B. Administer antibiotics as ordered	Infectious process will be minimized
Glucose metabolism, alteration in: potential for hyperglycemia/hypoglycemia Etiology *Hyperglycemia* Stress Epinephrine Iatrogenic *Hypoglycemia* Cold stress Inadequate glucose intake	**Hyperglycemia** Chemstrip ≥120 Glycosuria ≥1+ **Hypoglycemia** Chemstrip ≤40 Temperature instability Jitteriness	A. Assess Chemstrip and send blood glucose on admission B. Monitor Chemstrip q.30min. until stable, then q.2h. C. Assess temperature on admission, q.1h. until stable, then q.2h. D. Obtain report of all medications and fluids administered in OR	A. See SCP earlier in this chapter: Glucose and calcium metabolism, alterations in B. Increase IV glucose as ordered if Chemstrip ≤40 C. Decrease IV glucose as ordered if Chemstrip ≥240 or glycosuria ≥1+	Chemstrip will be between 40-120

Continued.

Neonate, Care of: after cardiac surgery—cont'd

NURSING DIAGNOSIS/ PATIENT PROBLEM	DEFINING CHARACTERISTICS	NURSING ORDERS		EXPECTED OUTCOMES
		ASSESSMENT	INTERVENTIONS	
Calcium metabolism, alteration in: hypocalcemia (potential) **Etiology** Stress Administration of citrated blood Metabolic acidosis treated with sodium bicarbonate	Muscle twitching/jitteriness Compromised myocardial function Ca level <8 mg%	A. Assess calcium level on admission B. See SCP earlier in this chapter: Glucose and calcium metabolism, alterations in	See SCP earlier in this chapter: Glucose and calcium metabolism, alterations in	Ca stable at 8-10 mg%
Parenting, alteration in **Etiology** Hospitalization of infant with life-threatening illness	Verbal/nonverbal expression of fear/ anxiety of intensive care environment Parents verbalize that infant may be in pain or that staff is hurting infant Parents blame themselves for infant's condition Parents verbalize guilt feelings for having a ''less than perfect infant'' Parents verbalize fear that infant will die	A. Assess level of comprehension B. Assess level of anxiety C. Assess existing support systems D. Assess knowledge of illness/condition E. Assess previous experience with hospitalized family members	A. Explain to parents 1. Infant's current condition 2. Equipment used 3. Immediate treatment B. Encourage visits and telephone calls C. Encourage parents to touch infant and to bring toys, clothes for infant D. Encourage verbalization of fears/anxieties E. Explain arrangements available to allow parents to stay overnight F. Refer to parent support group when appropriate	Parents will verbalize an understanding of infant's illness/condition and possible outcome
Etiology Possible inability of parents to visit	Mother too ill to visit Infant transported from another hospital Parents have transportation difficulties Single parent or substitute visits by relatives Attempt by father to ''protect'' mother from facts about infant's condition Financial situation makes it impossible for parents to remain close to infant	A. Assess mother's condition 1. Ability to come to special care nursery 2. Probable discharge date if infant in another hospital B. Assess distance parents live from hospital C. Assess availability of transportation D. If mother cannot visit, assess her knowledge of infant's condition	A. Send picture of infant to mother B. Encourage telephone calls C. Facilitate communication between parents D. Arrange accommodations if parents live a long distance from hospital E. Arrange for hospital to call family if long distance calls present a financial problem F. Refer to social worker G. Encourage attendance at parent support group	Optimal parenting role will be achieved

Parenting in Special Care Nursery

NURSING DIAGNOSIS/ PATIENT PROBLEM	DEFINING CHARACTERISTICS	NURSING ORDERS		EXPECTED OUTCOMES
		ASSESSMENT	INTERVENTIONS	

Parenting, alteration in
 Etiology
 Separation/hospitalization of infant
	Expresses verbal/nonverbal fear/anxiety with intensive care environment
	 Exhibits reluctance to look at infant
	 Verbalizes concern that infant may be in pain
	 Asks inappropriate questions
	 Holds unrealistic view of infant's condition/illness
	 Blames self for infant's condition
	 Does not demonstrate parental attachment behaviors
	 Verbalizes resentment toward infant
	 Verbalizes guilt feelings for having a ''less than perfect infant''
	 Does not visit or call regularly
	 Delays in naming infant
		Assess parents'
		 A. Level of comprehension
		 B. Developmental stage
		 C. Feelings regarding impact of pregnancy on the family
		 D. Level of anxiety
		 E. Existing support systems
		 F. Cultural background
		 G. Knowledge of illness or conditions
			A. Explain to parents
			   1. Reason for admission
			   2. Equipment used
			   3. Immediate treatment
			 B. Familiarize parents with staff of special care nursery
			 C. Encourage reading of parent booklet to clarify questions
			 D. Inform parents of 24-hour calling and visitation policy. Encourage frequent visiting and/or calling
			 E. Explain the infant's prognosis if one is projected (e.g., surgical intervention, long-term treatment with medication, close medical follow-up)
			 F. Offer additional support systems such as
			   1. Social service
			   2. Dysfunctional child center
			   3. Parent support group
			   4. Parent CPR classes
			 G. Encourage verbalization of perception regarding infant
			 H. Encourage parents to touch, kiss, and talk to infant. Allow them to hold infant if possible
			 I. Encourage parents to take pictures, or give them pictures of infant
			 J. Encourage participation in basic caretaking skills: diapering, bathing, and applying lotion
			 K. Promote parents' verbalization of feelings and use of support systems
			 L. Show parents movie: *A Joyful Tear* (available through Ross Laboratories)
				A. Parents will demonstrate increased comfort with staff and environment as evidenced by
				   1. Establishment of a calling/ visiting pattern
				   2. Verbalization of concerns/ fears
				   3. Asking appropriate questions
				 B. Parents will verbalize an understanding of illness/ condition and possible outcomes
				 C. Maternal/paternal bonding initiated as evidenced by
				   1. Increased calls and visits
				   2. Holding, touching infant
				   3. Verbalization of concern for infant
				   4. Bringing toys, clothing
				   5. Verbalization of incorporation of infant into family structure
				   6. Naming of infant

Originated by **Sandra P. Orr, RN, BS**
Resource person: **Martina Evans, RN, BS**

Continued.

Parenting in Special Care Nursery—cont'd

NURSING DIAGNOSIS/ PATIENT PROBLEM	DEFINING CHARACTERISTICS	NURSING ORDERS		EXPECTED OUTCOMES
		ASSESSMENT	INTERVENTIONS	

Parenting, alteration in—cont'd
Etiology
Inability of parent(s) to visit
	Mother extremely ill
	Infant transported from other hospital
	No visiting/telephone calls 24 to 48 hours after admission
	Transportation difficulties
	Single parent visiting and/or substitute visiting by relatives
		A. Assess mother's condition after delivery
		  1. Check maternal history and type of delivery
		  2. Obtain report of course of labor
		  3. Follow up on mother's condition
		B. Assess where parents live and modes of transportation
		C. Assess economic situation for financial ability to call/ visit
			A. Take or send infant's pictures to parents
			B. Encourage calling if visiting is impossible
			C. Send parent booklet
			D. Take infant to see mother if infant's condition allows
			E. Arrange to call parents at scheduled times if they are unable to call
				Parental infant bonding will be initiated as evidenced by
				A. Enthusiasm over pictures or requests for more
				B. Verbalization of concern for infant
				C. Verbalization of desire to see infant/interest in infant
				D. Anticipation of telephone calls from hospital or an established calling pattern

Etiology
Anxiety regarding impending discharge of infant
	Decrease in telephone contacts
	Change or decrease in visiting
	Increased anxiety with impending discharge
	Parents do not return telephone calls or are unable to be reached
	Lack of interest in learning care required to take infant home
		A. Identify primary caretaker
		B. Assess parental support system
		C. Evaluate previous degree of involvement with infant
		D. Determine parental plans for integrating infant into family structure
		E. Assess need for referrals to other support services
		  1. Visiting nurse
		  2. Dysfunctional child center
		  3. Social service
		  4. CPR class
		  5. Comprehensive care clinic
		  6. Retinal clinic
		  7. Follow-up by primary nurses
			A. Begin discharge planning at admission using the discharge planning tool
			B. Incorporate parents into infant's care early after admission
			C. Document calls and visits on flow sheets, and follow up during interdisciplinary and discharge-planning rounds
			D. Encourage and facilitate open communication between health care workers and parents
			E. Make referrals for follow up as needed
			F. Encourage participation in discharge classes
			G. Encourage parents to spend *extended* periods of time with infant
			H. Provide demonstration of special treatments/medications
				Before infant's discharge parents will demonstrate parental/infant bonding behavior
				A. Verbalization of feelings/fears
				B. Increased confidence in caretaking activities and administration of special treatments/ medications

Presurgical Care of Infant

NURSING DIAGNOSIS/ PATIENT PROBLEM	DEFINING CHARACTERISTICS	NURSING ORDERS		EXPECTED OUTCOMES
		ASSESSMENT	INTERVENTIONS	
Fluid volume deficit: potential **Etiology** NPO Nasogastric or orogastric tube to gravity drainage	Dry skin and mucous membrane Reduced skin turgor Depressed anterior fontanel Decreased urine output Weight loss Increased serum sodium	Assess hydration status A. Serum and urine blood status B. Presence of edema C. Vital signs	A. Maintain parenteral therapy as ordered to provide _____ ml/kg/day B. Administer fluid replacement as ordered C. Monitor strict I & O every _____ hours D. Report urine output of <1 ml/kg/hour for 2 consecutive hours E. Weigh every _____ F. Monitor urine specific gravity, urine Labstix at least q.8h. G. Replace nasogastric drainage as ordered H. Monitor electrolytes, serum and urine osmolarity as ordered	Infant will show signs of fluid balance as evidenced by A. Normal laboratory studies B. Urine output of at least 1 ml/kg/hour C. Urine specific gravity of _____ D. Balanced I & O E. Moist mucous membranes F. Stable vital signs G. Normal skin turgor
Nutrition, alteration in: less than body requirements **Etiology** NPO Total parenteral nutrition	Weight loss Reduced fatty tissue Sunken orbits Abnormal Chemstrip bG and blood sugar Restless Irritable Vomiting Documented inadequate caloric intake	A. Assess growth pattern according to Dancis curve B. Monitor caloric intake	A. Provide _____ cal/kg/day with ordered fluids B. Weigh every _____ C. Monitor Chemstrip bG and blood sugar	Caloric requirement of infant is met as evidenced by A. Weight gain of _____ (according to Dancis curve) B. Normal Chemstrip bG and blood sugar
Injury, potential for: infection **Etiology** Interrupted skin integrity (e.g., abdominal wall defect) Prematurity	Failure to do well Nonspecific respiratory distress Lethargy Temperature instability Poor feeder	A. Monitor vital signs and temperature every _____ B. Monitor results of CBC, blood, urine, and surface cultures C. Assess variability of vital signs D. Note activity and subtle symptoms of infection such as poor temperature control, irritability, lethargy, cyanosis, dyspnea, poor feeding, vomiting, and pallor	A. Observe routine handwashing between infants B. Restrict people with any infections (including colds, GI or GU symptoms, skin infections) from nursery C. Ascertain that equipment is cleaned as described in the procedure manual D. Perform daily skin and umbilical cord care E. Maintain a neutral thermal environment	Risk of infection will be minimized as evidenced by infant's A. Improved activity B. Stable temperature

Originated by **Mayda T. Roseta, RN**
Resource person: **Martina Evans, RN, BS**

Continued.

Presurgical Care of Infant—cont'd

NURSING DIAGNOSIS/ PATIENT PROBLEM	DEFINING CHARACTERISTICS	NURSING ORDERS		EXPECTED OUTCOMES
		ASSESSMENT	INTERVENTIONS	

Temperature instability: potential
Etiology
Open wound
Prematurity
	Infant's skin temperature < 36.4° C and axillary temperature > 36.8° C	A. Note warmth, coolness, and color of skin
		B. Check axillary temperature
			A. Maintain neutral thermal environment through the use of
			  1. Isolettes—add humidity as needed
			  2. Radiant warmers—for infants requiring close observation
			  3. Body hoods as needed—monitor temperature of hood every _____ and maintain temperature at _____
			  4. Clear plastic wrap over infant's bed—for extremely premature infants
			  5. Warmed blankets and extra clothing
			B. See SCP later in this chapter: Thermoregulation in low birth weight infant
				Infant's skin temperature will be maintained between 36.4°-36.8° C

Injury, potential for
Etiology
Transport
	Occurrence or exacerbation of
	  Temperature
	  Fluid overload/deficit
	  Cyanosis
	  Apnea
		A. Monitor temperature and heart rate every _____ during transport
		B. Note respiratory status
			A. Transport infant, covered with prewarmed blankets, in radiant warmer
			B. Bring emergency transport box
			C. Ascertain that the O_2 tank has been checked
			D. Provide ventilatory support as needed: FIO_2 _____, bag at _____ min
			E. Maintain parenteral fluids
				Infant will be transported safely without complications

Parent's knowledge deficit
Etiology
Infant's condition
	Anxious
	Asks repetitive questions
	Hostile—may even refuse to sign consent
	Silent
	Inconsistent visiting patterns
	Focuses on equipment instead of infant
		A. Assess level of knowledge
		B. Note
		  1. Patterns of communication between parents and family members
		  2. Resources
		  3. Strengths and weaknesses
		C. Observe how parents relate to infant
			A. Ask the physician/surgeon to explain the surgery to the parents or guardian
			B. Explain the routine preoperative and postoperative procedures in the nursery
			C. Foster close communication between health care team and parents
			D. Support parents in coping with their feelings of apprehension, anxiety, or guilt
			E. Encourage parent participation in the care of infant
			F. Keep parents informed of infant's progress; encourage them to ask questions
			G. Emphasize positive aspects of infant's status
				A. The parents will be able to verbalize purpose and potential outcomes of surgery
				B. The parents will be able to
				  1. Express their anger or apprehension
				  2. Ask questions
				  3. Visit or call at least once a day
				  4. Touch the baby more often and with ease
				  5. Express their feelings about the quality of care infant is receiving

Stimulation of Infant in Special Care Nursery

NURSING DIAGNOSIS/ PATIENT PROBLEM	DEFINING CHARACTERISTICS	NURSING ORDERS		EXPECTED OUTCOMES
		ASSESSMENT	INTERVENTIONS	
Sensory-perceptual, alteration: visual **Etiology** Excessive or insufficient environmental stimuli	No eye-to-eye contact Gazes without focus Unattentive	A. Review patient's history for possible neurologic deficits B. Assess infant's level of receptiveness 1. Is infant in an alert state? (i.e., bright eyes, follows voice with head and eyes) 2. Is infant using time-out signals? (e.g., sighs, looks away, yawns, skin color or respiratory rate changes)	A. Encourage establishment of eye-to-eye contact when possible. Minimize bright lights whenever possible B. Use appropriate visual tools 1. Organize visual field to remove excess items 2. Create a black-and-white visual tool (colorful visuals can be used for infants term and older) 3. Present a visual mobile, preferably black and white geometric shapes. Encourage reaching behavior (extension of toes and fingers) in term and older infants 4. Make big, funny faces at infant (motor imitation at term)	Optimal ability for infant to benefit from appropriate visual stimulation will be achieved
Sensory-perceptual alteration: tactile **Etiology** Excessive or insufficient environmental stimuli	Cries inappropriately Responds only when procedures are done Easily stimulated— hyperactive Hypoactive	Assess for presence or absence of Defining Characteristics	A. Lightly stroke the infant's whole body with your warm hands in a head-to-toe direction (enhances myelination) B. Provide alternative textures for head-to-toe stroking (e.g., cotton, sheepskin, velvet, smooth/rough, flat/raised, warm/cold, sticky/slick, wet/dry) C. Provide pacifier for sucking	Optimal ability of infant to benefit from tactile stimulation will be achieved
Sensory-perceptual alteration: auditory **Etiology** Insufficient or excessive environmental stimuli	Does not turn head toward noise stimulus (accurate localization at 3 months) Lack of body response to noise Decreased alertness	A. See previous assessments for "Sensory-perceptual, alteration in: visual" B. Review patient's medication history for possible ototoxic medication usage	A. Talk to infant. Encourage parents to talk to infant. Use maternal/paternal voices (tape recorded if prolonged hospitalization) while infant is awake or asleep. Use adult or baby talk conversation, preferably slow speech with many inflections B. Use items emitting agreeable sounds (e.g., music boxes, radios, ticking clocks) C. Call infant by name. Speak to infant while handling D. Hold infant close so your heartbeat can be heard (e.g., carry in a strap-on infant sack) E. Minimize excessive auditory stimulation 1. Lower monitor noises when possible 2. Avoid excessive conversation around infant bed (i.e., during reports, rounds) 3. Carefully handle equipment, cabinet drawers, and doors 4. Keep water drained out of O_2 tubing	Infant's ability to benefit from appropriate auditory stimulation will be maximized

Originated by **Phyllis Lawlor-Klean, RN, BSN**
Resource persons: **Diane Gallagher, RN, BSN**
　　　　　　　　Martina Evans, RN, BS

Continued.

Stimulation of Infant in Special Care Nursery—cont'd

NURSING DIAGNOSIS/ PATIENT PROBLEM	DEFINING CHARACTERISTICS	NURSING ORDERS		EXPECTED OUTCOMES
		ASSESSMENT	INTERVENTIONS	
Sensory-perceptual alteration: vestibular functions **Etiology** Excessive or insufficient environmental stimuli	Poor growth and development Absent or decreased grasp reflex	A. Review patient's history for possible muscular or neurologic deficits B. Plot weight gain along Dancis curve for appropriate growth curve	A. Use oscillating water bed. Limit oscillations of bed to 10/min for 10 min with rest period B. Use front-to-back rocking. Lift head from supine to upright position along with side-to-side body movement C. Use infant swing or rocker for slow, rocking, rhythmic movement D. Perform passive flexion and extension of hips, arms, and legs several times per day E. Place a holdable object (e.g., a ball) in infant's hand; encourage infant to close fist around object (grasp reflex fully developed at 32 weeks gestation)	Infant's ability to benefit from appropriate vestibular stimulation will be maximized
Sensory-perceptual alteration: olfactory and gustatory **Etiology** Excessive or insufficient environmental stimuli	Unresponsive to feeding needs Lack of hand-mouth contact Poor suck reflex	Assess for absence or presence of Defining Characteristics	A. Provide mother's milk as often as available. Allow infant to smell breast-milk container B. Place infant's hand or pacifier in mouth. Position it so it cannot fall out when sucking movements are observed C. Place infant in anatomical position D. Offer a taste of milk in pacifier with tube feeding	Infant's ability to benefit from appropriate olfactory and gustatory stimulation will be maximized
Parenting, alteration in: potential **Etiology** Related to infant's hospitalization Knowledge deficit	Excessive questions Increased anxiety Failure to name infant Excessive or infrequent telephone-calling patterns Verbal/nonverbal expressions regarding infant's condition	A. Assess degree of parental understanding B. Assess parent support system 1. Two-parent family 2. Other family members 3. Friends/peers C. Assess growth and development of infant D. Assess extent of parent involvement with infant	A. Instruct in techniques for the interventions of visual, tactile, auditory, vestibular, olfactory, and gustatory stimulation B. Instruct parents on cues displaying that infant is attentive 1. Slows or stops sucking 2. Face brightens 3. Opens eyes 4. Looks at or turns toward you or object 5. Stretches fingers or toes toward you or object 6. Stops movement or squirming C. Explain infant's time-out signals (cues that infant has had enough stimulation) 1. Begins to move arms and legs about 2. Squirms 3. Looks away from you or object 4. Starts to cry 5. Becomes irritable	Parents will be able to care for infant

Stimulation of Infant in Special Care Nursery—cont'd

NURSING DIAGNOSIS/ PATIENT PROBLEM	DEFINING CHARACTERISTICS	NURSING ORDERS		EXPECTED OUTCOMES
		ASSESSMENT	INTERVENTIONS	

			D. Explain recognizable signs of effective stimulation
			  1. Consistent weight gain
			  2. Longer periods of wakefulness following feedings
			  3. Establishment of regular sleep pattern
			  4. Infant recognizes parents and smiles sooner
			E. Provide parents with handout regarding Interventions *A, B, C,* and *D* for review at their leisure	

Thermoregulation in Low Birth Weight Infant

NURSING DIAGNOSIS/ PATIENT PROBLEM	DEFINING CHARACTERISTICS	NURSING ORDERS		EXPECTED OUTCOMES
		ASSESSMENT	INTERVENTIONS	

Injury, potential for
Etiology
Temperature fluctuation related to prematurity or illness
	Intrinsic factors
	Hyperthermia
	Body temperature >37° C
	Tachycardia
	Fluid/electrolyte imbalance
	Tachypnea
	Sweating
	Convulsions
	Irritability
	
	Hypothermia
	Pale or blue skin
	Body temperature <36.4° C
	Loss of or failure to gain weight
	Apneic spell
	Hypoxia
	Hypoglycemia
	CO_2 retention
	Convulsions
	Irritability
	Fluid/electrolyte imbalance
		A. Assess the following criteria to select the appropriate neutral thermal environment
		  1. Weight
		  2. Gestational age
		  3. Treatment
		  4. Patient activity
		B. Check infant's axillary temperature including vital signs, q.2-3h.
		  1. If temperature probe is used, assess correlation between skin temperature and axillary temperature
		  2. Assess infant's temperature as related to environmental temperature
		  3. Maintain skin temperature between 36.4°-36.8° C
		C. Assess for signs of hyperthermia/hypothermia as described in Defining Characteristics
			Infant weight <1 kg
			A. Place infant under radiant warmer
			  1. A Servo control service must be attached securely to baby's skin
			  2. Adjust temperature dial to desired temperature (36.5°-37.0° C, not to exceed 37.5° C)
			  3. Verify appropriate alarm functions
			B. Minimize insensible water loss through the following actions
			  1. Use humidity hood over body, and maintain temperature of hood between 34.0°-38° C
			  2. Drape plastic wrap over radiant warmer
			C. Cover infant's head with a hat
			D. Minimize handling
			E. If the plastic wrap or body hood has to be removed during a procedure, supplement heat source with a heat lamp positioned approximately 2-3 feet from infant
			
			Infant weight 1-1.5 kg
			A. Adjust Isolette temperature based on weight/age temperature chart
			B. Attach skin temperature probe monitor as needed
				Minimized effects of cold/heat stress will be evidenced by maintenance of a neutral thermal environment

Originated by **Vanida Komutanon, RN**
Resource person: **Diane Gallagher, RN, BSN**

Continued.

Thermoregulation in Low Birth Weight Infant—cont'd

NURSING DIAGNOSIS/ PATIENT PROBLEM	DEFINING CHARACTERISTICS	NURSING ORDERS		EXPECTED OUTCOMES
		ASSESSMENT	INTERVENTIONS	
Injury, potential for—cont'd		D. If infant weight ≤1 kg, assess for increased insensible fluid loss 1. Inappropriate weight loss (i.e., > 15% of birth weight within first 3 days of life) 2. Decreased urine output as evidenced by a. Sp. gr. > 1.010 b. Output < 2 ml/kg/hour c. Hypernatremia	C. Warm linen before use D. If O_2 is used, hood temperature should be equal to Isolette temperature but not <34° C E. Dress infant appropriately. If observation is required use booties, hat, and diaper only; otherwise, dress in hat and shirt F. Use following techniques during procedure 1. Work through portholes as much as possible 2. Use heat lamp when infant is exposed to external environment during procedures (heat lamp should be positioned 2-3 feet from infant) G. Do not bathe any infant who requires an external heat source H. Move infant to radiant warmer if resuscitation is required or if infant's condition becomes unstable **Infant weight 1.5 kg** A. Transfer a newly admitted infant to a bassinet after his/her condition has stabilized B. Dress in hat, booties, T-shirt, and diaper; cover with 2-3 blankets C. Delay routine bathing until temperature/condition is stable for at least 3 hours D. Wean from Isolette if an older, growing premature infant (see Interventions next section)	
Injury, potential for **Etiology** Temperature fluctuations (extrinsic factors)	**Hyperthermia** Body temperature >37° C Tachycardia Fluid/electrolyte imbalance Tachypnea Sweating Convulsion Irritability **Hypothermia** Pale or blue skin Body temperature <36.4° C Loss of or failure to gain weight Apneic spell Hypoxia Hypoglycemia CO_2 retention Convulsion	A. Assess infant's potential for heat loss in the environment based on principles of 1. Conduction (cold sheets, scale, X-ray plate) 2. Convection (Exposure to room temperature, drafts; temperature of O_2 administered (32°-35° C); room temperature (24° C); humidity (50%) 3. Radiation (assess proximity	**Care of infant in Isolette** A. Warm Isolette to appropriate temperature before use B. Keep portholes closed as much as possible C. Wean infant as tolerated 1. Decrease bed temperature 0.5° C if infant is able to maintain axillary temperature of 36.4° C 2. Unplug bed and open portholes when Isolette temperature reaches 26° C 3. Move to bassinet if temperature is stable and weight gain satisfactory D. If O_2 therapy or ventilation is needed, maintain O_2 temperature equal to Isolette temperature but not <34°-37° C E. Parenteral fluids should be warmed to room temperature	Minimized effects of cold/heat stress will be evidenced by maintenance of a neutral thermal environment

Thermoregulation in Low Birth Weight Infant—cont'd

NURSING DIAGNOSIS/ PATIENT PROBLEM	DEFINING CHARACTERISTICS	NURSING ORDERS		EXPECTED OUTCOMES
		ASSESSMENT	INTERVENTIONS	

	Irritability
	Fluid/electrolyte imbalance
		of infant to cold windows or cold incubator walls)
		4. Evaporation (Wet soak, wet linen, or wet infant)
		B. Assess for heat excess related to
		  1. Excessive handling
		  2. Inappropriate environmental temperature
			1. Run hyperalimentation fluid through IV tubing to facilitate warming
			2. Do not warm hyperalimentation in Isolette or under radiant warmer near infant
			F. Place warm sheet between infant and scale when infant is weighed
			G. Position infant's bed away from sunlight/cold draft
			
			Care of infant in Isolette or radiant warmer during parental visits
			A. Explain infant's thermoregulation needs to parents
			B. Establish time limit for infant's ability to tolerate room temperature
			C. Bundle infant before visit
			D. Use temperature probe if baby is under a radiant warmer
			
			Care of transported infant
			A. Warm transport Isolette before using
			B. If radiant warmer is used for the transport, cover infant with warm linen and a hat
			C. Use heat packs as necessary
			
			Care of the hypothermic infant
			A. Provide infant with appropriate environmental support
			  1. If infant is in a bassinet, move to Isolette
			  2. If infant is in an Isolette, move to radiant warmer (see "Interventions" for Care of infant <1 kg this section) or use heat lamp
			B. Attach skin temperature probe as necessary
			C. Monitor temperature every hour until stable
			
			Care of the hyperthermic infant
			A. Alleviate source of hyperthermia, i.e., bed temperature, bundling
			B. Cool slowly
			  1. Do not use alcohol or cold water
			  2. Wipe infant gently with tepid cloth
			  3. Adjust radiant warmer temperature; gradually decrease by 0.5° C/20 min
			C. Attach skin temperature probe to monitor temperature	

Tracheoesophageal Fistula with Esophageal Atresia: preoperative care

NURSING DIAGNOSIS/ PATIENT PROBLEM	DEFINING CHARACTERISTICS	NURSING ORDERS		EXPECTED OUTCOMES
		ASSESSMENT	INTERVENTIONS	
Airway clearance, ineffective **Etiology** Accumulation of excessive mucus and saliva in the nose, mouth, and blind pouch Bronchial infection	Constant drooling of secretions Intermittent cyanosis Tachypnea Nasal flaring Retractions Coarse breath sounds	A. Assess and document amount, color, and odor of secretions B. Assess respiratory status using Defining Characteristics C. Assess and document changes in vital signs: heart rate, respiratory rate, BP, and temperature	A. Place a no. 10 sump tube in the blind pouch, and attach it to continuous low suctioning with Gomco drainage pump as ordered by physician B. Irrigate the sump tube with ____ ml normal saline every ____ hours to ascertain tube patency C. Perform oral, nasal, and endotracheal suctioning every ____ hours as indicated D. Position the infant on his/her abdomen as tolerated or with the head of bed elevated 45 degrees E. Administer antibiotics as ordered F. Maintain ventilatory assistance as ordered	Patent airway will be evidenced by A. Decreased accumulation of secretions B. Decreased intermittent cyanosis
Breathing pattern, ineffective: potential **Etiology** Decreased lung expansion Atelectasis	Tachypnea Nasal flaring Substernal retractions Increased respiratory rate and heart rate Abnormal blood gases (arterial or capillary) Abnormal chest x-ray examination Diminished breath sounds	A. Assess and document 1. Respiratory rate 2. Presence of nasal flaring and retractions 3. Presence of cyanosis 4. Quality of breath sounds B. Assess and document changes in vital signs C. Assess the infant's tolerance to various positions D. Note pattern of serial chest x-ray examinations	A. Position the patient ____ for an optimal breathing pattern B. Perform chest physiotherapy with suctioning every ____, as indicated C. Monitor and document blood gases (arterial or capillary) every ____ D. Maintain ventilatory assistance as ordered	Optimal breathing pattern will be maintained

Originated by **Margaret Bell, RN**
Resource persons: **Karen Kavanaugh, RN, MSN**
Martina Evans, RN, BS

Tracheoesophageal Fistula with Esophageal Atresia: preoperative care—cont'd

NURSING DIAGNOSIS/ PATIENT PROBLEM	DEFINING CHARACTERISTICS	NURSING ORDERS		EXPECTED OUTCOMES
		ASSESSMENT	INTERVENTIONS	
Nutrition, alteration in: less than body requirements **Etiology** NPO	Weight loss Restlessness Irritability Documented inadequate caloric intake	A. Assess weight pattern in comparison to the Dancis growth curve B. Assess and document calorie intake	A. Administer ____ cal/kg/day ____ ml/kg/day with ordered fluids B. Weigh every day C. Monitor urine Labstix every ____ hours D. Monitor Chemstrip bG every ____ hours	Optimal caloric intake will be met as evidenced by A. Minimized weight loss B. Normal Chemstrip and blood sugar
Fluid volume deficit: potential **Etiology** Use of radiant warmer Loss of fluid through sump tube Inadequate amount of maintenance fluids for infant's weight and gestational age	Low urine output Elevated urine specific gravity Thick secretions Increased sodium Poor tissue turgor Weight loss Depressed fontanel	A. Assess hydration status using Defining Characteristics B. Assess thermal environment	A. Monitor weight every day B. Maintain strict I & O; report urine output of <1 ml/kg/hour to physician C. Monitor specific gravity with Labstix every voiding D. Monitor and document electrolytes every ____ hours; report abnormal findings to physician E. Administer parenteral fluids as ordered to provide ____ ml/kg/ 24 hours F. Administer fluid replacement as ordered G. Maintain optimal neutral thermal environment	Fluid balance will be maintained
Knowledge deficit: of parents **Etiology** Unfamiliarity with infant's condition	Verbal and nonverbal expressions of fear/anxiety with intensive care environment Unrealistic view of infant's illness Inappropriate response to infant Requests for information	A. Assess parent's knowledge of disease entity B. Assess parental bonding pattern	A. Encourage parents to 1. Visit and call frequently 2. Verbalize their concerns and feelings 3. Participate in their infant's care by demonstrating simple tasks (such as diapering and applying lotion) 4. Attend parent's group sessions B. With appropriate physicians, provide parents with information concerning 1. Unit policies 2. Etiology and nature of defect 3. Special needs of infant 4. Expected outcomes regarding infant's condition C. Refer parents to social worker	Parents will verbalize an understanding of the nature and sequelae of the infant's problem

Continued.

Tracheoesophageal Fistula with Esophageal Atresia: preoperative care—cont'd

NURSING DIAGNOSIS/ PATIENT PROBLEM	DEFINING CHARACTERISTICS	NURSING ORDERS		EXPECTED OUTCOMES
		ASSESSMENT	INTERVENTIONS	
Parenting, alteration in **Etiology** Separation/hospitalization of infant Inability of parent(s) to visit	Expresses verbal/nonverbal fear/anxiety with intensive care environment Exhibits reluctance to look at infant Verbalizes infant may be in pain or staff is hurting infant Asks inappropriate questions Holds unrealistic view of infant's condition/illness Blame themselves for infant's condition Absence of parental attachment behaviors Verbalizes resentment toward infant Verbalizes guilt feelings for having a "less than perfect infant" Does not visit or call regularly Delays in naming infant	Assess for presence of Defining Characteristics	See SCP earlier in this chapter: Parenting in special care nursery	Alteration in parenting will be minimized

Index

Cynthia Whyte